Practical Pulmonary
and Critical Care Medicine

LUNG BIOLOGY IN HEALTH AND DISEASE

Executive Editor

Claude Lenfant

Former Director, National Heart, Lung, and Blood Institute
National Institutes of Health
Bethesda, Maryland

Practical Pulmonary and Critical Care Medicine

Disease Management

Edited by

Zab Mosenifar
Cedars–Sinai Medical Center
Los Angeles, California, U.S.A.

Guy W. Soo Hoo
VA Greater Los Angeles Healthcare System
Geffen School of Medicine at UCLA
Los Angeles, California, U.S.A.

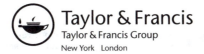

Taylor & Francis
Taylor & Francis Group
New York   London

Published in 2006 by
Taylor & Francis Group
270 Madison Avenue
New York, NY 10016

© 2006 by Taylor & Francis Group, LLC

No claim to original U.S. Government works
Printed in the United States of America on acid-free paper
10 9 8 7 6 5 4 3 2 1

International Standard Book Number-10: 0-8247-2597-2 (Hardcover)
International Standard Book Number-13: 978-0-8247-2597-6 (Hardcover)
Library of Congress Card Number 2005044634

Library of Congress Cataloging-in-Publication Data

Practical pulmonary and critical care medicine / edited by Zab Mosenifar, Guy W. Soo Hoo
      p. ; cm. -- (Lung biology in health and disease ; v. 213-214)
    Includes bibliographical references and index.
    Contents: v. 1. Respiratory failure-- v. 2. Disease management.
    ISBN-13: 978-0-8493-6663-5 (v. 1 : alk. paper)
    ISBN-10: 0-8493-6663-1 (v. 1 : alk. paper)
    ISBN-13: 978-0-8247-2597-6 (v. 2 : alk. paper)
    ISBN-10: 0-8247-2597-2 (v. 2 : alk. paper)
    1. Lungs--Diseases. 2. Respiratory intensive care. I. Mosenifar, Zab, 1951- II. Soo Hoo, Guy W. III. Series.
    [DNLM: 1. Lung Diseases--therapy. 2. Acute Disease--therapy. 3. Critical Care--methods. WF 600 P8947 2006]

RC941.P73 2006
616.2'4--dc22   2005044634

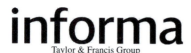

informa
Taylor & Francis Group
is the Academic Division of Informa plc.

**Visit the Taylor & Francis Web site at
http://www.taylorandfrancis.com**

Introduction

Surely, all of us would certainly concur with the first sentence of the Preface prepared by Drs. Mosenifar and Soo Hoo: "Over the past decade, the pace of progress in medicine has been astounding. New developments in diagnosis, management, and therapeutics occur at a breathtaking rate." On the other hand, one could argue with the time frame, that is, why only the past decade? This is a significant point, especially when it comes to pulmonary and critical care. Pulmonary medicine started to blossom many, many decades ago but especially during the last 30 years or so. Critical care started its course, to what it is today, with the development of the oxygen electrode (and later oximetry) and with the recognition of the value of blood pH measurements in the late 1950s. At the same time, the use of ventilators and respiratory assist devices became more common.

However, in reality it matters little when progress began. Today, what counts is that new developments are being introduced at such a fast pace that progress may exceed the ability to fully transfer and utilize all this knowledge in the practice of medicine. Sure enough, tertiary hospitals have the facilities and work force to adjust to and quickly adapt to changes as they occur. On the other hand, hospitals which are community based and distant from academic centers may find it more difficult to take full advantage of the newer approaches for the management of pulmonary patients and/or critical care situations.

What could be considered a dual standard between tertiary and community hospitals is well recognized today, and has raised concerns of policy makers, politicians, and medical leaders. The question is frequently raised about how fast, and how well, research advances are translated into the practice of medicine, including pulmonary and critical care medicine.

This monograph, *Practical Pulmonary and Critical Care Medicine: Disease Management* and its companion volume titled *Practical Pulmonary and Critical Care Medicine: Respiratory Failure* represent important steps to minimize translation difficulties. Indeed, they both present a very practical approach to pulmonary and critical care medicine. This volume examines a number of situations—both pulmonary and non-pulmonary—that require the use of "tools" described in the companion volume. The other volume addresses, and very carefully describes, the "tools" to provide the most optimal care and management of respiratory failure. Together, these volumes will not only enrich the knowledge of the readers, but also will provide a wealth of practical information that has the potential to positively impact on the care of their patients.

The editors, Dr. Zab Mosenifar and Dr. Guy W. Soo Hoo, have assembled contributors with outstanding expertise and a wealth of practical experience, coming from institutions/environments with large patient populations, and a wide variety of cases and medical situations. They share their very practical and real experiences throughout the volumes.

As the Executive Editor of the series of monographs Lung Biology in Health and Disease, I am proud to present these two volumes and to express my most sincere thanks to the editors and the authors.

Claude Lenfant, MD
Gaithersburg, Maryland, U.S.A.

Preface

Over the past decade, the pace of progress in medicine has been astounding. New developments in diagnosis, management, and therapeutics occur at a breathtaking rate. A new disease emerges and, aided by the ease of transcontinental travel, threatens to become the next pandemic. And just as quickly, the causative agent is identified with diagnostics and therapeutics soon to follow. Old diseases have their mysteries unraveled, and targeted therapeutics provide hope where there was once despair. Some conditions come under control in less than a generation's span, while others plod along inexorably to the end, with little available to alter their course.

Just as the conditions of disease have changed, so have the conduits for information. The speed and availability of electronic databases now allow access to vast warehouses of information at the click of a mouse or flick of a stylus. Where once the houseofficer carried a worn copy of a spiral bound manual, handheld computers are now the essential accessories. The grand old textbooks have followed suit, available in versions abbreviated to fit file-size limits or available in their own electronic internet based versions. This electronic world not only allows but mandates frequent content changes. Information can be updated daily and even more frequently if necessary. The online resource is now predominant in an arena that was once the domain of the print journal. Whereas attendance at national or international meetings once offered the latest developments, this information can now be accessed from a remote site and disseminated at near-instantaneous speed, certainly before one can return home.

Why then, in this information rich era, would there be a need for this book? First of all, even though there is instant access and availability to volumes of information, there remains a dearth of practical information. No one functions in the vacuum of cyberspace or isolation of an information warehouse. Everyone faces the limitations of available technology, restricted formularies, time pressures, and treatment preferences. In addition to the wealth of knowledge, one requires the wisdom of experience and expediency of practical management. The best technology or therapeutic is only as effective as the treatment that can be instituted by the lone practitioner. Treatment available only to the few or the very specialized usually has no role in general management.

Filling this void is the guiding premise of this book. Even if mutations threaten to render current antimicrobials ineffective or new disease entities emerge, there remains a need for comprehensive and effective supportive care. This care is best provided not by the disease specialist, but by physicians who carry a broader perspective while also maintaining focus on the most pressing problems. In the new lexicon of medicine, this is the hospitalist or intensivist.

This has required the intensivist to assume many roles in patient management, but none more important than as the functional equivalent of a chief executive with oversight over total management. This has required familiarity with areas where they are not generally considered expert, and reliance on a multi-disciplinary approach to care. These sections in the text are authored by experts in the area who provide a broad overview but highlight those issues most important in managing critically ill patients. This brings the intensivist's view to the specialist's world.

Practical Pulmonary and Critical Care is divided into two volumes. The first volume focuses on immediate management and diagnosis. This second volume covers frequently encountered disease conditions such as decompensated asthma, chronic obstructive pulmonary disease (COPD), pneumonia, acute respiratory distress syndrome, hemoptysis, acute coronary syndrome and heart failure, and provides in-depth coverage on management. Consideration is given to therapy both as primary conditions and as secondary complicating conditions. This includes pneumonia, pulmonary embolism, sepsis, neurologic and neuromuscular conditions, gastrointestinal bleeding, and renal failure. For example, renal replacement therapy is viewed not only in terms of a presenting symptom or condition, but also in its role in the management of the patient with acute gastrointestinal bleeding or sepsis. It is a unique perspective that focuses not only on supportive care, but also on management to facilitate recovery.

There is also coverage on management issues that have previously not been given much consideration. This includes chapters on nutrition, sedation, infection control, and bioethics. In the past decade, these topics have emerged in the realm of the patient care as they can adversely affect patient outcome and duration of stay. These are often considered to be supportive or ancillary issues, but they are not optional for optimal patient care. And there is also coverage on an aspect of patient management that has only recently been recognized as crucial for quality patient care, the use of the electronic health record in patient care. This has evolved beyond being a repository for patient notes, to being an indispensable component of patient care. It is now recognized that medical errors and/or inefficiencies are linked to inaccessible or illegible medical records, a problem that is almost fully remedied by electronic order entry, decision support systems, near instantaneous access to prior history, medications, and medical references. The systems can also provide safeguards against dosing errors or deleterious drug interactions. Although these systems are available, they are underutilized.

In summary, we present a reference that uses its scientific foundations to provide a focus on the practical and efficient management of critically ill patients. It is this perspective that not only defines this book, but hopefully lends an enduring quality to its content. A paper-based textbook may not have the allure of electronic media, but instead can provide a roadmap and framework for efficient and pragmatic care. Once in place, additional information can only enhance the work and final product. We share a common goal to enhance the recovery of patients from a critical illness. We hope this book can contribute to that end result.

Zab Mosenifar
Guy W. Soo Hoo

Contributors

David L. Balfe *Division of Pulmonary and Critical Care Medicine, Cedars–Sinai Medical Center, Los Angeles, California, U.S.A.*

Vikas Bhalla *Division of Cardiology, La Jolla VA Medical Center and University of California, San Diego School of Medicine, La Jolla, California, U.S.A.*

Bojan Cercek *Division of Cardiology, Cedars–Sinai Medical Center, Geffen School of Medicine at UCLA, Los Angeles, California, U.S.A.*

Kuang-Yuh Chyu *Division of Cardiology, Cedars–Sinai Medical Center, Geffen School of Medicine at UCLA, Los Angeles, California, U.S.A.*

Stanley N. Cohen *Stroke Prevention Program, Sunrise Hospital and Medical Center, Las Vegas, Nevada, U.S.A.*

Joanna Duffney *VA Greater Los Angeles Healthcare System and Geffen School of Medicine at UCLA, Los Angeles, California, U.S.A.*

Peter F. Fedullo *Division of Pulmonary and Critical Care Medicine, University of California San Diego, La Jolla, California, U.S.A.*

Matthew Bidwell Goetz   *VA Greater Los Angeles Healthcare System and Geffen School of Medicine at UCLA, Los Angeles, California, U.S.A.*

Jesse Hall   *Department of Medicine, Section of Pulmonary and Critical Care, University of Chicago Hospitals, Chicago, Illinois, U.S.A.*

D. Kyle Hogarth   *Department of Medicine, Section of Pulmonary and Critical Care, University of Chicago Hospitals, Chicago, Illinois, U.S.A.*

Catherine Lee Hough   *Division of Pulmonary and Critical Care Medicine, Harborview Medical Center, University of Washington, Seattle, Washington, U.S.A.*

Leonard D. Hudson   *Division of Pulmonary and Critical Care Medicine, Harborview Medical Center, University of Washington, Seattle, Washington, U.S.A.*

Nader Kamangar   *Division of Pulmonary and Critical Care, Olive View–UCLA Medical Center, Geffen School of Medicine at UCLA, Los Angeles, California, U.S.A.*

Eric C. Kleerup   *Division of Pulmonary, Critical Care Medicine and Hospitalists, UCLA Medical Center and Geffen School of Medicine at UCLA, Los Angeles, California, U.S.A.*

Jeffrey A. Kraut   *VA Greater Los Angeles Healthcare System and Geffen School of Medicine at UCLA, Los Angeles, California, U.S.A.*

Hsin-Yi Lee   *Department of Imaging, VA Greater Los Angeles Healthcare System and Geffen School of Medicine at UCLA, Los Angeles, California, U.S.A.*

Michael I. Lewis   *Division of Pulmonary and Critical Care Medicine, Cedars–Sinai Medical Center, Geffen School of Medicine at UCLA, Los Angeles, California, U.S.A.*

Alan Maisel   *Division of Cardiology, La Jolla VA Medical Center and University of California, San Diego School of Medicine, La Jolla, California, U.S.A.*

Paul E. Marik   *Division of Pulmonary/Critical Care Medicine, Thomas Jefferson University Hospital and Jefferson Medical College, Philadelphia, Pennsylvania, U.S.A.*

Sunit D. Mistry   *Division of Pulmonary and Critical Care Medicine, Cedars–Sinai Medical Center, Geffen School of Medicine at UCLA, Los Angeles, California, U.S.A.*

Rekha Murthy   *Hospital Epidemiology, Cedars–Sinai Medical Center and Geffen School of Medicine at UCLA, Los Angeles, California, U.S.A.*

Gordon V. Ohning *Department of Medicine, VA Greater Los Angeles Healthcare System-West Los Angeles, California; CURE Digestive Diseases Research Center, Center for Neurovisceral Sciences and Women's Health, Geffen School of Medicine at UCLA, Los Angeles, California, U.S.A.*

Silverio Santiago *Pulmonary and Critical Care Section, West Los Angeles Healthcare Center, VA Greater Los Angeles Healthcare System and Geffen School of Medicine at UCLA, Los Angeles, California, U.S.A.*

Paul Schneider *VA Greater Los Angeles Healthcare System, Geffen School of Medicine at UCLA, Los Angeles, California, U.S.A.*

Scott Selco *Stroke Program, Sunrise Hospital and Medical Center, Las Vegas, Nevada, U.S.A.*

Anna Somerto *Department of Medicine, Cedars–Sinai Medical Center, Los Angeles, California, U.S.A.*

Guy W. Soo Hoo *Pulmonary and Critical Care Section, West Los Angeles Healthcare Center, VA Greater Los Angeles Healthcare System and Geffen School of Medicine at UCLA, Los Angeles, California, U.S.A.*

Sanjay Vadgama *Pulmonary and Critical Care Section, West Los Angeles Healthcare Center, VA Greater Los Angeles Healthcare System, and Geffen School of Medicine at UCLA, Los Angeles, California, U.S.A.*

Behran Vaghaiwalla *VA Greater Los Angeles Healthcare System and Geffen School of Medicine at UCLA, Los Angeles, California, U.S.A.*

Timothy L. Williamson *Division of Pulmonary and Critical Care Medicine, University of Kansas Medical Center, Kansas City, Kansas, U.S.A.*

Richard G. Wunderink *Division of Pulmonary and Critical Care, Northwestern University Feinberg School of Medicine, Chicago, Illinois, U.S.A.*

Contents

1

Practical Management of the Patient with Acute Lung Injury

CATHERINE LEE HOUGH and LEONARD D. HUDSON

Division of Pulmonary and Critical Care Medicine
Harborview Medical Center, University of Washington
Seattle, Washington, U.S.A.

I. Introduction

In 1967, the first description of acute respiratory distress in adults, by Ashbaugh and Petty (1), launched a new field of clinical and laboratory research. Over the last four decades, much has been learned about the natural history, pathogenesis, epidemiology, and treatment of patients with acute lung injury (ALI) and the acute respiratory distress syndrome (ARDS) (2). Despite this increasing body of knowledge, mortality rates remained high, and no interventional trials demonstrated a convincing mortality benefit, until recently.

Within the last decade, survival of patients with ALI has dramatically improved (3–5). In the most recent National Institutes of Health/National Heart Lung and Blood Institute (NIH/NHLBI) ARDS Clinical Trials Network (ARDSnet) studies of patients with both early and late ALI, mortality decreased to 30% (6,7). During this period of time, there have been significant advances in the treatment of critically ill patients (8–13), including the first intervention that has been shown to improve the survival of patients with ALI (14). In this chapter, we will offer suggestions for the practical management of patients with ALI within the context of evidence-based clinical literature, particularly focusing on studies that included patient-centered outcomes, most importantly survival.

II. Definition and Recognition of ALI

Early reports and studies used varying definitions of ARDS. In 1994, the American–European Consensus Conference (AECC) of 1994 convened to establish a common definition. By the AECC criteria, ALI is defined as acute hypoxemic respiratory failure with fulfillment of three diagnostic criteria: bilateral infiltrates on chest radiograph, a ratio of arterial partial pressure of oxygen to fractional inspired oxygen ($P_aO_2{:}F_iO_2$) ≤ 300, and absence of evidence of left atrial hypertension (15). ARDS is a subset of ALI, defined by more severe hypoxemia ($P_aO_2{:}F_iO_2 \leq 200$) (15). Diagnosis of ALI therefore requires a chest radiograph, an arterial blood gas measurement, and an assessment of left atrial pressure by either a clinical estimate or pulmonary artery catheter measurement. Altered pulmonary mechanics, such as decreased lung compliance, are common in ALI (16) but are not included in the case definition of ALI. ALI is a complication of some acute illness or injury. Although an underlying risk condition such as sepsis is not required for the diagnosis, the presence of an acknowledged risk condition makes the criteria of ALI more specific for the pathological finding of diffuse alveolar damage.

Recent epidemiologic studies estimate an incidence of over 50 cases of ALI per 100,000 persons in the population per year (17,18). ALI is therefore a common disorder, with an incidence rate in the same range as lung cancer and colorectal cancer (19). However, there is a perception that ALI is much less common—even rare—as evidenced by the inclusion of the "adult respiratory distress syndrome" on the website of the National Organization for Rare Diseases (20,21). Two recent epidemiological studies revealed that only a fraction of patients who meet the definition of ALI are diagnosed with the syndrome in their medical records (22,23). This observation is important as we make recommendations for the practical management of patients with ALI, for the first step in management of a disease is recognition. In an observational study of recognition and treatment of ALI, documentation of ALI in the medical record was strongly associated with the use of a life-saving ventilator strategy (23).

III. Management of the Underlying Acute Condition

There are a number of risk factors associated with the development of ALI, including sepsis, trauma, pneumonia, aspiration, pancreatitis, multiple blood transfusions, inhalation injuries, fat emboli, and cardiopulmonary bypass (24,25). Presence of a specific risk factor is not part of the definition of ALI, but recognition and appropriate treatment of the predisposing acute condition is a crucial component of management of the ALI patient (26). Most patients who do not survive ALI die either from their initial acute insult or multiple organ dysfunction (27,28). Additionally, severity of ALI correlates to the degree of systemic inflammation (29). Management of the underlying inflammatory condition is crucial for pulmonary and patient outcomes.

For example, studies have shown that early, goal-directed resuscitation improves outcomes in sepsis (10) and trauma (30), including decreasing the days of multiple organ dysfunction, which includes ALI. Patients with sepsis have improved outcomes with early, appropriate antibiotic use (31) and early surgical treatment of abdominal sources of infection (32). Use of recombinant activated protein C has been shown to decrease days of ALI and improve outcomes of patients with severe sepsis (12). Intensive control of hyperglycemia has been shown to reduce multiple organ failure, length of ICU stay, and mortality among ICU patients (11). Management of acute pancreatitis with prophylactic broad spectrum antibiotics (33–35) and early jejunal feeding (36) have also been associated with improved patient outcomes, including decreased days of multiple organ failure.

Pneumonia is one of the most common risk factors for ALI (24,25). The importance of early antibiotic therapy targeted at the suspected organisms has been addressed in several recent consensus conferences that discussed the treatment of both community- and hospital-acquired pneumonia (37,38). Attempted identification of the infectious etiology of pneumonia is an important early step in the management of ALI patients, including a search for less common organisms. Sputum, blood, and bronchoalveolar lavage cultures, along with serologies and lavage and tissue histopathology, may be useful in identification of the culprit organism, particularly if patients have risk factors for less common infections, such as Pneumocystis carinii, Legionella pneumophila, and mycobacterial, viral, or fungal disease. Bronchoscopy has been shown to be safe and well tolerated, even in ALI patients with severe hypoxemia (39). Diagnosis and management of ventilator-associated pneumonia, a common complication of ALI, is covered later in this chapter.

In approximately 10% of ALI cases, no risk factor is identified (25). In a greater number, "pneumonia" is cited as the risk factor but no culprit organism is identified. It has recently been suggested that in these instances, a bronchoalveolar lavage and, potentially, lung biopsy are warranted to exclude an acute, noninfectious lung disease that mimics ALI (40). These "mimics" fulfill the diagnostic criteria of ALI, but may have different treatments and outcomes. These noninfectious diseases include acute eosinophilic pneumonia, acute cryptogenic organizing pneumonia, diffuse alveolar hemorrhage, acute hypersensitivity pneumonitis, and acute interstitial pneumonia (Hammon-Rich syndrome). The bronchoalveolar lavage and histopathologic findings are described and compared to those of ALI in Table 1.

The timing and indications for lung biopsy in ALI are not well studied and there have been no "official" recommendations. A recent study reviewed the findings, changes in treatment, and outcomes of 57 patients with ALI on whom lung biopsies were performed (41). Lung biopsies were preceded by bronchoalveolar lavage in 77% of cases. In this study, 60% of biopsies revealed diffuse alveolar damage, the classic pathologic finding of ALI. The most common alternative pathologic findings included specific infections in eight patients (including three cases of cytomegalovirus), diffuse alveolar hemorrhage in five patients, cryptogenic organizing pneumonia in five patients, and bronchiolitis in three patients. Findings on lung biopsy led to a change in treatment in

Table 1   ALI Imitators: Lavage and Histopathologic Findings

Disease	BAL findings	Histopathologic findings
Acute eosinophilic pneumonia	Eosinophilia[a] (20% or greater)	Diffuse alveolar damage with interstitial eosinophilic infiltration
Acute cryptogenic organizing pneumonia	Cellular and nonspecific	Organizing pneumonia with proliferative bronchiolitis
Diffuse alveolar hemorrhage	Progressive hemorrhagic return, hemosiderin-laden macrophages	Pulmonary capillaritis, hemorrhage, diffuse alveolar damage
Acute hypersensitivity pneumonitis	Lymphocytosis (>20%, with CD4 : CD8 ratio <1), may see neutrophilia	Loosely formed noncaseating granulomata, foamy histiocytes, and bronchocentric monocytosis

[a]BAL findings are diagnostic.
Source: From Refs. 40, 152–154.

60% of patients. There were complications of the operative procedure in 22 of the 57 patients, with one death, two hemothoraces, and 12 persistent air leaks. The overall mortality of the cohort was 53%, with no statistically significant difference in the mortality of patients with diffuse alveolar damage on biopsy versus other findings.

In summary, identification and treatment of the acute inflammatory process that is the risk factor for ALI is an important first step in patient management. Maintaining tissue perfusion and treating infection in patients with sepsis, pneumonia, trauma, and pancreatitis are crucial to limiting organ dysfunction and maximizing survival. For patients who meet criteria for ALI but have no clear inciting disorder, further evaluation beginning with bronchoalveolar lavage is safe and is recommended. Surgical lung biopsy may be considered in unexplained cases of ALI in which bronchoscopic evaluation is nondiagnostic.

IV. Mechanical Ventilation

A. Background

Patients with ALI present with hypoxemic respiratory failure. Alveolar flooding, inactivation of surfactant, and atelectasis all occur in the acute phase of ALI. These factors lead to intrapulmonary shunt and ventilation–perfusion mismatches that contribute to hypoxemia. Although hypercarbia is not usual in early ALI, the minute ventilation is nearly always markedly elevated for the level of PCO_2. Ventilation is adversely affected by microthromboses in the pulmonary capillary bed that increase dead space. Work of breathing is increased by atelectasis and lung edema that reduce pulmonary compliance. Without mechanical ventilation, many patients would die from respiratory insufficiency. Mechanical ventilation is the mainstay of supportive treatment of patients with ALI; studies of treatment of ALI patients have focused on methods and goals of mechanical ventilation.

Until recently, mechanical ventilation was used in patients with ALI with the support goals of correcting hypoxemia and hypercarbia and reducing work of breathing. Large tidal volumes were often used to overcome atelectasis. High minute ventilations were used to minimize the patient's work of breathing and to prevent or reverse hypercarbia and respiratory acidosis. High levels of positive end–expiratory pressure (PEEP) were used to recruit lung and decrease intrapulmonary shunt, often resulting in improvements in oxygenation and compliance. More recently, intermittent large-volume, high-pressure breaths (recruitment maneuvers) have been recommended in attempts to expand or recruit atelectatic lung with concomitant improvement of oxygenation and lung compliance. Different modes and methods of ventilation have been tried, also with the primary goal of normalizing aberrant oxygenation and ventilation. Generally, physiologic endpoints were used as outcome measures in clinical studies of ALI, with the expectation that improvement of oxygenation, ventilation, or compliance would translate to improved patient outcomes, such as resolution of lung injury and mortality.

In the mid-1980s, imaging studies of patients using computed tomography revealed that the lung injury of ALI is not evenly distributed throughout the lung, despite the homogenous appearance of the chest radiograph. Instead, there is a heterogeneous appearance, with areas of normal-appearing lung juxtaposed with patchy areas of edema, consolidation, and atelectasis in a predominant distribution in the dependent portions of the lung (42,43). Because of this marked reduction in volume of normal lung, delivering normal or supra-normal tidal volumes to an ALI patient was shown to lead to over-distension of previously unaffected lung and subsequent lung injury.

At the same time, laboratory studies gathered mounting evidence that larger tidal volumes and higher transpulmonary pressures were detrimental to the lung (44). In animal models, larger tidal volume ventilation could create lung injury in normal lungs (45), as well as increase lung inflammation, edema formation, bacterial translocation, and organ dysfunction in animals with injured lungs (46–48). It was also suggested that hypercapnia might be lung protective in the setting of lung injury, rather than detrimental (49–51). In humans with ARDS, so-called permissive hypercapnia with respiratory acidosis appeared to be well-tolerated (50,51).

Over the last 10 years, there have been a series of clinical trials designed to assess the effect of different strategies of mechanical ventilation on mortality of patients with ALI. The success of such studies has required the development of multi-institutional collaborations, such as the NIH/NHLBI ARDSnet. ARDSnet and other multinational collaborations have greatly advanced the knowledge of practical management of the ALI patient and have provided an increasingly solid evidence base with which to evaluate different management strategies. In the following section, we will review the clinical studies of tidal volume, PEEP, recruitment maneuvers, and ventilator mode in order to make recommendations about practical ventilator management for patients with ALI.

B. Tidal Volume

In the early 1990s, there were two observational studies that found a low mortality rate among ALI patients treated with a lung protective strategy of ventilation (52,53). Since then, there have been five randomized controlled trials that compared strategies of ventilation including larger tidal volumes and physiologic goals of normocarbia ("traditional ventilation strategies") with strategies including smaller tidal volumes and permissive hypercapnia ("lung protective strategies") in order to reach the goals of decreased lung stretch and lung protection (14,54–57).

Three of the five studies were underpowered to show any difference in mortality between the study groups (54–56). Two studies showed a significant improvement in survival in the study group assigned to the lung protective strategy. The first was a small single-center study performed in Brazil by Amato and colleagues comparing a lung protective strategy that included tidal volumes of 6 mL/kg of predicted body weight, permissive hypercapnia, and higher levels of PEEP to a more traditional strategy that included tidal volumes of 12 mL/kg, attempted normalization of arterial carbon dioxide levels, and lower levels of PEEP (57). Amato et al. found a marked reduction in 28-day mortality in the lung protective group: 38% compared with 71% ($p = 0.001$). While the results were tantalizing, concerns were raised about the generalizability of these results, particularly given the small sample size (53 subjects), the unexpectedly high mortality in the control group, and the single-center nature of the study with an unusual population. Despite the difference in 28-day mortality, there was no difference in survival to hospital discharge.

The largest study of lung protective ventilation was conducted by ARDSnet and included 861 patients recruited at 10 university centers across the United States. This study compared a lung protective strategy that included tidal volumes of 6 mL/kg predicted body weight (PBW; formula listed in Table 2), end-inspiratory plateau pressure limitation at 30 cmH$_2$O, and permissive hypercapnia to a traditional strategy that included tidal volumes of 12 mL/kg PBW and plateau pressure limitation at 50 cmH$_2$O. The approach to oxygenation was the same in both groups according to a PEEP/F_iO$_2$ "ladder" (Table 2), as was the approach to weaning. Patients with elevated intracranial pressures and those with sickle hemoglobinopathy were excluded due to concerns of adverse effects of acidosis in these populations.

Survival to hospital discharge was significantly higher in the study group randomized to the lung protective strategy. Mortality in this group was 31%,

Table 2 Guide to the ARDSnet Protocol

Identify patients with ALI	• Bilateral infiltrates on CXR
	• $P_aO_2:F_iO_2$ <300
	• No evidence of left atrial hypertension
Calculate predicted body weight PBW (kg)	• Men: 50 + 2.3 [(height in inches) − 60]
	• Women: 45.5 + 2.3 [(height in inches) − 60]
Choose ventilator mode	• Assist control (volume cycled)
Set tidal volume (Vt)	• Reduce Vt by 1 mL/kg every 1–2 hr until Vt = 6 mL/kg PBW
	• Measure inspiratory plateau pressure (Pplat) every 4 hr and after changes in ventilator settings
	• If Pplat >30 cmH$_2$O, decrease Vt to 5 or 4 mL/kg
	• If Pplat <25 cmH$_2$O and Vt <6 mL/kg, increase Vt by 1 mL/kg PBW
Set respiratory rate (RR)	• With first change in Vt, set RR to match minute ventilation
	• Adjust RR with setting changes to maintain RR <35 and pH 7.30–7.45
	• Do not increase RR if P_aCO_2 < 25
Inspiratory:expiratory ratio	• 1:1–1.3 (not inverse ratio)
Oxygenation:	• Goal P_aO_2: 55–80 mmHg, goal S_aO_2: 88–95%
Setting F_iO_2 and PEEP	• Use F_IO_2: PEEP ladder below (PEEP in cmH$_2$O)

F_iO_2	0.3–0.4	0.4	0.5	0.5	0.6	0.7	0.7	0.7	0.8	0.9	0.9	1.0
PEEP	5	8	8	10	10	10	12	14	14	16	16	18–25

Managing acidosis	• If pH < 7.30, increase RR until pH > 7.30 or RR > 35
	• If pH < 7.30 and RR = 35, consider bicarbonate
	• If pH < 7.15, may increase Vt (Pplat may exceed 30)
Weaning	• Start weaning by pressure support when all of the following criteria are present:
	• F_iO_2 ≤0.40
	• PEEP ≤8 cmH$_2$O
	• No neuromuscular blockade
	• Inspiratory efforts are present
	• Systolic blood pressure >90 mmHg
	• No vasopressor use

Source: From Ref. 62.

compared with 39.8% in the traditional strategy study group, an improvement in survival of 22% ($p = 0.007$). There was also a significant increase in the number of ventilator-free days and organ-failure free days in the lung protective group.

The results of the ARDSnet study have led to excitement and heated debate (58–61). While the study demonstrated that ventilation with 6 mL/kg PBW is superior to 12 mL/kg PBW, critics have commented that we still do not know if 6 mL/kg is better than 7 mL/kg or 8 mL/kg, since these tidal volumes were not directly compared (59). However, the mortality in the 6 mL/kg PBW study group was the lowest of any randomized controlled trial of ALI patients, considerably lower than the mortality of previous study groups ventilated with 7–8 mL/kg tidal volumes (54–56). It has also been questioned if patients with low plateau pressures need to have tidal volumes lowered down to 6 mL/kg PBW if plateau pressure is less than 30 cmH$_2$O at higher tidal volumes. While not a primary question addressed by the ARDSnet study, a subset analysis demonstrated that the mortality benefit of the lung protective strategy existed across all strata of plateau pressure, and that the subjects with the lowest quartile of plateau pressure at baseline and with plateau pressures considerably less than 30 cmH$_2$O when randomized to the traditional strategy had higher mortality than subjects in the same group (lowest quartile of plateau pressure) ventilated with 6 mL/kg PBW (62).

The ARDSnet lung protective protocol offers the best evidence in medicine to management of ALI patients to date and should be considered the standard of clinical care as well as the control group ventilation method to which all future clinical trials are tested. It is important to remember that the survival advantage of the ARDSnet lung protective protocol is the result of an entire strategy. Unfortunately, there is evidence that practice has been slow to change after the publication of these results (63). Effective employment of this strategy requires a multidisciplinary effort that involves physicians, nurses, and respiratory therapists alike, and will likely be improved by protocolizing aspects of care that are essential to using these ARDSnet lung protective protocols.

For example, calculation of predicted body weight requires assessment of patient height, which is not done in many facilities. The use of PBW, calculated from height, is thought to be important in order to reproduce the survival benefit of the ARDSnet trial. In North America, a tidal volume of 6 mL/kg based on *measured* body weight (MBW) approximates a tidal volume of 5 mL/kg PBW on the average. If MBW were used as a basis for calculating tidal volume, some patients would be ventilated with tidal volumes considerably higher than those used in the treatment group of the ARDSnet trial. Routine measurement and documentation of plateau pressure is necessary according to the ARDSnet protocol, yet a recent county-wide review of records in 17 hospitals found that five hospitals did not have a single record of plateau pressure among the ALI patients' charts reviewed, and only 10 of the 17 hospitals had plateau pressure recorded at any time for all ALI patients (64). The next step to improving mortality of ALI patients is the successful implementation of the ARDSnet protocol, which is summarized in Table 2, and is available in full at www.ardsnet.org.

C. PEEP

The acute phase of ALI is marked by abnormalities in surfactant production and metabolism (2,65–67). Without the effects of surfactant to reduce surface tension in alveoli, there is widespread alveolar collapse at end-expiration, leading to atelectasis (68). The use of lower tidal volumes is associated with an increase in atelectasis (69). Atelectasis is responsible for many of the pathologic findings in ALI: diffuse infiltrates on chest radiography, intrapulmonary shunt and hypoxemia, reduced lung compliance, and work of breathing. In addition, it has been demonstrated that atelectasis subjects the lungs to mechanical stress. The stress caused by repetitive opening and closing of alveoli and respiratory bronchioles has been termed "atelectrauma" (70), and is thought to be a significant contributor to ventilator-induced lung injury (71). Additionally, the juxtaposition of open lung units and atelectatic units leads to stretch injury and high transalveolar pressures in the open units during inspiration, which is another mechanical cause of lung injury (72).

The application of PEEP is effective in recruiting atelectatic lung regions and preventing repetitive closing and re-opening of alveoli and respiratory units between end-expiration and inspiration (73,74). By aerating previously nonaerated regions, PEEP decreases intrapulmonary shunt, improves oxygenation, and improves lung compliance (1). This effect may be more marked in patients with nonpulmonary risk factors for ALI, such as sepsis or pancreatitis, as opposed to pneumonia (75). By improving oxygenation with PEEP, the fractional inspired oxygen can often be reduced and the chances of worsening lung injury due to potential oxygen toxicity are limited (76,77). However, these beneficial effects of PEEP come at a cost. Increasing intrathoracic pressure decreases venous return and can adversely affect cardiac output. Increasing transalveolar pressure may increase the risk for further lung injury and barotrauma, and has been shown to increase pulmonary edema formation.

There are many animal studies that demonstrate the beneficial effects of PEEP. Studies have shown that the application of PEEP attenuates the effects of large tidal volume respiration on the development of lung injury (44,45) and improves pulmonary compliance. In human studies, PEEP in combination with lung-protective tidal volumes reduces systemic inflammation (29). Despite 30 years of laboratory research of PEEP, clinical research with patient-centered outcomes is extremely limited. While it is clear that ALI patients benefit from PEEP, the method of ascertainment of the optimal level of PEEP for an individual patient remains unclear. There are reports of tailoring PEEP to maximize compliance, which can be done using pressure–volume curves, stepwise incremental PEEP curves (78), or stepwise decremental PEEP curves (79,80). Computed tomography can be used during a PEEP titration to visually determine the amount of PEEP associated with maximal recruitment without hyperinflation (81). It has also been proposed that the effect of PEEP on oxygenation can be used for determination of optimal PEEP (82). Unfortunately, there are problems with reproducibility, resource availability, interobserver variability, and lack of clinical proof of concept for each of these methods that significantly limit their potential efficacy and ability to be used outside of the research arena as a part of general community care. The randomized controlled trial by Amato et al. (57) used two different PEEP strategies and assessed their effects on mortality.

Since this investigation compared a low tidal volume, high PEEP strategy to a traditional tidal volume, low PEEP strategy, it is impossible to discern whether the improved 28-day mortality was more a result of the lung-protective tidal volumes or the higher PEEP.

In February of 2002, the ARDSnet randomized controlled trial comparing a lower PEEP strategy to higher PEEP was stopped after enrolling 550 patients because of lack of efficacy (6). In this investigation, both study groups were ventilated according to the protocol of the ARDSnet low tidal volume strategy, with goal tidal volumes of 6 mL/kg and a plateau pressure target of less than 30 cmH$_2$O. The lower PEEP study group had PEEP and F_1O_2 set according to the same algorithm used in the tidal volume trial, as shown in Table 3. The higher PEEP study group was treated by an algorithm that used higher PEEP and lower F_iO_2. Both groups had a PaO2 goal of 55–80 mmHg, with instructions to lower PEEP/F_iO_2 according to the algorithm for P_aO_2 >80, and to raise PEEP/F_iO_2 for P_aO_2 <55.

The trial had 89% power to detect a 10% mortality difference between the study groups. Despite achieving the goal separation of PEEP between the study groups of 6 cmH$_2$O, there was no difference in the primary outcome of hospital mortality or any of the secondary outcome measures (ventilator-free days, organ-failure free days, ICU free days, and barotraumas) between the groups. Notably, the mortality was the lowest of any large ALI study to date: 25.2% in the lower PEEP study group and 27.1% in the higher PEEP study group, supporting the conclusion of the original ARDSnet trial that lower tidal volumes result in better survival. Although the physiologic rationale for higher PEEP is compelling, there is no strategy that has been clinically proven to be superior to the levels of PEEP and F_1O_2 used in the ARDSnet tidal volume trial (and the lower PEEP group of the PEEP trial).

D. Ventilator Mode

Patients with ALI are ventilated primarily using volume-cycled modes (volume assist control and intermittent mandatory ventilation) (83). Assist control is the mode that was used in the ARDSnet tidal volume trial, since this mode is readily available and ensures delivery of constant tidal volumes. Patients with ALI can also be ventilated with pressure-cycled modes, although these modes do not deliver consistent tidal volumes since changes in lung compliance are reflected in changes in tidal volume when pressure is held constant. Pressure-cycled modes offer a faster inspiratory flow than volume modes, which has been postulated to provide better aeration of the ALI lung. However, clinical studies comparing oxygenation and ventilation between pressure-cycled and volume-cycled modes found no difference (84). Similarly, there has been no convincing evidence to support the use of inverse-ratio ventilation, which gives more time for inspiration than exhalation. In the absence of clinical evidence demonstrating a mortality benefit of a ventilator mode compared with a volume-cycled mode according to the ARDSnet tidal volume protocol, we suggest that ALI patients should be ventilated with a volume-cycled mode as the current standard of care.

E. Recruitment Maneuvers

The application of a constant level of PEEP represents one method to attempt to recruit atelectatic lung regions in patients with ALI. Another approach is to perform periodic maneuvers with high tidal volumes, high levels of PEEP, or both in an attempt to open deaerated lung with the goal of increasing oxygenation and compliance. There have not been any studies of recruitment maneuvers designed to look at patient-centered outcomes, such as mortality or ventilator-free days. Smaller physiologic studies had conflicting results, with some showing an improvement in oxygenation and compliance lasting for a hour or more after the recruitment maneuver (69,85,86), while others showed no improvement at all (87). Recruitment maneuvers may be less efficacious in settings where the lung is already well recruited, such as when high levels of PEEP are used (87) or the patient is in the prone position (88), and more efficacious in settings where the lung is derecruited, such as after endotracheal suctioning (89).

In addition to the potential positive effects of recruitment maneuvers, such as improved lung aeration, oxygenation, and compliance, there are also potential detrimental effects. Performance of recruitment maneuvers is associated with decreases in oxygen saturation and systemic blood pressure, but these effects appear to be short-lived; there is no evidence that recruitment maneuvers lead to pneumothoraces (87). However, the ALI lung is susceptible to injury by extremes of pressure and volume, and it is possible that recruitment maneuvers lead to barotrauma or volutrauma. The current studies do not provide enough evidence to balance the potential risks and benefits of recruitment maneuvers, so we do not recommend their use in standard care of the ALI patient. However, there may be select patients with particularly poor compliance or oxygenation who could benefit from recruitment maneuvers.

F. Summary

Mechanical ventilation provides life-saving support for many patients with ALI. At the same time, mechanical ventilation can cause lung injury that leads to multiple organ dysfunction and death. Ventilation of ALI patients with the lung protective strategy used in the ARDSnet tidal volume trial that includes volume-cycled ventilation with tidal volumes of 6 mL/kg predicted body weight or less, plateau pressure limits of 30 cmH$_2$O, permissive hypercapnia (if it occurs with the lower tidal volume), and a moderate combination of PEEP and F_iO_2 is the recommended strategy. This should be the standard of care, and the control to which future clinical trials of mechanical ventilation strategies should be compared.

V. Prone Positioning

Prone positioning has been consistently shown to result in improved oxygenation in the great majority (two-thirds to three-quarters) of patients with ALI/ARDS. What is not known is whether this improvement in gas exchange is associated with improved patient-centered outcomes. Unlike other therapies that improve oxygenation, prone positioning has some underlying rationale that suggests a mechanism by which it could reduce ventilator-induced lung injury. There is much less of a pleural pressure gradient from the top to the bottom of the lung when animals are ventilated in the prone, compared to the supine, position. This is particularly striking in animals with existing lung injury. Therefore, it might be expected that nondependent lung regions would not be as susceptible to over-distention and dependent lung regions might not be as susceptible to collapse and cyclic opening and closure when ventilated in the prone, compared to the supine, position. Again, there has been no convincing demonstration to date in a clinical trial that this theoretic advantage translates to better survival.

Two randomized controlled trials of prone positioning in patients with ARDS have been conducted, only one of which has been published at the time of this publication. Gattinoni et al. (90) in a relatively large multi-center trial compared prone positioning for at least six hours per day to being maintained in the supine position. They showed a persistent oxygenation benefit in the prone position that was still demonstrated after 10 days in the patients remaining on mechanical ventilation. However, there was no difference in mortality between the two groups. A post-hoc analysis found that patients with more severe oxygenation abnormalities on study entrance had improved outcomes with prone positioning. This study was important as the first one which systematically examined the prone position in ARDS. Importantly, placing the patient in the prone position daily was not associated with an excess of complications, compared to controls. The study has been criticized for the relatively short time per day that the patients were kept prone, perhaps explaining the negative results.

A Spanish multi-center trial has been done, being stopped before reaching target enrollment because of difficulty in recruiting patients for the study. In this study, the results of which have been presented orally at an international meeting, patients randomized to the prone position were maintained prone for 18 hours or more per day. There was a strong trend for better survival in the prone position group, but the results were not significant at the $p = 0.05$ level. These results have stimulated further interest in study of the prone position. Both studies were initiated before the ARDSnet tidal volume study results were available, so neither used a lung protective ventilation protocol in the control patients. Currently, an Italian multi-center trial has been started in which patients randomized to prone positioning will be kept in that position for the great majority of the day, and all patients will be ventilated with the ARDSnet ventilation protocol.

Accidental extubation and removal of central lines are potential risks during the procedure of turning the patient between the supine and the prone position. In the study by Gattinoni and colleagues, these events did not occur more frequently in the patients randomized to the prone position (and turned twice daily) than patients maintained in the supine position, demonstrating that proning can be done safely if care is taken. We recommend that one individual, usually a respiratory therapist, be responsible only for maintaining the airway during turning. A special proning bed is commercially available, which allows proning to be safely done by one nurse. Proning can be safely carried out without such a bed, but three or more care-givers are usually required for position changes. Facial edema usually develops in the prone position; this may be lessened by maintaining a slight reverse Trendelenberg position. Skin breakdown can occur, especially over pressure points, but usually can be avoided with careful positioning. Spinal trauma and open abdominal surgical wounds are contraindications to proning. Closed surgical wounds and obesity are not contraindications.

Currently, we reserve use of the prone position for patients with a severe oxygenation abnormality. In these patients, we try to initiate the prone position as early as possible and leave patients prone unless they need to be turned supine for nursing care or procedures. Until we have more definitive data, we cannot recommend routine use of the prone position.

VI. Pharmacologic Therapies

As understanding of the pathophysiology of ALI has advanced, candidates for pharmacologic therapies with the potential to improve outcomes have emerged. There have been studies of corticosteroids and other anti-inflammatory drugs based on the recognition of the importance of inflammation in the pathogenesis of ALI. Interest in improving ventilation–perfusion matching and decreasing pulmonary artery pressures led to trials of inhaled nitric oxide and other vasodilators. Discovery of the abnormalities of surfactant synthesis and metabolism was followed by multiple studies of exogenous surfactant preparations. In this section, we will review the randomized controlled trials performed in investigation of these agents and make recommendations based on the results of these studies.

A. Nitric Oxide

Nitric oxide is an endogenous vasodilator that has a prominent role in vascular smooth muscle relaxation and in regulating systemic and pulmonary regional blood flow. It is an appealing candidate for an inhaled therapy in ALI, given its ability to promote increased perfusion of ventilated lung units without significant hemodynamic effects (91). There have been a number of randomized controlled trials of inhaled nitric oxide in patients with ALI (92–96). Single-center studies showed proof of concept: inhaled nitric oxide led to improved oxygenation (93,94). Subsequent multi-center randomized controlled trials (92,95), including a recently published study of 385 patients (96), have supported the finding that inhaled nitric oxide improves oxygenation. However, in all studies, there is no difference in mortality or ventilator-free days between subjects receiving inhaled nitric oxide and those randomized to placebo. We do not recommend the use of inhaled nitric oxide as a standard therapy for patients with ALI. It has been suggested that inhaled nitric oxide may be used as a rescue therapy for patients who are difficult to oxygenate with maximal F_1O_2 and PEEP (2), particularly those with right heart failure (26), but there is no evidence from clinical studies to support this recommendation. Studies of other vasodilators have not shown benefit in animal models of ALI (97,98) or human studies (99–101).

B. Corticosteroids

Inflammation, both local and systemic, plays an important role in the pathogenesis and recovery from ALI (29,102). Corticosteroids have myriad anti-inflammatory effects and have been studied in patients with risk factors for ALI as a possible preventative therapy (103), and for treatment of patients with early (103,104) and late (105) ALI. In the studies in early sepsis and ALI, there was no decrease in ALI incidence, severity, or mortality with treatment using high doses of corticosteroids. In fact, there was a concerning increase in mortality in the steroid arm in some of the trials. We do not recommend using high dose corticosteroids as a therapy for ALI early in the course, for there is no evidence supporting its use and some evidence demonstrating harm.

Since persistent inflammation is thought to play a role in the fibro-proliferative phase of ALI that leads to persistent lung injury, corticosteroids have also been studied in ALI patients with continuing lung injury for 1 week or more after first developing ALI. One small single-center study by Meduri et al. (105) noted promising results of longer-term treatment with corticosteroids in late ALI. This protocol used 2 mg/kg/day of methylprednisolone for the first 14 study days, then reduced the dose by 50% per week for an additional two weeks, and then tapered steroids off over a final four days. ARDSnet recently completed a trial of corticosteroids for late ALI. Enrollment of 180 patients was completed in November 2003 and 180-day outcomes are nearly completely collected. This study used a similar protocol to Meduri, differing by a more rapid taper off steroids after 48 hours of extubation. The results of this trial are highly anticipated since this is likely to be a definitive study of the role for corticosteroids in late ALI. Incomplete results presented orally at a national meeting indicated steroid treated patients were able to be weaned from mechanical ventilation earlier, but more patients were returned to mechanical ventilation compared to the control patients. There was no difference in 60-day mortality between the two groups. At the present time, there is not sufficient evidence to recommend the use of corticosteroids for late ALI.

C. Surfactant Therapy

Decreased production and increased inactivation of surfactant is thought to play an important role in the pathogenesis of ALI and is likely the primary contributor to widespread atelectasis. Surfactant-replacement therapy has been successful in newborns with respiratory distress syndrome (106), a condition marked by insufficient surfactant as the primary defect. There have been randomized controlled trials of a number of different surfactant preparations, including bovine surfactant, synthetic phosphatidylcholine-based surfactant (Exosurf®) and recombinant surfactant protein C-based surfactant (Venticute®). In the pilot study of Exosurf, there were no differences in the physiologic parameters between treatment groups, but there was a trend towards survival (107). In the large multi-center randomized controlled trial of 725 patients that followed, there was no difference in physiology or survival between patients treated with Exosurf and placebo (108). The pilot study of Venticute showed no beneficial effects associated with drug treatment (109). This was followed up with two multi-centered randomized controlled trials of a total of 448 patients, which demonstrated that Venticute improved oxygenation during administration but did not decrease time of mechanical ventilation or mortality (110). The pilot study of bovine surfactant was more promising, with significant improvements in oxygenation and a trend of improved survival (111). With improvements in synthetic surfactant formulations and delivery systems, it is possible that there will be a way to deliver surfactant to the distal airspaces in the future that will improve outcomes of ALI. At this time, the use of aerosolized surfactant in any form cannot yet be recommended.

VII. Fluid Management

The early pathogenesis of ALI is marked by edema formation, as the alveolar capillary bed increases in permeability and protein-rich edema fluid floods the alveolar spaces. Alveolar fluid accumulation is directly associated with filling pressures (hydrostatic forces), since competing oncotic forces are reduced by increased capillary permeability and the decreased oncotic gradient between capillary and interstitium. Decreasing filling pressures can markedly reduce edema formation and improve oxygenation (1,112). As such, optimal fluid management for patients with ALI has been an ongoing controversy for decades.

A. "Wet" or "Dry"?

What is the evidence in support of fluid-restrictive management in ALI? There have been a number of animal studies demonstrating that the reduction of pulmonary artery pressure (either by vasodilators, diuretics or ultra-filtration) improved physiologic end-points such as edema formation, gas exchange, and lung compliance (97,113–117). However, there are significant risks to a management strategy that decreases circulating volume, including decreased cardiac output, decreased tissue perfusion, and increased end-organ dysfunction. Since most deaths of patients with ALI are a result of multiple organ failure and not respiratory failure (27), and improved pulmonary physiology is not always associated with improved patient outcomes (6,14,90,92), basing a clinical strategy on these animal studies is not reasonable.

While opinion papers on fluid management are plentiful (118–123), there are no published randomized controlled trials comparing different strategies of fluid management in patients with ALI. There have been two retrospective studies in ALI patients that showed that patients who die with ALI are more likely to have net fluid gain than are survivors (124), and that patients who die are less likely to have reductions in pulmonary capillary wedge pressure than are survivors (125). Cause-and-effect relationships between fluid management and patient outcome cannot be made from these studies, which really only tell us that sicker patients are treated with more fluids. Two additional studies use measurement of extra-vascular lung water as a guide to clinical management of fluid administration, vasopressors and diuretics in ICU patients with pulmonary artery catheters, and either infiltrates on chest radiograph (126) or hypotension (127). Over 50% of subjects in each study had congestive heart failure; the subgroups of patients described with ARDS were underpowered to demonstrate an effect on oxygenation or mortality.

ARDSnet is currently conducting a randomized controlled clinical trial of fluid management in ALI with the primary outcome of mortality. This study, entitled the Fluid and Catheter Treatment Trial (FACTT), is a factorial designed study comparing liberal versus conservative fluid management and guidance of treatment decisions with and without pulmonary artery catheterization. The goal enrollment of FACTT is 1000 patients, which provides 90% power to detect a 10% absolute difference in mortality. As of October 2005, enrollment has reached the target. The hope is that this will be a definitive study leading to the development of a standard of care of fluid management in the near future.

While awaiting study results, there is little evidence to offer guidance of practice. We know that early, goal-directed fluid resuscitation of patients in shock improves outcomes (10), and that attempts to increase cardiac output and oxygen delivery to supra-physiologic in ICU patients do not decrease mortality (128,129). It is logical but unproven that appropriate fluid management of patients with ALI attempts to maintain organ perfusion while avoiding fluid overload. The role of the pulmonary artery catheter in guiding fluid management in patients with ALI also remains unclear (130–132).

VIII.   Protecting ALI Patients from the ICU

Compared with others in the ICU, ALI patients have a longer duration of mechanical ventilation and ICU stay. Providing the best supportive care is important in reducing the mortality of ALI patients and ensuring the best quality of life for survivors (133). Recommendations for the best supportive care, as substantiated by recent randomized controlled trials, are discussed in the other sections of this edition and in a recent review (134). The diagnosis, treatment, and prevention of ventilator associated pneumonia are complicated and especially important in ALI patients; we have included a review of this topic. There is also an overview of ventilator associated pneumonia included in the chapter on pneumonia in the ICU.

IX. Ventilator-Associated Pneumonia

Ventilator-associated pneumonia (VAP) is a common complication in mechanically ventilated, critically ill patients and especially those with ALI. VAP is associated with increased mortality, increased morbidity including prolongation of hospital stay, and increased economic costs. Two large one-day point prevalence studies in European ICUs found a point prevalence for hospital-acquired pneumonia of 10% and 9%, with a three-fold higher risk of hospital-acquired pneumonia in ventilated as compared to nonventilated critically ill patients. The incidence of VAP (VAP development at any time during the hospitalization) is usually 20–28%. VAP incidence is higher in patients with ALI/ARDS than in other ventilated patients. The mortality associated with VAP is two to four times higher than in similar patients without this condition. Several studies suggest that duration of mechanical ventilation, ICU length of stay, and hospital length of stay are from 25% to 100% longer in patients with VAP than matched control patients without VAP (135).

Several risk factors have been associated with VAP. These risk factors can be roughly divided into two groups: characteristics associated with the host and factors associated with medical interventions. These risk factors are summarized in Table 3.

The major risk in terms of pathogenesis is probably not the ventilator but the presence of the endotracheal tube. Most investigators believe that the major pathogenetic mechanism is the micro-aspiration of colonized upper airway or gastric secretions. Since the early 1970s, it has been known that the flora of the stomach and upper airway changes over several days following the onset of critical illness

Table 3 Risk Factors for Ventilator-Associated Pneumonia

Host factors	Intervention factors
Serum albumin <2.2	Paralysis, continuous sedation
Age >60 yr	>4 units blood products
ARDS, COPD, coma	Mechanical ventilation >2 days
Burns, trauma	Frequent ventilator circuit changes
Multi-organ failure	Reintubation
Large volume gastric aspiration	Nasogastric tube
Gastric and tracheal colonization	Supine position
	Prior or no antibiotic therapy

Abbreviations: ARDS, acute respiratory distress syndrome; COPD, chronic obstructive pulmonary disease.
Source: Adapted from Ref. 135.

with the emergence of potential pathogens. Changes in gastric colonization often precede the changes in upper airway colonization. Modern endotracheal tubes with high-volume, low-pressure cuffs minimize tracheal mucosal injury but allow continual leakage of small quantities of secretions past small invaginations in the cuff. Attention to preventing VAP has focused on preventing colonization of the stomach and minimizing the change of aspiration, especially by nursing the patient in the semi-recumbent position. VAP can also occur by the blood-borne route related to line infections or other causes of bacteremia.

Diagnosis of VAP can be difficult and is particularly problematic in the patient with ALI. It is well documented that the inflammatory condition of ALI can cause fever, leukocytosis, and purulent respiratory secretions. Since diffuse pulmonary infiltrates are already present, new infiltrates related to pneumonia are difficult to appreciate. And this is a difficult area to study because of the lack of a "gold standard" for diagnosis. Some clarity has been added through a series of investigations, especially those of Fagon and Chastre, using quantitative cultures of specimens from the lower respiratory tract obtained through a fiberoptic bronchoscope. These studies produced the hypothesis that quantitative cultures above a certain cut-off value can identify patients with VAP, whereas culture amounts lower than the arbitrary cut-off are not associated with clinical pneumonia, and these patients do not require treatment with antibiotics. The critical values that have been established are 10^3 colony forming units (cfu)/mL for bronchoalveolar lavage (BAL) and 10^4 cfu/mL for protected specimen brush (PSB) (13).

These authors tested this hypothesis in a multi-center randomized con-trolled trial in which patients suspected of having VAP were randomized to either an approach which utilized fiberoptic bronchoscopy in obtaining speci-mens for quantitative cultures or one in which this was not performed but all other clinical and laboratory data, including culture results, were available to the clin-ician. The approach using quantitative cultures resulted in better outcomes (lower mortality) with less use of antibiotics. This study suggests that patients suspected of having VAP, including those with new infiltrates, fever, and leukocytosis, but who do not meet quantitative culture criteria for pneumonia, do not need to be treated with antibiotics. They usually have atelectasis or other conditions accounting for these clinical findings. One of the advantages of this approach is that nondiagnostic quantitative culture results should prompt a search for causes of the fever other than pneumonia.

We should be clear that no approach has achieved the establishment of being the standard of care, at least in North America, and experts continue to debate the best strategy for diagnosis of VAP. Even though some doubt remains regarding the optimal approach, we believe that the best current evidence supports the use of quantitative cultures to determine the presence of VAP and its treatment. We recommend their use, therefore, in intubated patients in hospitals that have the laboratory capability of performing quantitative cultures of respir-atory tract specimens. This is clearest for patients who have not been treated with antibiotics, but also appears to be applicable to those patients who have been on an antibiotic regimen for several days without changes. Since recent changes in antibiotic therapy render the results less interpretable, it is mandatory that, if this approach is to be undertaken, access to obtaining specimens from the lower respiratory tract must be available within a short period of time, certainly no longer than a few hours. Antibiotics should be withheld until fiberoptic bronchoscopy is done and then started either guided by direct smear results of the obtained specimens or empirically while awaiting the culture results.

Streptococcus pneumoniae is much less frequent as a cause of VAP than of community-acquired pneumonia, whereas *Staphylococcus aureus* (SA), including methacillin resistant staphylococcus aureus (MRSA) and Gram-negative bacilli, including Pseudomonas and Acinetobacter, are more common as causative pathogens. Guidelines have been developed by several societies to help guide initial empiric antibiotic therapy. The most important factor in this decision, however, is knowledge of the local hospital's pattern of causative organisms and their antibiotic resistance pattern, since these patterns vary by region and by institution. The guidelines are based on whether Pseudomonas, Acinetobacter, or MRSA are likely to be etiologic. If a Gram-negative bacillus is likely, then double coverage is warranted. If MRSA is considered likely, then vancomycin can be added (136).

A recent trial in France compared eight days of therapy to 15 days of therapy with antibiotics. With the exception of pneumonia due to Pseudomonas, the outcome was just as effective with eight days of therapy. In the case of pneumonia due to Pseudomonas, there was no difference in mortality between the two groups, but patients treated for eight days were more likely to have a clinical recurrence. We recommend eight days of therapy except when the pneumonia is caused by Pseudomonas, in which case either a longer antibiotic course or increased vigilance for recurrent infection are reasonable approaches (137).

Several strategies have been suggested to reduce the incidence of VAP. Most of these strategies have been tested in relatively small trials and do not reach the level of IA evidence, the highest level of evidence basis. Some of the strategies, however, have been found to have consistent results in small studies, have not been associated with toxicity, and are inexpensive. These can be recommended for implementation (138,139).

The most important strategy for preventing VAP appears to be nursing the patient in the semi-recumbent (45°) position. Two trials measured gastroesophageal reflux and aspiration events as surrogate outcomes and showed a decrease in both. A third trial found a statistically significant reduction in VAP in patients nursed with the head of the bed elevated to 45°, compared to those patients nursed in the supine position (140). Based on these studies, it is recommended that all critically ill patients be nursed in a semi-recumbent position unless there is a specific contraindication to this.

Patients who are mechanically ventilated are known to be at risk for stress gastric ulceration. Early studies suggested that antacids and possible H2 blockers, which reduce the gastric acidity in an attempt to decrease stress ulceration, were associated with increased risk for VAP. Sucralfate, which protects the mucosa from stress ulceration but does not affect gastric pH, was associated with lower rates of VAP, a finding which was confirmed by additional studies. However, a recent large well-designed trial of 1200 ventilated patients found that H2 blockers were more effective than sucralfate in preventing gastrointestinal bleeding but failed to find a difference in VAP incidence between the two (141). H2 blockers are more expensive than sucralfate but are easier to administer. With our current state of knowledge, therefore, one can choose between H2 blockers and sucralfate as the means of reducing stress ulceration in mechanically ventilated patients.

Finally, several studies have shown that more frequent changes of ventilator circuits are associated with a higher incidence of VAP development. Current recommendations are to change ventilator circuits no more frequently than weekly, unless they are obviously contaminated. There is no clear evidence favoring any specific form of enteral feeding as being advantageous in reducing the incidence of VAP.

X.   Caring for Survivors of ALI

As the mortality of patients with ALI declines, more patients become survivors of ALI every year. Understanding the issues that confront ALI survivors is important in providing care to this population. Over the last decade, a number of studies have contributed to our knowledge about survivors of critical illness in general and ALI in particular.

Although ALI is characterized by severe lung dysfunction, several studies have demonstrated by pulmonary function testing that lung function returns to the normal range in most survivors by the end of the first year of recovery (133,142). While many survivors have respiratory symptoms at hospital discharge, most resolve over the first year as well. A small subset has worsening of shortness of breath; it is important to evaluate these patients for upper airway obstruction associated with tracheal stenosis, since this can be effectively treated in most (133,143).

For those who survive the acute illness, long-term survival is not decreased for those with ALI compared with controls matched for severity of illness and primary risk factor for ALI (sepsis or trauma) (144). However, compared to these controls, there is a persistent impairment of health-related quality of life among ALI survivors (145). The precise etiology of this impairment in quality of life is not known, but studies have revealed problems with weakness and musculoskeletal function (133,146), cognitive dysfunction (147), depression (148), post-traumatic stress disorder (149), and difficulty returning to full-time employment (133,150). Studies are currently ongoing to investigate the potential of post-hospital interventions (such as antidepressants, occupational and physical therapy, and rehabilitation) to improve long-term health related quality of life among survivors. Patient and family education may also be important in helping survivors understand that the road to recovery is a long one; one recent study showed that providing information and reassurance decreased anxiety among ALI survivors (151). Information and peer support may be available through individual hospitals, and is available through patient-based organizations such as the ARDS Foundation (www.ardsil.com) and the ARDS Support Center (www.ards.org).

XI. Summary

Practical management of the patient with ALI should focus on protecting the patient from the perils of supportive care. We can improve survival and decrease ventilator-induced lung injury by identifying patients with ALI, using low tidal volume ventilation, and introducing the systems changes needed to correctly apply the ARDSnet protocol. There is no high-quality evidence that a different strategy of PEEP, recruitment maneuvers, prone positioning, or ventilator modes other than volume-cycle offer significant benefits over the ARDSnet lung protective ventilation protocol, nor that any pharmacologic interventions specifically improve ALI outcomes. Instead, we need to focus on providing the best supportive care to help ALI patients survive their hospital stay. We need to educate patients and their primary care providers about the long-term sequelae of ALI. Finally, we need to continue to perform clinical research in ALI and work to incorporate these results into our clinical practices.

References

1. Ashbaugh DG, Bigelow DB, Petty TL, Levine BE. Acute respiratory distress in adults. Lancet 1967; 2(7511):319–323.
2. Ware LB, Matthay MA. The acute respiratory distress syndrome. N Engl J Med 2000; 342(18):1334–1349.
3. Milberg JA, Davis DR, Steinberg KP, Hudson LD. Improved survival of patients with acute respiratory distress syndrome (ARDS): 1983–1993. J Am Med Assoc 1995; 273(4):306–309.
4. Steinberg KP, Hudson LD. Acute lung injury and acute respiratory distress syndrome. The clinical syndrome. Clin Chest Med 2000; 21(3):401–417, vii.
5. Abel SJ, Finney SJ, Brett SJ, Keogh BF, Morgan CJ, Evans TW. Reduced mortality in association with the acute respiratory distress syndrome (ARDS). Thorax 1998; 53(4):292–294.
6. Brower RG, Lanken PN, MacIntyre N, Matthay MA, Morris A, Ancukiewicz M, Schoenfeld D, Thompson BT. Higher versus lower positive end-expiratory pressures in patients with the acute respiratory distress syndrome. N Engl J Med 2004; 351(4):327–336.

7. ARDSNetwork. Update on the late steroids rescue study (LaSRS). In: American Thoracic Society International Conference, Orlando, Florida, 2003.

8. Kress JP, Pohlman AS, O'Connor MF, Hall JB. Daily interruption of sedative infusions in critically ill patients undergoing mechanical ventilation. N Engl J Med 2000; 342(20):1471–1477.

9. Kollef MH, Shapiro SD, Silver P, St John RE, Prentice D, Sauer S, Ahrens TS, Shannon W, Baker-Clinkscale D. A randomized, controlled trial of protocol-directed versus physician-directed weaning from mechanical ventilation. Crit Care Med 1997; 25(4):567–574.

10. Rivers E, Nguyen B, Havstad S, Ressler J, Muzzin A, Knoblich B, Peterson E, Tomlanovich M. Early goal-directed therapy in the treatment of severe sepsis and septic shock. N Engl J Med 2001; 345(19):1368–1377.

11. van den Berghe G., Wouters P, Weekers F, Verwaest C, Bruyninckx F, Schetz M, Vlasselaers D, Ferdinande P, Lauwers P, Bouillon R. Intensive insulin therapy in the critically ill patients. N Engl J Med 2001; 345(19):1359–1367.

12. Bernard GR, Vincent JL, Laterre PF, LaRosa SP, Dhainaut JF, Lopez-Rodriguez A, Steingrub JS, Garber GE, Helterbrand JD, Ely EW, et al. Efficacy and safety of recombinant human activated protein C for severe sepsis. N Engl J Med 2001; 344(10):699–709.

13. Fagon JY, Chastre J, Wolff M, Gervais C, Parer-Aubas S, Stephan F, Similowski T, Mercat A, Diehl JL, Sollet JP, et al. Invasive and noninvasive strategies for management of suspected ventilator-associated pneumonia. A randomized trial. Ann Intern Med 2000; 132(8):621–630.

14. Brower R, Matthay M, Morris A, Schoenfeld D, Thompson BT, Wheeler A, Network TARDS. Ventilation with lower tidal volumes as compared with traditional tidal volumes for acute lung injury and the acute respiratory distress syndrome. The Acute Respiratory Distress Syndrome Network. N Engl J Med 2000; 342(18):1301–1308.

15. Bernard GR, Artigas A, Brigham KL, Carlet J, Falke K, Hudson L, Lamy M, Legall JR, Morris A, Spragg R. The American-European Consensus Conference on ARDS. Definitions, mechanisms, relevant outcomes, and clinical trial coordination. Am J Respir Crit Care Med 1994; 149(3 Pt 1):818–824.

16. Lamy M, Fallat RJ, Koeniger E, Dietrich HP, Ratliff JL, Eberhart RC, Tucker HJ, Hill JD. Pathologic features and mechanisms of hypoxemia in adult respiratory distress syndrome. Am Rev Respir Dis 1976; 114(2):267–284.

17. Goss CH, Brower RG, Hudson LD, Rubenfeld GD. Incidence of acute lung injury in the United States. Crit Care Med 2003; 31(6):1607–1611.

18. Rubenfeld GD, Caldwell ES, Martin DM. The incidence of acute lung injury in adults in the US: results of the King County Lung Injury Project. Am J Respir Crit Care Med 2002; 165(Abstracts):A96.

19. Weir HK, Thun MJ, Hankey BF, Ries LA, Howe HL, Wingo PA, Jemal A, Ward E, Anderson RN, Edwards BK. Annual report to the nation on the status of cancer, 1975–2000, featuring the uses of surveillance data for cancer prevention and control. J Natl Cancer Inst 2003; 95(17):1276–1299.

20. Rubenfeld GD. Epidemiology of acute lung injury. Crit Care Med 2003; 31(suppl 4):S276–S284.

21. Index of 1,000 Rare Diseases, N.O.f.R. Diseases, Editor, 2004.

22. Mahoney AM, Caldwell E, Hudson LD, Rubenfeld GD. Barriers to physician recognition of acute lung injury. Am J Respir Crit Care Med 2003; 167(7):A738.

23. Dedhiya P, Mikkelsen R, Kalhan R, Gaughan C, Lanken PN, Fuchs BD. Early clinician recognition of acute lung injury may increase use of lung protective ventilation. Am J Respir Crit Care Med 2004; 169(7):A5175.

24. Pepe PE, Potkin RT, Reus DH, Hudson LD, Carrico CJ. Clinical predictors of the adult respiratory distress syndrome. Am J Surg 1982; 144(1):124–130.

25. Hudson LD, Milberg JA, Anardi D, Maunder RJ. Clinical risks for development of the acute respiratory distress syndrome. Am J Respir Crit Care Med 1995; 151(2 Pt 1):293–301.

26. Brower RG, Ware LB, Berthiaume Y, Matthay MA. Treatment of ARDS. Chest 2001; 120(4):1347–1367.

27. Montgomery AB, Stager MA, Carrico CJ, Hudson LD. Causes of mortality in patients with the adult respiratory distress syndrome. Am Rev Respir Dis 1985; 132(3):485–489.

28. Stapleton RD, Wang BM, Hudson LD, Rubenfeld GD, Caldwell ES, Steinberg KP. Causes and timing of mortality in patients with the acute respiratory distress syndrome (ARDS). Am J Respir Crit Care Med 2001; 163:A449.

29. Ranieri VM, Suter PM, Tortorella C, De Tullio R, Dayer JM, Brienza A, Bruno F, Slutsky AS. Effect of mechanical ventilation on inflammatory mediators in patients with acute respiratory distress syndrome: a randomized controlled trial. J Am Med Assoc 1999; 282(1):54–61.

30. Chang MC, Meredith JW, Kincaid EH, Miller PR. Maintaining survivors' values of left ventricular power output during shock resuscitation: a prospective pilot study. J Trauma 2000; 49(1):26–33; discussion 34–37.

31. Garnacho-Montero J, Garcia-Garmendia JL, Barrero-Almodovar A, Jimenez-Jimenez FJ, Perez-Paredes C, Ortiz-Leyba C. Impact of adequate empirical anti-biotic therapy on the outcome of patients admitted to the intensive care unit with sepsis. Crit Care Med 2003; 31(12):2742–2751.

32. Anderson ID, Fearon, KC, Grant IS. Laparotomy for abdominal sepsis in the critically ill. Br J Surg 1996; 83(4):535–539.

33. Le Mee J, Paye F, Sauvanet A, O'Toole D, Hammel P, Marty J, Ruszniewski P, Belghiti J. Incidence and reversibility of organ failure in the course of sterile or infected necrotizing pancreatitis. Arch Surg 2001; 136(12):1386–1390.

34. Bassi C, Mangiante G, Falconi M, Salvia R, Frigerio I, Pederzoli P. Prophylaxis for septic complications in acute necrotizing pancreatitis. J Hepatobiliary Pancreat Surg 2001; 8(3):211–215.

35. Hartwig W, Werner J, Uhl W, Buchler MW. Management of infection in acute pancreatitis. J Hepatobiliary Pancreat Surg 2002; 9(4):423–428.

36. Olah A, Pardavi G, Belagyi T, Nagy A, Issekutz A, Mohamed GE. Early nasojejunal feeding in acute pancreatitis is associated with a lower complication rate. Nutrition 2002; 18(3):259–262.

37. Bartlett J. Treatment of community-acquired pneumonia. Chemotherapy 2000; 46(suppl 1):24–31.

38. Markewitz BA, Mayer J, Sud PR, Campbell GD. Treatment of hospital-acquired penumonia. Semin Respir Infect 2000; 15(3):248–257.

39. Steinberg KP, Mitchell DR, Maunder RJ, Milberg JA, Whitcomb ME, Hudson LD. Safety of bronchoalveolar lavage in patients with adult respiratory distress syndrome. Am Rev Respir Dis 1993; 148(3):556–561.
40. Schwarz MI, Albert RK. "Imitators" of the ARDS: implications for diagnosis and treatment. Chest 2004; 125(4):1530–1535.
41. Patel SR, Karmpaliotis D, Ayas NT, Mark EJ, Wain J, Thompson BT, Malhotra A. The role of open-lung biopsy in ARDS. Chest 2004; 125(1):197–202.
42. Maunder RJ, Shuman WP, McHugh JW, Marglin SI, Butler J. Preservation of normal lung regions in the adult respiratory distress syndrome. Analysis by computed tomography. J Am Med Assoc 1986; 255(18):2463–2465.
43. Gattinoni L, Presenti A, Torresin A, Baglioni S, Rivolta M, Rossi F, Scarani F, Marcolin R, Cappelletti G. Adult respiratory distress syndrome profiles by computed tomography. J Thorac Imaging 1986; 1(3):25–30.
44. Dreyfuss D, Basset G, Soler P, Saumon G. Intermittent positive-pressure hyperventilation with high inflation pressures produces pulmonary microvascular injury in rats. Am Rev Respir Dis 1985; 132(4):880–884.
45. Webb HH, Tierney DF. Experimental pulmonary edema due to intermittent positive pressure ventilation with high inflation pressures. Protection by positive end-expiratory pressure. Am Rev Respir Dis 1974; 110(5):556–565.
46. Corbridge TC, Wood LD, Crawford GP, Chudoba MJ, Yanos J, Sznajder JI. Adverse effects of large tidal volume and low PEEP in canine acid aspiration. Am Rev Respir Dis 1990; 142(2):311–315.
47. Tremblay L, Valenza F, Ribeiro SP, Li J, Slutsky AS. Injurious ventilatory strategies increase cytokines and c-fos m-RNA expression in an isolated rat lung model. J Clin Invest 1997; 99(5):944–952.
48. Parker JC, Hernandez LA, Peevy KJ. Mechanisms of ventilator-induced lung injury. Crit Care Med 1993; 21(1):131–143.
49. Laffey JG, Engelberts D, Kavanagh BP. Buffering hypercapnic acidosis worsens acute lung injury. Am J Respir Crit Care Med 2000; 161(1):141–146.
50. Kavanagh B. Normocapnia vs hypercapnia. Minerva Anestesiol 2002; 68(5):346–350.
51. Sinclair SE, Kregenow DA, Lamm WJ, Starr IR, Chi EY, Hlastala MP. Hypercapnic acidosis is protective in an in vivo model of ventilator-induced lung injury. Am J Respir Crit Care Med 2002; 166(3):403–408.
52. Hickling KG, Henderson SJ, Jackson R. Low mortality associated with low volume pressure limited ventilation with permissive hypercapnia in severe adult respiratory distress syndrome. Intensive Care Med 1990; 16(6):372–377.
53. Hickling KG, Walsh J, Henderson S, Jackson R. Low mortality rate in adult respiratory distress syndrome using low-volume, pressure-limited ventilation with permissive hypercapnia: a prospective study. Crit Care Med 1994; 22(10):1568–1578.
54. Brower RG, Shanholtz CB, Fessler HE, Shade DM, White P, Jr., Wiener CM, Teeter JG, Dodd-o JM, Almog Y, Piantadosi S. Prospective, randomized, controlled clinical trial comparing traditional versus reduced tidal volume ventilation in acute respiratory distress syndrome patients. Crit Care Med 1999; 27(8):1492–1498.
55. Brochard L, Roudot-Thoraval F, Roupie E, Delclaux C, Chastre J, Fernandez-Mondejar E, Clementi E, Mancebo J, Factor P, Matamis D, et al. Tidal volume reduction for prevention of ventilator-induced lung injury in acute respiratory distress syndrome. Am J Respir Crit Care Med 1998; 158(6):1831–1838.

56. Stewart TE, Meade MO, Cook DJ, Granton JT, Hodder RV, Lapinsky SE, Mazer CD, McLean RF, Rogovein TS, Schouten BD, et al. Evaluation of a ventilation strategy to prevent barotrauma in patients at high risk for acute respiratory distress syndrome. N Engl J Med 1998; 338(6):355–361.

57. Amato MB, Barbas CS, Medeiros DM, Magaldi RB, Schettino GP, Lorenzi-Filho G, Kairalla RA, Deheinzelin D, Munoz C, Oliveira R, et al. Effect of a protective-ventilation strategy on mortality in the acute respiratory distress syndrome. N Engl J Med 1998; 338(6):347–354.

58. Tobin MJ, Culmination of an era in research on the acute respiratory distress syndrome. N Engl J Med 2000; 342(18):1360–1361.

59. Eichacker PQ, Gerstenberger EP, Banks SM, Cui X, Natanson C. Meta-analysis of acute lung injury and acute respiratory distress syndrome trials testing low tidal volumes. Am J Respir Crit Care Med 2002; 166(11):1510–1514.

60. Brower RG, Matthay M, Schoenfeld D. Meta-analysis of acute lung injury and acute respiratory distress syndrome trials. Am J Respir Crit Care Med 2002; 166(11):1515–1517.

61. Stewart TE. Controversies around lung protective mechanical ventilation. Am J Respir Crit Care Med 2002; 166(11):1421–1422.

62. Brower RG. Mechanical ventilation in acute lung injury and ARDS. Tidal volume reduction. Crit Care Clin 2002; 18(1):1–13, v.

63. Weinert CR, Gross CR, Marinelli WA. Impact of randomized trial results on acute lung injury ventilator therapy in teaching hospitals. Am J Respir Crit Care Med 2003; 167(10):1304–1309.

64. Akhtar SR, Weaver J, Pierson DJ, Rubenfeld GD. Practice variation in respiratory therapy documentation during mechanical ventilation. Chest 2003; 124(6):2275–2282.

65. Petty TL, Silvers GW, Paul GW, Stanford RE. Abnormalities in lung elastic properties and surfactant function in adult respiratory distress syndrome. Chest 1979; 75(5):571–574.

66. Petty TL, Reiss OK, Paul GW, Silvers GW, Elkins ND. Characteristics of pulmonary surfactant in adult respiratory distress syndrome associated with trauma and shock. Am Rev Respir Dis 1977; 115(3):531–536.

67. Seeger W, Gunther A, Walmrath HD, Grimminger F, Lasch HG. Alveolar surfactant and adult respiratory distress syndrome. Pathogenetic role and therapeutic prospects. Clin Investig 1993; 71(3):177–190.

68. Bachofen H, Schurch S, Urbinelli M, Weibel ER. Relations among alveolar surface tension, surface area, volume, and recoil pressure. J Appl Physiol 1987; 62(5):1878–1887.

69. Richard JC, Maggiore SM, Jonson B, Mancebo J, Lemaire F, Brochard L. Influence of tidal volume on alveolar recruitment. Respective role of PEEP and a recruitment maneuver. Am J Respir Crit Care Med 2001; 163(7):1609–1613.

70. Tremblay LN, Slutsky AS. Ventilator-induced injury: from barotrauma to biotrauma. Proc Assoc Am Physicians 1998; 110(6):482–488.

71. Amato MB, Barbas CS, Medeiros DM, Schettino Gde P, Lorenzi Filho G, Kairalla RA, Deheinzelin D, Morais C, Fernandes Ede O, Takagaki TY, et al. Beneficial effects of the "open lung approach" with low distending pressures in acute respiratory distress syndrome. A prospective randomized study on mechanical ventilation. Am J Respir Crit Care Med 1995; 152(6 Pt 1):1835–1846.

72. Mead J, Takishima T, Leith D. Stress distribution in lungs: a model of pulmonary elasticity. J Appl Physiol 1970; 28(5):596–608.

73. Thompson BT, Hayden D, Matthay MA, Brower R, Parsons PE. Clinicians' approaches to mechanical ventilation in acute lung injury and ARDS. Chest 2001; 120(5):1622–1627.

74. Carmichael LC, Dorinsky PM, Higgins SB, Bernard GR, Dupont WD, Swindell B, Wheeler AP. Diagnosis and therapy of acute respiratory distress syndrome in adults: an international survey. J Crit Care 1996; 11(1):9–18.

75. Gattinoni L, Pelosi P, Suter PM, Pedoto A, Vercesi P, Lissoni A. Acute respiratory distress syndrome caused by pulmonary and extrapulmonary disease. Different syndromes Am J Respir Crit Care Med 1998; 158(1):3–11.

76. Tierney DF. Oxygen toxicity. West J Med 1979; 130(3):227–229.

77. Fisher AB. Oxygen therapy. Side effects and toxicity. Am Rev Respir Dis 1980; 122(5 Pt 2):61–69.

78. Suter PM, Fairley B, Isenberg MD. Optimum end-expiratory airway pressure in patients with acute pulmonary failure. N Engl J Med 1975; 292(6):284–289.

79. Hickling KG. The pressure-volume curve is greatly modified by recruitment. A mathematical model of ARDS lungs. Am J Respir Crit Care Med 1998; 158(1): 194–202.

80. Hickling KG. Best compliance during a decremental, but not incremental, positive end-expiratory pressure trial is related to open-lung positive end-expiratory pressure: a mathematical model of acute respiratory distress syndrome lungs. Am J Respir Crit Care Med 2001; 163(1):69–78.

81. Gattinoni L, Pelosi P, Crotti S, Valenza F. Effects of positive end-expiratory pressure on regional distribution of tidal volume and recruitment in adult respiratory distress syndrome. Am J Respir Crit Care Med 1995; 151(6):1807–1814.

82. Ranieri VM, Eissa NT, Corbeil C, Chasse M, Braidy J, Matar N, Milic-Emili J. Effects of positive end-expiratory pressure on alveolar recruitment and gas exchange in patients with the adult respiratory distress syndrome. Am Rev Respir Dis 1991; 144(3 Pt 1):544–551.

83. Esteban A, Anzueto A, Alia I, Gordo F, Apezteguia C, Palizas F, Cide D, Goldwaser R, Soto L, Bugedo G, et al. How is mechanical ventilation employed in the intensive care unit An international utilization review. Am J Respir Crit Care Med 2000; 161(5):1450–1458.

84. Lessard MR, Guerot E, Lorino H, Lemaire F, Brochard L. Effects of pressure-controlled with different I : E ratios versus volume-controlled ventilation on respiratory mechanics, gas exchange, and hemodynamics in patients with adult respiratory distress syndrome. Anesthesiology 1994; 80(5):983–991.

85. Lapinsky SE, Aubin M, Mehta S, Boiteau P, Slutsky AS. Safety and efficacy of a sustained inflation for alveolar recruitment in adults with respiratory failure. Intensive Care Med 1999; 25(11):1297–1301.

86. Tusman G, Bohm SH, Vazquez de Anda GF, do Campo JL, Lachmann B. 'Alveolar recruitment strategy' improves arterial oxygenation during general anaesthesia. Br J Anaesth 1999; 82(1):8–13.

87. Brower RG, Morris A, MacIntyre N, Matthay MA, Hayden D, Thompson T, Clemmer T, Lanken PN, Schoenfeld D. Effects of recruitment maneuvers in patients with acute lung injury and acute respiratory distress syndrome ventilated

with high positive end-expiratory pressure. Crit Care Med 2003; 31(11):2592–2597.

88. Lim CM, Jung H, Koh Y, Lee JS, Shim TS, Lee SD, Kim WS, Kim DS, Kim WD. Effect of alveolar recruitment maneuver in early acute respiratory distress syndrome according to antiderecruitment strategy, etiological category of diffuse lung injury, and body position of the patient. Crit Care Med 2003; 31(2):411–418.

89. Maggiore SM, Lellouche F, Pigeot J, Taille S, Deye N, Durrmeyer X, Richard JC, Mancebo J, Lemaire F, Brochard L. Prevention of endotracheal suctioning-induced alveolar derecruitment in acute lung injury. Am J Respir Crit Care Med 2003; 167(9):1215–1224.

90. Gattinoni L, Tognoni G, Pesenti A, Taccone P, Mascheroni D, Labarta V, Malacrida R, Di Giulio P, Fumagalli R, Pelosi P, et al. Effect of prone positioning on the survival of patients with acute respiratory failure. N Engl J Med 2001; 345(8):568–573.

91. Frostell CG, Blomqvist H, Hedenstierna G, Lundberg J, Zapol WM. Inhaled nitric oxide selectively reverses human hypoxic pulmonary vasoconstriction without causing systemic vasodilation. Anesthesiology 1993; 78(3):427–435.

92. Dellinger RP, Zimmerman JL, Taylor RW, Straube RC, Hauser DL, Criner GJ, Davis K, Jr., Hyers TM, Papadakos P. Effects of inhaled nitric oxide in patients with acute respiratory distress syndrome: results of a randomized phase II trial. Inhaled Nitric Oxide in ARDS Study Group. Crit Care Med 1998; 26(1):15–23.

93. Michael JR, Barton RG, Saffle JR, Mone M, Markewitz BA, Hillier K, Elstad MR, Campbell EJ, Troyer BE, Whatley RE, et al. Inhaled nitric oxide versus conventional therapy: effect on oxygenation in ARDS. Am J Respir Crit Care Med 1998; 157(5 Pt 1):1372–1380.

94. Troncy E, Collet JP, Shapiro S, Guimond JG, Blair L, Ducruet T, Francoeur M, Charbonneau M, Blaise G. Inhaled nitric oxide in acute respiratory distress syndrome: a pilot randomized controlled study. Am J Respir Crit Care Med 1998; 157(5 Pt 1):1483–1488.

95. Lundin S, Mang H, Smithies M, Stenqvist O, Frostell C. Inhalation of nitric oxide in acute lung injury: results of a European multicentre study. The European Study Group of Inhaled Nitric Oxide. Intensive Care Med 1999; 25(9):911–919.

96. Taylor RW, Zimmerman JL, Dellinger RP, Straube RC, Criner GJ, Davis K, Jr., Kelly KM, Smith TC, Small RJ. Low-dose inhaled nitric oxide in patients with acute lung injury: a randomized controlled trial. J Am Med Assoc 2004; 291(13):1603–1609.

97. Prewitt RM, Wood LD. Effect of sodium nitroprusside on cardiovascular function and pulmonary shunt in canine oleic acid pulmonary edema. Anesthesiology 1981; 55(5):537–541.

98. Bishop MJ, Kennard S, Artman LD, Cheney FW. Hydralazine does not inhibit canine hypoxic pulmonary vasoconstriction. Am Rev Respir Dis 1983; 128(6):998–1001.

99. Bone RC, Slotman G, Maunder R, Silverman H, Hyers TM, Kerstein MD, Ursprung JJ. Randomized double-blind, multicenter study of prostaglandin E1 in patients with the adult respiratory distress syndrome. Prostaglandin E1 Study Group. Chest 1989; 96(1):114–119.

100. Radermacher P, Santak B, Wust HJ, Tarnow J, Falke KJ. Prostacyclin for the treatment of pulmonary hypertension in the adult respiratory distress syndrome: effects on pulmonary capillary pressure and ventilation-perfusion distributions. Anesthesiology 1990; 72(2):238–244.

101. Abraham E, Baughman R, Fletcher E, Heard S, Lamberti J, Levy H, Nelson L, Rumbak M, Steingrub J, Taylor J, et al. Liposomal prostaglandin E1 (TLC C-53) in acute respiratory distress syndrome: a controlled, randomized, double-blind, multicenter clinical trial. TLC C-53 ARDS Study Group. Crit Care Med 1999; 27(8):1478–1485.

102. Pittet JF, Mackersie RC, Martin TR, Matthay MA. Biological markers of acute lung injury: prognostic and pathogenetic significance. Am J Respir Crit Care Med 1997; 155(4):1187–1205.

103. Bone RC, Fisher CJ, Jr., Clemmer TP, Slotman GJ, Metz CA. Early methylprednisolone treatment for septic syndrome and the adult respiratory distress syndrome. Chest 1987; 92(6):1032–1036.

104. Bernard GR, Luce JM, Sprung CL, Rinaldo JE, Tate RM, Sibbald WJ, Kariman K, Higgins S, Bradley R, Metz CA, et al. High-dose corticosteroids in patients with the adult respiratory distress syndrome. N Engl J Med 1987; 317(25):1565–1570.

105. Meduri GU, Headley AS, Golden E, Carson SJ, Umberger RA, Kelso T, Tolley EA. Effect of prolonged methylprednisolone therapy in unresolving acute respiratory distress syndrome: a randomized controlled trial. J Am Med Assoc 1998; 280(2):159–165.

106. Long W, Thompson T, Sundell H, Schumacher R, Volberg F, Guthrie R. Effects of two rescue doses of a synthetic surfactant on mortality rate and survival without bronchopulmonary dysplasia in 700- to 1350-gram infants with respiratory distress syndrome. The American Exosurf Neonatal Study Group I. J Pediatr 1991; 118(4 Pt 1):595–605.

107. Weg JG, Balk RA, Tharratt RS, Jenkinson SG, Shah JB, Zaccardelli D, Horton J, Pattishall EN. Safety and potential efficacy of an aerosolized surfactant in human sepsis-induced adult respiratory distress syndrome. J Am Med Assoc 1994; 272(18):1433–1438.

108. Anzueto A, Baughman RP, Guntupalli KK, Weg JG, Wiedemann HP, Raventos AA, Lemaire F, Long W, Zaccardelli DS, Pattishall EN. Aerosolized surfactant in adults with sepsis-induced acute respiratory distress syndrome. Exosurf Acute Respiratory Distress Syndrome Sepsis Study Group. N Engl J Med 1996; 334(22):1417–1421.

109. Spragg RG, Lewis JF, Wurst W, Hafner D, Baughman RP, Wewers MD, Marsh JJ. Treatment of acute respiratory distress syndrome with recombinant surfactant protein C surfactant. Am J Respir Crit Care Med 2003; 167(11):1562–1566.

110. Spragg RG, Lewis JF, Walmrath HD, Johannigman J, Bellingan G, Laterre PF, Witte MC, Richards GA, Rippin G, Rathgeb F, et al. Effect of recombinant surfactant protein C-based surfactant on the acute respiratory distress syndrome. N Engl J Med 2004; 351(9):884–892.

111. Gregory TJ, Steinberg KP, Spragg R, Gadek JE, Hyers TM, Longmore WJ, Moxley MA, Cai GZ, Hite RD, Smith RM, et al. Bovine surfactant therapy for patients with acute respiratory distress syndrome. Am J Respir Crit Care Med 1997; 155(4):1309–1315.

112. Bone RC. Treatment of adult respiratory distress syndrome with diuretics, dialysis, and positive end-expiratory pressure. Crit Care Med 1978; 6(3):136–139.

113. Prewitt RM, McCarthy J, Wood LD. Treatment of acute low pressure pulmonary edema in dogs: relative effects of hydrostatic and oncotic pressure, nitroprusside, and positive end-expiratory pressure. J Clin Invest 1981; 67(2):409–418.

114. Molloy WD, Lee KY, Girling L, Prewitt RM. Treatment of canine permeability pulmonary edema: short-term effects of dobutamine, furosemide, and hydralazine. Circulation 1985; 72(6):1365–1371.

115. Sznajder JI, Zucker AR, Wood LD, Long GR. The effects of plasmapheresis and hemofiltration on canine acid aspiration pulmonary edema. Am Rev Respir Dis 1986; 134(2):222–228.

116. Allen SJ, Drake RE, Katz J, Gabel JC, Laine GA. Elevation of superior vena caval pressure increases extravascular lung water after endotoxemia. J Appl Physiol 1987; 62(3):1006–1009.

117. Berner ME, Teague WG, Jr., Scheerer RG, Bland RD. Furosemide reduces lung fluid filtration in lambs with lung microvascular injury from air emboli. J Appl Physiol 1989; 67(5):1990–1996.

118. Schuster DP. The case for and against fluid restriction and occlusion pressure reduction in adult respiratory distress syndrome. New Horiz 1993; 1(4): 478–488.

119. Schuster DP. Fluid management in ARDS: "keep them dry" or does it matter Intensive Care Med 1995; 21(2):101–103.

120. Hyers TM. ARDS: the therapeutic dilemma. Chest 1990; 97(5):1025.

121. Hudson LD. Fluid management strategy in acute lung injury. Am Rev Respir Dis 1992; 145(5):988–989.

122. Sporn P. Keep the lung dry—sense or nonsense? Acta Anaesthesiol Scand Suppl 1996; 109:63–65.

123. Eklund J. Management of the fluid balance in prevention and therapy of ARDS. Acta Anaesthesiol Scand Suppl 1991; 95:102–104; discussion 104–105.

124. Simmons RS, Berdine GG, Seidenfeld JJ, Prihoda TJ, Harris GD, Smith JD, Gilbert TJ, Mota E, Johanson WG, Jr. Fluid balance and the adult respiratory distress syndrome. Am Rev Respir Dis 1987; 135(4):924–929.

125. Humphrey H, Hall J, Sznajder I, Silverstein M, Wood L. Improved survival in ARDS patients associated with a reduction in pulmonary capillary wedge pressure. Chest 1990; 97(5):1176–1180.

126. Mitchell JP, Schuller D, Calandrino FS, Schuster DP. Improved outcome based on fluid management in critically ill patients requiring pulmonary artery catheterization. Am Rev Respir Dis 1992; 145(5):990–998.

127. Eisenberg PR, Hansbrough JR, Anderson D, Schuster DP. A prospective study of lung water measurements during patient management in an intensive care unit. Am Rev Respir Dis 1987; 136(3):662–668.

128. Hayes MA, Timmins AC, Yau EH, Palazzo M, Hinds CJ, Watson D. Elevation of systemic oxygen delivery in the treatment of critically ill patients. N Engl J Med 1994; 330(24):1717–1722.

129. Gattinoni L, Brazzi L, Pelosi P, Latini R, Tognoni G, Pesenti A, Fumagalli R. A trial of goal-oriented hemodynamic therapy in critically ill patients. SvO2 Collaborative Group. N Engl J Med 1995; 333(16):1025–1032.

130. Richard C, Warszawski J, Anguel N, Deye N, Combes A, Barnoud D, Boulain T, Lefort Y, Fartoukh M, Baud F, et al. Early use of the pulmonary artery catheter and outcomes in patients with shock and acute respiratory distress syndrome: a randomized controlled trial. J Am Med Assoc 2003; 290(20):2713–2720.

131. Marinelli WA, Weinert CR, Gross CR, Knoedler JP, Jr., Bury CL, Kangas JR, Leatherman JW. Right heart catheterization in acute lung injury: an observational study. Am J Respir Crit Care Med 1999; 160(1):69–76.

132. Connors AF, Jr., Speroff T, Dawson NV, Thomas C, Harrell FE, Jr., Wagner D, Desbiens N, Goldman L, Wu AW, Califf RM, et al. The effectiveness of right heart catheterization in the initial care of critically ill patients. SUPPORT Investigators. J Am Med Assoc 1996; 276(11):889–897.

133. Herridge MS, Cheung AM, Tansey CM, Matte-Martyn A, Diaz-Granados N, Al-Saidi F, Cooper AB, Guest CB, Mazer CD, Mehta S, et al. One-year outcomes in survivors of the acute respiratory distress syndrome. N Engl J Med 2003; 348(8):683–693.

134. Vincent JL. Evidence-based medicine in the ICU: important advances and limitations. Chest 2004; 126(2):592–600.

135. Chastre J, Fagon JY. Ventilator-associated pneumonia. Am J Respir Crit Care Med 2002; 165(7):867–903.

136. Rello J, Paiva JA, Baraibar J, Barcenilla F, Bodi M, Castander D, Correa H, Diaz E, Garnacho J, Llorio M, et al. International Conference for the Development of Consensus on the Diagnosis and Treatment of Ventilator-associated Pneumonia. Chest 2001; 120(3):955–970.

137. Chastre J, Wolff M, Fagon JY, Chevret S, Thomas F, Wermert D, Clementi E, Gonzalez J, Jusserand D, Asfar P, et al. Comparison of 8 vs 15 days of antibiotic therapy for ventilator-associated pneumonia in adults: a randomized trial. J Am Med Assoc 2003; 290(19):2588–2598.

138. Collard HR, Saint S, Matthay MA. Prevention of ventilator-associated pneumonia: an evidence-based systematic review. Ann Intern Med 2003; 138(6): 494–501.

139. Tablan OC, Anderson LJ, Besser R, Bridges C, Hajjeh R. Guidelines for preventing health-care—associated pneumonia, 2003: recommendations of CDC and the Healthcare Infection Control Practices Advisory Committee. MMWR Recomm Rep 2004; 53(RR 3):1–36.

140. Drakulovic MB, Torres A, Bauer TT, Nicolas JM, Nogue S, Ferrer M. Supine body position as a risk factor for nosocomial pneumonia in mechanically ventilated patients: a randomised trial. Lancet 1999; 354(9193):1851–1858.

141. Cook D, Guyatt G, Marshall J, Leasa D, Fuller H, Hall R, Peters S, Rutledge F, Griffith L, McLellan A, et al. A comparison of sucralfate and ranitidine for the prevention of upper gastrointestinal bleeding in patients requiring mechanical ventilation. Canadian Critical Care Trials Group. N Engl J Med 1998; 338(12):791–797.

142. McHugh LG, Milberg JA, Whitcomb ME, Schoene RB, Maunder RJ, Hudson LD. Recovery of function in survivors of the acute respiratory distress syndrome. Am J Respir Crit Care Med 1994; 150(1):90–94.

143. Elliott CG, Rasmusson BY, Crapo RO. Upper airway obstruction following adult respiratory distress syndrome. An analysis of 30 survivors. Chest 1988; 94(3):526–530.

144. Davidson TA, Rubenfeld GD, Caldwell ES, Hudson LD, Steinberg KP. The effect of acute respiratory distress syndrome on long-term survival. Am J Respir Crit Care Med 1999; 160(6):1838–1842.

145. Davidson TA, Caldwell ES, Curtis JR, Hudson LD, Steinberg KP. Reduced quality of life in survivors of acute respiratory distress syndrome compared with critically ill control patients. J Am Med Assoc 1999; 281(4):354–360.

146. Angus DC, Musthafa AA, Clermont G, Griffin MF, Linde-Zwirble WT, Dremsizov TT, Pinsky MR. Quality-adjusted survival in the first year after the acute respiratory distress syndrome. Am J Respir Crit Care Med 2001; 163(6):1389–1394.

147. Hopkins RO, Weaver LK, Pope D, Orme JF, Bigler ED, Larson LV. Neuropsychological sequelae and impaired health status in survivors of severe acute respiratory distress syndrome. Am J Respir Crit Care Med 1999; 160(1):50–56.

148. Weinert CR, Gross CR, Kangas JR, Bury CL, Marinelli WA. Health-related quality of life after acute lung injury. Am J Respir Crit Care Med 1997; 156(4 Pt 1):1120–1128.

149. Schelling G, Stoll C, Haller M, Briegel J, Manert W, Hummel T, Lenhart A, Heyduck M, Polasek J, Meier M, et al. Health-related quality of life and posttraumatic stress disorder in survivors of the acute respiratory distress syndrome. Crit Care Med 1998; 26(4):651–659.

150. Rothenhausler HB, Ehrentraut S, Stoll C, Schelling G, Kapfhammer HP. The relationship between cognitive performance and employment and health status in long-term survivors of the acute respiratory distress syndrome: results of an exploratory study. Gen Hosp Psychiatry 2001; 23(2):90–96.

151. Jones C, Skirrow P, Griffiths RD, Humphris GH, Ingleby S, Eddleston J, Waldmann C, Gager M. Rehabilitation after critical illness: a randomized, controlled trial. Crit Care Med 2003; 31(10):2456–2461.

152. Philit F, Etienne-Mastroianni B, Parrot A, Guerin C, Robert D, Cordier JF. Idiopathic acute eosinophilic pneumonia: a study of 22 patients. Am J Respir Crit Care Med 2002; 166(9):1235–1239.

153. King TE, Jr., Mortenson RL. Cryptogenic organizing pneumonitis. The North American experience. Chest 1992; 102(suppl 1):8S–13S.

154. Lynch DA, Rose CS, Way D, King TE, Jr. Hypersensitivity pneumonitis: sensitivity of high-resolution CT in a population-based study. Am J Roentgenol 1992; 159(3):469–472.

2

Critical Care for Acute Severe Asthma

ERIC C. KLEERUP

Division of Pulmonary, Critical Care Medicine and Hospitalists
UCLA Medical Center and Geffen School of Medicine at UCLA
Los Angeles, California, U.S.A.

Plenty of bronchodilators, enough corticosteroids, oxygen, and the kitchen sink summarizes the treatment of severe asthma exacerbations—the devil is in the details.

I. Guidelines

National and international guidelines and recent reviews detail the treatment of asthma exacerbations in the emergency department and hospital (1–8).

II. Definition

Exacerbations are a relatively abrupt and severe departure from the smaller random variation of symptoms generally seen in well-controlled asthma. In more poorly-controlled asthmatics, the extremes of daily random variation may be sufficient to be called exacerbations. Typical symptoms of an exacerbation are similar to, but more severe than, the usual chronic symptoms: dyspnea, wheezing, cough, nocturnal awakening, and exercise limitation. Severe exacerbations may be seen in even mild intermittent asthmatics.

Classifying acute severe exacerbations by the speed of onset may be useful (9–11). Rapid-onset exacerbations, less than three hours, are often caused by an acute profound exposure or have no identifiable cause (Table 1) and comprise 11–14% of severe exacerbations (10–12). Bronchoconstriction with neutrophilic infiltration of the airways and minimal mucous production are primarily present (13). Fortunately, although more severe airway obstruction is present, rapid-onset exacerbations may resolve as quickly as they appear (10–12). Slow-onset exacerbations are characterized by a gradual deterioration of function

Table 1   Triggers of Acute Asthma Exacerbations

Sudden-onset <3 hr (14% of severe exacerbations)
   Respiratory allergens
   Exercise
   Psychosocial stress
   Medications: β-blockers, aspirin, inhalational anesthesia
   Metabisulfite
   Inhaled heroin or cocaine (nasal or smoked)
Slow-onset >3 hr
   Respiratory viruses
   Bacterial infection (sinus source?)
   Gradual deterioration of asthma

Source: From Refs. 12, 14–21.

and increase of symptoms, often over days, with increasing use of bronchodilators, nonadherence to chronic controller medications, and failure of the patient to recognize the severity. Upper respiratory tract infections are the most common trigger. Eosinophils infiltrate the walls, the epithelium sloughs off, and large amounts of viscous mucous are present in the airways (13). Hospitalization is more common (odds ratio 3.9) (10,11). Often, slow-onset exacerbations resolve slowly and require prolonged hospitalization. Severe airflow obstruction, somewhat arbitrarily, is an initial peak expiratory flow (PEF) or FEV_1 less than 50% predicted or personal best or deterioration during intensive Emergency Department (ED) treatment (Fig. 1) (22).

III. Pathophysiology

Asthma is a chronic inflammatory disorder of the airways in which many cells and cellular elements play a role. The chronic inflammation causes an associated increase in airway hyperresponsiveness that leads to recurrent episodes of wheezing, breathlessness, chest tightness, and coughing, particularly at night or in the early morning. These episodes are usually associated with widespread but variable airflow obstruction that is often reversible either spontaneously or with treatment (Global Initiative for Asthma, GINA) (7).

The immediate (early) bronchoconstriction following antigen exposure results from IgE-dependent release of preformed mediators from mast cells, including histamine, prostaglandins, and leukotrienes. Nonatopic triggers cause bronchoconstriction from a variety of mechanisms, including direct contraction of smooth muscle, stimulation of local and central neural reflexes, unopposed action of constrictor mediators, and mediator release from cytokine "primed" inflammatory cells.

Like chronic asthma, TH-2 lymphocytes control inflammation in acute exacerbations (23). These $CD4^+$ T-helper cells are activated as evidenced by surface markers including: interleukin-2 receptor (IL-2R), class II

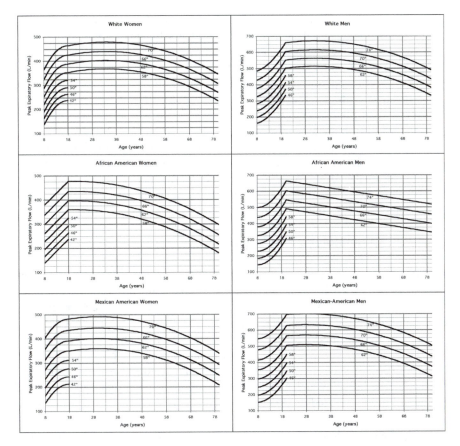

Figure 1 Predicted peak expiratory flow for men and women, based on age, height, and ethnicity. *Source:* From Ref. 22.

histocompatibility antigen (HLA-DR), and "very late activation" antigen (VLA-1) (24). In acute exacerbations, an influx of neutrophils occurs early and persists, while activated eosinophils infiltrate somewhat more slowly (>24 hours). Goblet cells and intraluminal mucous are also increased, but the time course is unclear (25). Proinflammatory cytokines (IL-1beta, IL-5, IL-6, TNF alpha) and chemokines (MCP-1, MIP-alpha, and RANTES) and metalloproteinase 9 (MMP9) are increased in BAL during acute severe asthma (26–29). Interleukin-5 (IL-5) and eosinophils are increased in acute exacerbations and decrease with corticosteroids (30). IL-5, MCP-3, eotaxin, and RANTES may contribute to eosinophil chemotaxis (28). Eotaxin localized in macrophages increases with acute exacerbations but is not altered by corticosteroids (30).

Charcot-Leyden crystals in sputum are formed in eosinophils, basophils, and possibly neutrophils from an autocrystallizing protein (galectin-10) perhaps involved in modulating adhesion and differentiation of myeloid precursor cells (31,32). Lipids may contribute to the "mucus" plugs in which only 25% of the material is mucin (33,34). Curschmann's spirals consist of high-viscosity mucous from the lumen of smaller bronchi, bronchioles, and the ducts of the seromucous bronchial glands (35).

No specific polymorphism or haplotype of the $\beta2$-adrenergic receptor is associated with fatal/near-fatal asthma (36). There is evidence for contributions of platelet activating factor (37), thromboxane A2, and cysteinyl leukotrienes (38) in acute severe asthma attacks.

Hypoxemia during acute asthma attacks is due to ventilation-perfusion (VA/Q) inequality and is characterized by a marked bimodal blood flow distribution to normal and low VA/Q populations (39). This is an exaggeration of the pattern seen in asthmatics in general. Respiratory arrest and, likely, death in asthma are due to asphyxia rather than cardiac arrhythmias (40).

IV. Epidemiology and Triggers

In 2002, 16 million (7.5%, 95% CI 7.3–7.7) U.S. adults self-reported current asthma as diagnosed by a healthcare professional, but the prevalence among racial/ethnic minority populations ranged from 3.1% to 14.5%, compared with 7.6% among whites (41). Among current asthmatics, 18.4% (95% CI 16.4–20.4) were seen in the ED, 28.5% (95% CI 26.3–30.8) reported urgent visits and 51.1% (95% CI 48.4–53.9) had asthma attacks in the proceeding 12 months. Non-Hispanic black (37.2%), Hispanic (26.0%), American Indian/Alaska Native (20.4%), and Asian (18.8%) asthmatics had higher than average ED usage. In the proceeding 30 days, asthma symptoms were present in 75.1% (95% CI 73.1–77.2) of asthmatics.

In practice, admission of adults to the hospital occurs in 49% of severe exacerbations (PEF <50% predicted) and 4% of mild to moderate exacerbations (42). Admission in severe exacerbations is correlated with final ED peak flow, female sex, nonwhite race, severity of chronic illness and severity of exacerbation. Risk factors for death are the primary indicator for admission in mild to moderate exacerbations. Of those discharged from the ED, 5% relapse in 72 hours. In children, admission is associated with severity of symptoms, intensity of therapy both before and during ED visit, previous admission for asthma, recent use of inhaled corticosteroids and low peak flows, but PEF is infrequently (inappropriately 23% overall) measured (43). Those admitted with severe life-threatening asthma, compared to those with acute asthma admitted to the general medical ward, are more likely to have had previous severe life-threatening asthma (OR 2.04), hospitalization in the last year (OR 1.86), and not be using inhaled corticosteroids in the two weeks preceding the attack (OR 0.69) (44). Both groups have similar sociodemographic criteria, ongoing asthma care, and no evidence of increased physical, economic, or other barriers to health care. Death from asthma is proceeded by a severe life threatening asthma attack 22–24% of the time, but 33% of deaths have previously mild

asthma, and 32% have no prior hospitalizations (45,46). The higher hospitalization rate in urban areas is primarily due to increased frequency of severe
attacks (47,48). Most of the apparent increase in risk due to second and third
line drugs is due to confounding by more severe disease (49,50). There remain
questions about fenoterol (removed from the market) specifically (51). After
adjusting for clinical severity (OR 9.33; 95% CI 2.84–30.7), metered dose
inhaler β-agonists are no longer a statistically significant risk factor
(OR = 2.08, 95% CI 0.78–5.50) for life-threatening asthma or fatality (52).
However, utilization of β-agonists is a marker for severity— ≥ 13 prescriptions
of short-acting β-agonists during the previous year carries a relative risk of
51.6 (95% CI 7.9–345) for death and 7 to12 prescriptions a relative risk 16.2
(95% CI 2.6–101) (53). Even in the higher risk group, regular use of inhaled
corticosteroids results in a 60% reduction in death. Patient factors persist in
deaths due to asthma including factors such as poor compliance, lack of PEF
measurements, increasing or overuse (>1.4 canisters/month) of reliever
medication without inhaled corticosteroids, and psychosocial problems,
notably depression and denial (54–57).

High-risk female patients are admitted twice as often as high-risk male
patients and tend to have longer admissions, but once admitted, require similar
medical, intensive care unit (ICU), or intubation interventions (58). Uninsured
patients have consistently poorer quality of care than insured patients, but no
differences in short-term patient outcomes by type of insurance is found (59).
Obesity (body mass index) does not seem to be a risk factor (60).

V. Assessment

The Global Initiative for Asthma (GINA) guidelines give a rubric for assessing
the severity of exacerbations (Table 2). The correlation of the severity measured
by the various signs and symptoms are unknown, but can be assumed to be poor
and vary from one individual to another. The presence of several parameters, but
not necessarily all, indicates the general classification of the exacerbation. Not
surprisingly, those patients presenting with the most severe obstruction ($<30\%$
predicted) and having the least response to therapy ($<35\%$ improvement or
$<40\%$ predicted) in the first 60 minutes are at the highest risk for prolonged
ED therapy and/or hospitalization (61). Severity of the exacerbation after one
hour of treatment is a better predictor of hospitalization and ICU admission
than severity at presentation (62). However, there is no combination of findings
that is perfect or even adequate to predict which asthmatics will benefit from
admission or ICU care (Table 3) (63). Patient-reported symptoms and severity
are especially poor, indicating the need for objective measures of airflow
obstruction (64–66). Wheezing of moderate to severe intensity, higher pitch
wheezing, wheezing throughout expiration, and combination inspiratory and
expiratory wheezing all indicate lower PEF in general, but are insufficient to

Table 2 Severity of Asthma Exacerbation Modified from GINA and British Guidelines

	Mild	Moderate	Severe	Life threatening
Respiratory findings				
Breathlessness	Walking Can lie down Talks in sentences	Talking Prefers sitting Talks in phrases	At rest Hunched forward Talks in words only	
In infant		Softer shorter cry and difficulty feeding	Stops feeding	
Respiratory rate	Increased <2 months >60 2–12 months >50 1–5 years >40 6–8 years >30	Increased	>30/min	
Accessory muscles and suprasternal or intracostal retractions	Usually not, perhaps increased scalene contractions	Usually	Usually	Paradoxical thoraco-abdominal movement
Wheeze	Usually not	Loud	Usually loud	Absence due to lack of air movement
PEF or FEV_1 after initial bronchodilator (% predicted or personal best)	>80%	60–80%	<60% or <100 L/min or duration of initial response <2 hr	<25–33% predicted or personal best initially or <40% or after initial therapy
Oxygenation (on room air)	S_pO_2 >95% P_aO_2 normal, test not usually needed	S_pO_2 91–95% P_aO_2 >60 mmHg	$S_pO_2 \leq 90\%$ $P_aO_2 \leq 60$ mmHg	$P_aO_2 \leq 60$ mmHg on supplemental O_2

	$P_aCO_2 \leq 45$ mmHg, often lower than 35	$P_aCO_2 \leq 45$ mmHg	$P_aCO_2 > 45$ mmHg	
Hypoventilation (hypercapnea develops more readily in young children)				
Other findings				
Alertness	May be agitated	Usually agitated	Usually agitated	Drowsy or confused, coma
Pulse	<100/min 2–12 months <160 1–2 years <120 2–8 years <110	100–120/min	>120/min	Bradycardia Arrhythmia
Pulsus paradoxus	Absent, <10 mmHg, not palpable	May be present, 10–25 mmHg (10–20 mmHg in children)	Often present, >25 mmHg (>20 mmHg in children)	May be absent due to respiratory muscle fatigue

Abbreviation: PEF, peak expiratory flow.
Source: From Refs. 6 and 7.

Table 3 Criteria for Disposition Within the Emergency Department and Hospital

Criteria for continuous monitoring
    Inadequate or deteriorating response to therapy within one to two hours of treatment
    Persisting severe airflow limitation (PEF <30% predicted or personal best)
    Past history of severe asthma, particularly if hospitalization and admission to the ICU
        was required
    Presence of factors indicating high risk of asthma related death
    Prolonged symptoms before current ED visit
    Inadequate access at home to medical care and medications
    Difficult home conditions
    Difficulty obtaining transport to hospital in the event of further deterioration
Criteria for hospitalization
    Pre-treatment FEV_1 or PEF below 25% predicted or personal best
    Post-treatment FEV_1 or PEF below 40% predicted or personal best
Criteria for intensive care unit admission
    Severe asthma with lack of response to initial therapy or worsening despite adequate
        therapy
    Presence of confusion, drowsiness, loss of consciousness or other signs of impending
        respiratory arrest
    Impending respiratory arrest: primarily a clinical judgement, hypoxemia
        (P_aO_2 >60 mmHg) despite supplemental oxygen and/or P_aCO_2 > 42 mmHg

Abbreviations: PEF, peak expiratory flow; ED, emergency department.
Source: From Ref. 7.

classify severity of airways obstruction (67). Accessory muscle use correlates
with lung function and S_aO_2 (68).

    Children with $S_pO_2 \leq 88\%$ are 32 times more likely to be admitted than
those with a saturation of 100% (69). As a cut point, $\leq 88\%$ (odds ratio 12),
$\leq 91\%$ (4.6), or $\leq 94\%$ (2.7) are not useful alone. $S_pO_2 > 92\%$ is associated
with respiratory failure ($P_aCO_2 > 45$ mmHg) in only 4.2% of cases (70). Pulsus
paradoxus >15 mmHg after 30 minutes of treatment may predict admission
(sensitivity 0.42, specificity 0.89, odds ratio 3.9) (71). Physicians tend to underestimate initial airways obstruction by 8.1 $\pm$ 16.0% predicted, and knowledge of
the pulmonary function test result changes management in 20.4% of patients in
the ED (72). An $FEV_1 < 25\%$ or a PEF <20% predicted accurately indicates a
severe asthma exacerbation (73). An increase in FEV_1 or PEF >60% predicted
after therapy negates the need for hospitalization in most cases. Younger children
and some adults may have difficulty in performing adequate PEF measurements
during acute exacerbations, even after treatment (74). Inferior lead T-wave inversion on ECG due to right ventricular pressure overload may relate to severity of
asthma attack (75). Slow onset exacerbations often take longer to resolve, but
sudden onset exacerbations may be equally severe. An assessment driven treatment algorithm may shorten hospital stays and decrease costs (76). Risk
factors for severe asthma exacerbations and death should also be considered in

the assessment. In asthmatics admitted to the ICU in England, Wales, and Northern Ireland, Acute Physiology and Chronic Health Evaluation (APACHE) II score predicted mechanical ventilation with an odds ratio of 1.05/point (1.02–1.08) increase and death with an odds ratio of 1.10/point (95% CI 1.05–1.04) increase (77). An increased risk of mechanical ventilation in the first 24 hours was present, after adjustment for APACHE II score, due to neurologic insult in first 24 hours (OR $\geq$10.75; 95% CI 4.23–27.31), P_aCO_2 from arterial blood gas with the lowest pH/$\geq$5kPa ($\geq$37.5 mmHg) (5.22; 4.02–6.77), and CPR within 24 hours prior to admission (3.65; 1.81–7.36). An increased risk of death during hospitalization was present, after adjustment for APACHE II score, due to CPR within 24 hours prior to admission (6.40; 3.91–10.46), neurologic insult in first 24 hours (OR 1.81; 1.04–3.14), age/10 years (1.51; 1.32–1.74), and P_aCO_2 from arterial blood gas with the lowest pH/$\geq$5kPa ($\geq$37.5 mmHg) (1.38; 1.08–1.77). In the absence of hypercapnia (<5.7 kPa, 42.8 mmHg), 34.8% required mechanical ventilation, but 65.0% with modest hypercapnia (5.7–8.2 kPa, 42.8–61.5 mmHg) and 88.2% with more severe hypercapnia (>8.2 kPa, 61.5 mmHg). One-third of ICU admissions fell into each hypercapnia category. Hospital mortality showed a similar progression, 3.8%, 10.9%, and 16.5%, with progressive hypercapnia. At minimum, aggressive intervention and close monitoring is necessary if the P_aCO_2 is >42 mmHg.

VI. Therapy

A. Beta Agonists

Bronchodilators remain the mainstay of treatment in the ED and ICU. Inhaled β2-agonists reverse bronchospasm in most asthmatics presenting for acute exacerbations. Unfortunately, not all individuals respond adequately or, sometimes, seemingly at all to initial doses. In general, the degree of efficacy reflects the dosage and potency of the β-agonist and the severity of airflow present at presentation. A Cochrane review of nebulized β-agonists (5–30 mg/2 hours, 15 mg in children) in the ED favored continuous over intermittent, especially for severe patients, with a relative risk for admission of 0.68 (95% CI 0.5–0.9) (78). In the first hours, differences in FEV_1 and PEF were not apparent; by two to three hours, they were significant, and by four to six hours, there was again no difference. Keeping carefully to the same dose with intermittent and continuous nebulization, there may be less differences (79,80). However, it is possible that asthmatics with lower initial PEF respond better to continuous, rather than intermittent, nebulized β-agonist in the first and second hours of treatment (81). Preliminary studies show levalbuterol (Xopenex®) to be more effective than racemic albuterol at four times the dose (82). Formoterol and albuterol are equivalent in onset of bronchodilation, but the former has a long duration of action (83). Severe patients may benefit from delivery of B2-agonists in nebulizers driven by heliox rather than air, and this does not seem detrimental (84).

The inspiratory flow, although reduced in acute exacerbations, remains adequate for the Turbuhaler® and Diskus® dry powder devices (85).

Intravenous salbutamol (same as albuterol, not available in the U.S.) boluses 250 μg (5 μg/kg in children) repeated two to six times, up to every two minutes, have been used after failure of inhaled β2-agonists and additional treatment (86). In children failing three nebulized treatments, salbutamol 15 μg/kg over 20 minutes was not better than aminophylline (87). Continuous infusion of salbutamol 5 μg/kg/min × 1–2 hours, followed by 1 μg/kg/min and, if an inadequate response, 10 μg/kg/min × 1 hour, followed by 2 μg/kg/min, has been used, but the range of doses in general use is wide (88,89). Initial intravenous terbutaline doses of 2.5–10 μg/min, increasing to a maximum of 17.5–80 μg/min, are used in obstetrics, and the airway effects are comparable to salbutamol. In children, diastolic hypotension was noted with doses of 0.4–1.0 μg/kg/min, but not when the dose was above 2 μg/kg/min (90). Terbutaline intravenously 6 μg/kg hourly twice (equivalent to 0.1 μg/kg/min) was equal in effect to 0.1 mg/kg nebulized twice hourly (91). The β1, β2-agonist, isoproterenol has also been used intravenously (92). Epinephrine, traditionally used subcutaneously or nebulized, has additional α-adrenergic effects. Administered as an aerosol, it may selectively constrict the pulmonary vessels, resulting in a decrease in bronchial mucosal congestion.

In ED management, no advantage of intravenous β-agonist over other deliveries was seen, and an increased rate of adverse event was found (93). Although endotracheal tubes impair delivery of aerosols, there are no comparisons of intravenous and nebulized routes in intubated patients and no comparisons to other bronchodilators or placebo (94). Higher doses are generally used in intubated patients based on the assumed inefficiency of delivery. Humidification, nebulizer triggering, and ventilator model affect delivery (95). Inspiratory time and flow rate affect nebulized, but not MDI, delivery (96). Many ED studies show no difference between MDI and nebulized albuterol; however, very little information is available for asthmatics on ventilators. An individual titration of 4–28 or even 40 puffs, following intrinsic positive end-expiratory pressure or expiratory resistance is reasonable (97). Interactions with the ventilator triggering and volume measurement must be considered during nebulization through a ventilator circuit.

B. Anticholinergics

In the pediatric ED, the addition of ipratropium to less than 0.15 mg/kg q 20 min albuterol may provide an additive benefit (98–100), as have two meta-analyses (101,102), but others have shown no additional benefit (103). Twice the nebulized albuterol (104) or intravenous salbutamol (105) resulted in more improvement than ipratropium. For the reverse question, in hospitalized patients, ipratropium 0.5–1 mg produced 56–71% of the maximal bronchodilation of ipratropium and terbutaline 5 mg together (106,107). Ipratropium could be considered a β-agonist sparing agent, but there is little information on use in the ICU or whether it is truly additive to high doses of β-agonists. Initial doses of 250–500 μg nebulized, or four puffs (80 μg) with a spacer every 20 minutes, or continuous nebulization of 1–1.5 mg/hr followed by similar doses every three to four hours are appropriate. Adverse effects of ipratropium are minimal.

C. Corticosteroids

In acute asthma, corticosteroids improve outcomes compared to placebo (108–110). Doses of over 80 mg/day methylprednisolone, 100 mg/day prednisone, and 400 mg/day hydrocortisone confer no advantage in hospitalized asthmatics (111). Doses as low as 40 mg qd of prednisolone appear equivalent to 60 mg q 6 for 24 hours followed by 60 qd assessed at 24 hours, discharge, and 30 days (81). There are no adequate studies of asthmatics with impending respiratory failure or intubated. Pharmacologically, an initial intravenous loading dose is rational, but may be obviated by the speed with which a PO dose can be obtained and administered. In some ED exacerbations, high doses of inhaled corticosteroids (flunisolide 1 mg bid, budesonide 1.6 mg qid) may be adequate, but there are no studies of nebulized corticosteroids (112–114). Acute psychiatric reactions, acute myopathy and rhabdomyolysis, fluid and electrolyte disturbance, hypertension, peptic ulcer disease, and manifestation of latent diabetes may be dependent on systemic corticosteroid dosage. If methylprednisolone or prednisone is used in adrenally suppressed patients, consider adding fludrocortisone for additional mineralocorticoid effect.

D. Oxygen

Oxygen is vital. Hypoxemia is present only in more severe exacerbations and is generally easy to treat with supplemental oxygen. Very high F_IO_2 may be detrimental to ventilation (P_aCO_2) (115). Difficulty in oxygenation may indicate concomitant disease, such as pneumonia or pulmonary embolus.

E. Magnesium

In the ED, magnesium sulfate 2 g IV improves FEV_1 if the presenting FEV_1 is <25% predicted (42). Most ED studies use similar doses. Two meta analyses concluded IV magnesium may be helpful in ED treatment only of more severe asthmatics (116,117), and another found no effect (11). In intubated asthmatics, 3.6 g/hr or 10–20 g within one hour resulted in bronchodilation (118,119), and rapid infusion of 2 g magnesium over two minutes prevented impending respiratory failure in two cases (120). Although nebulized $MgSO_4$ is a bronchodilator, there is no information on the treatment of acute severe asthma. In obstetrics, initial doses of 4–6 g IV over 20 min followed by 2–4 g/hr with a maximum dosage of 20 g/48 hr are used for relaxation of uterine contractions. At high doses, serum concentrations should be monitored; toxicity may be seen at >4 mEq/L.

F. Methylxanthines

Aminophylline reverses bronchospasm less than β2-agonists (121). In the ED, adding aminophylline to β2-agonists, ipratropium, and corticosteroids does not appear to add much (122). In patients with low initial PEF, aminophylline as a first line agent is less likely to succeed than β2-agonists (123). A serum level is imperative before IV aminophylline in any patient who *might* be taking theophylline. A careful history for multiple doses of sustained release theophylline just before admission is also critical to avoid iatrogenic toxicity or even mortality. Patients with serum levels over 7.5 mg/L before aminophylline infusion are unlikely to benefit (124). In some studies of aminophylline as an add-on, there are less admissions and perhaps less intubations (125,126). Aminophylline causes more nausea, vomiting, and palpitations/arrhythmias. In the pediatric ICU, symptoms may improve sooner, but aminophylline does not reduce the length of stay (127).

The clearance/metabolism of theophylline is complex and cannot be readily predicted (128–130). The half-life in nonsmoking asthmatic adults ranges from 3–12.8 hours (children 1.5–9.5) (131). Clearance is decreased (theophylline levels increased) with congestive heart failure, COPD, cor pulmonale, liver disease, and in geriatric patients. Clearance is increased in cigarette or marijuana smokers. zileuton, zafirlukast, influenza vaccines, oral contraceptives, thyroid hormones, paroxetine, cimetidine, HIV protease inhibitors, azole antifungals, thiabendazole, quinolones, erythromycin, clarithromycin, telithromycin, troleandomycin, calcium channel blockers, mexiletine, propafenone, propranolol, ticlopidine, rofecoxib, high-dose allopurinol, methotrexate, aprepitant, fluvoxamine, ropivacaine, tacrine, and interferon alfa may decrease clearance and increase levels of theophylline. Rifampin, rifapentine, moricizine, modafinil, barbiturates, carbamazepine, and phenytoin may increase clearance and decrease levels. Theophylline and derivatives may decrease the effectiveness of lithium and adenosine (in cardiac stress tests) and increase the effectiveness of warfarin. Theophylline may be additive or synergistic to the toxicities of cardiac glycosides, sympathomimetics, pentoxifylline, and caffeine.

It is reasonable to consider aminophylline in patients who have persistent bronchospasm after adequate doses of β2-agonists, anticholinergics, and corticosteroids, but the magnitude of benefit, if any, is unclear.

G. Anesthetics, Sedatives, and Paralytic Agents

General anesthesia has long been considered a last resort for status asthmaticus. After halothane 1% for 30 minutes, P_aCO_2 and peak inspiratory pressure decreased, VD/VT, mean pulmonary arterial pressure, and heart rate decreased, and arterial pH increased without change in cardiac index in 12 asthmatics requiring mechanical ventilation (132). Isoflurane (133–140), sevoflurane (141,142), and enflurane (134) behave similarly and may have less risk of rhythm disorders. These inhaled agents appear to directly relax the smooth muscle, similar to their better-studied effects on uterine smooth muscle. Practical issues limit the use in the ICU for any significant duration, and typical anesthesia ventilators may be inadequate (143).

As an adjunct to allow mechanical ventilation, especially with permissive hypercapnia, sedatives and paralytic agents have an obvious role. Their role as therapeutic agents is less clear. Barbiturates [thiopental (144)] and perhaps benzodiazepines [propofol (145,146)] and narcotics [fentanyl (147)] reduce peak airway pressure and P_aCO_2 and increase arterial pH. Sedatives and other respiratory depressants should not be used outside the ICU setting. Ketamine, a dissociative anesthetic, improved clinical asthma scores, respiratory rate, and oxygenation within 10 minutes after a loading dose of 1 mg/kg intravenously (i.v.), followed by a continuous infusion of 0.75 mg/kg/hr (12.5 μg/kg/min) for one hour in pediatric asthmatics refractory to initial therapy in the ED, but not intubated (148). Ketamine has been used in both adult and pediatric mechanically ventilated asthmatics (145, 149–156). In almost half the adults over the age of 30, discontinuation of ketamine may be accompanied by delirium, excitement, or visual disturbances, sometimes days or weeks later.

Systemic paralytic agents may require higher doses and be associated with more prolonged weakness in asthmatics than other ICU patients (157). High subarachnoid blocks might be efficacious, but can be accompanied by profound hypotension (158,159).

H. Heliox

Heliox, helium/oxygen blends, are temporizing measures without direct therapeutic effect on asthma. Heliox has been traditionally used for upper airway obstruction. It does allow a reduced work of breathing, which may stave off respiratory failure while other agents improve asthma. The lower density of helium, as opposed to nitrogen, allows more of the airway to have laminar airflow. The bulk flow of gas under laminar conditions is approximately the square of turbulent flow. The density of helium is 14.3% of nitrogen, but the viscosity or thickness is 111.2%, resulting in somewhat worse flow in airways with laminar flow conditions already. All caregivers should use extreme caution if helium and oxygen are blended at the bedside rather than using premixed tanks of heliox (usually F_IO_2 0.3, balance He), because it is possible to inadvertently administer hypoxemic gas mixtures. Blenders are generally calibrated for air/oxygen and give erroneous results with helium/oxygen. Measurement of oxygen concentrations in the presence of helium requires paramagnetic gas analyzers. In general, heliox is used to reduce the work of breathing and avert intubation (160,161). It may reduce inspiratory and expiratory airway resistance, as evidenced by pulsus paradoxus and PEF respectively (162,161). During mechanical ventilation, it may lower peak pressures, auto-/intrinsic positive end-expiratory pressure (PEEP), and A-a gradient (163–165). It is reasonable, and perhaps beneficial, to administer nebulized bronchodilators with heliox (166,167). Helium concentrations under 60% are probably not helpful. Since most cases improve with *therapeutic* measures, it is unclear in practice and studies who benefits from heliox as a *temporizing* measure (168). Heliox should likely be reserved for those patients on the edge of intubation or failing a permissive hypercapnia ventilation strategy.

I. Mechanical Ventilation

Increased airway resistance in acute asthma increases dynamic hyperinflation and intrinsic PEEP, which may result in barotrauma even without mechanical ventilation. A flow-dependent increase in resistance, perhaps due to turbulence, noncompliant airways, and/or "reflex" bronchoconstriction, occurs in status asthmaticus, which contrasts with the decrease seen in most other forms of respiratory failure (169). Ventilator strategies to minimize the dynamic hyperinflation, including noninvasive positive pressure ventilation, hypoventilation (permissive hypercapnia), pressure support ventilation, increase of expiratory time, and promotion of patient–ventilator synchrony, significantly decrease the morbidity and mortality of the disease (Table 4).

Noninvasive positive pressure ventilation, begun at 10 cmH_2O inspiratory pressure and 0 cmH_2O expiratory pressure and typically increased to 18/4, reverses gas exchange abnormalities in severe asthma exacerbations with hypercapnia (177). Allowing the patient to determine the I:E and respiratory rate with pressure support ventilation may result in better synchrony with the ventilator and lower peak airway pressures (178,179). Use of PEEP at low values (5 cm H_2O) may help overcome ventilator asynchrony (172).

Permissive hypercapnia is safe and effective for asthma (170,171,173). Infused bicarbonate to compensate for respiratory acidosis may even preclude the need for mechanical ventilation, but has not been widely studied (180). External chest compression to augment passive expiration during mechanical ventilation is probably unnecessary with a permissive hypercapnia strategy (181). Measuring intrinsic PEEP as a surrogate for end expiratory volume may be useful in optimizing ventilation. Measuring plateau pressure in unsedated patients may be difficult, but the set pressure on pressure-regulated breaths may be a useful surrogate. Often sedation with benzodiazepine and/or narcotic drips may be needed to meet the ventilatory goals; paralytics are seldom necessary with adequate sedation. Paralytics may reduce CO_2 production, much of which may come from respiratory muscles. In the extreme, hypothermia (30°C) has been used to reduce CO_2 production (182). Partial liquid perfluorocarbon ventilation has been reported (183).

J. Fluids

Mild dehydration, <5%, may be common in acute asthma, and modest rehydration may be reasonable (2 cc/kg/hr) (184). Excessive fluid may lead to

Table 4 Ventilator Strategy for Asthma

Adequate inspiratory flow to meet inspiratory demands
  Shorten inspiratory time
  Pressure regulated breath (pressure assist control, pressure support ventilation, pressure
    regulated volume control)
  Avoid small endotrachial tubes
  Anesthesia ventilators may be inadequate
  Evaluate for patient inspiratory effort or negative deflections on pressure–time tracings
Minimize dynamic hyperinflation (intrinsic PEEP)
  Increase expiratory time (slow rate 6–14)
  Decrease minute ventilation
  Accept hypercapnea (typically PCO_2 50–60 mmHg, but occasionally much higher,
    augmenting bicarbonate if pH $\leq$7.15–7.30)
  Measure intrinsic PEEP in well sedated or paralyzed patients
Maintain end inspiratory plateau pressure <30 cmH$_2$O
  Pressure regulated breath (pressure assist control, pressure support ventilation, pressure
    regulated volume control)
  Measure plateau pressure in well sedated of paralyzed patients, or use pressure regulated
    peak pressure as a surrogate
Oxygen sufficient to maintain S_pO_2 >88–90%
Promote patient–ventilator synchrony
  PEEP (set) 5 cmH$_2$O
  Adequate sedation and occasionally pharmacologic paralysis
  Consider pressure support ventilation
Rest fatigued muscles for at least 24 hr
  Full support ventilator mode initially

Abbreviation: PEEP, positive end-expiratory pressure.
Source: Adapted from Refs. 170–175.

pulmonary edema. Dead space ventilation may decrease with intravascular volume expansion (185). Inappropriate antidiuretic hormone (ADH) secretion may occur during acute asthma attacks (186).

K. Mucolytics, DNase, and Chest Physical Therapy

Mucous plugging and impaction is commonly seen in fatal asthma. DNase (187,188), mucolytics, and bronchoscopy (189–191) may be helpful in selected cases, based on anecdotal reports. Although a pneumothorax has been attributed to chest physical therapy, it might help in selected cases (192,193). Acetyl-cysteine may cause severe bronchospasm, but can be combined with β2-agonists (194). In the extreme, unilateral hyperinflation from the ball-valve effect of a mucous plug may shift the mediastinum, mimicking tension pneumothorax, and be cured by bronchoscopic removal (195).

L. Leukotrienes

There are no studies of anti-leukotrienes in very severe asthma exacerbations, and their role is therefore unclear. Montelukast IV (7 or 14 mg) or PO (10 mg) bronchodilates rapidly as an addition to albuterol alone in moderate to severe ED asthmatic exacerbations (196). It appears that higher doses, up to 500 mg IV, are safe, but not more efficacious in stable asthmatics (197).

M. Nitric Oxide

Ventilation improved (PCO_2 decreased) after administration of nitric oxide in very limited studies of severely hypercapnic asthmatics on mechanical ventilation (198,199).

N. EcMO

Reducing the necessary ventilation in the lung to zero is possible with extracorporal membrane oxygenation (EcMO, or extracorporal lung assist, EcLA), but in itself is not therapeutic for asthma. In refractory cases with cardiovascular collapse or extensive barotrauma, EcMO may be useful as a temporizing measure to avoid death (200–206).

VII. Contributing Comorbidities, Sequelae, and Medication Side Effects

Studies of outpatient deaths in asthmatics suggest that oral and nebulized β-agonists and theophylline may exacerbate pre-existing cardiovascular disease, especially acute coronary insufficiency and congestive cardiomyopathy, resulting in death (207). Certainly avoiding the combination of increased respiratory muscle work, hypoxemia, and β-agonist stimulation should be considered in those at high risk for acute coronary events (208,209). However, withholding inhaled β-agonists is not appropriate, even in the face of acute myocardial infarction complicating asthma exacerbations. Tachycardia is a cardinal feature of asthma exacerbations, and heart rate and blood pressure decrease—a therapeutic response—more after nebulized than intravenous salbutamol (albuterol) in children, rather than increase as perhaps expected (210). Multifocal atrial tachycardia is present in 8% of patients with a theophylline serum level 10–20 mg/L and in 16% with a level over 20, and may herald sudden cardiac death (211). Asthma comorbidity in long QT syndrome patients increased the risk of cardiac events (212), perhaps due to otherwise trivial prolongation of QT due to beta agonists. Rarely catecholamine-induced myocarditis can reduce ventricular function, and it may be more common with infused isoproterenol (213–215). Peripheral vasoconstriction and transient tissue hypoperfusion from intravenous and subcutaneous sympathomemetics may result in lactic acidosis (216–218). High doses of albuterol result in slight decreases (0.7 mEq/L) in serum potassium, which could be significant in patients with preexisting cardiovascular disease or hypokalemia (219).

Aspirin or other nonsteroidal antiinflammatory agents may be the trigger for up to 8% of acute exacerbations of asthma requiring mechanical ventilation, reflecting the 5–10% of asthmatics with aspirin-intolerance (16). Blockade of the cyclo-oxygenase pathway may shunt precursors to the leukotriene pathway, triggering asthma. Leukotriene receptor blockers (but not 5-lipoxygenase inhibitors) may be useful in aspirin-intolerant asthma and perhaps during acute exacerbations triggered by aspirin or other cyclooxygenase inhibitors (220,221). Pretreatment with inhaled prostaglandin E2, albuterol, and perhaps the prostaglandin E1-analog misoprostol is successful in blunting aspirin-induced broncho-constriction and could be useful in acute attacks (222). Laryngeal edema, angioedema, and anaphylaxis should also be considered in acute aspirin-induced asthma exacerbations.

Barotrauma before, during, and after mechanical ventilation includes pneumothorax with or without tension, pneumomediastinum, pulmonary interstitial emphysema, subcutaneous emphysema, coronary air embolism pneumoretroperitoneum, and pneumoperitoneum (183,202,223,224).

Pregnancy may contribute causatively to asthma, and occasionally severe exacerbations are relieved by delivery (225,226). In general, management of exacerbations during pregnancy is similar to other exacerbations (227). In practice, pregnant women presenting to the ED with asthma exacerbations receive corticosteroids less often (44% vs. 66%) and are 2.9 times more likely to report a continuing exacerbation at two weeks (228). Of particular concern is oxygenation, because the P_aO_2 supplied to the fetus (umbilical vein) is 10–15 mmHg less than the uterine venous blood. Maternal P_aO_2 above 70 mmHg is adequate (229). Budesonide (Pulmicort Turbuhaler® and Pulmicort Respules®), terbutaline (Brethine®), ipratropium (Atrovent®), nedocromil (Tilade®), cromolyn (Intal®), omalizumab (Xolair®), montelukast (Singulair®) and zafirlukast (Accolate®) have category B ratings for use during pregnancy. Systemic corticosteroids should be used when needed.

Mucous plugs may obstruct or narrow the lumen of endotracheal tubes (230). Pulmonary embolus or deep vein thrombosis may be a precipitating event for bronchospasm or the sequelae of immobility in the ICU. Stress ulcers and acute gastrointestinal bleeding risk are increased by corticosteroids and ICU stays. Prophylaxis for deep vein thrombosis and stress ulcers is appropriate for asthmatics in the ICU. Acute chest syndrome in sickle cell disease may be more common and severe in patients with concomitant asthma (231). Since viruses are the most common infectious triggers, antibiotics are indicated only if a chest X-ray suggests pneumonia (*M. pneumoniae* and *C. pneumoniae*, especially in children) (232,233). As in chronic treatment, allergic bronchopulmonary aspergillosis may complicate acute exacerbations of asthma and require higher doses of corticosteroids and anti-fungal therapy.

Rarely, dose dependent bronchospasm, angioedema, or urticaria due to intravenous steroids have been reported (234). Overt or subclinical adrenal atrophy and insufficiency may be manifested during tapers of corticosteroids, or during acute therapy as mineralocorticoid insufficiency (235,236). Corticosteroid associated or exacerbated diabetes mellitus is common at high doses, but less so at the moderate doses recommended above. Acute myopathy due to corticosteroids (237,238), the combination of corticosteroids and paralytic agents (239–242), or prolonged paralysis after paralytic agents (243–245) may complicate acute asthma care. Recovery to functional independence generally occurs over the first month (246). Rarely frank rhabdomyolysis may be present (247–250). Hyperthyroidism may present with recurrent asthma exacerbations, causing and many of the symptoms to be attributed incorrectly to asthma therapy (251). Subconjunctival hemorrhage affects as much a 5% of acute severe asthma attacks (252).

Fixed dilation of one or both pupils due to aerosolized anticholinergic agents may be mistaken for serious intracranial pathology (253). Rarely subarachnoid hemorrhage has been reported in severe asthma; the pathophysiologic mechanism is unclear (254,255). Anxiety and panic disorders may coexist or complicate recovery from asthma exacerbations (256). Unfortunately, brain death and other hypoxemic sequelae can be present on presentation to the ED; they are fortunately rare within the hospital.

VIII. Recovery

In-hospital death should be rare with the exception of those presenting with cardiac arrest, hypoxic encephalopathy, or brain death. In the UK, the mortality of patients admitted to the ICU for asthma was 7.1% in the ICU and 9.8% overall during hospitalization (257). In asthmatics who die, the following were more likely present on presentation: older age, African-American and other non-Caucasian race, female sex, neurologic insult or CPR within 24 hours before admission, higher APACHE II score, higher heart rate, higher P_aCO_2, and lower pH (258,259). These are the same factors that relate to receipt of mechanical ventilation after admission. Preventable causes of death include administration of aminophylline without a known blood level, sedation outside the ICU setting, inadequate treatment with steroids, and inadequate asthma clinical assessment or action (260–262). Duration of hospital stay is longer with female sex, endotracheal intubation, administration of neuromuscular blockade for >24 hours, inhaled corticosteroid use prior to ICU admission, and increasing APACHE II score (263,264). However, avoiding these interventions does not necessarily shorten hospital stays or improve morbidity and mortality. Time to achieve recovery is proportional to the degree of airways obstruction at presentation (265,266). Resolution of hyperinflation may lag behind PEF resolution, perhaps indicating persistent small airways obstruction (267).

Environmental tobacco smoke exposure in the month following hospitalization increases β-agonist use and symptomatic days (268). Mortality after discharge from an intubation-requiring attack is high: 13% in Singapore (269), 10.1% at one year and 22.6% after six years in France, (48), and 4.5% in children in Australia (270). Lack of prescription of inhaled corticosteroids or prescription of ipratropium on discharge or PCO_2 >46 mmHg increase the risk of death from all causes after discharge (271).

IX. Prevention

Prevention of severe exacerbations, ED visits, hospitalizations, and death in asthma is complex, but likely simplifies to good asthma treatment and education, and also compliance with an inhaled corticosteroid regimen. The risk of death decreases 21% with each additional canister/year of inhaled corticosteroid, beginning at a mean of 1.18 canisters/year in patients who die (272). Written

Table 5 Differential Diagnosis for Severe Airway Obstruction

COPD including parenchymal destruction and small airways disease
RADS: high level exposure to a corrosive gas, vapor, or fume
Bronchiectasis including cystic fibrosis
Bronchiolitis: viral, nitrogen dioxide and other insoluble corrosive gases, obliterative, constrictive, respiratory bronchiolitis with interstitial lung disease
Sarcoidosis
Bronchopulmonary dysplasia
Pseudomembranous aspergillus, herpetic tracheobronchitis
LAM
Allergic bronchopulmonary aspergillosis
  Churg-Strauss syndrome
Anaphylaxis and urticaria-angioedema
Fixed airway obstruction: subglottic or tracheal stenosis, Schwannoma, carcinoid, lung cancer, head and neck tumor, mediastinal tumors, papillary carcinomatosis, tracheal chondroma, tubular adenoma or leimyoma, mediastinal fibrosis, inflammatory pseudotumour of the trachea (some may be variable at times)
Variable extra-thoracic upper airway obstruction: vocal cord spasm or dysfunction, epiglotitis, retropharyngeal abscess, hemorrhagic vocal cord lesions, cricoarytenoid arthritis, Wegner's granulomatosis, laryngoceal, tonsilar abscess
Misplacement of endotracheal tube (although capnography may be misleading)
Foreign bodies, aspiration, trauma
Mucous plugs and endobronchial casts
Pulmonary edema from congestive heart failure or renal failure
Pulmonary embolus
Tropical eosinophilia, parasitic infections, larva migrans syndrome
Herniation of abdominal contents into the thoracic cavity through a diaphragmatic hernia
Diaphragmatic flutter (high-frequency, pulsatile contractions of the thorax and abdominal wall)

Abbreviations: COPD, Chronic obstructive pulmonary disease; RADS, Reactive airways dysfunction syndrome; LAM, Lymphangioleimyomatosis.
Source: From Refs. 195, 275–291.

Table 6   Summary of Treatment

Bronchodilators
   Continuous nebulized albuterol at 15 mg/hr [children 7.5 mg/hr] and ipratropium at
      1.5 mg/hr [1 mg/hr] for the first one to two hours and continued at half dose until
      improved then converted to metered dose inhaler.
Corticosteroids
   Methylprednisolone 40 mg IV (perhaps 125 mg if impending respiratory failure)
      [children 0.5 or 1 mg/kg] once, followed by prednisone 40 (perhaps 80) [0.5 or
      1 mg/kg], PO if possible, divided two to four times daily or methylprednisolone
      20 mg (perhaps 40) [0.25 or 0.5 mg/kg] q6 hr. Add fludrocortisone 0.1 mg qd in any
      patient on oral corticosteroids in the past 12 months.
Oxygen
   Sufficient to maintain $S_pO_2 > 92\%$.
Consider
   Alternative diagnoses
   Magnesium sulfate 6 g IV over 20 min followed by 2 g/hr for four hours, reduced if
      renal failure. Proportional for children.
   Heliox (F_1O_2 0.3, balance He)
   Intravenous salbutamol (not available in the US) 250 μg/min [5 μg/kg/min in
      children] × 1–2 hr, followed by 50 μg/min [1 μg/kg/min] If no response,
      rebolused and continued at twice the dose.
   OR intravenous terbutaline 100 μg/min [2 μg/kg/min in children] × 1–2 hr,
      followed by 50 μg/min [1 μg/kg/min] If no response, rebolused and continued at
      twice the dose.
   Aminophylline hydrous 6 mg/kg lean body weight over 30 min followed by
      0.7 mg/kg/hr [children 0.5–9 yr 1.2 mg/kg/hr, 9–16 yr 1.0 mg/kg/hr] for next
      12 hours and reduced to 0.5 mg/kg/hr [children 0.5–9 yr 1 mg/kg/hr, 9–16 yr
      0.8 mg/kg/hr] following. Adjust dose for age, smoking and imperatively, if the
      patient has taken any recent theophylline. Monitor blood levels.
   Intubation and mechanical ventilation with permissive hypercapnea
   Sedatives, narcotics—only in the ICU, usually after intubation
   Montelukast
   Paralytic agents
   Bronchoscopy if radiographic evidence of segmental or lobar mucous plugs
   Anesthetic agents
   Nitric oxide
Discharge
   Oral steroid burst
   Inhaled corticosteroid at high dose often with long-acting β2-agonist
   Adequate rescue medication
   Plan for exacerbations
   Good follow-up

action plans are associated with a 70% reduction in the risk of death (273). The use of oral steroids for an attack of asthma reduced the risk of death by 90% (273). True adherence to guideline-based management of asthmatics would significantly reduce morbidity and mortality. Each exacerbation represents a new chance to get the patient back on track, and the more severe the exacerbation the more critical this is. Aggressive management after the diagnosis of potentially fatal asthma, the occurrence of major asthma events that place the patient at high risk for a death from asthma, may prevent future mortality (274).

X. Differential Diagnosis

All that wheezes is not asthma. Diseases that are not asthma may not respond to asthma therapy. Part of noting a lack of response to initial therapy of asthma exacerbation is being certain the diagnosis is asthma (Table 5). Usually the distinction between asthma and COPD is fairly obvious based on history. In the 5–10% of individuals with both, or if there is uncertainty, management as for asthma is usually successful.

Vocal cord spasm (spastic dysphonia, adductor dystonia) is paradoxical adduction of the vocal cords primarily during inspiration, which may be visualized during indirect laryngoscopy. In general, upper airway obstruction produces stridor—inspiratory wheeze loudest at the throat, but transmitted to the lungs. Spirometry often shows an inspiratory plateau or very irregular flow–volume curves with abrupt cutoffs (292). The true incidence is unknown, but case series report more women, military recruits, and outdoor athletes, especially those with social or performance stress (293–297). Etiologies include (1) brainstem compression, (2) cortical or upper motor neuron injury, (3) nuclear or lower motor neuron injury, (4) movement disorder, (5) gastroesophageal reflux, (6) factitious or malingering disorder, and (7) somatization/conversion disorder (298). Therapy with acid reflux suppression, speech therapy, psychotherapy/biofeedback, or botulinum toxin injection of the vocal cord adductor muscles may be helpful (297,299,300). Intubation eliminates the airway resistance immediately.

XI. Summary

Quick intensive assessment and intervention with inhaled bronchodilators, systemic corticosteroids, and oxygen is effective in most cases of acute severe asthma presenting to the ED (Table 6). For those who fail initial therapy, more of the same, support with mechanical ventilation, and additional less well-proven therapies are appropriate. Adequate discharge planning and follow-up are essential to insure longer-term success.

References

1. Beveridge RC, Grunfeld AF, Hodder RV, Verbeek PR. Guidelines for the emergency management of asthma in adults. CAEP/CTS Asthma Advisory Committee. Canadian Association of Emergency Physicians and the Canadian Thoracic Society. CMAJ 1996; 155:25–37.
2. Rowe BH, Edmonds ML, Spooner CH, Camargo CA. Evidence-based treatments for acute asthma. Respir Care 2001; 46:1380–1390; discussion 1390–1391.
3. Werner HA. Status asthmaticus in children: a review. Chest 2001; 119:1913–1929.
4. L'Her E. [Revision of the 3rd Consensus Conference in Intensive Care and Emergency Medicine in 1988: management of acute asthmatic crisis in adults and chidren (excluding infants)]. Rev Mal Respir 2002; 19:658–665.
5. Papiris S, Kotanidou A, Malagari K, Roussos C. Clinical review: severe asthma. Crit Care 2002; 6:30–44.
6. British guideline on the management of asthma. Thorax 2003; 58 (suppl 1):i, 1–94.
7. Clark TJH. Global initiative for asthma: global strategy for asthma management and prevention, NHLBI/WHO workshop report, Updated 2003. Bethesda, MD: US Department of Health and Human Services Publication NIH/NHLBI 02–3659, 2003:197.
8. McFadden ER. Acute severe asthma. American Journal of Respiratory and Critical Care Medicine 2003; 168:740–759.
9. Picado C. Classification of severe asthma exacerbations: a proposal. Eur Respir J 1996; 9:1775–1778.
10. Woodruff PG, Emond SD, Singh AK, Camargo CA Jr. Sudden-onset severe acute asthma: clinical features and response to therapy. Acad Emerg Med 1998; 5:695–701.
11. Rodrigo GJ, Rodrigo C. Rapid-onset asthma attack: a prospective cohort study about characteristics and response to emergency department treatment. Chest 2000; 118:1547–1552.
12. Barr RG, Woodruff PG, Clark S, Camargo CA Jr. Sudden-onset asthma exacerbations: clinical features, response to therapy, and 2-week follow-up. Multicenter Airway Research Collaboration (MARC) investigators. Eur Respir J 2000; 15:266–273.
13. Sur S, Crotty TB, Kephart GM, Hyma BA, Colby TV, Reed CE, Hunt LW, Gleich GJ. Sudden-onset fatal asthma. A distinct entity with few eosinophils and relatively more neutrophils in the airway submucosa? Am Rev Respir Dis 1993; 148:713–719.
14. Ordaz VA, Castaneda CB, Campos CL, Rodriguez VM, Saenz JG, Rios PC. Asthmatic exacerbations and environmental pollen concentration in La Comarca Lagunera (Mexico). Rev Alerg Mex 1998; 45:106–111.
15. Landau SN, Kyff JV. Risks of inhalational anesthesia. Crit Care Med 1987; 15:801–802.
16. Picado C, Castillo JA, Montserrat JM, Agusti-Vidal A. Aspirin-intolerance as a precipitating factor of life-threatening attacks of asthma requiring mechanical ventilation. Eur Respir J 1989; 2:127–129.
17. Stevenson DD, Simon RA. Sensitivity to ingested metabisulfites in asthmatic subjects. J Allergy Clin Immunol 1981; 68:26–32.
18. Averbach M, Casey KK, Frank E. Near-fatal status asthmaticus induced by nasal insufflation of cocaine. South Med J 1996; 89:340–341.

19. Cygan J, Trunsky M, Corbridge T. Inhaled heroin-induced status asthmaticus: five cases and a review of the literature. Chest 2000; 117:272–275.
20. Tatum AM, Greenberger PA, Mileusnic D, Donoghue ER, Lifschultz BD. Clinical, pathologic, and toxicologic findings in asthma deaths in Cook County, Illinois. Allergy Asthma Proc 2001; 22:285–291.
21. Oehling A, Gamboa PM. The viral factor in childhood asthma. Allerg Immunol (Paris) 1987; 19:13–17.
22. Hankinson JL, Odencrantz JR, Fedan KB. Spirometric reference values from a sample of the general U.S. population. Am J Respir Crit Care Med 1999; 159:179–187.
23. Azzawi M, Johnston PW, Majumdar S, Kay AB, Jeffery PK. T lymphocytes and activated eosinophils in airway mucosa in fatal asthma and cystic fibrosis. Am Rev Respir Dis 1992; 145:1477–1482.
24. Corrigan CJ, Hartnell A, Kay AB. T lymphocyte activation in acute severe asthma. Lancet 1988; 1:1129–1132.
25. Aikawa T, Shimura S, Sasaki H, Ebina M, Takishima T. Marked goblet cell hyperplasia with mucus accumulation in the airways of patients who died of severe acute asthma attack. Chest 1992; 101:916–921.
26. Lemjabbar H, Gosset P, Lamblin C, Tillie I, Hartmann D, Wallaert B, Tonnel AB, Lafuma C. Contribution of 92 kDa gelatinase/type IV collagenase in bronchial inflammation during status asthmaticus. Am J Respir Crit Care Med 1999; 159:1298–1307.
27. Tillie-Leblond I, Pugin J, Marquette CH, Lamblin C, Saulnier F, Brichet A, Wallaert B, Tonnel AB, Gosset P. Balance between proinflammatory cytokines and their inhibitors in bronchial lavage from patients with status asthmaticus. Am J Respir Crit Care Med 1999; 159:487–194.
28. Tillie-Leblond I, Hammad H, Desurmont S, Pugin J, Wallaert B, Tonnel AB, Gosset P. CC chemokines and interleukin-5 in bronchial lavage fluid from patients with status asthmaticus. Potential implication in eosinophil recruitment. Am J Respir Crit Care Med 2000; 162:586–592.
29. Tonnel AB, Gosset P, Tillie-Leblond I. Characteristics of the inflammatory response in bronchial lavage fluids from patients with status asthmaticus. Int Arch Allergy Immunol 2001; 124:267–271.
30. Park SW, Kim do J, Chang HS, Park SJ, Lee YM, Park JS, Chung IY, Lee JH, Park CS. Association of interleukin-5 and eotaxin with acute exacerbation of asthma. Int Arch Allergy Immunol 2003; 131:283–290.
31. Ackerman SJ, Liu L, Kwatia MA, Savage MP, Leonidas DD, Swaminathan GJ, Acharya KR. Charcot-Leyden crystal protein (galectin-10) is not a dual function galectin with lysophospholipase activity but binds a lysophospholipase inhibitor in a novel structural fashion. J Biol Chem 2002; 277:14859–14868.
32. Abedin MJ, Kashio Y, Seki M, Nakamura K, Hirashima M. Potential roles of galectins in myeloid differentiation into three different lineages. J Leukoc Biol 2003; 73:650–656.
33. Bhaskar KR, O'Sullivan DD, Coles SJ, Kozakewich H, Vawter GP, Reid LM. Characterization of airway mucus from a fatal case of status asthmaticus. Pediatr Pulmonol 1988; 5:176–182.
34. Sheehan JK, Richardson PS, Fung DC, Howard M, Thornton DJ. Analysis of respiratory mucus glycoproteins in asthma: a detailed study from a patient who died in status asthmaticus. Am J Respir Cell Mol Biol 1995; 13:748–756.

35. Antonakopoulos GN, Lambrinaki E, Kyrkou KA. Curschmann's spirals in sputum: histochemical evidence of bronchial gland ductal origin. Diagn Cytopathol 1987; 3:291–294.

36. Weir TD, Mallek N, Sandford AJ, Bai TR, Awadh N, Fitzgerald JM, Cockcroft D, James A, Liggett SB, Pare PD. beta2-Adrenergic receptor haplotypes in mild, moderate and fatal/near fatal asthma. Am J Respir Crit Care Med 1998; 158:787–791.

37. Rodriguez-Roisin R. Acute severe asthma: pathophysiology and pathobiology of gas exchange abnormalities. Eur Respir J 1997; 10:1359–1371.

38. Oosaki R, Mizushima Y, Kawasaki A, Kashii T, Mita H, Shida T, Akiyama K, Kobayashi M. Urinary excretion of leukotriene E4 and 11-dehydrothromboxane B2 in patients with spontaneous asthma attacks. Int Arch Allergy Immunol 1997; 114:373–378.

39. Rodriguez-Roisin R, Ballester E, Roca J, Torres A, Wagner PD. Mechanisms of hypoxemia in patients with status asthmaticus requiring mechanical ventilation. Am Rev Respir Dis 1989; 139:732–739.

40. Molfino NA, Nannini LJ, Martelli AN, Slutsky AS. Respiratory arrest in near-fatal asthma. N Engl J Med 1991; 324:285–288.

41. Asthma prevalence and control characteristics by race/ethnicity—United States, 2002. Morb Mortal Wkly Rep 2004; 53:145–148.

42. Weber EJ, Silverman RA, Callaham ML, Pollack CV, Woodruff PG, Clark S, Camargo CA, Jr. A prospective multicenter study of factors associated with hospital admission among adults with acute asthma. Am J Med 2002; 113:371–378.

43. Pollack CV, Jr., Pollack ES, Baren JM, Smith SR, Woodruff PG, Clark S, Camargo CA, Jr. A prospective multicenter study of patient factors associated with hospital admission from the emergency department among children with acute asthma. Arch Pediatr Adolesc Med 2002; 156:934–940.

44. Kolbe J, Fergusson W, Vamos M, Garrett J. Case—control study of severe life threatening asthma (SLTA) in adults: demographics, health care, and management of the acute attack. Thorax 2000; 55:1007–1015.

45. Robertson CF, Rubinfeld AR, Bowes G. Pediatric asthma deaths in Victoria: the mild are at risk. Pediatr Pulmonol 1992; 13:95–100.

46. Richards GN, Kolbe J, Fenwick J, Rea HH. Demographic characteristics of patients with severe life threatening asthma: comparison with asthma deaths. Thorax 1993; 48:1105–1109.

47. McConnochie KM, Russo MJ, McBride JT, Szilagyi PG, Brooks AM, Roghmann KJ. Socioeconomic variation in asthma hospitalization: excess utilization or greater need? Pediatrics 1999; 103:e75.

48. Boudreaux ED, Emond SD, Clark S, Camargo CA Jr. Acute asthma among adults presenting to the emergency department: the role of race/ethnicity and socioeconomic status. Chest 2003; 124:803–812.

49. Garrett JE, Lanes SF, Kolbe J, Rea HH. Risk of severe life threatening asthma and beta agonist type: an example of confounding by severity. Thorax 1996; 51:1093–1099.

50. Rea HH, Garrett JE, Lanes SF, Birmann BM, Kolbe J. The association between asthma drugs and severe life-threatening attacks. Chest 1996; 110:1446–1451.

51. Pearce N, Beasley R, Crane J, Burgess C, Jackson R. End of the New Zealand asthma mortality epidemic. Lancet 1995; 345:41–44.

52. Tanihara S, Nakamura Y, Matsui T, Nishima S. A case-control study of asthma death and life-threatening attack: their possible relationship with prescribed drug therapy in Japan. J Epidemiol 2002; 12:223–228.

53. Lanes SF, Garcia Rodriguez LA, Huerta C. Respiratory medications and risk of asthma death. Thorax 2002; 57:683–686.

54. Suissa S, Ernst P, Boivin JF, Horwitz RI, Habbick B, Cockroft D, Blais L, McNutt M, Buist AS, Spitzer WO. A cohort analysis of excess mortality in asthma and the use of inhaled beta-agonists. Am J Respir Crit Care Med 1994; 149:604–610.

55. Suissa S, Ernst P, Spitzer WO. Beta-agonist use and death from asthma. J Am Med Assoc 1994; 271:821–822.

56. Innes NJ, Reid A, Halstead J, Watkin SW, Harrison BD. Psychosocial risk factors in near-fatal asthma and in asthma deaths. J R Coll Physicians Lond 1998; 32:430–434.

57. Bucknall CE, Slack R, Godley CC, Mackay TW, Wright SC. Scottish Confidential Inquiry into Asthma Deaths (SCIAD), 1994–1996. Thorax 1999; 54:978–984.

58. Trawick DR, Holm C, Wirth J. Influence of gender on rates of hospitalization, hospital course, and hypercapnea in high-risk patients admitted for asthma: a 10-year retrospective study at Yale-New Haven Hospital. Chest 2001; 119:115–119.

59. Ferris TG, Blumenthal D, Woodruff PG, Clark S, Camargo CA. Insurance and quality of care for adults with acute asthma. J Gen Intern Med 2002; 17:905–913.

60. Thomson CC, Clark S, Camargo CA Jr. Body mass index and asthma severity among adults presenting to the emergency department. Chest 2003; 124: 795–802.

61. Fanta CH, Rossing TH, McFadden ER Jr. Emergency room of treatment of asthma. Relationships among therapeutic combinations, severity of obstruction and time course of response. Am J Med 1982; 72:416–422.

62. Kelly AM, Kerr D, Powell C. Is severity assessment after one hour of treatment better for predicting the need for admission in acute asthma? Respir Med 2004; 98:777–781.

63. Baker MD. Pitfalls in the use of clinical asthma scoring. Am J Dis Child 1988; 142:183–185.

64. Veen JC, Smits HH, Ravensberg AJ, Hiemstra PS, Sterk PJ, Bel EH. Impaired perception of dyspnea in patients with severe asthma. Relation to sputum eosinophils. Am J Respir Crit Care Med 1998; 158:1134–1141.

65. Jang AS, Choi IS. Increased perception of dyspnea by inhalation of short acting beta2 agonist in patients with asthma of varying severity. Ann Allergy Asthma Immunol 2000; 84:79–83.

66. Cydulka RK, Emerman CL, Rowe BH, Clark S, Woodruff PG, Singh AK, Camargo CA, Jr. Differences between men and women in reporting of symptoms during an asthma exacerbation. Ann Emerg Med 2001; 38:123–128.

67. Shim CS, Williams MH Jr. Relationship of wheezing to the severity of obstruction in asthma. Arch Intern Med 1983; 143:890–892.

68. Kerem E, Canny G, Tibshirani R, Reisman J, Bentur L, Schuh S, Levison H. Clinical-physiologic correlations in acute asthma of childhood. Pediatrics 1991; 87:481–486.

69. Keahey L, Bulloch B, Becker AB, Pollack CV Jr, Clark S, Camargo CA, Jr. Initial oxygen saturation as a predictor of admission in children presenting to the emergency department with acute asthma. Ann Emerg Med 2002; 40: 300–307.

70. Carruthers DM, Harrison BD. Arterial blood gas analysis or oxygen saturation in the assessment of acute asthma? Thorax 1995; 50:186–188.

71. Wright RO, Steele DW, Santucci KA, Natarajan R, Jay GD. Continuous, noninvasive measurement of pulsus paradoxus in patients with acute asthma. Arch Pediatr Adolesc Med 1996; 150:914–918.

72. Emerman CL, Cydulka RK. Effect of pulmonary function testing on the management of acute asthma. Arch Intern Med 1995; 155:2225–2228.

73. Corre KA, Rothstein RJ. Assessing severity of adult asthma and need for hospitalization. Ann Emerg Med 1985; 14:45–52.

74. Gorelick MH, Stevens MW, Schultz T, Scribano PV. Difficulty in obtaining peak expiratory flow measurements in children with acute asthma. Pediatr Emerg Care 2004; 20:22–26.

75. Efthimiou J, Hassan AB, Ormerod O, Benson MK. Reversible T-wave abnormality in severe acute asthma: an electrocardiographic sign of severity. Respir Med 1991; 85:195–202.

76. McDowell KM, Chatburn RL, Myers TR, O'Riordan MA, Kercsmar CM. A cost-saving algorithm for children hospitalized for status asthmaticus. Arch Pediatr Adolesc Med 1998; 152:977–984.

77. Gupta D, Keogh B, Chung KF, Ayres JG, Harrison DA, Goldfrad C, Brady AR, Rowan K. Characteristics and outcome for admissions to adult, general critical care units with acute severe asthma: a secondary analysis of the ICNARC Case Mix Programme Database. Critical Care 2004; 8:R112–R121.

78. Camargo C Jr, Spooner C, Rowe B. Continuous versus intermittent beta-agonists in the treatment of acute asthma. Cochrane Database Syst Rev 2003; 4: CD001115.

79. Colacone A, Wolkove N, Stern E, Afilalo M, Rosenthal TM, Kreisman H. Continuous nebulization of albuterol (salbutamol) in acute asthma. Chest 1990; 97:693–697.

80. Besbes-Ouanes L, Nouira S, Elatrous S, Knani J, Boussarsar M, Abroug F. Continuous versus intermittent nebulization of salbutamol in acute severe asthma: a randomized, controlled trial. Ann Emerg Med 2000; 36:198–203.

81. Innes NJ, Stocking JA, Daynes TJ, Harrison BD. Randomised pragmatic comparison of UK and US treatment of acute asthma presenting to hospital. Thorax 2002; 57:1040–1044.

82. Nowak RM, Emerman CL, Schaefer K, Disantostefano RL, Vaickus L, Roach JM. Levalbuterol compared with racemic albuterol in the treatment of acute asthma: results of a pilot study. Am J Emerg Med 2004; 22:29–36.

83. Avila-Castanon L, Casas–Becerra B, Del Rio-Navarro BE, Velazquez-Armenta Y, Sienra-Monge JJ. Formoterol vs. albuterol administered via Turbuhaler system in the emergency treatment of acute asthma in children. Allergol Immunopathol (Madr) 2004; 32:18–20.

84. Xie L, Liu Y, Chen L, Hao F, Jin G, Zhao H. Inhaling beta(2)-agonist with heliox-driven in bronchial asthma. Chin Med J (Engl) 2003; 116:1011–1015.

85. Bentur L, Mansour Y, Hamzani Y, Beck R, Elias N, Amirav I. Measurement of inspiratory flow in children with acute asthma. Pediatr Pulmonol 2004; 38:304–307.

86. Sellers WF, Messahel B. Rapidly repeated intravenous boluses of salbutamol for acute severe asthma. Anaesthesia 2003; 58:680–683.

87. Roberts G, Newsom D, Gomez K, Raffles A, Saglani S, Begent J, Lachman P, Sloper K, Buchdahl R, Habel A. Intravenous salbutamol bolus compared with an aminophylline infusion in children with severe asthma: a randomised controlled trial. Thorax 2003; 58:306–310.
88. Browne GJ, Wilkins BH. Use of intravenous salbutamol in acute severe asthma. Anaesthesia 2003; 58:729–732.
89. Habashy D, Lam LT, Browne GJ. The administration of beta2-agonists for paediatric asthma and its adverse reaction in Australian and New Zealand emergency departments: a cross-sectional survey. Eur J Emerg Med 2003; 10:219–224.
90. Stephanopoulos DE, Monge R, Schell KH, Wyckoff P, Peterson BM. Continuous intravenous terbutaline for pediatric status asthmaticus. Crit Care Med 1998; 26:1744–1748.
91. Van Renterghem D, Lamont H, Elinck W, Pauwels R, Van der Straeten M. Intravenous versus nebulized terbutaline in patients with acute severe asthma; a double-blind randomized study. Ann Allergy 1987; 59:313–316.
92. Victoria MS, Tayaba RG, Nangia BS. Isoproterenol infusion in the management of respiratory failure in children with status asthmaticus: experience in a small community hospital and review of the literature. J Asthma 1991; 28:103–108.
93. Travers A, Jones AP, Kelly K, Barker SJ, Camargo CA, Rowe BH. Intravenous beta2-agonists for acute asthma in the emergency department. Cochrane Database Syst Rev 2001; CD002988.
94. Jones SL, Kittelson J, Cowan JO, Flannery EM, Hancox RJ, McLachlan CR, Taylor DR. The predictive value of exhaled nitric oxide measurements in assessing changes in asthma control. Am J Respir Crit Care Med 2001; 164:738–743.
95. Miller DD, Amin MM, Palmer LB, Shah AR, Smaldone GC. Aerosol delivery and modern mechanical ventilation: in vitro/in vivo evaluation. Am J Respir Crit Care Med 2003; 168:1205–1209.
96. Hess DR, Dillman C, Kacmarek RM. In vitro evaluation of aerosol bronchodilator delivery during mechanical ventilation: pressure-control vs. volume control ventilation. Intensive Care Med 2003; 29:1145–1150.
97. Georgopoulos D, Kondili E, Prinianakis G. How to set the ventilator in asthma. Monaldi Arch Chest Dis 2000; 55:74–83.
98. Schuh S, Johnson DW, Callahan S, Canny G, Levison H. Efficacy of frequent nebulized ipratropium bromide added to frequent high-dose albuterol therapy in severe childhood asthma. J Pediatr 1995; 126:639–645.
99. Qureshi F, Zaritsky A, Lakkis H. Efficacy of nebulized ipratropium in severely asthmatic children. Ann Emerg Med 1997; 29:205–211.
100. Benito Fernandez J, Mintegui Raso S, Sanchez Echaniz J, Vazquez Ronco MA, Pijoan Zubizarreta JI. [Efficacy of early administration of nebulized ipratropium bromide in children with asthmatic crisis.] An Esp Pediatr 2000; 53:217–222.
101. Lanes SF, Garrett JE, Wentworth CE, 3rd, Fitzgerald JM, Karpel JP. The effect of adding ipratropium bromide to salbutamol in the treatment of acute asthma: a pooled analysis of three trials. Chest 1998; 114:365–372.
102. Stoodley RG, Aaron SD, Dales RE. The role of ipratropium bromide in the emergency management of acute asthma exacerbation: a metaanalysis of randomized clinical trials. Ann Emerg Med 1999; 34:8–18.

103. Craven D, Kercsmar CM, Myers TR, O'Riordan M A, Golonka G, Moore S. Ipratropium bromide plus nebulized albuterol for the treatment of hospitalized children with acute asthma. J Pediatr 2001; 138:51–58.

104. Timsit S, Sannier N, Bocquet N, Cojocaru B, Wille C, Boursiquot C, Garel D, Marcombes F, Cheron G. [Benefits of ipratropium bromide in the management of asthmatic crises in the emergency department.] Arch Pediatr 2002; 9:117–125.

105. Browne GJ, Trieu L, Van Asperen P. Randomized, double-blind, placebo-controlled trial of intravenous salbutamol and nebulized ipratropium bromide in early management of severe acute asthma in children presenting to an emergency department. Crit Care Med 2002; 30:448–453.

106. Whyte KF, Gould GA, Jeffrey AA, Airlie MA, Flenley DC, Douglas NJ. Dose of nebulized ipratropium bromide in acute severe asthma. Respir Med 1991; 85:517–520.

107. Teale C, Morrison JF, Muers MF, Pearson SB. Response to nebulized ipratropium bromide and terbutaline in acute severe asthma. Respir Med 1992; 86:215–218.

108. Fanta CH, Rossing TH, McFadden ER Jr. Glucocorticoids in acute asthma. A critical controlled trial. Am J Med 1983; 74:845–851.

109. Younger RE, Gerber PS, Herrod HG, Cohen RM, Crawford LV. Intravenous methylprednisolone efficacy in status asthmaticus of childhood. Pediatrics 1987; 80:225–230.

110. Gleeson JG, Loftus BG, Price JF. Placebo controlled trial of systemic corticosteroids in acute childhood asthma. Acta Paediatr Scand 1990; 79:1052–1058.

111. Manser R, Reid D, Abramson M. Corticosteroids for acute severe asthma in hospitalised patients. Cochrane Database Syst Rev 2001: CD001740.

112. Volovitz B, Bentur L, Finkelstein Y, Mansour Y, Shalitin S, Nussinovitch M, Varsano I. Effectiveness and safety of inhaled corticosteroids in controlling acute asthma attacks in children who were treated in the emergency department: a controlled comparative study with oral prednisolone. J Allergy Clin Immunol 1998; 102:605–609.

113. Edmonds ML, Camargo CA Jr, Pollack CV Jr, Rowe BH. Early use of inhaled corticosteroids in the emergency department treatment of acute asthma. Cochrane Database Syst Rev 2003; CD002308.

114. Nakanishi AK, Klasner AK, Rubin BK. A randomized controlled trial of inhaled flunisolide in the management of acute asthma in children. Chest 2003; 124:790–794.

115. Chien JW, Ciufo R, Novak R, Skowronski M, Nelson J, Coreno A, McFadden ER, Jr. Uncontrolled oxygen administration and respiratory failure in acute asthma. Chest 2000; 117:728–733.

116. Alter HJ, Koepsell TD, Hilty WM. Intravenous magnesium as an adjuvant in acute bronchospasm: a meta-analysis. Ann Emerg Med 2000; 36:191–197.

117. Rowe BH, Bretzlaff JA, Bourdon C, Bota GW, Camargo CA Jr. Intravenous magnesium sulfate treatment for acute asthma in the emergency department: a systematic review of the literature. Ann Emerg Med 2000; 36:181–190.

118. Okayama H, Okayama M, Aikawa T, Sasaki M, Takishima T. Treatment of status asthmaticus with intravenous magnesium sulfate. J Asthma 1991; 28:11–17.

119. Sydow M, Crozier TA, Zielmann S, Radke J, Burchardi H. High-dose intravenous magnesium sulfate in the management of life-threatening status asthmaticus. Intensive Care Med 1993; 19:467–471.

120. Schiermeyer RP, Finkelstein JA. Rapid infusion of magnesium sulfate obviates need for intubation in status asthmaticus. Am J Emerg Med 1994; 12: 164–166.

121. Magnussen H, Jorres R, Hartmann V. Bronchodilator effect of theophylline preparations and aerosol fenoterol in stable asthma. Chest 1986; 90:722–725.

122. Parameswaran K, Belda J, Rowe BH. Addition of intravenous aminophylline to beta2-agonists in adults with acute asthma. Cochrane Database Syst Rev 2000; CD002742.

123. Nakahara Y, Murata M, Suzuki T, Ohtsu F, Nagasawa K. Significance of the thera-peutic range of serum theophylline concentration in the treatment of an attack of bronchial asthma. Biol Pharm Bull 1996; 19:710–715.

124. Janson C, Boman G, Boe J. Which patients benefit from adding theophylline to beta 2-agonist treatment in severe acute asthma? Ann Allergy 1992; 69:107–110.

125. Wrenn K, Slovis CM, Murphy F, Greenberg RS. Aminophylline therapy for acute bronchospastic disease in the emergency room. Ann Intern Med 1991; 115:241–247.

126. Yung M, South M. Randomised controlled trial of aminophylline for severe acute asthma. Arch Dis Child 1998; 79:405–410.

127. Ream RS, Loftis LL, Albers GM, Becker BA, Lynch RE, Mink RB. Efficacy of IV theophylline in children with severe status asthmaticus. Chest 2001; 119:1480–1488.

128. Kolski GB, Levy J, Anolik R. The use of theophylline clearance in pediatric status asthmaticus. I. Interpatient and intrapatient theophylline clearance variability. Am J Dis Child 1987; 141:282–287.

129. Levy J, Kolski GB. The use of theophylline clearance in pediatric status asthmati-cus. II. The choice of appropriate dose for the intravenous theophylline infusion. Am J Dis Child 1987; 141:288–291.

130. Kurland G, Anderson DA, Mitsuoka JC, Marquardt ED. Prediction of intravenous theophylline dosage based on a single, nonsteady-state concentration: a clinical study of childhood status asthmaticus. Pediatrics 1988; 82:880–883.

131. McEvoy GK. AHFS Drug Information 2000. Bethesda, MD: American Society of Health-System Pharmacists, 2000.

132. Saulnier FF, Durocher AV, Deturck RA, Lefebvre MC, Wattel FE. Respiratory and hemodynamic effects of halothane in status asthmaticus. Intensive Care Med 1990; 16:104–107.

133. Bierman MI, Brown M, Muren O, Keenan RL, Glauser FL. Prolonged isoflurane anesthesia in status asthmaticus. Crit Care Med 1986; 14:832–833.

134. Parnass SM, Feld JM, Chamberlin WH, Segil LJ. Status asthmaticus treated with isoflurane and enflurane. Anesth Analg 1987; 66:193–195.

135. Johnston RG, Noseworthy TW, Friesen EG, Yule HA, Shustack A. Isoflurane therapy for status asthmaticus in children and adults. Chest 1990; 97:698–701.

136. Otte RW, Fireman P. Isoflurane anesthesia for the treatment of refractory status asthmaticus. Ann Allergy 1991; 66:305–309.

137. Best A, Wenstone R, Murphy P. Prolonged use of isoflurane in asthma. Can J Anaesth 1994; 41:452–453.

138. Maltais F, Sovilj M, Goldberg P, Gottfried SB. Respiratory mechanics in status asthmaticus. Effects of inhalational anesthesia. Chest 1994; 106:1401–1406.

139. Miyagi T, Gushima Y, Matsumoto T, Okamoto K, Miike T. Prolonged isoflurane anesthesia in a case of catastrophic asthma. Acta Paediatr Jpn 1997; 39:375–378.
140. Rice M, Hatherill M, Murdoch IA. Rapid response to isoflurane in refractory status asthmaticus. Arch Dis Child 1998; 78:395–396.
141. Mori N, Nagata H, Ohta S, Suzuki M. Prolonged sevoflurane inhalation was not nephrotoxic in two patients with refractory status asthmaticus. Anesth Analg 1996; 83:189–191.
142. Que JC, Lusaya VO. Sevoflurane induction for emergency cesarean section in a parturient in status asthmaticus. Anesthesiology 1999; 90:1475–1476.
143. Mutlu GM, Factor P, Schwartz DE, Sznajder JI. Severe status asthmaticus: management with permissive hypercapnia and inhalation anesthesia. Crit Care Med 2002; 30:477–480.
144. Grunberg G, Cohen JD, Keslin J, Gassner S. Facilitation of mechanical ventilation in status asthmaticus with continuous intravenous thiopental. Chest 1991; 99:1216–1219.
145. Conti G, Ferretti A, Tellan G, Rocco M, Lappa A. Propofol induces bronchodilation in a patient mechanically ventilated for status asthmaticus. Intensive Care Med 1993; 19:305.
146. Parmar M, Sansome A. Propofol-induced bronchodilation in status asthmaticus? Anaesthesia 1995; 50:1003–1004.
147. Gerson JI. Intravenous fentanyl for the treatment of status asthmaticus. Crit Care Med 1989; 17:382–383.
148. Petrillo TM, Fortenberry JD, Linzer JF, Simon HK. Emergency department use of ketamine in pediatric status asthmaticus. J Asthma 2001; 38:657–664.
149. Rock MJ, Reyes de la Rocha S, L'Hommedieu CS, Truemper E. Use of ketamine in asthmatic children to treat respiratory failure refractory to conventional therapy. Crit Care Med 1986; 14:514–516.
150. Strube PJ, Hallam PL. Ketamine by continuous infusion in status asthmaticus. Anaesthesia 1986; 41:1017–1019.
151. L'Hommedieu CS, Arens JJ. The use of ketamine for the emergency intubation of patients with status asthmaticus. Ann Emerg Med 1987; 16:568–571.
152. Turnpenny PD, Nash SF. Ketamine in severe acute asthma. Arch Emerg Med 1991; 8:291–292.
153. Roy TM, Pruitt VL, Garner PA, Heine MF. The potential role of anesthesia in status asthmaticus. J Asthma 1992; 29:73–77.
154. Achar MN, Achar KN. Efficacy of ketamine infusion in refractory asthma complicated by acute myocardial infarction. Anaesth Intensive Care 1993; 21:115–117.
155. Hemming A, MacKenzie I, Finfer S. Response to ketamine in status asthmaticus resistant to maximal medical treatment. Thorax 1994; 49:90–91.
156. Nehama J, Pass R, Bechtler-Karsch A, Steinberg C, Notterman DA. Continuous ketamine infusion for the treatment of refractory asthma in a mechanically ventilated infant: case report and review of the pediatric literature. Pediatr Emerg Care 1996; 12:294–297.
157. de Lemos JM, Carr RR, Shalansky KF, Bevan DR, Ronco JJ. Paralysis in the critically ill: intermittent bolus pancuronium compared with continuous infusion. Crit Care Med 1999; 27:2648–2655.

158. Pakulski C, Swiniarski A, Jaszczyk G. High subarachnoid block for severe bronchospasm. Eur J Anaesthesiol 2000; 17:594–595.

159. Kotsev S, Morais RJ. High spinal block for bronchospasm. Eur J Anaesthesiol 2001; 18:486.

160. Shiue ST, Gluck EH. The use of helium-oxygen mixtures in the support of patients with status asthmaticus and respiratory acidosis. J Asthma 1989; 26:177–180.

161. Kudukis TM, Manthous CA, Schmidt GA, Hall JB, Wylam ME. Inhaled helium-oxygen revisited: effect of inhaled helium-oxygen during the treatment of status asthmaticus in children. J Pediatr 1997; 130:217–224.

162. Manthous CA, Hall JB, Caputo MA, Walter J, Klocksieben JM, Schmidt GA, Wood LD. Heliox improves pulsus paradoxus and peak expiratory flow in non-intubated patients with severe asthma. Am J Respir Crit Care Med 1995; 151:310–314.

163. Gluck EH, Onorato DJ, Castriotta R. Helium-oxygen mixtures in intubated patients with status asthmaticus and respiratory acidosis. Chest 1990; 98:693–698.

164. Schaeffer EM, Pohlman A, Morgan S, Hall JB. Oxygenation in status asthmaticus improves during ventilation with helium-oxygen. Crit Care Med 1999; 27:2666–2670.

165. George R, Berkenbosch JW, Fraser RF II, Tobias JD. Mechanical ventilation during pregnancy using a helium-oxygen mixture in a patient with respiratory failure due to status asthmaticus. J Perinatol 2001; 21:395–398.

166. Anderson M, Svartengren M, Bylin G, Philipson K, Camner P. Deposition in asthmatics of particles inhaled in air or in helium-oxygen. Am Rev Respir Dis 1993; 147:524–528.

167. Garner SS, Wiest DB, Bradley JW, Lesher BA, Habib DM. Albuterol delivery by metered-dose inhaler in a mechanically ventilated pediatric lung model. Crit Care Med 1996; 24:870–874.

168. Rodrigo GJ, Rodrigo C, Pollack CV, Rowe B. Use of helium-oxygen mixtures in the treatment of acute asthma: a systematic review. Chest 2003; 123:891–896.

169. Prezant DJ, Aldrich TK, Karpel JP, Park SS. Inspiratory flow dynamics during mechanical ventilation in patients with respiratory failure. Am Rev Respir Dis 1990; 142:1284–1287.

170. Menitove SM, Goldring RM. Combined ventilator and bicarbonate strategy in the management of status asthmaticus. Am J Med 1983; 74:898–901.

171. Darioli R, Perret C. Mechanical controlled hypoventilation in status asthmaticus. Am Rev Respir Dis 1984; 129:385–387.

172. Broux R, Foidart G, Mendes P, Saad G, Fatemi M, D'Orio V, Marcelle R. Use of PEEP in management of life-threatening status asthmaticus: a method for the recovery of appropriate ventilation-perfusion ratio. Appl Cardiopulm Pathophysiol 1991; 4:79–83.

173. Cox RG, Barker GA, Bohn DJ. Efficacy, results, and complications of mechanical ventilation in children with status asthmaticus. Pediatr Pulmonol 1991; 11:120–126.

174. Slutsky AS. Mechanical ventilation. American College of Chest Physicians' Consensus Conference. Chest 1993; 104:1833–1859.

175. Ventilation with lower tidal volumes as compared with traditional tidal volumes for acute lung injury and the acute respiratory distress syndrome. The Acute Respiratory Distress Syndrome Network. N Engl J Med 2000; 342:1301–1308.

176. Adnet F, Plaisance P, Borron SW, Levy A, Payen D. Prolonged severe hypercapnia complicating near fatal asthma in a 35-year-old woman. Intensive Care Med 1998; 24:1335–1338.

177. Meduri GU, Cook TR, Turner RE, Cohen M, Leeper KV. Noninvasive positive pressure ventilation in status asthmaticus. Chest 1996; 110:767–774.

178. Tokioka H, Saito S, Takahashi T, Kinjo M, Saeki S, Kosaka F, Hirakawa M. Effectiveness of pressure support ventilation for mechanical ventilatory support in patients with status asthmaticus. Acta Anaesthesiol Scand 1992; 36:5–9.

179. Wetzel RC. Pressure-support ventilation in children with severe asthma. Crit Care Med 1996; 24:1603–1605.

180. Mansmann HC Jr, Abboud EM, McGeady SJ. Treatment of severe respiratory failure during status asthmaticus in children and adolescents using high flow oxygen and sodium bicarbonate. Ann Allergy Asthma Immunol 1997; 78:69–73.

181. Fisher MM, Whaley AP, Pye RR. External chest compression in the management of acute severe asthma—a technique in search of evidence. Prehospital Disaster Med 2001; 16:124–127.

182. Browning D, Goodrum DT. Treatment of acute severe asthma assisted by hypothermia. Anaesthesia 1992; 47:223–225.

183. Jamadar DA, Kazerooni EA, Hirschl RB. Pneumomediastinum: elucidation of the anatomic pathway by liquid ventilation. J Comput Assist Tomogr 1996; 20:309–311.

184. Potter PC, Klein M, Weinberg EG. Hydration in severe acute asthma. Arch Dis Child 1991; 66:216–219.

185. Manthous CA, Goulding P. The effect of volume infusion on dead space in mechanically ventilated patients with severe asthma. Chest 1997; 112:843–846.

186. Shimura N, Arisaka O. Urinary arginine vasopressin in asthma: consideration of fluid therapy. Acta Paediatr Jpn 1990; 32:197–200.

187. Greally P. Human recombinant DNase for mucus plugging in status asthmaticus. Lancet 1995; 346:1423–1424.

188. Durward A, Forte V, Shemie SD. Resolution of mucus plugging and atelectasis after intratracheal rhDNase therapy in a mechanically ventilated child with refractory status asthmaticus. Crit Care Med 2000; 28:560–562.

189. Millman M, Goldstein IM, Millman F, Goodman AH, Van Campen S, Mercandetti AJ. Bronchial asthma, the tough case. Ann Allergy 1985; 54:77–80.

190. Munakata M, Abe S, Fujimoto S, Kawakami Y. Bronchoalveolar lavage during third-trimester pregnancy in patients with status asthmaticus: a case report. Respiration 1987; 51:252–255.

191. Henke CA, Hertz M, Gustafson P. Combined bronchoscopy and mucolytic therapy for patients with severe refractory status asthmaticus on mechanical ventilation: a case report and review of the literature. Crit Care Med 1994; 22:1880–1883.

192. Asher MI, Douglas C, Airy M, Andrews D, Trenholme A. Effects of chest physical therapy on lung function in children recovering from acute severe asthma. Pediatr Pulmonol 1990; 9:146–151.

193. Echeverria Zudaire L, Tomico Del Rio M, Bracamonte Bermejo T, Garcia Cuartero B. Status asthmaticus: is respiratory physiotherapy necessary? Allergol Immunopathol (Madr) 2000; 28:290–291.

194. Falliers CJ, Cato A. Controlled trial of bronchodilator-mucolytic aerosols, combined and separate. Ann Allergy 1978; 40:77–83.

195. Niederman MS, Gambino A, Lichter J, Weinblatt M, Fein AM. Tension ball valve mucus plug in asthma. Am J Med 1985; 79:131–134.

196. Camargo CA Jr, Smithline HA, Malice MP, Green SA, Reiss TF. A randomized controlled trial of intravenous montelukast in acute asthma. Am J Respir Crit Care Med 2003; 167:528–533.

197. Impens N, Reiss TF, Teahan JA, Desmet M, Rossing TH, Shingo S, Zhang J, Schandevyl W, Verbesselt R, Dupont AG. Acute bronchodilation with an intravenously administered leukotriene D4 antagonist, MK-679. Am Rev Respir Dis 1993; 147:1442–1446.

198. Rishani R, El-Khatib M, Mroueh S. Treatment of severe status asthmaticus with nitric oxide. Pediatr Pulmonol 1999; 28:451–453.

199. Nakagawa TA, Johnston SJ, Falkos SA, Gomez RJ, Morris A. Life-threatening status asthmaticus treated with inhaled nitric oxide. J Pediatr 2000; 137:119–122.

200. MacDonnell KF, Moon HS, Sekar TS, Ahluwalia MP. Extracorporeal membrane oxygenator support in a case of severe status asthmaticus. Ann Thorac Surg 1981; 31:171–175.

201. Lukomskii GI, Alekseeva ME, Vaisberg LA, Pavliutenkov MG, Sagalovich MA, Sevost'ianov DA, Karasev AB, Pisarevskii AA. [Extracorporeal elimination of CO_2 as a component of the intensive therapy of status asthmaticus]. Anesteziol Reanimatol 1990; 6–8.

202. Mabuchi N, Takasu H, Ito S, Yamada T, Arakawa M, Hatta M, Katsuya H. Successful extracorporeal lung assist (ECLA) for a patient with severe asthma and cardiac arrest. Clin Intensive Care 1991; 2:292–294.

203. Shapiro MB, Kleaveland AC, Bartlett RH. Extracorporeal life support for status asthmaticus. Chest 1993; 103:1651–1654.

204. Sakai M, Ohteki H, Doi K, Narita Y. Clinical use of extracorporeal lung assist for a patient in status asthmaticus. Ann Thorac Surg 1996; 62:885–887.

205. Yamaguchi T, Kohrogi H, Kawano O, Sakurai K, Kukita I, Sato T, Okamoto K, Terasaki H, Suga M, Ando M. [Endobronchial treatments made possible by extracorporeal lung assist in a patient in status asthmaticus refractory to mechanical ventilation]. Nihon Kyobu Shikkan Gakkai Zasshi 1996; 34: 241–246.

206. Kukita I, Okamoto K, Sato T, Shibata Y, Taki K, Kurose M, Terasaki H, Kohrogi H, Ando M. Emergency extracorporeal life support for patients with near-fatal status asthmaticus. Am J Emerg Med 1997; 15:566–569.

207. Suissa S, Hemmelgarn B, Blais L, Ernst P. Bronchodilators and acute cardiac death. Am J Respir Crit Care Med 1996; 154:1598–1602.

208. Mikhail MS, Hunsinger SY, Goodwin SR, Loughlin GM. Myocardial ischemia complicating therapy of status asthmaticus. Clin Pediatr (Phila) 1987; 26:419–421.

209. Salpeter SR, Ormiston TM, Salpeter EE. Cardiovascular effects of beta-agonists in patients with asthma and COPD: a meta-analysis. Chest 2004; 125:2309–2321.

210. Edmunds AT, Godfrey S. Cardiovascular response during severe acute asthma and its treatment in children. Thorax 1981; 36:534–540.

211. Bittar G, Friedman HS. The arrhythmogenicity of theophylline. A multivariate analysis of clinical determinants. Chest 1991; 99:1415–1420.

212. Rosero SZ, Zareba W, Moss AJ, Robinson JL, Hajj Ali RH, Locati EH, Benhorin J, Andrews ML. Asthma and the risk of cardiac events in the Long QT syndrome. Long QT Syndrome Investigative Group. Am J Cardiol 1999; 84:1406–1411.

213. Page R, Gay W, Friday G, Fireman P. Isoproterenol-associated myocardial dysfunction during status asthmaticus. Ann Allergy 1986; 57:402–404, 429–430.

214. Nino AF, Berman MM, Gluck EH, Conway MM, Fisher JP, Dougherty JE, Rossi MA. Drug-induced left ventricular failure in patients with pulmonary disease. Endomyocardial biopsy demonstration of catecholamine myocarditis. Chest 1987; 92:732–736.

215. Maguire JF, O'Rourke PP, Colan SD, Geha RS, Crone R. Cardiotoxicity during treatment of severe childhood asthma. Pediatrics 1991; 88:1180–1186.

216. Murphy FT, Manown TJ, Knutson SW, Eliasson AH. Epinephrine-induced lactic acidosis in the setting of status asthmaticus. South Med J 1995; 88:577–579.

217. Manthous CA. Lactic acidosis in status asthmaticus: three cases and review of the literature. Chest 2001; 119:1599–1602.

218. Yousef E, McGeady SJ. Lactic acidosis and status asthmaticus: how common in pediatrics? Ann Allergy Asthma Immunol 2002; 89:585–588.

219. Del Rio-Navarro B, Gazca-Aguilar A, Quibrera Matienzo JA, Rodriguez Galvan Y, Sienra-Monge JJ. Metabolic and electrocardiographic effects of albuterol in pediatric asthmatic patients treated in an emergency room setting. Allergol Immunopathol (Madr) 1999; 27:18–23.

220. Pauls JD, Simon RA, Daffern PJ, Stevenson DD. Lack of effect of the 5-lipoxygenase inhibitor zileuton in blocking oral aspirin challenges in aspirin-sensitive asthmatics. Annals of Allergy, Asthma, and Immunology 2000; 85:40–45.

221. Yoshida S, Sakamoto H, Ishizaki Y, Onuma K, Shoji T, Nakagawa H, Hasegawa H, Nakabayashi M, Amayasu H. Efficacy of leukotriene receptor antagonist in bronchial hyperresponsiveness and hypersensitivity to analgesic in aspirin-intolerant asthma. Clinical and Experimental Allergy 2000; 30:64–70.

222. Szczeklik A, Mastalerz L, Nizankowska E, Cmiel A. Protective and bronchodilator effects of prostaglandin E and salbutamol in aspirin-induced asthma. Am J Respir Crit Care Med 1996; 153:567–571.

223. Shennib HF, Barkun AN, Matouk E, Blundell PE. Surgical decompression of a tension pneumomediastinum. A ventilatory complication of status asthmaticus. Chest 1988; 93:1301–1302.

224. Lantsberg L, Rosenzweig V. Pneumomediastinum causing pneumoperitoneum. Chest 1992; 101:1176.

225. Gelber M, Sidi Y, Gassner S, Ovadia Y, Spitzer S, Weinberger A, Pinkhas J. Uncontrollable life-threatening status asthmaticus—an indicator for termination of pregnancy by cesarean section. Respiration 1984; 46:320–322.

226. Greenberger PA, Patterson R. The outcome of pregnancy complicated by severe asthma. Allergy Proc 1988; 9:539–543.

227. Gardner MO, Doyle NM. Asthma in pregnancy. Obstet Gynecol Clin North Am 2004; 31:385–413, vii.

228. Cydulka RK, Emerman CL, Schreiber D, Molander KH, Woodruff PG, Camargo CA Jr. Acute asthma among pregnant women presenting to the emergency department. Am J Respir Crit Care Med 1999; 160:887–892.

229. Longo LD, G.A. N. Fetal and newborn respiratory gas exchange. In: Crystal R, West JB, Barnes PJ, Weibel ER, eds. The Lung: Scientific Foundations. Vol. 2. New York: Raven, 1992:2141–2149.

230. Bernard SA, Jones BM. Endotracheal tube obstruction in a patient with status asthmaticus. Anaesth Intensive Care 1991; 19:121–123.

231. Boyd JH, Moinuddin A, Strunk RC, DeBaun MR. Asthma and acute chest in sickle-cell disease. Pediatr Pulmonol 2004; 38:229–232.

232. Biscardi S, Lorrot M, Marc E, Moulin F, Boutonnat-Faucher B, Heilbronner C, Iniguez JL, Chaussain M, Nicand E, Raymond J, et al. Mycoplasma pneumoniae and asthma in children. Clin Infect Dis 2004; 38:1341–1346.

233. Rodrigues RG. Steroids and antibiotics for treatment of acute asthma exacerbations in African-American children. J Natl Med Assoc 2004; 96:945–947.

234. Judson MA, Sperl PL. Status asthmaticus with acute decompensation with therapy in a 27-year-old woman. Chest 1995; 107:563–565.

235. Karalus NC, Mahood CB, Dunn PJ, Speed JF. Adrenal function in acute severe asthma. NZ Med J 1985; 98:843–846.

236. Busuttil A. Adrenal atrophy at autopsy in two asthmatic children. Am J Forensic Med Pathol 1991; 12:36–39.

237. Kaplan PW, Rocha W, Sanders DB, D'Souza B, Spock A. Acute steroid-induced tetraplegia following status asthmaticus. Pediatrics 1986; 78:121–123.

238. Lacomis D, Smith TW, Chad DA. Acute myopathy and neuropathy in status asthmaticus: case report and literature review. Muscle Nerve 1993; 16:84–90.

239. Griffin D, Fairman N, Coursin D, Rawsthorne L, Grossman JE. Acute myopathy during treatment of status asthmaticus with corticosteroids and steroidal muscle relaxants. Chest 1992; 102:510–514.

240. Waclawik AJ, Sufit RL, Beinlich BR, Schutta HS. Acute myopathy with selective degeneration of myosin filaments following status asthmaticus treated with methyl-prednisolone and vecuronium. Neuromuscul Disord 1992; 2:19–26.

241. Blackie JD, Gibson P, Murree-Allen K, Saul WP. Acute myopathy in status asthmaticus. Clin Exp Neurol 1993; 30:72–81.

242. Road J, Mackie G, Jiang TX, Stewart H, Eisen A. Reversible paralysis with status asthmaticus, steroids, and pancuronium: clinical electrophysiological correlates. Muscle Nerve 1997; 20:1587–1590.

243. Kupfer Y, Okrent DG, Twersky RA, Tessler S. Disuse atrophy in a ventilated patient with status asthmaticus receiving neuromuscular blockade. Crit Care Med 1987; 15:795–796.

244. Tanigaki T, Kondo T, Ohta Y, Yamabayashi H. Transient neuromuscular impairment resulting from prolonged inhalation of halothane and enflurane. Chest 1990; 98:1012–1013.

245. Danon MJ, Carpenter S. Myopathy with thick filament (myosin) loss following prolonged paralysis with vecuronium during steroid treatment. Muscle Nerve 1991; 14:1131–1139.

246. David WS, Roehr CL, Leatherman JW. EMG findings in acute myopathy with status asthmaticus, steroids and paralytics. Clinical and electrophysiologic correlation. Electromyogr Clin Neurophysiol 1998; 38:371–376.

247. Barrett SA, Mourani S, Villareal CA, Gonzales JM, Zimmerman JL. Rhabdomyolysis associated with status asthmaticus. Crit Care Med 1993; 21:151–153.

248. Bando T, Fujimura M, Noda Y, Ohta G, Matsuda T. Rhabdomyolysis following status asthmaticus. Respiration 1996; 63:309–311.

249. Goh AY, Chan PW. Acute myopathy after status asthmaticus: steroids, myo-relaxants or carbon dioxide? Respirology 1999; 4:97–99.

250. Li AM, Li CC, Chik KW, Shing MM, Fok TF. Rhabdomyolysis following status asthmaticus. J Paediatr Child Health 2001; 37:409–410.

251. Settipane GA, Hamolsky MW. Status asthmaticus associated with hyperthyroidism. N Engl Reg Allergy Proc 1987; 8:323–326.

252. Rodriguez-Roisin R, Torres A, Agusti AG, Ussetti P, Agusti-Vidal A. Subconjunctival haemorrhage: a feature of acute severe asthma. Postgrad Med J 1985; 61:579–581.

253. Nakagawa TA, Guerra L, Storgion SA. Aerosolized atropine as an unusual cause of anisocoria in a child with asthma. Pediatr Emerg Care 1993; 9:153–154.

254. Rodrigo C, Rodrigo G. Subarachnoid hemorrhage following permissive hypercapnia in a patient with severe acute asthma. Am J Emerg Med 1999; 17:697–699.

255. Edmunds SM, Harrison R. Subarachnoid hemorrhage in a child with status asthmaticus: significance of permissive hypercapnia. Pediatr Crit Care Med 2003; 4:100–103.

256. Park SJ, Sawyer SM, Glaun DE. Childhood asthma complicated by anxiety: an application of cognitive behavioural therapy. J Paediatr Child Health 1996; 32:183–187.

257. Gupta D, Keogh B, Chung KF, Ayres JG, Harrison DA, Goldfrad C, Brady AR, Rowan K. Characteristics and outcome for admissions to adult, general critical care units with acute severe asthma: a secondary analysis of the ICNARC Case Mix Programme Database. Crit Care 2004; 8:R112–R121.

258. Afessa B, Morales I, Cury JD. Clinical course and outcome of patients admitted to an ICU for status asthmaticus. Chest 2001; 120:1616–1621.

259. Mannino DM, Homa DM, Akinbami LJ, Moorman JE, Gwynn C, Redd SC. Surveillance for asthma—United States, 1980–1999. MMWR Surveill Summ 2002; 51:1–13.

260. Eason J, Markowe HL. Controlled investigation of deaths from asthma in hospitals in the North East Thames region. Br Med J (Clin Res Ed) 1987; 294:1255–1258.

261. Rothwell RP, Rea HH, Sears MR, et al. Lessons from the national asthma mortality study: deaths in hospital. NZ Med J 1987; 100:199–202.

262. Eason J, Markowe HL. Aminophylline toxicity—how many hospital asthma deaths does it cause? Respir Med 1989; 83:219–226.

263. Khadadah ME, Onadeko BO, Mustafa HT, Metwali KE. Clinical features and outcome of management of severe acute asthma (status asthmaticus) in the intensive care unit of a tertiary medical center. Singapore Med J 2000; 41: 214–217.

264. Gehlbach B, Kress JP, Kahn J, DeRuiter C, Pohlman A, Hall J. Correlates of prolonged hospitalization in inner-city ICU patients receiving noninvasive and invasive positive pressure ventilation for status asthmaticus. Chest 2002; 122:1709–1714.

265. Gupta A, Chaubal CC, Manoria PC, Jain SC, Misra NP. Patterns of recovery of pulmonary functions in severe acute bronchial asthma. Indian J Chest Dis Allied Sci 1989; 31:171–175.

266. Klaustermeyer WB, Kinney JL. Nomograms to follow recovery rate in status asthmaticus in a veteran population. Mil Med 1998; 163:177–179.

267. Jenkins PF, Benfield GF, Smith AP. Predicting recovery from acute severe asthma. Thorax 1981; 36:835–841.

268. Abulhosn RS, Morray BH, Llewellyn CE, Redding GJ. Passive smoke exposure impairs recovery after hospitalization for acute asthma. Arch Pediatr Adolesc Med 1997; 151:135–139.

269. Tan WC, Lim KP, Ng TP, Chao TC, Ong YY, Chee YC. Long-term outcome and disease control in near-fatal asthma. Ann Acad Med Singapore 1999; 28:384–388.

270. Shugg AW, Kerr S, Butt WW. Mechanical ventilation of paediatric patients with asthma: short and long term outcome. J Paediatr Child Health 1990; 26:343–346.

271. Guite HF, Dundas R, Burney PG. Risk factors for death from asthma, chronic obstructive pulmonary disease, and cardiovascular disease after a hospital admission for asthma. Thorax 1999; 54:301–307.

272. Suissa S, Ernst P, Benayoun S, Baltzan M, Cai B. Low-dose inhaled corticosteroids and the prevention of death from asthma. N Engl J Med 2000; 343:332–336.

273. Abramson MJ, Bailey MJ, Couper FJ, Driver JS, Drummer OH, Forbes AB, McNeil JJ, Haydn Walters E. Are asthma medications and management related to deaths from asthma? Am J Respir Crit Care Med 2001; 163:12–18.

274. Greenberger PA, Patterson R. The diagnosis of potentially fatal asthma. N Engl Reg Allergy Proc 1988; 9:147–152.

275. Bardana EJ Jr. Reactive airways dysfunction syndrome (RADS): guidelines for diagnosis and treatment and insight into likely prognosis. Ann Allergy Asthma Immunol 1999; 83:583–586.

276. Soto-Aguilar MC, deShazo RD, Waring NP. Anaphylaxis. Why it happens and what to do about it. Postgrad Med 1987; 82:154–160, 162–164, 167–170.

277. Aijaz F, Salam AU, Muzaffar S, Akbani Y, Hasan SH. Inflammatory pseudotumour of the trachea: report of a case in an eight-year-old child. J Laryngol Otol 1994; 108:613–616.

278. Weiner DJ, Weatherly RA, DiPietro MA, Sanders GM. Tracheal schwannoma presenting as status asthmaticus in a sixteen-year-old boy: airway considerations and removal with the CO_2 laser. Pediatr Pulmonol 1998; 25:393–397.

279. Irwin RS. A 55year-old man admitted to the medical ICU with the diagnosis of status asthmaticus responds poorly to intensive asthma therapy. Chest 2000; 117:892–893.

280. Marcus MG, Semel LJ. An unusual case of epiglottitis in a patient with asthma. Pediatr Emerg Care 1988; 4:124–126.

281. Murray DM, Lawler PG. All that wheezes is not asthma. Paradoxical vocal cord movement presenting as severe acute asthma requiring ventilatory support. Anaesthesia 1998; 53:1006–1011.

282. Hume L. A wheeze by any other name? Pediatr Nurs 2002; 28:390–391.

283. Chan YK, Zuraidah S, Tan PS. Use of capnography delaying the diagnosis of tracheal intubation. Anaesthesia 1998; 53:1207–1208.

284. Cox RG. Bronchospasm and confirmation of tracheal tube placement. Anaesthesia 1999; 54:498–499.

285. Noizet O, Leclerc F, Leteurtre S, Brichet A, Pouessel G, Dorkenoo A, Fourier C, Cremer R. Plastic bronchitis mimicking foreign body aspiration that needs a specific diagnostic procedure. Intensive Care Med 2003; 29:329–331.

286. Fletcher D, Mainardi JL, Brun-Buisson C, Lemaire F, Brochard L. Cardiac asthma presenting as status asthmaticus: deleterious effect of epinephrine therapy. Intensive Care Med 1990; 16:466–468.

287. Caksen H, Odabas D, Arslan S. A case of chronic renal failure misdiagnosed as status asthmaticus. J Emerg Med 2002; 22:103–104.

288. Liesching T, O'Brien A. Significance of a syncopal event. Pulmonary embolism. Postgrad Med 2002; 111:19–20.

289. Nesme P, Deniaud F, Perol M, Guerin JC. [Larva migrans syndrome: a rare differential asthma diagnosis.] Rev Pneumol Clin 1998; 54:225–227.

290. Singer JI. Herniation of abdominal contents simulating status asthmaticus. Pediatr Emerg Care 1987; 3:250–252.

291. Harrison P, Onorato DJ. Diaphragmatic flutter emulating recalcitrant asthma. South Med J 1997; 90:234–236.

292. Vlahakis NE, Patel AM, Maragos NE, Beck KC. Diagnosis of vocal cord dysfunction: the utility of spirometry and plethysmography. Chest 2002; 122:2246–2249.

293. Newman KB, Mason UG III, Schmaling KB. Clinical features of vocal cord dysfunction. Am J Respir Crit Care Med 1995; 152:1382–1386.

294. Morris MJ, Deal LE, Bean DR, Grbach VX, Morgan JA. Vocal cord dysfunction in patients with exertional dyspnea. Chest 1999; 116:1676–1682.

295. Powell DM, Karanfilov BI, Beechler KB, Treole K, Trudeau MD, Forrest LA. Paradoxical vocal cord dysfunction in juveniles. Arch Otolaryngol Head Neck Surg 2000; 126:29–34.

296. Rundell KW, Spiering BA. Inspiratory stridor in elite athletes. Chest 2003; 123:468–474.

297. Tisch SH, Brake HM, Law M, Cole IE, Darveniza P. Spasmodic dysphonia: clinical features and effects of botulinum toxin therapy in 169 patients—an Australian experience. J Clin Neurosci 2003; 10:434–438.

298. Maschka DA, Bauman NM, McCray PB Jr, Hoffman HT, Karnell MP, Smith RJ. A classification scheme for paradoxical vocal cord motion. Laryngoscope 1997; 107:1429–1435.

299. Sullivan MD, Heywood BM, Beukelman DR. A treatment for vocal cord dysfunction in female athletes: an outcome study. Laryngoscope 2001; 111:1751–1755.

300. Earles J, Kerr B, Kellar M. Psychophysiologic treatment of vocal cord dysfunction. Ann Allergy Asthma Immunol 2003; 90:669–671.

3

Management of Patients with Chronic Obstructive Pulmonary Disease in the Critical Care Unit

GUY W. SOO HOO

Pulmonary and Critical Care Section, West Los Angeles Healthcare Center
VA Greater Los Angeles Healthcare System and Geffen School
  of Medicine at UCLA
Los Angeles, California, U.S.A.

I. Introduction

The burden of chronic obstructive pulmonary disease (COPD) on the health care system is enormous. COPD is currently the fourth leading cause of death in the United States. It is predicted to be the fifth (currently 12th) leading cause of DALY (Disability adjusted life year = the sum of years lost because of premature morbidity and mortality, and years of life lived with disability adjusted for the severity of disability) in the world by 2020 (1). Since 1979, deaths attributed to COPD have increased 118%, and *this is the only condition in which the death rate has continued to rise* (2,3). Over 16 million patients are afflicted with COPD in the United States, with annual health care utilization including 17 million office visits, 700,000 hospitalizations, and direct costs of care estimated to exceed $14 billion annually (indirect costs exceed $10 billion) (4). When compared with other conditions, COPD accounts for 5% of all office visits to physicians and over 13% of all hospitalizations (5,6).

II. Definitions: COPD Exacerbation

Hospitalization of these patients is usually due to worsening of their respiratory status, often referred to as a COPD exacerbation. However, there are many causes of respiratory deterioration in patients with COPD, including heart failure, pneumonia, pneumothorax, or pulmonary embolism. These distinct conditions are considered and treated differently from a COPD exacerbation. Exacerbations of COPD have been and continue to be defined on clinical grounds. A frequently utilized definition included the presence of increased dyspnea, sputum purulence, and sputum production, with a type I exacerbation defined by the presence of all three criteria, type II by two of the three, and type III by one plus another from a list of other symptoms (recent upper respiratory tract infection, fever, wheezing, cough, or 20% increase from baseline in respiratory rate or heart rate) (7). However, these criteria were used in the context of an evaluation of antibiotic therapy, and infection is only one process that may lead to a COPD exacerbation.

There have been continued efforts to refine the criteria used to define an exacerbation. Part of the difficulty lies in the recognition that the clinical entity is difficult to define since its pathogenesis is poorly understood (8). Attempts to improve the definition have led to modifications that acknowledge the inherent variability in the condition, using the need for changes in treatment as an objective indicator of a change in status. The importance of a consensus definition is obvious since it would allow a framework to accurately determine the prevalence of the condition, improve the accuracy of diagnosis and therapy, and to assess the response to therapy (9). The most recent synthesis defines an exacerbation as "a sustained worsening of the patient's symptoms from his or her usual stable state that is beyond normal day-to-day variations and is acute in onset. Commonly reported symptoms are worsening breathlessness, cough, increased sputum production, and change in sputum color. The change in these symptoms often necessitates a change in medication" (10). This is also the definition used in the American Thoracic Society/European Respiratory Society position paper on the diagnosis and treatment of patients with COPD (11).

It is also recognized that there may be significant overlap in patients with asthma as opposed to COPD (12). It is generally not difficult to diagnose the condition in prototypical patients, with asthma generally affecting younger patients, causing intermittent airflow obstruction manifested by marked bronchial hyper-reactivtiy and active inflammatory component. Patients with COPD are generally older smokers, with progressive airflow obstruction and less intense bronchial hyper-reactivity or inflammation. However, patients may manifest components of both conditions. Some of this confusion is manifest in the similarities in approach and management of these patients. Similar classes of medications are used, despite differences in pathophysiology of these conditions (13).

III. Causes: COPD Exacerbation

The most frequently recognized causes of a COPD exacerbation include tracheo-bronchitis (bacterial and/or viral) and the noxious components of air pollution, but about a third of cases have no identified cause (14,15). It is important to recognize that as many as half of the exacerbations are not reported and therefore do not come to medical attention (16). Unlike asthma, measures of peak expiratory flow and spirometry (FEV_1) may be insensitive in identifying these episodes, or with median changes of $<5\%$ in magnitude (17).

Bacterial infections or acute bronchitis have long been recognized as a cause of a COPD exacerbation. The benefit of antimicrobial therapy in its management provides support for this premise (7). However, bacteria can be isolated from sputum during periods of clinical stability, and bacterial isolates represent colonization of the airway in a quarter or more of patients (18,19). The most frequent isolates include *Hemophilus influenzae*, *Streptococcus pneumoniae*, and *Moraxella catarrhalis*, but Pseudomonas has also been isolated. These are the same organisms isolated during clinical exacerbations, highlighting the need for clinical correlation with any bacterial isolate. In patients with greater severity of illness or those requiring mechanical ventilation, a greater proportion of enteric gram negative bacilli, such as *Pseudomonas*, *Stenotrophomonas*, or *Enterobacter* have been noted (20–22). Mycoplasma, Legionella and Chlamydia are atypical pathogens that have also been implicated in COPD exacerbations, but of uncertain overall significance given the difficulties in their routine diagnosis (23,24). Knowledge of the most likely infectious causes of an exacerbation is important, as it provides the basis for empiric antibiotic therapy. In one series, half of the COPD exacerbations were associated with a bacterial infection (25).

The role of viral infections in COPD exacerbations has been under increased study. They are underdiagnosed since viral cultures are not routinely obtained in these patients. A viral respiratory infection may produce many of the same clinical features seen with a COPD exacerbation, including bronchoconstriction, mucus hypersecretion, and epithelial injury leading to dyspnea and change in sputum quality (26,27). Viral infections may also predispose to secondary bacterial infection (28). Viruses were detected in almost 40% of COPD exacerbations in one cohort study (29). Viruses were more frequently isolated from COPD patients during an exacerbation than periods of clinical stability (30). Patients with viruses isolated had higher levels of inflammatory markers and a longer duration of exacerbation. The most frequently isolated viruses include rhinovirus, respiratory syncytial virus, picornavirus, coronavirus, and influenzae virus (29,31–33).

The noxious gases (ozone, sulfur dioxide, nitrogen dioxide), diesel, and small particulates (PM_{10}) that comprise air pollution have also been linked to COPD exacerbations. These materials can worsen lung function in normal subjects causing bronchospasm and inflammation under experimental and natural conditions, and the effect on those with compromised respiratory status may be more severe (34). Worsening air quality has been linked to increased emergency room visits, hospitalization, and death in those with underlying chronic lung disease (35–37).

IV. Pathophysiologic Mechanisms

Irrespective of the inciting factor, patients develop symptoms that include all of the cardinal features of a COPD exacerbation. They become dyspneic, often with increased sputum production and a change in sputum color. The pathophysiologic changes that contribute to these symptoms have undergone increased scrutiny over the past few years, resulting in a better understanding of the mechanisms of disease. However, much remains to be elucidated.

Inflammation is a key component in patients with COPD, with increased indices of inflammation noted during both periods of stability and during exacerbations, and with the severity of inflammation correlating with the severity of lung function (38–40). This inflammatory response increases during a COPD exacerbation and most noticeably during exacerbations associated with bacterial infection (41,42). Neutrophils are the predominant cell isolated from respiratory secretions, but there is also a proportionately greater increase in eosinophils (38,43,44). This occurs in the setting of chronic airway inflammation and increased lymphocytes ($CD4^+$ and $CD8^+$) (45). Associated with the increase in cells is an increase in inflammatory markers or mediators (neutrophil elastase, myeloperoxidase, leukotriene B_4, endothelin-1), inflammatory cytokines (IL-6, IL-8, TNF_α), fibrinogen, and albumin leakage noted in sputum analysis (29,41,46–49). These markers of inflammation markedly decrease with treatment and eradication of bacteria, providing further support for the role of bacteria in exacerbations. Similar findings have been noted with viral infections, although the observed changes in inflammatory markers have been limited to fibrinogen and IL-6. Another indicator of inflammation, sputum color (green) and purulence, has also been found to correlate with neutrophils and increase in inflammatory mediators (50,51).

This increased inflammatory response results in airflow limitation by bronchospasm; increased airway mucus and the increased cellular components may also limit airway caliber. Narrowing of the airways creates ventilation-perfusion (V/Q) inequalities, hypoxemia, and hypercapnia (52). This increases the load to the ventilatory system, and one of the compensatory responses is tachypnea. These patients are often already hyperinflated, and tachypnea only worsens their hyperinflation. Patients breathe on the less compliant portion of the pressure–volume curve, further increasing the work of breathing and decreasing muscle efficiency. Decreased exhalation time creates more air trapping, leading to higher end-expiratory lung volumes. This results in worsening of existing dynamic hyperinflation and intrinsic positive end expiratory pressure ($PEEP_i$). This eventually leads to an unsustainable breathing pattern, ventilatory muscle fatigue, and eventual ventilatory failure (53). Although there is a wide spectrum in the severity of illness, this is the type of patient with COPD often encountered in the critical care unit.

V. Clinical Course

In addition to the above changes that occur during a COPD exacerbation, other features in more severe episodes may presage respiratory failure. These include pursed lips breathing pattern, use of the accessory muscles of respiration (including the use of abdominal muscles and active expiration), paradoxical abdominal movement, pulsus paradox, lethargy, confusion, cyanosis, and worsening peripheral edema. As clinical signs, a single finding may not be cause for alarm, but multiple findings in a patient who also meets the definition of a COPD exacerbation should be of concern. Although some patients can be treated at home as outpatients (54), the risk of respiratory failure should always be a consideration. Clinical features may help identify patients best treated in a hospitalized setting. These features are summarized in Table 1.

A review of the clinical course of patients hospitalized with a severe COPD exacerbation and respiratory failure provides a better perspective in the management of these patients. It should be noted that there is a wide range of reported morbidity and mortality of these patients, partly related to study design, cohort, and period effect. There also appears to have been a decline over the past decade or so in morbidity and mortality rate, although this has not been uniformly noted. Early experience noted mortality to be about 28% in hospitalized patients, but mortality was over 40% in those requiring mechanical ventilation and as high as 80% in some series (55). More recent reports suggest that the mortality rate is in the 10–20% range with severe exacerbations (56–60), with a higher mortality rate in the 20–30+% range for those requiring intubation and mechanical ventilation (61). Chronic ventilator dependence was reported as 24% in one series, but another reported <5% requiring long term ventilation (59,62). The mortality in the ensuing year after an episode of respiratory failure can be quite high and has been reported in the 35–50% range after one year (63,64). As a frame of reference, COPD patients primarily treated in a ward setting, and therefore with a lower severity of illness, had an intubation rate of <10% and a mortality rate of only 4% in one study (65) and even lower (2.5%) in another cross sectional analysis (61).

Table 1   Indications for Hospitalization in COPD Exacerbations

---

High risk comorbid condition (pneumonia, cardiac arrhythmia, congestive heart failure, diabetes mellitus, renal or hepatic failure)
Inadequate response of symptoms to outpatient management
Marked increase in dyspnea
Inability to eat or sleep due to symptoms
Worsening hypoxemia
Worsening hypercapnia
Changes in mental status
Inability of patient to care for (lack of home support)
Uncertainty in diagnosis
Inadequate home care

Source: From Ref. 11.

A more detailed examination of the two largest databases provides further insight. Using a large database of patients used as the index population for APACHE III, the course of 362 admissions with COPD exacerbations was reviewed (66). The hospital mortality rate was 24%, but it was higher in patients >65 years of age, who experienced a 30% hospital mortality rate with a one year mortality rate of 59%. After controlling for the severity of illness, mechanical ventilation on admission was not an independent risk factor for survival, a finding also noted by others (63). However, intubation and mechanical ventilation was associated with higher ICU mortality (15.9% vs. 3.6%), ICU length of stay (11.1 ± 19.9 days vs. 4 ± 5.4 days), and hospital mortality (31.8% vs. 16.7%). The overall intubation rate was 47%. Survival curves were lower for those analyzed based on their initial P_aCO_2, with a one year mortality of 70% for those ≥50 mmHg compared to 54% in those <50 mmHg. In a five-hospital survey of 1016 patients with a COPD exacerbation and P_aCO_2 >50 mmHg (median $P_aCO_2 = 56$ mmHg) involved in the Study to Understand Prognosis and Preferences of Outcomes and Risks of Treatment (SUPPORT), the hospital mortality rate was 11% (67). However, it was 43% at one year and 49% at two years. The intubation rate was 34% and this as well as ICU admission were associated with an increased mortality rate at six months (43% and 37% respectively). Half of the patients were readmitted within six months. In their analysis, risk factors for death include the severity of the acute illness (severity of illness score, P_aO_2/F_IO_2), health status (advanced age, poor functional status), comorbid illness (congestive heart failure, cor pulmonale), and nutritional status (body mass index, serum albumin).

It has long been recognized that worsening acidosis is associated with increased risk of ventilatory failure, intubation, and mortality. Depending on the investigation, a threshold for requiring intubation lies somewhere between a pH < 7.23 and <7.26 (60,68–71). The risk is best demonstrated with declining pH, not changes in P_aO_2 or P_aCO_2, although these parameters are closely linked with pH. In a one-year survey of 983 COPD patients, acidosis was noted in 20% of those who did not require immediate intubation, and was the only factor associated with the need for ICU care (pH < 7.25) and intubation (pH < 7.30) (71). In our analysis of 138 episodes of hypercapnic respiratory failure (defined as a pH ≤ 7.35 and P_aCO_2 ≥50 mmHg), an initial pH < 7.25 was associated with a >50% intubation rate (72). A gradual increase in the intubation rate was noted with worsening pH and this is illustrated in Figure 1. It should be noted that this analysis excluded patients who were treated with noninvasive mechanical ventilation, as do most of the other analyses of this risk factor. However, the availability of noninvasive ventilatory support does not change the implications of progressive acidosis in these patients, but merely provides another option in their management. Management with noninvasive ventilation will be discussed in subsequent sections.

Other factors have been identified that increase the risk for ventilatory failure and poor outcome. As might be expected, these included a greater

INTUBATION RATE BY INITIAL
LEVEL OF ACIDOSIS

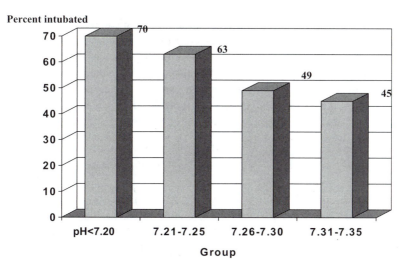

Figure 1 Percentage of COPD patients with hypercapnic respiratory acidosis requiring intubation based on initial pH range. *Source*: From Ref. 72.

severity of illness (APACHE II score) and measures of lower functional status, lower nutritional status, and poor lung function (spirometry) (73,74). However, these measures may not be easily accessible, and the arterial blood gas, with its pH determination, remains the easiest and most reliable measure in this regard.

In summary, patients hospitalized with an exacerbation of COPD are at increased risk for progression to frank respiratory failure, chronic ventilator dependence, and death. However, the need for mechanical ventilation is not an independent predictor of mortality. Features that predict the need for ventilatory support can help guide the focus and intensity of therapy. Progressive acidosis is the greatest risk factor and best predictor of respiratory failure.

VI. Treatment

Treatment of these patients should focus on the physiologic derangements and processes that contribute to their symptoms, with a primary goal of relief of symptoms and averting respiratory failure. As previous described, increased airways resistance, whether due to bronchospasm, infection or inflammation, is a key component of their dyspnea. This leads to changes in ventilatory pattern with increasing frequency and minute ventilation, development of dynamic hyperinflation, intrinsic PEEP, and increased work of breathing. There is also worsening of gas exchange, resulting in hypoxemia and/or hypercapnia that can progress to respiratory failure. Concerns about respiratory failure often drive the intensity of therapy. The severity of symptoms will dictate the optimal site for treatment. Table 2 outlines recommendations for management of these patients based on the severity and ideal location for treatment. Not surprisingly, patients with the greatest severity of illness are better managed in a critical care unit. The remainder of this chapter focuses on the hospitalized patient and specifically the patient requiring management in a critical care unit. The approach to management is often all-encompassing, since it may be difficult to identify a single

Table 2   Clinical History, Physical Findings, and Recommended Diagnostic Procedure in Patients with COPD Exacerbations Based on Location of Management

	Level I Home care	Level II Requires hospitalization	Level III ICU setting (or equivalent)
Clinical history			
Comorbid conditions[a]	+	+++	+++
History of frequent exacerbations	+	+++	+++
Severity of COPD	Mild/ moderate	Moderate/ severe	Severe
Physical findings			
Hemodynamic evaluation	Stable	Stable	Stable/unstable
Use of accessory muscles, tachypnea	Not present	++	+++
Persistent symptoms after initial therapy	No	++	+++
Diagnostic procedures			
Oxygen saturation	Yes	Yes	Yes
Arterial blood gases	No	Yes	Yes
Chest roentgenogram	No	Yes	Yes
Blood tests[b]	No	Yes	Yes
Serum drug concentrations[c]	If applicable	If applicable	If applicable
Sputum gram stain and culture	No[d]	Yes	Yes
Electrocardiogram	No	Yes	Yes

Key to symbols:
+Unlikely to be present.
++Likely to be present.
+++Very likely to be present.
[a]Comorbid conditions associate with poor prognosis in exacerbations: congestive heart failure, coronary artery disease, diabetes mellitus, renal and liver failure.
[b]Blood tests include: complete blood count, serum electrolytes, renal and liver function tests.
[c]Consider if the patient is using theophylline, warfarin, carbamazepine, digoxin.
[d]Consider if the patient has recently been on antibiotics.
Source: From Ref. 11.

area to target therapy. The individual components of comprehensive management are reviewed in detail.

VII. Bronchodilators

Although it is acknowledged that the airways obstruction in most patients with COPD is fixed, there is probably an element of reversibility. Inhaled broncho-dilators directed at relieving the bronchoconstriction associated with COPD exacerbations are a mainstay of therapy and are part of every consensus recommendation (1,8,10,11,75). Inhaled bronchodilators are superior to administration of bronchodilators via other routes and are associated with less systemic effects (76–78). Inhalation is the preferred method of drug delivery. In addition to decreasing airways resistance, bronchodilation also allows more complete exhalation, reducing air trapping and thereby the development and magnitude of dynamic hyperinflation (79). This benefit may occur without any demonstrable change in other spirometric measures such as FEV_1. Patients usually have ready access to bronchodilators as part of their maintenance therapy, and often increase use of these agents during periods of exacerbation. Increased bronchodilator use is often used as a proxy to signify worsening respiratory status, with decreased use representing control of symptoms.

Inhaled bronchodilators fall in two main classes of agents, sympathomimetics (β_2-agonists) and anticholinergic agents. Methylxanthines also have bronchodilating effects, but will be discussed separately. The bronchodilating effects of β_2-agonists are mediated by their action on bronchial smooth muscle, causing smooth muscle relaxation and reversing bronchoconstriction. Early formulations included nonspecific β-agents (epinephrine, isoproterenol), supplanted by more specific β_2-agents (isoethraine, metoproterenol), with subsequent formulations having longer duration of action (albuterol, terbutaline, pirbuterol, bitolterol). While many of these forumulations still exist, the predominant agent in use is albuterol (or salbutamol). The anticholinergics act by blocking muscarinic receptors, decreasing existing cholinergic mediated bronchomotor tone as well as cholinergic mediated bronchoconstriction. Of the three muscarinic receptors, the M_3 receptor is primarily responsible for mediating bronchoconstriction and mucus secretion. Ipratropium bromide is the predominant anticholinergic agent but is nonspecific in action, acting on all three muscarinic receptors. Tiotropium is a long-acting anticholinergic agent with greater affinity for the M_3 receptor and greater potency when compared to ipratropium. Table 3 provides a summary of the most frequently used bronchodilators.

These two different mechanisms and different sites of action allow a basis for the simultaneous use of both agents as well as the potential for additive effects when used in combination. However, there is not conclusive evidence favoring the benefit of combined therapy in an acute exacerbation. First of all, both β_2-agonists and anticholinergics have comparable bronchodilatory effects, with

Table 3 Commonly Used Bronchodilators in the Management of Patients with COPD Exacerbations

Bronchodilators	MDI dose (per puff) (recommended dose)	Nebulized dose (concentrations)	Frequency of administration	Comments
β_2-agonists				
Albuterol	90 μgm (2 puffs)	2.5–5.0 mg (0.5 mg/mL and 0.83 mg/mL concentrations)	Every 4–6 hr	Continuous nebulization either 15 mg over two hours or 10 mg over one hour
Albuterol HFA	90 μgm (2 puffs)		Every 4–6 hr	Non-CFC propellant
Levalbuterol		0.63–1.25 mg (0.31 mg/3 mL or 0.63 mg/3 mL or 1.25 mg/3 mL)	Every 6–8 hr	Supplied as unit doses Possibly less cardiac toxicity than albuterol
Pirbuterol	200 μgm (1–2 puffs)		Every 4–6 hr	Not evaluated in severe exacerbations
Dry powder inhalers				
Formoterol	12 μgm (1 capsule)		Every 12 hr	NOT recommended for acute relief of symptoms
Salmeterol	50 μgm (1 blister)		Every 12 hr	NOT recommended for acute relief of symptoms
Anticholinergics				
Ipratropium bromide (MDI)	18 μgm (2–4 puffs)	0.5–1.0 mg (0.25 mg/mL)	Every 4–6 hr	Often nebulized with albuterol
Tiotropium (DPI)	18 μgm (1 capsule)		Every 24 hr	NOT recommended for acute relief of symptoms

Notes: (1) Added benefit of long acting agents (salmeterol, formoterol, tiotropium) in acute exacerbations not established.
(2) Higher doses limited by systemic toxicity (cardiac tachyarrhythmias, tremors, palpitations, hypokalemia, insomnia).
(3) Paradoxical bronchospam rare, but reported, and may be related to medication preservatives.
Abbreviations: MDI: metered dose inhaler; HFA: hydrofluoroalkane; CFC: chlorofluorocarbon; DPI: dry powder inhaler.

neither demonstrated to be superior to the other in comparison, cross-over studies (80). In stable patients, when maximum bronchodilation has been achieved with one agent, the other has not been demonstrated to provide further bronchodila-tiion (81). There are several clinical studies that have failed to demonstrate an incremental benefit in a variety of outcome parameters, including spirometry, symptoms, and hospitalization with the addition of a second bronchodilator (usually an anticholinergic) to full doses of β_2-agonists (82–86). Others have demonstrated a proportionately greater improvement in FEV_1 or shorter duration of emergency room treatment with combination therapy (87,88), but the magnitude of differences is modest. This experience in patients with acute exacerbations contrasts with findings using combination therapy in patients with stable disease. Several studies have demonstrated that the combination of both a β_2-agonist and an anticholinergic results in greater bronchodilation as compared to either alone (89–91).

Despite the lack of definitive evidence, the two agents are often administered in combination during acute exacerbations. Recommendations to add a second agent if the first is ineffective are tempered by the realization that the overall benefit in this group of patients may be modest and slow to occur, making a trial of a single agent difficult to interpret (92). In patients who may have worsening bronchocontriction due to beta-blockers, the β_2-agonists are less effective than anticholinergic bronchodilators in management. Of course, if patients develop adverse effects to one class of agents, comparable benefit can be achieved with the alternate class as sole therapy.

The adverse effects of these medications are reflective of their mechanism of action. Although with greater stimulation of β_2-receptors, sympathomimetic agents also affect β_1-receptors. This may cause tachycardia, rapid atrial tachyarrhythmias, ventricular ectopy, and palpitations. In a meta-analysis of placebo controlled trials, a single dose of an inhaled β_2 agonist increased the heart rate by 9.1 beats/min (95% CI 5.3–12.9). (93). These agents also cause pulmonary vascular dilatation, which may worsen ventilation/perfusion relationships and cause transient hypoxemia (94). Other adverse effects include hypokalemia, tremor, and headache. Although these agents are important in relieving airway obstruction and dyspnea, there is potential for some cardiac toxicity, especially in those with underlying cardiac disease.

The anticholinergics agents (ipratropium, tiotropium) have much fewer adverse effects, primarily due to their minimal systemic absorption. Their effects are primarily limited to local symptoms (dry mouth, blurred vision) and rarely urinary retention. They are not associated with hypoxemia or tachycardia, but tachycardia can occur with the use of nebulized atropine. However, with the advent of ipratropium, atropine is now rarely, if ever, used as a bronchodilator. It should be noted that a rare patient will experience a paradoxical reaction, with wheezing and bronchoconstriction, to bronchodilator therapy. This may be due to the additives in bronchodilator solutions used to prevent bacterial growth (benzalkonium chloride) (95). Multiuse dropper bottles of albuterol and some unit dose vials are the most likely to contain these additives. The effect may become more evident with cumulative doses of medication. Sulfites were present in some older formulations (isoproterenol and isoethraine) that are no longer used.

In addition to combination therapy, bronchodilators are often administered in high doses during acute exacerbations. This likely reflects an extension of the experience in asthma, in which greater bronchodilatory benefit is seen with higher doses of albuterol delivered by continuous nebulization (96). There is not a consistent benefit of continuous nebulization compared to frequent intermittent doses (97–99). Greater bronchodilation has been noted in stable COPD patients with higher doses of albuterol and ipratropium bromide (100,101). In patients with acute exacerbations, greater bronchodilation was noted with frequent, high-dose inhaled albuterol (15 mg over two hours), but this was also associated with a greater incidence of adverse effects (tremor, palpitations) (102). No other clinical benefit was noted. As might be expected, once maximally bronchodilated, higher doses of bronchodilators are not likely to provide much additional benefit, but do increase the risk of adverse events. However, determination of maximal bronchodilation may be difficult, especially in the setting of uncertain drug delivery; therefore, frequent and high dose bronchodilators are often administered in lieu of reliable clinical markers of bronchodilatation.

In addition to the frequently used combination of albuterol and ipratropium, there are some other choices of bronchodilators that deserve comment. Albuterol represents a racemic mixture of two optical isomers, referred to as R and S enantiomers, of which bronchodilation occurs only with the R-enantiomer. The S-enantiomer may have adverse inflammatory effects, which in theory may antagonize the bronchodilatory effects of the R-enantiomer. This is the basis for a formulation of albuterol comprised only of the R-enantiomer, levalbuterol. The potential advantage to this formulation is greater potency at a lower dose, longer duration of action, and fewer systemic adverse effects (103). Levalbuterol is certainly comparable to racemic albuterol in terms of bronchodilation, but investigations to demonstrate additional benefits, including less systemic effects, have been inconclusive (104–106). It is more expensive on the order of 2.5–5 times the cost of albuterol.

Long acting β_2 agonists have become a mainstay in the management of stable COPD. Their role in acute exacerbations is unknown, but there is potential for added benefit due to their longer duration of action. They do provide bronchodilation comparable to the short acting agents in mild acute exacerbations, but it is unknown if there is additional benefit to that achieved with short acting β_2-agonist (107,108). The current formulations of salmeterol and formoterol are delivered using dry powder inhalers, which may provide more effective drug delivery than metered dose inhalers or nebulizers.

Effective bronchodilator therapy is dependent upon efficient delivery of medications to the airways. In the acute setting, the major modes of delivery have been with a metered dose inhaler, with or without a spacer, or with a wet nebulizer using either compressed air or oxygen. The major limitations of the metered dose inhaler are its requirements for patient coordination, slow, deep inhalation, and breath hold. This may be difficult in the patient with acute dyspnea. Spacer devices or holding chambers ameliorate the need for precise coordination and thereby allow more efficient drug delivery. Drug delivery with nebulizers is less dependent on patient coordination and may be more effective in patients with increased dyspnea. However, they require more personnel time and equipment, and are therefore more costly (109). Comparisons between the metered dose inhalers with spacers and nebulizers during exacerbations of COPD have only demonstrated very small differences, if present, in favor of nebulizer therapy (110,111). This was also the conclusion of a meta-analysis involving 507 patients, 89 with COPD (112), which found a small treatment difference favoring wet nebulizer delivery. However, this finding was not felt to be clinically or therapeutically significant. It was also noted that the doses in patients treated with metered dose inhalers were on the low side, and this may have been a more important determinant of the treatment difference as opposed to the mode of drug delivery. As it appears that the two methods are equivalent in efficiency of drug delivery, other considerations will dictate the modality utilized, including patient coordination and costs.

VIII. Antibiotics

As noted earlier, bacterial infections are a common cause of COPD exacerbations. However, it may be difficult to determine whether the exacerbation is due to a bacterial infection and whether organisms isolated from sputum represent a true pathogen or colonization. Isolation of bacteria from sputum occurs in 40–60% of all COPD exacerbations (113), and occurs both during periods of clinical stability as well as exacerbation. Bacteria may lead to exacerbations as a primary infection of the lower respiratory tract, as a secondary infection after a viral infection, or by contributing antigens that lead to bronchial hyperactivity and inflammation. Evidence that supports the role of bacteria include demonstration of higher bacterial load based on protected specimen brush cultures in patients with clinical exacerbations as opposed to stable patients (19). In a study of 40 patients, the percentage of stable patients exceeding thresholds of 10^3 CFU/mL and 10^4 CFU/mL were 25% and 5%, as opposed to those with exacerbations where this was noted in 52% and 24%, respectively. Molecular typing of sputum isolates during a longitudinal study identified new serotypes that were also associated with clinical COPD exacerbations (114). These involved serotypes of frequently isolated organisms, *H. influenzae*, *M. catarrhalis*, and *S. pneumoniae*, and this serotype change was noted in 33% of the exacerbations investigated. During clinical exacerbations, isolation of pathogenic organisms is also associated with increases in sputum inflammatory markers (IL-8, TNF-α, neutrophil elastase) (115). Purulent sputum color (green) is associated with a high percentage of bacteria isolation (84%), clearing of sputum color, and other markers of inflammation, including eradiation of bacteria with antibiotic therapy (50,116). There is also serologic evidence for infection (conversion) during exacerbations of COPD (117).

While this data provides support for the role of bacterial infection in COPD exacerbations, there exists considerable controversy on the role of antibiotics in the management of these patients (118,119). It would follow that if bacterial infections contributed to the symptoms and pathology associated with a COPD exacerbation, treatment of the infection should not only alleviate symptoms, but also provide evidence of improvement in key outcomes measures. In one of the largest outpatient trials, success defined by symptom resolution with antibiotics was modest (68% vs. 55%), but the percentage of patients with deterioration was halved (15% vs. 34%) (7). The duration of an exacerbation was reduced on average 2.2 days, and there was also more rapid improvement in peak expiratory flow rates. Patients with a type I exacerbation (increased dyspnea, sputum, and purulent sputum) were most likely to benefit from antibiotics, whereas no benefit was noted in those with only one of these symptoms (type III exacerbation).

In a meta-analysis of nine randomized, placebo-controlled antibiotic trials in COPD, a small benefit in favor of antibiotics was noted (0.22, CI 0.10–0.34), with 7/9 trials reporting benefit (120). There was also a summary increase in peak expiratory flow of 10.75 L/min (CI 4.96–16.54 L/min), based on six trials. In subgroup analyses, those with more severe infections were more likely to benefit from antibiotic therapy. In a subsequent placebo-controlled trial of outpatients with mild exacerbations treated with steroids, no difference was noted in the symptoms or peak flow rates with the addition of antibiotic therapy (121). Others have also reported that the benefit of antibiotic therapy in COPD exacerbations occurs in those with the most severe lung disease (122).

It should be noted that most of the antibiotic trials in COPD were completed prior to 1990 (1957–1992), before the emergence of current antibiotic resistance patterns and before the development of many currently available antimicrobial agents. Many of the tested regimens (i.e., ampicillin, tetracycline, trimethoprim-sulfamethoxazole) are no longer effective against current isolates. More enteric gram negative agents as well as Pseudomonas have been isolated during exacerbations, making it important to consider these potential pathogens and to provide adequate empiric antibiotic coverage during an exacerbation. Many newer broad spectrum antibiotics have become available in the past decade. However, most clinical trials have focused on comparison of newer agents against other newer classes of antibiotics. The main focus of these evaluations has been comparable efficacy, and these agents are all fairly effective as might be expected (123,124). These investigations also support shorter courses (5 days) of therapy (125). However, there may be differences in the duration of the exacerbation-free period between infectious exacerbations with different classes of agents, and this may represent the main difference between these many agents (126).

There is one placebo-controlled trial involving COPD patients with severe exacerbations, but not pneumonia, who required mechanical ventilation. In this placebo controlled trial, oral ofloxacin significantly reduced ICU (13.2% risk reduction; 95% CI 0.8–25.6) and hospital mortality (17.5% risk reduction; 95% CI 4.3–30.7), as well as duration of mechanical ventilation (6.4 $\pm$ 3.1 vs. 10.6 $\pm$ 5.1 days), ICU (9.4 $\pm$ 5.2 vs. 14.5 $\pm$ 6.0 days), and hospital stay (14.9 $\pm$ 7.4 vs. 24.5 $\pm$ 8.5 days) (127). The greatest impact was on the reduction of subsequent episodes of nosocomial pneumonia. Of note, there was not a significant improvement in the Kaplan–Meier survival curves. Management also differed from more mainstream treatment in that steroids were not administered and methylxanthines were used in almost two-thirds of patients. Initial respiratory isolates were representative of frequent isolates from COPD patients (*H. influenzae*, *M. catarrhalis*, *S. pneumoniae*). While these findings support the use of antibiotics in general, and specifically a fluoroquinolone in severely ill patients, only a minority of isolates may have required the extended antibiotic spectrum of the fluoroquinolone.

Nevertheless, increasing antibiotic resistance among frequently isolated pathogens necessitates consideration of the newer macrolides, fluoroquinolones, and cephalosporins as initial treatment (128,129). Retrospective reviews suggest clinical benefit with lower failure or relapse rates when using newer agents (130–132). Treatment earlier in the course of an exacerbation may also be of clinical benefit, although the benefit may be greater with macrolides, as opposed to fluroquinolones (133). Although antibiotic resistance patterns may necessitate the use of these agents, frequent use also promotes emergence of resistance, which limits their long term utility (134). As with all antibiotics, the key to their effectiveness requires recognition of likely local bacterial isolates, resistance patterns, and limitation of indiscriminate use. Antibiotics are effective in the management of COPD exacerbations, but it is important to recognize that not all exacerbations are due to bacterial infections. Major considerations in antibiotic selection are summarized in Table 4.

IX. Corticosteroids

In addition to bronchodilators and antibiotics, corticosteroids are the other frequently administered agent in the management of patients with exacerbations of COPD. The basis for treatment with corticosteroids is extrapolated in part from the favorable experience with corticosteroids in patients with asthma. Inflammation and bronchial hyperreactivity are features of both conditions, although to a lesser extent in COPD (135,136). The clinical response to corticosteroids in COPD patients is not as compelling as in asthma, and objective measures of improvement or inflammation may be difficult to demonstrate (137). In stable patients, only about 10% may improve with a course of corticosteroids (138). Nevertheless, in placebo-controlled trials, when added to

Table 4 Other Frequently Used Agents in the Management of Patients with COPD Exacerbations

	Doses (initial)	Maintenance	Comments
Antibiotics		Focus therapy against common pathogens *H. influenzae*, *S. pneumonia*, *M. catarrhalis*. Be cognizant of other potential pathogens, *P. aeruginosa*, *S. aureus*, Legionella, Chlamydia. Base antibiotic choices on local resistance patterns; older antibiotics (doxycycline, TMP-SMX, etc.) may also be effective in mild exacerbations. Severe exacerbations: Amoxicllin/clavulante, fluoroquinolone with activity against drug resistant *S. pneumoniae* (levofloxacin, gatifloxacin, moxifloxacin), azithromycin, clarithromycin, telithromycin, cephalosporin (second or third generation)	
Corticosteroids			
Prednisone	30–60 mg/day	Taper off over two weeks	Oral and parenteral dose equivalent in patients with intact gut function
Methylprednisolone	125 mg q 6 hr × 3 days or 0.5 mg/kg q 6 hr × 3 days	Convert to prednisone 60 mg/day and taper over a total of two weeks	1 mg prednisone = 0.8 mg methylprednisolone
Budesonide	Nebulized 2.0 mg q 6 hr × 3 days (0.5 mg/2 mL)	MDI dose (400 μgm/puff) 2000 μgm/d × 7 days (3 puffs q AM; 2 puffs q PM)	Efficacy likely limited to those with mild exacerbations
Methylxanthines			
Aminophylline	6 mg/kg IBW (loading) over 20 min	0.5–0.6 mg/kg/hr (35–45 mg/hr) 0.2–0.4 mg/kg/hr in CHF, hepatic failure, elderly (15–30 mg/hr)	Rarely used; fourth line agent Parenteral form, represents 80% theophylline by weight NEED TO MONITOR SERUM LEVELS
Theophylline	10 mg/kg/day (avg dose 400–800 mg) unless converting from aminophylline (see right)	Same	Oral dose is 80% of total aminophylline dose administered 2–3 ×/day NEED TO MONITOR SERUM LEVELS

Abbreviations: TMP-SMX: trimethoprim-sulfamethoxazole; IBW: ideal body weight.

antibiotics and bronchodilators, corticosteroids result in improvement in dyspnea, gas exchange, and spirometry, with fewer treatment failures and shorter duration of hospitalization (139–143). This represents the major findings of both placebo-controlled trials and a meta-analysis (144).

The benefit with corticosteroids appears confined to about the first three to five days of therapy. There may be sustained benefit over a longer time frame, but most investigations did not extend close monitoring beyond this point. The benefit of corticosteroid therapy over placebo was not demonstrable after about two weeks. With respect to spirometry, the maximal change in FEV_1 of 120 mL was noted by the first day of therapy (143) and is outlined in Figure 2. The magnitude of change is similar in studies that report change, and this represents about a three fold greater rate of change than those treated with placebo (142).

The decrease in treatment failures with corticosteroid therapy is not as well defined. In the largest study, this represented an intensification of therapy and consisted mainly of the use of open label systemic corticosteroids, and also included high dose inhaled corticosteroids or methylxanthines (143). The difference between study groups was modest (33% vs. 23% at one month). Intubation rates and death rates did not differ. Duration of hospitalization was reduced with

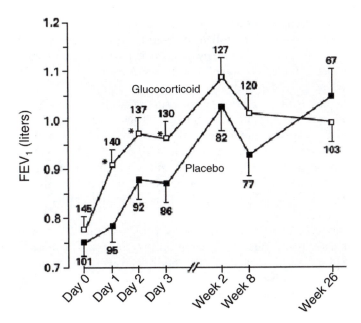

Figure 2 Improvement in spirometry of COPD patients treated with corticosteroids compared to nonsteroid treated controls. Improvement begins with treatment, persists for at least two months, but is no longer evident six months after treatment. *Source*: From Ref. 143.

corticosteroid therapy by one to two days in two separate studies (8.5 vs. 9.7 and 7 vs. 9) (142,143).

There remain some unresolved issues with the duration and dose of corti-costeroids. Treatment with corticosteroids can be limited to a two-week course of therapy. No differences in outcome measures were noted in a study that included an eight-week treatment arm. However, the benefit of fewer days of corticoster-oid therapy remains unknown. Comparison of a three-day versus 10-day course was notable for greater improvement in symptoms and spirometry with a 10-day course of therapy, but no change in the relapse rate (145). The impact on other outcome parameters is unknown since patients were hospitalized for the duration of the study (10 days). There is also no consensus on the optimal dose of corti-costeroids. The largest report on corticosteroids in COPD utilized a regimen of 500 mg of methylprednisolone per day (125 mg q six hours) for the first three days, followed by oral prednisone at 60 mg per day tapered over two weeks or eight weeks (143). Dose have ranged from as little as 30 mg of prednisolone per day to weight based regimens (0.5 mg/kg every six hours) with total daily doses of over 100 mg of methylprednisolone (142,146). The optimal dose remains to be defined, but is probably closer to 100 mg than 500 mg per day of methylprednisolone. No investigation has directly compared oral and parenteral corticosteroids in COPD patients, but there is no difference between these two routes in the treatment of asthma (147).

Inhaled corticosteroids can also be used in mild COPD exacerbations (148). In a randomized, placebo-controlled three-arm study, three days of nebulized budesonide (8 mg/day) followed by inhaled budesonide was compared with oral prednisone (60 mg/day) tapered over seven days. The budesonide group had improvement in spirometry and gas exchange compared to the placebo group, but the magnitude of changes did not match that seen with prednisone, although this was not statistically significant. There was a greater incidence of hyperglycemia with oral prednisone, as may be expected. It is important to emphasize that these were patients with a mild severity of illness with a mean pH = 7.41 or greater in all groups. The efficacy of this approach in patients with a greater acuity of illness remains to be determined, but this seems to be a viable option in selected patients. Dosing regimens for corticosteroid use are summarized in Table 4.

No discussion of corticosterioids is complete without mention of the adverse effects of therapy. Hyperglycemia and psychosis are the most commonly noted complications associated with short courses of high dose steroids. However, in practice, the dose and duration of corticosteroid therapy varies widely, with patients often receiving very high doses for extended periods of time. Severe fungal or viral infections, severe corticosteroid associated myopa-thy, and bowel perforation have all been attributed to the use of steroids, usually within the time frame of hospitalization for an acute illness (<3 weeks) (149–151). As with all complications, the risk is dose dependent. Infectious complications are not increased as long as the daily dose of prednisone is <10 mg/day or a cumulative dose of <700 mg (152). Osteoporosis and compression fractures are more commonly noted with long term use (153). There may also be an increase in mortality with long term use (154). As a general principle of steroid use, administration should be limited to the lowest dose for the shortest period of time.

X. Oxygen

Oxygen is an important adjunct in the management of acute exacerbations of COPD, especially in hypoxemic patients. However, its use has always been tempered by a concern that some COPD patients are more dependent on their hypoxic drive and have a blunted ventilatory response (relative hypoventilation) to hypercapnia. Excess supplemental oxygen may eliminate the hypoxic drive and worsen hypercapnia, leading to CO_2 narcosis and eventually respiratory arrest. The risks are especially cogent with the use of uncontrolled oxygen. Although this has been frequently cited as the mechanism leading to hyperoxic-induced hypercapnia, experimental data suggests other mechanisms of action. Investigators have not been able to correlate an increase in hypercapnia with decreasing minute ventilation. Instead, increasing hypercapnia is better explained by reversal of the changes of hypoxic vasoconstriction, with associated increases in ventilation/perfusion mismatch and dead space (155–157). Others have found significant hypoventilatiom as well as increasing dead space associated with hyperoxic-inducted hypercapnia in their group of COPD patients. Of note, those with CO_2 retention were more hypercapnic (56.3 ± 13.6 vs. 49.7 ± 8.3 mm-Hg) on initial evaluation (158).

Early experience with oxygen therapy may have influenced the concerns with supplemental oxygen. With uncontrolled oxygen, 30% of patients were reported to develop CO_2 narcosis with a >30 mm rise in P_aCO_2 (159). With controlled oxygen (precise $F_IO_2 = 0.24-0.28$) in a group of 27 patients, almost 60% had associated hypercapnia, but severe respiratory acidosis occurred only in three, with only one requiring mechanical ventilation, and there was one death (160). It should be noted that there is great individual variation in response to hyperoxia that is not easily predictable. In another series of 73 patients treated with controlled oxygen, 22% developed CO_2 narcosis, and 13 (18%) were intubated. Initial severe hypoxemia, or combined hypoxemia and acidemia (7.27 ± 0.04), but not the severity of lung function, seemed to predict the development of CO_2 narcosis (161). More recent experience suggests that the incidence of clinically significant CO_2 narcosis is low. In a series of 24 COPD patients, only three (12.5%) had an increase in $P_aCO_2 > 7.5$ mm-Hg, and only one became acidemia (pH < 7.25). None developed clinical CO_2 narcosis and none were intubated (162). In a trial that compared titration of oxygen to maintain a target P_aO_2 of either >50 mm-Hg or >70 mmHg, only patients in the low oxygen group required intubation (163). No patient in the high oxygen group developed CO_2 narcosis. This would also underscore the importance of correcting hypoxemia.

On the other hand, higher levels of P_aO_2 are associated with hypercapnia and acidemia. In a large prevalence analysis of 983 COPD patients, over 40% of those with a $P_aO_2 > 75$ mmHg were hypercapnic and academia (pH ≥ 7.30) (164). Figure 3 provides recommendations on the use of oxygen therapy in exacerbations of COPD.

In summary, hypoxemia has greater deleterious effects than hypercapnia, and its correction is of paramount importance in treatment. A portion of these patients are at risk for hyperoxia-induced hypercapnia, and this may be ameliorated by the use of controlled oxygen. The proportion of patients who retain significant CO_2 can vary greatly but is likely in the 10–20% range. Even if patients develop increasing hypercapnia, clinically significant respiratory acidosis and CO_2 narcosis are rare, as is frank respiratory failure. Fortunately, there is near universal improvement in the severity of hypercapnia and respiratory acidosis with a reduction in the amount of supplemental oxygen. There needs to be proper caution with the use of oxygen, but its administration should never be compromised because of concern of a possible, relatively infrequent complication.

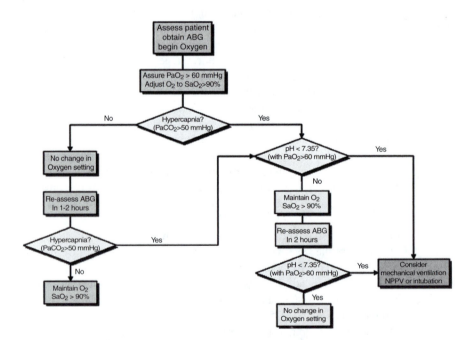

Figure 3 Suggested approach to the management of supplemental oxygen in COPD patients. *Source*: From Ref. 11.

XI. Methylxanthines (Theophylline)

Once a mainstay of therapy in COPD exacerbations, methylxanthines (theophylline or aminophylline) have been relegated to near-salvage therapy status in these patients. Current recommendations do not recommend their routine use and advocate their use only in patients with a poor or incomplete response to aerosolized brochodilators, with close attention to potential adverse medication effects (75). Clinical investigations and meta-analyses have been unable to demonstrate any clinically significant benefit of methylxanthines when added to standard therapy (nebulized bronchodilators, corticosteroids, and antibiotics) in COPD exacerbations (165,166). There is one randomized trial that supports the benefit of oral theophylline, but the study has only been published in abstract form (167).

Although used extensively as a bronchodilator, it is a relatively weak one, and provides little additional benefit above that obtained with nebulized bronchodilators. If there is a benefit with theophylline, it is unlikely to improve spirometric values of FEV_1 by more than 100 mL. There may be benefits of theophylline aside from bronchodilation. These include improvement in diaphragmatic contractility, reversal of diaphragm fatigue, anti-inflammatory effects, immunomodulation, and increasing respiratory drive (168–170). However, there is no clinical evidence that the effect of theophylline in these areas translates to a clinical benefit for patients with acute exacerbations of COPD. Admittedly, there is a relative paucity of high quality, prospective randomized, blinded evidence with this agent, and there may eventually be a role for its more frequent use in exacerbations. There is some data in stable patients that suggests additional benefit of theophylline when added to salmeterol (171).

The use of theophylline has always been tempered by its narrow therapeutic window, adverse side effects, and need to monitor serum levels. In the meta-analysis, increased adverse gastrointestinal effects (nausea, emesis) were noted in all of the placebo-controlled trials. More severe adverse effects include seizures, life threatening atrial and ventricular arrhythmias, and death. There is also a plethora of drug interactions, especially with macrolides (erythromycin and clarithromycin) and ciprofloxacin that may further increase the risk of toxicity (172). Theophylline metabolism is also decreased in elderly patients and those with congestive heart failure or liver disease, and should be used with caution in these patients. Increased metabolism occurs with cigarette smoking and medications (phenytoin, phenobarbital, carbamazepine), and dosing may need to be adjusted in these situations. Higher serum levels do not increase the efficacy of theophylline and only increase its toxicity. Serum levels in the 8–10 μmol/L range represent a reasonable goal for therapy. It should be noted that for patients initially treated with an aminophylline infusion, conversion to oral theophylline requires a reduction to 80% of the aminophylline dose. Failure to account for the dosing change can be another cause for toxicity. Table 4 provides a summary of recommended dosing regimens.

Despite its limited role and benefit, there remains significant interest in theophylline and related compounds. Theophylline is a nonspecific phosphodiesterase (PDE) inhibitor that mediates its effects by increasing cyclic adenosine monophosphate (cAMP) and cyclic guanosine monophosphate (cGMP) by inhibition of PDE3, PDE4, and PDE5. There has been a flurry of interest in PDE inhibitors, specifically PDE4 inhibitors that may improve the beneficial effects of theophylline, especially with respect to its anti-inflammatory effect while minimizing adverse effects. Cilomilast, a second generation PDE4 inhibitor, has undergone the most extensive evaluation to date, although the experience has been limited to patients with stable COPD (173,174). Roflumilast is the most potent PDE4 inhibitor under development (175). Although the incidence of adverse events may be decreased, nausea and headache remain prominent and may limit long term use. The other potential advantage of these agents is that they are administered orally, which may be useful in those unable to tolerate nebulizer treatments. Their role in the management of acute exacerbations remains to be investigated.

XII. Other Adjuncts (Helium–Oxygen, Magnesium, Mucolytics, Respiratory Stimulants)

The above comprise the major components of therapy in the treatment of exacerbations of COPD. These interventions are directed at not only relieving dyspnea and correcting gas exchange abnormalities, but also in averting progression of respiratory distress to frank respiratory failure. While discussed separately, they are usually administered simultaneously during treatment. There are a few other adjuncts to therapy that may be of benefit in these patients. These adjuncts are summarized in Table 5.

Table 5   Other Adjuncts in the Management of COPD Exacerbations

Therapy	Key points
Helium–oxygen	Decreases work of breathing
	Potential increase in drug delivery
	May decrease intubation rate or facilitate extubation
	Greatest benefit if helium–oxygen $>$70:30; therefore limited if F_1O_2 requirements $>$0.40
Magnesium	Potential additional bronchodilation
	Adjunct to standard bronchodilator therapy
	Experience in COPD limited
Mucolytics	No benefit demonstrated in acute exacerbations
	Caution with use of *N*-acetylcysteine (bronchospasm)
Respiratory stimulants	Not recommended for routine use
(doxapram, acetazolamide, medroxyprogesterone)	May provide some benefit in patients without options for noninvasive or invasive ventilation

A combination of helium and oxygen, heliox, may be a useful adjunct in the management. Heliox has no bronchodilatory or anti-inflammatory properties, but other physiologic effects may help facilitate the action of other therapeutics or reduce the potential for respiratory muscle fatigue and respiratory failure. The lower gas density of helium, in combination with oxygen, allows for a reduction in turbulent airflow, increasing laminar airflow through obstructed airways. However, the benefit of helium requires relatively high levels of the gas, preferably >70% and probably at least 60% (176). This tempers the benefit of heliox in patients who would require a $F_1O_2 > 40\%$. Additional details on the use of helium–oxygen can be found in the chapters on asthma and oxygen therapy.

The decreased turbulent flow with heliox reduces the work of breathing, with increased peak expiratory flows, improvement in hypercapnia, decreased pulsus paradoxus, decreased dyspnea, and reduced respiratory rate (177–179). The improved distribution of ventilation has the potential of increasing drug delivery to the distal airways (180). Most of the experience has been in patients with asthma, with experience accumulating in COPD patients. A retrospective review suggests that COPD patients treated with heliox have a lower intubation rate, a shorter ICU stay, and lower mortality (181). However, its use as a substitute for compressed air during nebulizer treatments did not result in any additional improvement in the spirometry of COPD patients during an exacerbation (182). Other investigations have utilizing heliox mixtures in conjuction with noninvasive ventilation. There is a reduction in the work of breathing indices with noninvasive ventilation using heliox, and the rate of resolution of hypercapnia, intubation rate, or ICU stay may be better but is not significantly different with heliox and noninvasive ventilation (183,184). There are added costs associated with heliox (acquisition and equipment), and these must be factored into its use. While there is certainly a basis for the potential benefit of heliox, experience is limited and not sufficient to currently recommend its routine use. However, it is a consideration in subgroups of COPD patients at risk for respiratory failure who have failed or are intolerant of conventional therapy.

Magnesium sulfate has bronchodilatory effects, probably mediated through smooth muscle relaxation. Most of the experience with magnesium has been in asthma patients and seems to provide the most benefit in those with most severe asthma (185). There has been limited experience in patients with COPD exacerbations, but there does appear to be an additional bronchodilatory effect with magnesium when used with nebulized albuterol in an emergency room setting (186). Administration of 1.2 g of magnesium significantly increased peak expiratory flow by an average of 25 L/min (compared to about 6 L/min with placebo), and was associated with fewer admissions, although this was not statistically significant. Its use in hospitalized COPD patients has not been evaluated.

Respiratory stimulants, like doxapram, have been used to treat COPD patients with hypercapnic respiratory failure with variable success. Doxapram is an analeptic agent that stimulates medullary respiratory centers and may also stimulate carotid chemoreceptors. It is administered intravenously and can increase tidal volume and minute ventilation with a reduction in hypercapnia (187). Its effect was found comparable to noninvasive ventilation in one small study, but short lived (188). There may have been more of a role for doxapram in the past when options were limited after patients who were not candidates for intubation had failed or were failing therapy. Noninvasive ventilation has emerged as the preferred treatment in these patients, relegating doxapram to use in isolated patients with no other viable options (189). Other respiratory stimulants, such as acetazolamide and medroxyprogesterone, may be effective in patients with chronic hypercapnia, but like doxapram, are among the last options in patients with acute exacerbations (190).

Other adjuncts of treatment designed to improve mucus clearance have not been found to shorten the course of COPD exacerbations. This includes the use of expectorants, mucolytics, and percussion chest physiotherapy (191,192). *N*-acetylcysteine, a mucolytic with antioxidant properties, has been the subject of intense study and may be beneficial in reducing COPD exacerbations, but there is no data in patients with acute exacerbations (193,194). There must be caution with nebulized administration given a risk of provoking bronchospasm, and it should be administered simultaneously with a bronchodilator (albuterol). While these agents cannot be recommended as part of routine therapy, some patients may experience improvement in symptoms, with a possible increased risk of significant adverse effects.

XIII. Noninvasive Ventilation

Noninvasive ventilation, defined as ventilatory support without an endotracheal tube, has emerged as a viable and often first option in the management of critically ill patients. It appears to be especially suited for the management of respiratory distress and respiratory failure in patients with decompensated COPD. The indications, patient selection, method of application, and other elements of management are discussed in detail in the chapter on noninvasive ventilation.

In general, noninvasive ventilation is best suited for those COPD patients with a moderate respiratory acidosis defined as a pH in the 7.25–7.35 range, although there is no firm consensus on these values (195,196). Other comorbidities may limit the effectiveness and success of noninvasive ventilation, and it is important to recognize these limiting factors. These factors include severe patient obtundation, inability to cooperate with the mask and ventilator, hemodynamic instability, excess secretions, gastrointestinal bleeding, and seizures (197). In these patients, noninvasive ventilation is not as effective at correcting gas exchange abnormalities, and should be bypassed to avoid undue delays in endotracheal intubation.

In those patients treated with noninvasive ventilation, improvement is usually evident within a short period of its application. Numerous investigators have noted significant improvement within an hour or two of its use, and the magnitude of improvement can also help identify those most likely to be successfully treated with noninvasive ventilation. If there is no significant improvement, it is likely patients will require intubation and mechanical ventilation. However, this is not a uniform experience, as some patients can be successfully managed, but with a slower rate of resolution of gas exchange abnormalities. Patients must be closely monitored, and successful therapy is also dependent on the experience and expertise of other medical staff (nursing and respiratory therapy) with noninvasive ventilation. The importance of these factors cannot be underestimated.

The success rate at avoiding intubation can vary widely from 50% to almost 90%, with an average success rate closer to 75%. In addition, noninvasive ventilation is effective in reducing the duration of hospitalization and mortality in these patients as well as the development of nosocomial pneumonia. It can also be successful in those patients who are not candidates or who do not wish to be endotracheally intubated (198). There is a role for it use even in those patients who require intubation. An early extubation approach using noninvasive ventilation as a weaning tool can successfully bridge patients to eventual discontinuation of mechanical ventilation. Patients successfully treated with noninvasive ventilation have lower one-year mortality rates, possibly related to avoidance of some of the adverse events associated with mechanical ventilation.

In summary, noninvasive ventilation is a reasonable first line intervention for COPD patients with progressive hypercapnia and respiratory failure, but patient selection and staff expertise are crucial for its successful application. It is important to recognize the limitations of noninvasive support so as not to delay intubation and mechanical ventilation.

XIV. Mechanical Ventilation

The course of patients with COPD exacerbations has been reviewed earlier in this chapter. Their severity of illness, specifically the degree of respiratory acidosis, is closely associated with the risk of subsequent respiratory failure and need for intubation, which in turn is associated with increased length of stay, ICU, hospital, and one-year mortality. About 20% of patients are acidemic on presentation, with >50% of those with a pH < 7.25 requiring intubation and hospital mortality ranging from 20–30+%.

During an exacerbation, there is increased outflow obstruction due to bronchoconstriction, inflammation, and mucus plugging, which leads to increased ventilatory requirements with subsequent air trapping and dynamic hyperinflation. This causes patients to breathe on the less compliant portion of the pressure–volume curve, increasing the work of breathing for an already mechanically disadvantaged, shortened diaphragm with less force generation capacity (199). The load may exceed the capacity of the respiratory muscles, leading to breathing patterns that cannot be sustained or which worsen existing dynamic hyperinflation, with ultimately less efficient breathing, hypercapnia, and eventual respiratory failure (200). The respiratory drive may be further impaired by either a blunted response to hypercapnia or hypoxia (due to hyperoxia), which further limits the ability to correct gas exchange abnormalities. Other factors, such as pneumonia or heart failure, may also contribute to the respiratory load and increase the likelihood or respiratory failure.

Further progression requires assisted ventilatory support, either as noninvasive ventilation or invasively via an endotracheal tube. The management of these patients during mechanical ventilation is similar to most patients, but there are a few areas that require special attention. Since increased airways obstruction and increased respiratory load are the primary causes of respiratory failure and lead to dynamic hyperinflation, treatment should decrease the air trapping and other conditions that increase the respiratory load. This approach has been discussed at length and includes bronchodilators, antibiotics, and steroids and occurs simultaneously with ventilatory support. There are some special considerations worth noting.

A. Dynamic Hyperinflation or Auto-PEEP

Since dynamic hyperinflation in a major cause of increased respiratory load and respiratory failure, it follows that this should also be a primary focus in the ventilator management of these patients. Dynamic hyperinflation usually reflects significant air trapping, with poorly emptying alveolar units leading to continued end-expiratory airflow and pressure. The latter is often referred to as $PEEP_i$, or auto-PEEP (201). While patients with obstructive lung disease are at the greatest risk for auto-PEEP, it may occur in other circumstances, with or without dynamic hyperinflation, in patients who may or may not have obstructive lung disease. This has been noted in patients with a high respiratory rate or minute ventilation, increased expiratory valve resistance, and increased abdominal contraction and expiratory muscle activity (202–205). The auto-PEEP may have the same adverse physiologic consequences on cardiac function and outflow as extrinsically applied PEEP, and in extreme circumstances, it can result in high intrathoracic pressures, decreased venous return, and hypotension. It can also contribute to further alveolar distension, increasing the risk for barotrauma. It can increase the work of breathing by acting as an inspiratory threshold, which must be overcome by the patient to trigger mechanical ventilation and can worsen the length–tension relationship of the diaphragm with further hyperinflation (206,207).

Although auto-PEEP is defined by its effects on patient–ventilator mechanics, its presence can be suspected by findings at the bedside. The initial description of auto-PEEP involved patients with COPD who become hypotensive shortly after intubation and mechanical ventilation. This is a not uncommon occurrence and may initially be interpreted as a consequence of relative hypovolemia and exposure to positive intrathoracic pressure. This also occurs in euvolemic patients; volume infusion may partially or fully correct the hypotension and should be administered before moving to the use of pressors. However, the timing in close proximity to intubation and mechanical ventilation should raise the index of suspicion for the presence of auto-PEEP. Other bedside findings include exhaled tidal volume readings that exceed set tidal volume, ineffective inspiratory efforts that do not trigger ventilator breaths (by visual exam or palpation), auscultatory evidence of persistent exhalation up to the next ventilator breath, and immediate improvement in hemodynamics with disconnection of the patient from the ventilator (208). The latter maneuver removes the effects of positive intrathoracic airway pressure and can be therapeutic as well as diagnostic. It should be noted that the physical signs of auto-PEEP are better at identifying its presence and should not be used to exclude this diagnosis. Bedside ventilator waveforms are available on most currently used ventilators, and inspection of expiratory flow waveforms may be helpful in detecting the presence of auto-PEEP. Expiratory flow is expected to cease prior to the next ventilator breath, but ineffective respiratory efforts or persistent flow would suggest continued flow, and therefore, pressure (or auto-PEEP) at the end of exhalation. Representative waveforms demonstrating auto-PEEP can be found in the chapters on modes of mechanical ventilation and monitoring during mechanical ventilation.

Once identified, additional maneuvers are required to measure the amount of auto-PEEP. The end-expiratory port occlusion method involves occlusion of the expiratory port and measurement of ≥ 0.5 second plateau prior to the next breath. The pressures in the lung and proximal airway equilibrate, and the reading on the ventilator manometer will be a reflection of the amount of auto-PEEP present in the system. As such, the pressures represent measures of mean alveolar pressure, especially in patients with COPD with inhomogenous lung and regional differences in end-expiratory lung volume (209). This is often referred to as static auto-PEEP. However, this maneuver may not be easy to perform nor accurately reflect the level of auto-PEEP. Patients must be sufficiently relaxed to cooperate with the maneuver, and some use sedatives or paralytics to facilitate measurement. The expiratory port may be difficult to identify or occlude in some ventilators. Some ventilator software packages automate this measurement, but patients may be too tachypneic or uncooperative to allow an accurate measurement. The method of measurement only reflects the contribution of airways in communication with the proximal airway. There is the potential that auto-PEEP may be underestimated if there are noncommunicating lung segments or airways that prematurely close (210).

The impact of auto-PEEP may also be assessed by its effect as an inspiratory threshold to breathing. Since auto-PEEP reflects the persistence of airflow at the end of exhalation, the change in pressure needed to reduce expiratory flow to zero and start lung inflation would also be representative of auto-PEEP. This measurement has been referred to as dynamic auto-PEEP to distinguish it from static auto-PEEP. However, dynamic auto-PEEP may also not provide an accurate measure of a patient's auto-PEEP. It is probably a more accurate measure of the lowest amount of regional auto-PEEP, especially in patients with inhomogeneous lungs. This is apparent in COPD patients, in whom the dynamic auto-PEEP may be only 75% or less of static auto-PEEP (211). Dynamic auto-PEEP usually requires an esophageal balloon for proper measurement, thereby further limiting its general detection (212). With both types of auto-PEEP, there may be further confounding by expiratory muscle activity, and there are methods of correcting for that contribution, although they both require measurement of gastric pressures (213,214). This expiratory muscle activity does not produce dynamic hyperinflation. From a clinical standpoint, dynamic auto-PEEP is a better measure of the pressure need to be generated to initiate inspiration, while the static auto-PEEP is a better reflection of its hemodynamic effects. An accurate measurement of static auto-PEEP would have the greatest impact on clinical management. Accordingly, the need for precise measurements of dynamic auto-PEEP has been questioned (215). The differences may only be a few centimeters of water pressure, and the efforts required would far exceed any clinical benefit of its measurement. Nevertheless, accurate measurement of auto-PEEP is important as a marker of dynamic hyperinflation, a marker of response to therapy, and a guide to the use of extrinsic PEEP in COPD.

The management of auto-PEEP in the mechanically ventilated patient highlights the general approach to patients with COPD and respiratory failure. There are a number of ventilator adjustments that may help minimize or attenuate the impact of auto-PEEP in COPD patients. Large tidal volumes contribute to air trapping, dynamic hyperinflation, and subsequent auto-PEEP (216). Although most extensively evaluated in patients with asthma, the same principles apply for patients with COPD. Using a technique to measure end-expiratory lung volume, these investigators noted increased air trapping as manifested by increasing end-expiratory lung volume with associated effects on blood pressure (hypotension) in a dose-response manner over three levels of minute ventilation (10, 16, 26 L) and three levels of set tidal volume (0.6, 1.0, 1.6 L). They noted over 4 L of end-expiratory lung volume in one patient, with barotrauma (pneumothoraces) a noteworthy complication in another. These changes were ameliorated at lower tidal volumes, and by maneuvers that increased expiratory time (lower minute ventilation and higher inspiratory flow rates). They found that tidal volumes in the 8–10 mg/kg range provided the optimal balance between ventilation, hyperinflation, and hemodynamics. These findings serve as guidelines to ventilator settings in these patients (lower tidal volumes, lower frequency rate, higher inspiratory flow rates). It should be noted that strategies that decrease inspiratory time (decreased duration of inspiratory pause, increased inspiratory flow rates) can cause tachypnea in COPD patients, but produce an increase in expiratory time, which in turn is beneficial in reducing the amount of auto-PEEP (217).

The other maneuver that may benefit these patients is the addition of extrinsic PEEP to counter auto-PEEP. This may be beneficial in the patient with severe airflow obstruction by increasing flow resistance, thereby keeping easily collapsible airways open. This would limit air trapping and allow continued exhalation from slowly emptying airways. Added PEEP would also decrease the difference between end-expiratory alveolar and central airway pressures. This pressure difference is another manifestion of auto-PEEP and must be overcome by the patient along with the set triggering sensitivity to initiate a ventilator breath. Reducing this difference would not only increase the ability of the patient to trigger a breath, but also decrease ventilatory drive and reduce the overall work of breathing (206,218). The benefit can be appreciated with as little as 5 cm H_2O of PEEP. It is important to recognize that the benefits of extrinsic PEEP are manifest as long as this added PEEP does not exceed auto-PEEP. If this occurs, the added PEEP will contribute to hyperinflation with its associated adverse effects and potential for barotrauma (218–220). This principle was demonstrated with bedside respiratory impedance plethysmography used to indirectly determine the amount of auto-PEEP in mechanically ventilated patients (221). Changes in end-expiratory thoracic gas volume with added PEEP were monitored and PEEP was added until there was an increase in the end-expiratory thoracic gas volume. This represented a condition in which extrinsic PEEP exceeded auto-PEEP, and the amount of auto-PEEP could be inferred as the level prior to the increase in end-expiratory thoracic gas volume. The changes noted with this noninvasive method of assessing auto-PEEP correlated well with expiratory port occlusion. Unfortunately, this is not a widely available method for measuring auto-PEEP.

This potential hazard of extrinsic PEEP mandates that there be accurate measurement of auto-PEEP. The limitations of the end-expiratory port occlusion method have been discussed, but it remains the most frequently used method of measuring auto-PEEP. Whether values are obtained manually or with the assistance of a extrinsic ventilator, PEEP applied is always less than measured auto-PEEP. The magnitude of auto-PEEP is subject to change with changes in the patient's underlying airway obstruction and must be monitored closely and frequently with changes in extrinsic PEEP as appropriate.

XV. Other Aspects

The main aspects in the ventilator management of these patients are outlined in Table 6. Additional areas of concern are as follows.

A. Drug Delivery (MDIs vs. Nebulizers)

As previously discussed, inhaled bronchodilators are an integral component in the management of COPD exacerbations. There has been considerable investigation in the optimal method of delivery of inhaled medications in mechanically

Table 6 Considerations in the Management of Mechanical Ventilation in COPD Patients

Ventilator management	
Parameter	*Management strategies*
Hypoxemia	Lowest F_1O_2 to achieve oxygen saturation 92–95%
Hypercapnia with respiratory acidosis	Ensure adequate minute ventilation limited by development of dynamic hyperinflation
	Avoid excess ventilation to prevent post-hypercapnic metabolic alkalosis
Dynamic hyperinflation	Reduce tidal volume to 8–10 mg/kg; accept increasing hypercapnia with pH $\geq$ 7.25
	Reduce respiratory rate to 6–10 breaths/min with goal of I:E of 1:3 or 1:4 lower
	Reduce minute ventilation to 8–10 L/min
	Increase inspiratory flow (limited by peak airway pressures and not as effective as decreasing respiratory rate)
	Adding extrinsic PEEP at a lower level than measured auto-PEEP
Bronchodilator delivery	Variable delivery based on delivery device (MDI vs. nebulizer) and techniques
	MDI with a spacer most efficient
	Increased delivery with coordinated breath actuation
	Tidal volumes >500 mg increase drug delivery
	Elbow nebulizer least efficient
	Differences between MDI or nebulizer drug delivery probably not clinically significant
	Higher doses may only increase toxicity without improving drug efficacy
	Potential costs savings with MDI delivery

ventilated patients, with much of the focus on the method of drug delivery. There is a wide range in the efficiency of aerosol deposition when comparing small volume nebulizers and meter-dose inhalers (MDIs). There are a multitude of factors that influence the drug deposition. Aerosol particles must have a mass median aerodynamic diameter between 1–6 μm in size for optimal deposition in the airways (222). Larger sized particles will end up in the oropharynx, endotracheal tube, or ventilator circuit. Humidity decreases aerosol deposition by about 40% but is a necessary component of ventilatory support (223). Placement of the nebulizer 30 cm or more from the endotracheal tube is more efficient that placement of the nebulizer between the endotracheal tube and ventilator Y connection, because the tubing serves as a drug reservoir (224). An MDI with a spacer provides greater drug delivery than an MDI with an elbow adaptor or nebulizer. Greater aerosol delivery is also noted when nebulization is synchronized with inspiratory airflow (versus continuous nebulization), tidal volumes >500 mL and longer duty cycles (T_I/T_{TOT}) (225). Most of these studies have been in test lungs. Although there may be greater drug delivery with MDIs, this does not necessarily translate into increased clinical efficacy.

Most clinical studies in mechanically ventilated COPD patients have evaluated the change in inspiratory resistance to bronchodilator therapy. If properly administered, there is no significant difference in inspiratory resistance between albuterol delivered using a MDI (four puffs or 0.4 mg) or a nebulizer (2.5 mg) (226). Higher doses did not further reduce inspiratory resistance, as four puffs were equally effective as eight, or 16 puffs (227). However, toxicity is increased at higher doses. Comparable changes in total respiratory resistance were noted in a study that evaluated a combination of fenoterol and ipratropium bromide delivered either by a MDI or nebulizer (228). Neither delivery method was more effective than the other, but respiratory resistance was partitioned, and it was found that MDI had a greater effect on airway resistance, whereas nebulizer therapy had a greater effect on tissue resistance. Breath-actuated delivery further improves drug delivery as noted in an aerosolized antibiotic study (229).

Although MDIs are more efficient with drug delivery in mechanically ventilated patients, there has been no demonstrated advantage in terms of clinical efficacy. Other aspects favor their use in mechanically ventilated patients. The aerosols produced by in-line nebulizers can be quite variable in size, and delivery can be influenced by ventilator settings. Most ventilators are programmed to deliver continuous nebulization, whereas delivery that is coordinated with inspiration is more efficient. There is a risk of bacterial contamination and nosocomial infection with the nebulizers. On the other hand, MDIs and an in-line spacer are easier to use, with drug delivery that is easier to coordinate with inspiration, probably requiring less time for administration with more reliable dosing. There may be some cost-savings advantage as well with MDIs (230). The importance of proper technique and administration cannot be underestimated, as both methods can be severely hampered by flaws in delivery (231).

While corticosteroids are usually administered systemically (parenteral or oral), inhaled coriticosteroids have been administered to ventilator-dependent COPD patients (232). High-dose inhaled fluticasone (2000 μgm) resulted in improvement in measures of auto-PEEP and respiratory resistance within six days of administration. This may be an option for therapy in those who cannot tolerate systemic corticosteroids.

B. Heliox During Mechanical Ventilation

Helium–oxygen has previously been discussed as an adjunct to avoid intubation or improve drug delivery. Its low density and ability to promote laminar flow with decreased airway turbulence and decreased work of breathing may also be beneficial in intubated patients. It can reduce dynamic hyperinflation and auto-PEEP in intubated patients, but its benefits are short lived and limited to the time the gas mixture is in use (233). There may also be some benefit in facilitating weaning in some patients as well (234). However, it is not easy to use in mechanically ventilated patients, requiring adjustments for flow and volume measurement as well as blenders for gas delivery (235). Despite theoretical advantages, its benefit in COPD remains to be determined.

C. Nutritional Support

Nutritional support is crucial to maintain sufficient muscle strength and to promote recovery in these patients. This is an intuitive concept, although difficult to confirm in patients with acute COPD exacerbations. Even in a prospective, randomized evaluation of aggressive nutritional supplementation (39 kcal/kg/day vs. 29 kcal/kg/day), both groups of COPD patients incurred negative nitrogen balance (with possible muscle wasting) due to concomitant corticosteroid use. Indices of muscle strength were unchanged, but there may be modest improvement in spirometry in high intake patients compared to patients with less caloric intake (236). There have been concerns that excessive hypercapnia as a result of high carbohydrate loads may contribute to acute or chronic respiratory failure in COPD patients with a limited capacity to increase their minute ventilation (237). This is more of a theoretical concern than an actual risk. Excess carbon dioxide production is actually associated with overfeeding, not diets with high carbohydrate composition (238). While feedings with higher fat and lower carbohydrate composition can reduce carbon dioxide production (239), these are more costly and not necessary as long as the patient is not receiving excess calories.

XVI. Weaning and Extubation

These aspects of management are covered in detail in respective chapters dealing with these topics. Management in COPD patients is similar to that of other patients with respiratory failure. In addition to commonly encountered obstacles to extubation, auto-PEEP may be a significant limiting factor. It can act as an inspiratory threshold, increasing the work required for each breath. The strategies discussed for reducing auto-PEEP are also relevant during weaning. However, there may be greater concern for chronic respiratory failure and ventilator dependence because of advanced underlying lung disease. There are a few strategies that may be considered for those at risk for ventilator dependence or to limit adverse events that may prolong duration of mechanical ventilation.

Early extubation and support with noninvasive ventilation has been one approach that may provide an advantage in the management of these patients. The benefit to this approach may be avoidance of complications of endotracheal intubation and mechanical ventilation, specifically ventilator associated pneumonia. This strategy is discussed in detail in the chapter on noninvasive ventilation. There is a survival advantage with early extubation, whether applied arbitrarily two days after intubation or after failure of three consecutive trials of spontaneous breathing (240–242). This approach is distinctly different from the use of noninvasive ventilation in post-extubation respiratory distress, where the success has been less impressive (243,244).

These patients often have compromised ventilatory muscle function due to a number of factors, including hyperinflation, impaired chest wall and diaphragm mechanics, and malnutrition. This often translates to decreased muscle strength, which further impairs their ability to be weaned from mechanical ventilation (245). They are at risk for chronic ventilator dependence. Inspiratory muscle training may be helpful for those with chronic respiratory failure, and this concept has been applied to patients requiring mechanical ventilation. Improvement in inspiratory muscle strength has been demonstratred, whether using resistance training or pressure threshold devices (246,247). This approach obviously requires weeks to months of training for success and has not undergone comparison with more common approaches to weaning.

In the rare patient, surgical intervention may be necessary to facilitate discontinuation of mechanical ventilation. These are typically patients with severe emphysema and hyperinflation with markedly impaired lung and chest wall mechanics. There are reports of patients undergoing bullectomy or lung volume reduction surgery to facilitate their weaning off the ventilator (248–250). Lung transplantation is an even less common, but reported, option (251). Obviously, this would be reserved for patients without any other options to chronic ventilator support and must be in facilities with the proper surgical expertise.

XVII. Response to Therapy

Resolution of gas exchange abnormalties, specifically hypercapnia and respiratory acidosis, along with signs of respiratory distress (accessory muscle use, abdominal paradox, etc.) and dyspnea, are the clinical features that accompany successful therapy. The time course of resolution of objective measures of a patient's respiratory status can be gleaned from therapeutic studies. Spirometry obtained during corticosteroid treatment demonstrates about a 100 mL improvement in FEV_1 over the first day, which is about the extent of improvement (143). Blood gases in hypercapnic patients not treated with assisted ventilation normalize over about three days of therapy (72). These are illustrated in Figures 2 and 4. There has been intense interest in exhaled gases and exhaled breath constituents as markers of inflammation and oxidative stress in these patients. Promising markers include nitric oxide and eicosanoids (LTB_4 and PGE_2) and 8-isoprostane, but these remain in the investigational stage (252–255).

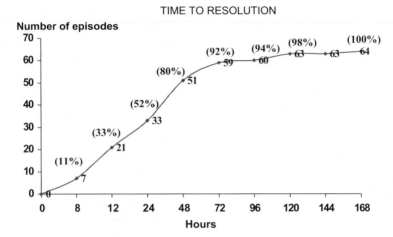

Figure 4 Time course of resolution of hypercapnic respiratory acidosis in COPD patients NOT requiring mechanical ventilation. *Source*: From Ref. 72.

XVIII. Chronic Ventilator Dependence and End-of-Life Care

While the focus has been on patients with acute exacerbations of their COPD, it would be remiss not to examine the issues of chronic ventilator dependence and end-of-life care in these patients. Factors leading to chronic ventilator dependence are also discussed in the chapters dealing with weaning and prolonged mechanical ventilation. Patients may not be able to discontinue mechanical ventilation and end up in a long-term acute care or chronic ventilator facility. This obviously increases associated health care costs, and patients may continue to require assistance with reduced quality of life indices even if they are able to be discharged home (256). In the experience of long term ventilator facilities, a third to half of their patients are eventually liberated off the ventilator, with chronic ventilator dependence in 15–30% (257–259).

It is this spector of chronic disability and severe disabling dyspnea that has led many to re-evaluate the goals of therapy in those patients with advanced COPD. Although most patients hospitalized with COPD exacerbations will recover to be discharged even if intubated, the long-term mortality is fairly high. Patients often return to a baseline that is fragile at best with severe, limiting dyspnea. They are at risk for recurrent exacerbations and episodes of respiratory failure. There has been somewhat of a reluctance to discuss palliative care and end-of-life issues, especially mechanical ventilation, with these patients. Part of this stems from the difficulty in predicting mortality in these patients.

Despite acknowledgement of advanced disease, it remains difficult for physicians to gauge the prognosis of patients with advanced chronic obstructive lung disease. Estimates for a prototypical COPD patient with a recent prolonged episode of mechanical ventilation including tracheostomy placement can vary widely from one month to five years, although most physicians would estimate less than a one-year survival (260). However, the need for intubation and mechanical ventilation to treat an acute exacerbation is NOT a predictor of short or long term mortality ($\leq$2 years) (60,261). The prospect of intubation may greatly influence the management offered to these patients, and there is also great variation in this decision among physicians for identical patients (262,263).

While the outcome of patients requiring mechanical ventilation is not predictable at the time of intubation, it is evident that the long-term mortality of these patients can be quite high and approaches 50% within two years (67). However, it is very difficult to identify those patients at greatest risk of death within a six-months time frame with current prediction criteria (264). Other measures such as dyspnea, quality of life measures, cor pulmonale, depression, other comorbidities, functional status, and six-minute walk distance may be helpful in identifying those with a increased one-year mortality (265–267).

Therefore, it is important to address end-of-life care and treatment preferences with these patients. This represents an underappreciated and often unmet need of these patients, especially when compared to patients with lung cancer who may have a similar prognosis (268). Patients with severe COPD often have severe, limiting dyspnea and disability with significant emotional and social needs. Surrogates may not be able to accurately reflect patient preferences and physicians may not clearly comprehend their preferences (269,270). This can also be a difficult topic of discussion and is often not broached, even in patients with the greatest impairment, until relatively late in the course of their disease (271,272). In addition to intubation and resuscitation, dyspnea, pain, and symptoms control are other topics that merit discussion and attention (273). These issues are probably addressed in less than half of these patients.

XIX. Conclusion

In summary, the increasing incidence of COPD will translate into an increasing healthcare burden for all physicians. Those whose disease cannot be managed as an outpatient will require hospitalization. Current management remains focused on averting frank respiratory failure with bronchodilators, corticosteroids, and antibiotics. Other adjuncts that may facilitate recovery include helium–oxygen mixtures and noninvasive ventilation. Once intubated, control of dynamic hyperinflation is crucial for recovery and eventual extubation. Noninvasive ventilation may facilitate discontinuation of mechanical ventilation. Additional markers may help better define and monitor the response to therapy, but these remain investigational at this time.

References

1. National Institutes of Health, World Health Organization. Executive summary: global strategy for the diagnosis, management, and prevention of chronic obstructive pulmonary disease: NHLBI/WHO Workshop, 2001:1–30.
2. Mannino DM, Homa DM, Akinbami LJ, Ford ES, Redd SC. Chronic obstructive pulmonary disease surveillance—United States, 1971–2000. MMWR Surveill Summ 2002; 51(6):1–16.
3. National Heart LBI, DoE. Morbidity and mortality 1998. Chartbook on cardiovascular, lung and blood diseases, 1998.
4. Wilson L, Devine EB, So K. Direct medical costs of chronic obstructive pulmonary disease: chronic bronchitis and emphysema. Respir Med 2000; 94(3):204–213.
5. Sullivan SD, Ramsey SD, Lee TA. The economic burden of COPD. Chest 2000; 117(suppl 2):5S–9S.
6. Centers for Disease Control and Prevention. National hospital discharge survey 1998.
7. Anthonisen NR, Manfreda J, Warren CP, Hershfield ES, Harding GK, Nelson NA. Antibiotic therapy in exacerbations of chronic obstructive pulmonary disease. Ann Intern Med 1987; 106(2):196–204.
8. Standards for the diagnosis and care of patients with chronic obstructive pulmonary disease. American Thoracic Society. Am J Respir Crit Care Med 1995; 152(5 Pt 2):S77–S121.
9. Rodriguez-Roisin R. Toward a consensus definition for COPD exacerbations. Chest 2000; 117(90052):398S–401S.
10. Chronic obstructive pulmonary disease. National clinical guideline on management of chronic obstructive pulmonary disease in adults in primary and secondary care. Thorax 2004; 59(suppl 1):1–232.
11. Celli BR, MacNee W. Standards for the diagnosis and treatment of patients with COPD: a summary of the ATS/ERS position paper. Eur Respir J 2004; 23(6):932–946.
12. Pauwels RA, Rabe KF. Burden and clinical features of chronic obstructive pulmonary disease (COPD). Lancet 2004; 364(9434):613–620.
13. Sciurba FC. Physiologic similarities and differences between COPD and asthma. Chest 2004; 126(suppl 2):117S–124S.
14. Voelkel NF, Tuder R. COPD: exacerbation. Chest 2000; 117(90052):376S–379S.
15. White AJ, Gompertz S, Stockley RA. Chronic obstructive pulmonary disease. 6: The aetiology of exacerbations of chronic obstructive pulmonary disease. Thorax 2003; 58(1):73–80.
16. Seemungal TA, Donaldson GC, Paul EA, Bestall JC, Jeffries DJ, Wedzicha JA. Effect of exacerbation on quality of life in patients with chronic obstructive pulmonary disease. Am J Respir Crit Care Med 1998; 157(5 Pt 1):1418–1422.
17. Seemungal TA, Donaldson GC, Bhowmik A, Jeffries DJ, Wedzicha JA. Time course and recovery of exacerbations in patients with chronic obstructive pulmonary disease. Am J Respir Crit Care Med 2000; 161(5):1608–1613.
18. Cabello H, Torres A, Celis R, El Ebiary M, Puig de la Bellacasa J, Xaubet A, Gonzalez J, Agusti C, Soler N. Bacterial colonization of distal airways in healthy

subjects and chronic lung disease: a bronchoscopic study. Eur Respir J 1997; 10(5):1137–1144.

19. Monso E, Ruiz J, Rosell A, Manterola J, Fiz J, Morera J, Aasina V. Bacterial infection in chronic obstructive pulmonary disease. A study of stable and exacerbated outpatients using the protected specimen brush. Am J Respir Crit Care Med 1995; 152(4):1316–1320.

20. Soler N, Torres A, Ewig S, Gonzalez J, Cellis R, El Ebiary M, Hernandez C, Rodrigurz-Roisin R. Bronchial microbial patterns in severe exacerbations of chronic obstructive pulmonary disease (COPD) requiring mechanical ventilation. Am J Respir Crit Care Med 1998; 157(5 Pt 1):1498–1505.

21. Eller J, Ede A, Schaberg T, Neiderman MS, Mauch H, Lode H. Infective exacerbations of chronic bronchitis: relation between bacteriologic etiology and lung function. Chest 1998; 113(6):1542–1548.

22. Miravitlles M, Espinosa C, Fernandez-Laso E, Martos JA, Maldonado JA, Gallego M. Relationship between bacterial flora in sputum and functional impairment in patients with acute exacerbations of COPD. Study Group of Bacterial Infection in COPD. Chest 1999; 116(1):40–46.

23. Lieberman D, Lieberman D, Ben Yaakov M, Lazarovich Z, Hoffman S, Ohana B, Friedman MG, Dvockin B, Leinonen M, Bolder I. Infectious etiologies in acute exacerbation of COPD. Diagn Microbiol Infect Dis 2001; 40(3):95–102.

24. Mogulkoc N, Karakurt S, Isalska B, Bayindir V, Celikel T, Korten V, Colpan N. Acute purulent exacerbation of chronic obstructive pulmonary disease and Chlamydia pneumoniae infection. Am J Respir Crit Care Med 1999; 160(1):349–353.

25. Groenewegen KH, Wouters EF. Bacterial infections in patients requiring admission for an acute exacerbation of COPD: a 1-year prospective study. Respir Med 2003; 97(7):770–777.

26. Hegele RG, Hayashi S, Hogg JC, Pare PD. Mechanisms of airway narrowing and hyperresponsiveness in viral respiratory tract infections. Am J Respir Crit Care Med 1995; 151(5):1659–1664.

27. Jacoby DB, Fryer AD. Interaction of viral infections with muscarinic receptors. Clin Exp Allergy 1999; 29(suppl 2):59–64.

28. Smith CB, Golden C, Klauber MR, Kanner R, Renzetti A. Interactions between viruses and bacteria in patients with chronic bronchitis. J Infect Dis 1976; 134(6):552–561.

29. Seemungal T, Harper-Owen R, Bhowmik A, Moric I, Sanderson G, Message S, Mccalium P, Meade TW, Jeffries DJ, Johnston SL et al. Respiratory viruses, symptoms, and inflammatory markers in acute exacerbations and stable chronic obstructive pulmonary disease. Am J Respir Crit Care Med 2001; 164(9):1618–1623.

30. Rohde G, Wiethege A, Borg I, Kauth M, Bauer TT, Gillissen A, Bufe A, Scholtze-Werninghaus G. Respiratory viruses in exacerbations of chronic obstructive pulmonary disease requiring hospitalisation: a case-control study. Thorax 2003; 58(1):37–42.

31. Smith CB, Golden CA, Kanner RE, Renzetti AD. Association of viral and Mycoplasma pneumoniae infections with acute respiratory illness in patients with chronic obstructive pulmonary diseases. Am Rev Respir Dis 1980; 121(2):225–232.

32. Greenberg SB, Allen M, Wilson J, Atmar RL. Respiratory viral infections in adults with and without chronic obstructive pulmonary disease. Am J Respir Crit Care Med 2000; 162(1):167–173.

33. Rohde G, Wiethege A, Borg I, Kanth M, Bauer TT, Gillissen A, Bufe A, Scholtze-Werninghaus G. Respiratory viruses in exacerbations of chronic obstructive pulmonary disease requiring hospitalisation: a case-control study. Thorax 2003; 58(1):37–42.

34. Gong H, Jr. Health effects of air pollution. A review of clinical studies. Clin Chest Med 1992; 13(2):201–214.

35. Sunyer J, Saez M, Murillo C, Castellsague J, Martinez F, Anto JM. Air pollution and emergency room admissions for chronic obstructive pulmonary disease: a 5-year study. Am J Epidemiol 1993; 137(7):701–705.

36. Sunyer J, Schwartz J, Tobias A, Macfarlane D, Garcia J, Anto JM. Patients with chronic obstructive pulmonary disease are at increased risk of death associated with urban particle air pollution: a case-crossover analysis. Am J Epidemiol 2000; 151(1):50–56.

37. Atkinson RW, Anderson HR, Sunyer J, Ayres J, Baccini M, Vonk JM, Boumghar A, Forastiere F, Forberg B, Touloumi G, et al. Acute effects of particulate air pollution on respiratory admissions: results from APHEA 2 project. Air Pollution and Health: a European Approach. Am J Respir Crit Care Med 2001; 164(10 Pt 1):1860–1866.

38. Maestrelli P, Saetta M, Di Stefano A, Calcagn, PG, Torato G, Ruggieri MP, Roggeri A, Mapp CE, Fabri LM. Comparison of leukocyte counts in sputum, bronchial biopsies, and bronchoalveolar lavage. Am J Respir Crit Care Med 1995; 152(6 Pt 1):1926–1931.

39. Di Stefano A, Capelli A, Lusuardi M, Balbo P, Vecchio C, Maestrelli P, Map CE, Fabbri LM, Donner CF, Saetta M. Severity of airflow limitation is associated with severity of airway inflammation in smokers. Am J Respir Crit Care Med 1998; 158(4):1277–1285.

40. Rutgers SR, Postma DS, ten Hacken NH, Kauffman HF, Der Mark TW, Koeter GH. Ongoing airway inflammation in patients with COPD who do not currently smoke. Chest 2000; 117(5 Supp 1):262S.

41. Sethi S, Muscarella K, Evans N, Klingman KL, Grant BJ, Murphy TF. Airway inflammation and etiology of acute exacerbations of chronic bronchitis. Chest 2000; 118(6):1557–1565.

42. Qiu Y, Zhu J, Bandi V, Atmar RL, Hattotuwa K, Guntupalli KK, Jeffrey PK. Biopsy neutrophilia, neutrophil chemokine, and receptor gene expression in severe exacerbations of chronic obstructive pulmonary disease. Am J Respir Crit Care Med 2003; 168(8):968–975.

43. Saetta M, Di Stefano A, Maestrelli P, Maestrelli P, Turato G, Ruggieri MP, Roggeri A, Calcagni P, Mopp CE, Ciaccia A, Fabbri LM. Airway eosinophilia in chronic bronchitis during exacerbations. Am J Respir Crit Care Med 1994; 150(6 Pt 1):1646–1652.

44. Saetta M, Turato G, Maestrelli P, Mapp CE, Fabbri LM. Cellular and structural bases of chronic obstructive pulmonary disease. Am J Respir Crit Care Med 2001; 163(6):1304–1309.

45. Turato G, Zuin R, Miniati M, baraldo S, Rea F, Beghe B, Monti S, Formichi B, Boschetto P, Harai S, et al. Airway inflammation in severe chronic obstructive

pulmonary disease: relationship with lung function and radiologic emphysema. Am J Respir Crit Care Med 2002; 166(1):105–110.

46. Bhowmik A, Seemungal TA, Sapsford RJ, Wedzicha JA. Relation of sputum inflammatory markers to symptoms and lung function changes in COPD exacerbations. Thorax 2000; 55(2):114–120.

47. Roland M, Bhowmik A, Sapsford RJ, Seemungal TA, Jeffries DJ, Warner TD, Wedzicha JA. Sputum and plasma endothelin-1 levels in exacerbations of chronic obstructive pulmonary disease. Thorax 2001; 56(1):30–35.

48. Aaron SD, Angel JB, Lunau M, Wright K, Fex C, Le Saux N, Dales RE. Granulocyte inflammatory markers and airway infection during acute exacerbation of chronic obstructive pulmonary disease. Am J Respir Crit Care Med 2001; 163(2):349–355.

49. White AJ, Gompertz S, Bayley DL, Hill SL, O'Brien C, Unsal I, Stockley RA. Resolution of bronchial inflammation is related to bacterial eradication following treatment of exacerbations of chronic bronchitis. Thorax 2003; 58(8):680–685.

50. Stockley RA, O'Brien C, Pye A, Hill SL. Relationship of sputum color to nature and outpatient management of acute exacerbations of COPD. Chest 2000; 117(6):1638–1645.

51. Stockley RA, Bayley D, Hill SL, Hill AT, Crooks S, Campbell EJ. Assessment of airway neutrophils by sputum colour: correlation with airways inflammation. Thorax 2001; 56(5):366–372.

52. Barbera JA, Roca J, Ferrer A, Felez MA, Diaz O, Roger N, Rodriguez-Roisin R. Mechanisms of worsening gas exchange during acute exacerbations of chronic obstructive pulmonary disease. Eur Respir J 1997; 10(6):1285–1291.

53. Schmidt GA, Hall JB. Acute or chronic respiratory failure. Assessment and management of patients with COPD in the emergency setting. J Am Med Assoc 1989; 261(23):3444–3453.

54. Ram FS, Wedzicha JA, Wright J, Greenstone M. Hospital at home for patients with acute exacerbations of chronic obstructive pulmonary disease: systematic review of evidence. BMJ 2004; 329(7461):315.

55. Hudson LD. Survival data in patients with acute and chronic lung disease requiring mechanical ventilation. Am Rev Respir Dis 1989; 140(2 Pt 2):S19–S24.

56. Fuso L, Incalzi RA, Pistelli R, Muzzolon R, Valente S, Pagliari G, Gliozzi F, Ciappi G. Predicting mortality of patients hospitalized for acutely exacerbated chronic obstructive pulmonary disease. Am J Med 1995; 98(3):272–277.

57. Breen D, Churches T, Hawker F, Torzillo PJ. Acute respiratory failure secondary to chronic obstructive pulmonary disease treated in the intensive care unit: a long term follow up study. Thorax 2002; 57(1):29–33.

58. Groenewegen KH, Schols AM, Wouters EF. Mortality and mortality-related factors after hospitalization for acute exacerbation of COPD. Chest 2003; 124(2):459–467.

59. Nevins ML, Epstein SK. Predictors of outcome for patients with COPD requiring invasive mechanical ventilation. Chest 2001; 119(6):1840–1849.

60. Moran JL, Green JV, Homan SD, Leeson RJ, Leppard PI. Acute exacerbations of chronic obstructive pulmonary disease and mechanical ventilation: a reevaluation. Crit Care Med 1998; 26(1):71–78.

61. Patil SP, Krishnan JA, Lechtzin N, Diette GB. In-hospital mortality following acute exacerbations of chronic obstructive pulmonary disease. Arch Intern Med 2003; 163(10):1180–1186.

62. Menzies R, Gibbons W, Goldberg P. Determinants of weaning and survival among patients with COPD who require mechanical ventilation for acute respiratory failure. Chest 1989; 95(2):398–405.

63. Breen D, Churches T, Hawker F, Torzillo PJ. Acute respiratory failure secondary to chronic obstructive pulmonary disease treated in the intensive care unit: a long term follow up study. Thorax 2002; 57(1):29–33.

64. Groenewegen KH, Schols AM, Wouters EF. Mortality and mortality-related factors after hospitalization for acute exacerbation of COPD. Chest 2003; 124(2):459–467.

65. Mushlin AI, Black ER, Connolly CA, Buonaccorso KM, Eberly SW. The necessary length of hospital stay for chronic pulmonary disease. J Am Med Assoc 1991; 266(1):80–83.

66. Seneff MG, Wagner DP, Wagner RP, Zimmerman JE, Knaus WA. Hospital and 1-year survival of patients admitted to intensive care units with acute exacerbation of chronic obstructive pulmonary disease. J Am Med Assoc 1995; 274:1852–1857.

67. Connors AF, Jr., Dawson NV, Thomas C, Harrell FE, Jr., Desbiens N, Fulkerson WJ, Kussin P, Bellamy P, Goldman L, Knaus WA. Outcomes following acute exacerbation of severe chronic obstructive lung disease. The SUPPORT investigators (Study to Understand Prognoses and Preferences for Outcomes and Risks of Treatments). Am J Respir Crit Care Med 1996; 154(4 Pt 1):959–967.

68. Sluiter HJ, Blokzijl EJ, van Dijl W, van Haeringen JR, Hilvering C, Steenhuis EJ. Conservative and respirator treatment of acute respiratory insufficiency in patients with chronic obstructive lung disease. A reappraisal. Am Rev Respir Dis 1972; 105(6):932–943.

69. Warren PM, Flenley DC, Millar JS, Avery A. Respiratory failure revisited: acute exacerbations of chronic bronchitis between 1961–68 and 1970–76. Lancet 1980; 1(8166):467–470.

70. Jeffrey AA, Warren PM, Flenley DC. Acute hypercapnic respiratory failure in patients with chronic obstructive lung disease: risk factors and use of guidelines for management. Thorax 1992; 47(1):34–40.

71. Plant PK, Owen JL, Elliott MW. One year period prevalence study of respiratory acidosis in acute exacerbations of COPD: implications for the provision of noninvasive ventilation and oxygen administration. Thorax 2000; 55(7):550–554.

72. Soo Hoo GW, Hakimian N, Santiago SM. Hypercapnic respiratory failure in COPD patients: response to therapy. Chest 2000; 117(1):169–177.

73. Vitacca M, Clini E, Porta R, Foglio K, Ambrosino N. Acute exacerbations in patients with COPD: predictors of need for mechanical ventilation. Eur Respir J 1996; 9(7):1487–1493.

74. Roberts CM, Lowe D, Bucknall CE, Ryland I, Kelly Y, Pearson MG. Clinical audit indicators of outcome following admission to hospital with acute exacerbation of chronic obstructive pulmonary disease. Thorax 2002; 57(2):137–141.

75. Pauwels RA, Buist AS, Ma P, Jenkins CR, Hurd SS. Global strategy for the diagnosis, management, and prevention of chronic obstructive pulmonary disease: National Heart, Lung, and Blood Institute and World Health Organization Global Initiative for Chronic Obstructive Lung Disease (GOLD): executive summary. Respir Care 2001; 46(8):798–825.

76. Bleecker ER, Britt EJ. Acute bronchodilating effects of ipratropium bromide and theophylline in chronic obstructive pulmonary disease. Am J Med 1991; 91(4):24S–27S.

77. Zehner WJ Jr, Scott JM, Iannolo PM, Ungaro A, Terndrup TE. Terbutaline vs. albuterol for out-of-hospital respiratory distress: randomized, double-blind trial. Acad Emerg Med 1995; 2(8):686–691.

78. Volta CA, Alvisi R, Marangoni E, Righini ER, Verri M, Ragazzi R, Alvisi V, Ferri E, Milic-Emili J. Responsiveness to intravenous administration of salbutamol in chronic obstructive pulmonary disease patients with acute respiratory failure. Intensive Care Med 2001; 27(12):1949–1953.

79. Tantucci C, Duguet A, Similowski T, Zelter M, Derenne JP, Milic-Emili J. Effect of salbutamol on dynamic hyperinflation in chronic obstructive pulmonary disease patients. Eur Respir J 1998; 12(4):799–804.

80. Karpel JP, Pesin J, Greenberg D, Gentry E. A comparison of the effects of ipratropium bromide and metaproterenol sulfate in acute exacerbations of COPD. Chest 1990; 98(4):835–839.

81. Easton PA, Jadue C, Dhingra S, Anthonisen NR. A comparison of the bronchodilating effects of a beta-2 adrenergic agent (albuterol) and an anticholinergic agent (ipratropium bromide), given by aerosol alone or in sequence. N Engl J Med 1986; 315(12): 735–739.

82. Moayyedi P, Congleton J, Page RL, Pearson SB, Muers MF. Comparison of nebulised salbutamol and ipratropium bromide with salbutamol alone in the treatment of chronic obstructive pulmonary disease. Thorax 1995; 50(8):834–837.

83. Koutsogiannis Z, Kelly AM. Does high dose ipratropium bromide added to salbutamol improve pulmonary function for patients with chronic obstructive airways disease in the emergency department? Aust N Z J Med 2000; 30(1): 38–40.

84. Patrick DM, Dales RE, Stark RM, Laliberte G, Dickinson G. Severe exacerbations of COPD and asthma. Incremental benefit of adding ipratropium to usual therapy. Chest 1990; 98(2):295–297.

85. O'Driscoll BR, Taylor RJ, Horsley MG, Chambers DK, Bernstein A. Nebulised salbutamol with and without ipratropium bromide in acute airflow obstruction. Lancet 1989; 1(8652):1418–1420.

86. Lloberes P, Ramis L, Montserrat JM, Serra J, Campistol J, Picado C, Agusti-Vidal A. Effect of three different bronchodilators during an exacerbation of chronic obstructive pulmonary disease. Eur Respir J 1988; 1(6):536–539.

87. Cydulka RK, Emerman CL. Effects of combined treatment with glycopyrrolate and albuterol in acute exacerbation of chronic obstructive pulmonary disease. Ann Emerg Med 1995; 25(4):470–473.

88. Shrestha M, O'Brien T, Haddox R, Gourlay HS, Reed G. Decreased duration of emergency department treatment of chronic obstructive pulmonary disease exacerbations with the addition of ipratropium bromide to β-agonist therapy. Ann Emerg Med 1991; 20(11):1206–1209.

89. COMBIVENT Inhalation Aerosol Study Group. In chronic obstructive pulmonary disease, a combination of ipratropium and albuterol is more effective than either agent alone. An 85-day multicenter trial. Chest 1994; 105(5):1411–1419.

90. Gross N, Tashkin D, Miller R, Oren J, Coleman W, Linberg S. Inhalation by nebulization of albuterol-ipratropium combination (Dey combination) is superior to either agent alone in the treatment of chronic obstructive pulmonary disease. Dey Combination Solution Study Group. Respiration 1998; 65(5):354–362.

91. Campbell S. For COPD a combination of ipratropium bromide and albuterol sulfate is more effective than albuterol base. Arch Intern Med 1999; 159(2):156–160.

92. BTS guidelines for the management of chronic obstructive pulmonary disease. The COPD Guidelines Group of the Standards of Care Committee of the BTS. Thorax 1997; 52(suppl 5):S1–S28.

93. Salpeter SR, Ormiston TM, Salpeter EE. Cardiovascular effects of beta-agonists in patients with asthma and COPD: a meta-analysis. Chest 2004; 125(6): 2309–2321.

94. Gross NJ, Bankwala Z. Effects of an anticholinergic bronchodilator on arterial blood gases of hypoxemic patients with chronic obstructive pulmonary disease. Comparison with a beta-adrenergic agent. Am Rev Respir Dis 1987; 136(5): 1091–1094.

95. Asmus MJ, Sherman J, Hendeles L. Bronchoconstrictor additives in bronchodilator solutions. J Allergy Clin Immunol 1999; 104(2 Pt 2):S53–S60.

96. Shrestha M, Bidadi K, Gourlay S, Hayes J. Continuous vs. intermittent albuterol, at high and low doses, in the treatment of severe acute asthma in adults. Chest 1996; 110(1):42–47.

97. Khine H, Fuchs SM, Saville AL. Continuous vs. intermittent nebulized albuterol for emergency management of asthma. Acad Emerg Med 1996; 3(11):1019–1024.

98. Reisner C, Kotch A, Dworkin G. Continuous versus frequent intermittent nebuliza-tion of albuterol in acute asthma: a randomized, prospective study. Ann Allergy Asthma Immunol 1995; 75(1):41–47.

99. Rodrigo GJ, Rodrigo C. Continuous vs. intermittent beta-agonists in the treatment of acute adult asthma: a systematic review with meta-analysis. Chest 2002; 122(1):160–165.

100. Vathenen AS, Britton JR, Ebden P, Cookson JB, Wharrad HJ, Tattersfield AE. High-dose inhaled albuterol in severe chronic airflow limitation. Am Rev Respir Dis 1988; 138(4):850–855.

101. Gross NJ, Petty TL, Friedman M, Skorodin MS, Silvers GW, Donohue JF. Dose response to ipratropium as a nebulized solution in patients with chronic obstructive pul-monary disease. A three-center study. Am Rev Respir Dis 1989; 139(5):1188–1191.

102. Emerman CL, Cydulka RK. Effect of different albuterol dosing regimens in the treatment of acute exacerbation of chronic obstructive pulmonary disease. Ann Emerg Med 1997; 29(4):474–478.

103. Costello J. Prospects for improved therapy in chronic obstructive pulmonary disease by the use of levalbuterol. J Allergy Clin Immunol 1999; 104(2 Pt 2): S61–S68.

104. Datta D, Vitale A, Lahiri B, ZuWallack R. An evaluation of nebulized levalbuterol in stable COPD. Chest 2003; 124(3):844–849.

105. Hendeles L, Hartzema A. Levalbuterol is not more cost-effective than albuterol for COPD. Chest 2003; 124(3):1176–1178.

106. Truitt T, Witko J, Halpern M. Levalbuterol compared to racemic albuterol: efficacy and outcomes in patients hospitalized with COPD or asthma. Chest 2003; 123(1): 128–135.

107. Cazzola M, Califano C, Di Perna F, D'Amato M, Terzano C, Matera MG, D'Amato G, Marsico SA. Acute effects of higher than customary doses of salmeterol and salbutamol in patients with acute exacerbation of COPD. Respir Med 2002; 96(10):790–795.

108. Cazzola M, D'Amato M, Califano C, Di Perna F, Calderaro E, Matera MG, D'Amato G. Formoterol as dry powder oral inhalation compared with salbutamol metered-dose inhaler in acute exacerbations of chronic obstructive pulmonary disease. Clin Ther 2002; 24(4):595–604.

109. Jasper AC, Mohsenifar Z, Kahan S, Goldberg HS, Koerner SK. Cost-benefit comparison of aerosol bronchodilator delivery methods in hospitalized patients. Chest 1987; 91(4): 614–618.

110. Berry RB, Shinto RA, Wong FH, Despars JA, Light RW. Nebulizer vs. spacer for bronchodilator delivery in patients hospitalized for acute exacerbations of COPD. Chest 1989; 96(6):1241–1246.

111. Maguire GP, Newman T, DeLorenzo LJ, Brown RB, Stone D. Comparison of a hand-held nebulizer with a metered dose inhaler-spacer combination in acute obstructive pulmonary disease. Chest 1991; 100(5):1300–1305.

112. Turner MO, Patel A, Ginsburg S, FitzGerald JM. Bronchodilator delivery in acute airflow obstruction. A meta-analysis. Arch Intern Med 1997; 157(15): 1736–1744.

113. Sethi S, Murphy TF. Bacterial infection in chronic obstructive pulmonary disease in 2000: a state-of-the-art review. Clin Microbiol Rev 2001; 14(2):336–363.

114. Sethi S, Evans N, Grant BJ, Murphy TF. New strains of bacteria and exacerbations of chronic obstructive pulmonary disease. N Engl J Med 2002; 347(7):465–471.

115. Sethi S, Muscarella K, Evans N, Klingman KL, Grant BJ, Murphy TF. Airway inflammation and etiology of acute exacerbations of chronic bronchitis. Chest 2000; 118(6):1557–1565.

116. White AJ, Gompertz S, Bayley DL, Hill SL, O'Brien C, Unsal I, Stockley RA. Resolution of bronchial inflammation is related to bacterial eradication following treatment of exacerbations of chronic bronchitis. Thorax 2003; 58(8):680–685.

117. Yi K, Sethi S, Murphy TF. Human immune response to nontypeable Haemophilus influenzae in chronic bronchitis. J Infect Dis 1997; 176(5):1247–1252.

118. Hirschmann JV. Do bacteria cause exacerbations of COPD? Chest 2000; 118(1):193–203.

119. Murphy TF, Sethi S, Niederman MS. The role of bacteria in exacerbations of COPD: a constructive view. Chest 2000; 118(1):204–209.

120. Saint S, Bent S, Vittinghoff E, Grady D. Antibiotics in chronic obstructive pulmonary disease exacerbations. A meta-analysis. J Am Med Assoc 1995; 273(12):957–960.

121. Sachs AP, Koeter GH, Groenier KH, van der WD, Schiphuis J, Meyboom-de Jong B. Changes in symptoms, peak expiratory flow, and sputum flora during treatment with antibiotics of exacerbations in patients with chronic obstructive pulmonary disease in general practice. Thorax 1995; 50(7):758–763.

122. Allegra L, Blasi F, de Bernardi B, Cosentini R, Tarsia P. Antibiotic treatment and baseline severity of disease in acute exacerbations of chronic bronchitis: a re-evaluation of previously published data of a placebo-controlled randomized study. Pulm Pharmacol Ther 2001; 14(2):149–155.

123. Chodosh S, McCarty J, Farkas S, Drehobl M, Tosiello R, Shan M, Aneiro L, Kowalsky S. Randomized, double-blind study of ciprofloxacin and cefuroxime axetil for treatment of acute bacterial exacerbations of chronic bronchitis. The Bronchitis Study Group. Clin Infect Dis 1998; 27(4):722–729.

124. Chodosh S, Schreurs A, Siami G, Barkman HW, Jr., Anzueto A, Shan M, Moesken H, Stack T, Kowalsky S. Efficacy of oral ciprofloxacin vs. clarithromycin for treatment of acute bacterial exacerbations of chronic bronchitis. The Bronchitis Study Group. Clin Infect Dis 1998; 27(4):730–738.

125. Amsden GW, Baird IM, Simon S, Treadway G. Efficacy and safety of azithromycin vs. levofloxacin in the outpatient treatment of acute bacterial exacerbations of chronic bronchitis. Chest 2003; 123(3):772–777.

126. Anzueto A, Rizzo JA, Grossman RF. The infection-free interval: its use in evaluating antimicrobial treatment of acute exacerbation of chronic bronchitis. Clin Infect Dis 1999; 28(6):1344–1345.

127. Nouira S, Marghli S, Belghith M, Besbes L, Elatrous S, Abroug F. Once daily oral ofloxacin in chronic obstructive pulmonary disease exacerbation requiring mechanical ventilation: a randomised placebo-controlled trial. Lancet 2001; 358(9298):2020–2025.

128. Sethi S. Infectious exacerbations of chronic bronchitis: diagnosis and management. J Antimicrob Chemother 1999; 43(suppl A):97–105.

129. Fogarty CM, Kohno S, Buchanan P, Aubier M, Baz M. Community-acquired respiratory tract infections caused by resistant pneumococci: clinical and bacteriological efficacy of the ketolide telithromycin. J Antimicrob Chemother 2003; 51(4):947–955.

130. Destache CJ, Dewan N, O'Donohue WJ, Campbell JC, Angelillo VA. Clinical and economic considerations in the treatment of acute exacerbations of chronic bronchitis. J Antimicrob Chemother 1999; 43(suppl A):107–113.

131. Grossman R, Mukherjee J, Vaughan D, Eastwood C, Cook R, LaForge J, Lampron N. A 1-year community-based health economic study of ciprofloxacin vs. usual antibiotic treatment in acute exacerbations of chronic bronchitis: the Canadian Ciprofloxacin Health Economic Study Group. Chest 1998; 113(1):131–141.

132. Adams SG, Melo J, Luther M, Anzueto A. Antibiotics are associated with lower relapse rates in outpatients with acute exacerbations of COPD. Chest 2000; 117(5): 1345–1352.

133. Sin DD, Tu JV. Outpatient antibiotic therapy and short term mortality in elderly patients with chronic obstructive pulmonary disease. Can Respir J 2000; 7(6):466–471.

134. Davidson R, Cavalcanti R, Brunton JL, Bast DJ, de Azavedo JC, Kibsey P, Fleming C, Low OE. Resistance to levofloxacin and failure of treatment of pneumococcal pneumonia. N Engl J Med 2002; 346(10): 747–750.

135. Sunyer J, Anto JM, Sabria J, Roca J, Morell F, Rodriguez-Roisin R, Rodrigo MJ. Relationship between serum IgE and airway responsiveness in adults with asthma. J Allergy Clin Immunol 1995; 95(3):699–706.

136. Tashkin DP, Altose MD, Bleecker ER, Connett JE, Kanner RE, Lee WW, Wise R. The lung health study: airway responsiveness to inhaled methacholine in smokers with mild to moderate airflow limitation. The Lung Health Study Research Group. Am Rev Respir Dis 1992; 145(2 Pt 1):301–310.

137. Keatings VM, Jatakanon A, Worsdell YM, Barnes PJ. Effects of inhaled and oral glucocorticoids on inflammatory indices in asthma and COPD. Am J Respir Crit Care Med 1997; 155(2):542–548.

138. Callahan CM, Dittus RS, Katz BP. Oral corticosteroid therapy for patients with stable chronic obstructive pulmonary disease. A meta-analysis. Ann Intern Med 1991; 114(3):216–223.

139. Albert RK, Martin TR, Lewis SW. Controlled clinical trial of methylprednisolone in patients with chronic bronchitis and acute respiratory insufficiency. Ann Intern Med 1980; 92(6):753–758.

140. Bullard MJ, Liaw SJ, Tsai YH, Min HP. Early corticosteroid use in acute exacerbations of chronic airflow obstruction. Am J Emerg Med 1996; 14(2):139–143.

141. Thompson WH, Nielson CP, Carvalho P, Charan NB, Crowley JJ. Controlled trial of oral prednisone in outpatients with acute COPD exacerbation. Am J Respir Crit Care Med 1996; 154(2 Pt 1):407–412.

142. Davies L, Nisar M, Pearson MG, Costello RW, Earis JE, Calverley PM. Oral corticosteroid trials in the management of stable chronic obstructive pulmonary disease. QJM 1999; 92(1):395–400.

143. Niewoehner DE, Erbland ML, Deupree RH, Collins D, Gross NJ, Light RW, Anderson P, Morgan NA. Effect of systemic glucocorticoids on exacerbations of chronic obstructive pulmonary disease. Department of Veterans Affairs Cooperative Study Group. N Engl J Med 1999; 340(25): 1941–1947.

144. Singh JM, Palda VA, Stanbrook MB, Chapman KR. Corticosteroid therapy for patients with acute exacerbations of chronic obstructive pulmonary disease: a systematic review. Arch Intern Med 2002; 162(22):2527–2536.

145. Sayiner A, Aytemur ZA, Cirit M, Unsal I. Systemic glucocorticoids in severe exacerbations of COPD. Chest 2001; 119(3):726–730.

146. Albert RK, Martin TR, Lewis SW. Controlled clinical trial of methylprednisolone in patients with chronic bronchitis and acute respiratory insufficiency. Ann Intern Med 1980; 92(6):753–758.

147. Becker JM, Arora A, Scarfone RJ, Spector ND, Fontana-Penn ME, Gracely E, Joffe MD, Goldsmith DP, Malatack JJ. Oral versus intravenous corticosteroids in children hospitalized with asthma. J Allergy Clin Immunol 1999; 103(4): 586–590.

148. Maltais F, Ostinelli J, Bourbeau J, Tonnel AB, Jacquemet N, Haddon J, Rouleau M, Boukhana U, Martinot JB, Duroux P. Comparison of nebulized budesonide and oral prednisolone with placebo in the treatment of acute exacerbations of chronic obstructive pulmonary disease: a randomized controlled trial. Am J Respir Crit Care Med 2002; 165(5):698–703.

149. Kwong FK, Sue MA, Klaustermeyer WB. Corticosteroid complications in respiratory disease. Ann Allergy 1987; 58(5):326–330.

150. Wiest PM, Flanigan T, Salata RA, Shlaes DM, Katzman M, Lederman MM. Serious infectious complications of corticosteroid therapy for COPD. Chest 1989; 95(6):1180–1184.

151. McEvoy CE, Niewoehner DE. Adverse effects of corticosteroid therapy for COPD. A critical review. Chest 1997; 111(3):732–743.

152. Stuck AE, Minder CE, Frey FJ. Risk of infectious complications in patients taking glucocorticosteroids. Rev Infect Dis 1989; 11(6):954–963.

153. Walsh LJ, Wong CA, Oborne J, Cooper S, Lewis SA, Pringle M, Hubbard R, Tattersfield AE. Adverse effects of oral corticosteroids in relation to dose in patients with lung disease. Thorax 2001; 56(4):279–284.

154. Schols AM, Wesseling G, Kester AD, de Vries G, Mostert R, Slangen J, Wouters EF. Dose dependent increased mortality risk in COPD patients treated with oral glucocorticoids. Eur Respir J 2001; 17(3): 337–342.

155. Aubier M, Murciano D, Milic-Emili J, Touaty E, Daghfous J, Pariente R, Derenne JP. Effects of the administration of O2 on ventilation and blood gases in patients with chronic obstructive pulmonary disease during acute respiratory failure. Am Rev Respir Dis 1980; 122(5):747–754.

156. Aubier M, Murciano D, Fournier M, Milic-Emili J, Pariente R, Derenne JP. Central respiratory drive in acute respiratory failure of patients with chronic obstructive pulmonary disease. Am Rev Respir Dis 1980; 122(2):191–199.

157. Sassoon CS, Hassell KT, Mahutte CK. Hyperoxic-induced hypercapnia in stable chronic obstructive pulmonary disease. Am Rev Respir Dis 1987; 135(4): 907–911.

158. Robinson TD, Freiberg DB, Regnis JA, Young IH. The role of hypoventilation and ventilation-perfusion redistribution in oxygen-induced hypercapnia during acute exacerbations of chronic obstructive pulmonary disease. Am J Respir Crit Care Med 2000; 161(5):1524–1529.

159. Campbell EJ. The J. Burns Amberson Lecture. The management of acute respiratory failure in chronic bronchitis and emphysema. Am Rev Respir Dis 1967; 96(4):626–639.

160. Smith JP, Stone RW, Muschenheim C. Acute respiratory failure in chronic lung disease. Observations on controlled oxygen therapy. Am Rev Respir Dis 1968; 97(5):791–803.

161. Bone RC, Pierce AK, Johnson RL, Jr. Controlled oxygen administration in acute respiratory failure in chronic obstructive pulmonary disease: a reappraisal. Am J Med 1978; 65(6):896–902.

162. Moloney ED, Kiely JL, McNicholas WT. Controlled oxygen therapy and carbon dioxide retention during exacerbations of chronic obstructive pulmonary disease. Lancet 2001; 357(9255):526–528.

163. Gomersall CD, Joynt GM, Freebairn RC, Lai CK, Oh TE. Oxygen therapy for hypercapnic patients with chronic obstructive pulmonary disease and acute respiratory failure: a randomized, controlled pilot study. Crit Care Med 2002; 30(1):113–116.

164. Plant PK, Owen JL, Elliott MW. One year period prevalence study of respiratory acidosis in acute exacerbations of COPD: implications for the provision of noninvasive ventilation and oxygen administration. Thorax 2000; 55(7):550–554.

165. Rice KL, Leatherman JW, Duane PG, Snyder LS, Harmon KR, Abel J, Niewoehner DE. Aminophylline for acute exacerbations of chronic obstructive pulmonary disease. A controlled trial. Ann Intern Med 1987; 107(3):305–309.

166. Barr RG, Rowe BH, Camargo CA, Jr. Methylxanthines for exacerbations of chronic obstructive pulmonary disease: meta-analysis of randomised trials. BMJ 2003; 327(7416):643.

167. Black PN Ram FS, Poole PJ, Bagg W, Stewart J, Black PN. Randomised, controlled trial of theophylline for the treatment of exacerbations of COPD. Am J Respir Crit Care Med 2000; 161(3):A489.

168. Peleman RA, Kips JC, Pauwels RA. Therapeutic activities of theophylline in chronic obstructive pulmonary disease. Clin Exp Allergy 1998; 28(suppl 3):53–56.

169. Barnes PJ. Theophylline: new perspectives for an old drug. Am J Respir Crit Care Med 2003; 167(6):813–818.

170. Murciano D, Aubier M, Lecocguic Y, Pariente R. Effects of theophylline on dia-phragmatic strength and fatigue in patients with chronic obstructive pulmonary disease. N Engl J Med 1984; 311(6):349–353.

171. ZuWallack RL, Mahler DA, Reilly D, Church N, Emmett A, Rickard K, Knobil K. Salmeterol plus theophylline combination therapy in the treatment of COPD. Chest 2001; 119(6):1661–1670.

172. Lam A, Newhouse MT. Management of asthma and chronic airflow limitation. Are methylxanthines obsolete? Chest 1990; 98(1):44–52.

173. Gamble E, Grootendorst DC, Brightling CE, Troy S, Qiu Y, Zhu J, Parker D, Martin D, Majumdar S, Vignola AM et al. Antiinflammatory effects of the phos-phodiesterase-4 inhibitor cilomilast (Ariflo) in chronic obstructive pulmonary disease. Am J Respir Crit Care Med 2003; 168(8):976–982.

174. Compton CH, Gubb J, Nieman R, Edelson J, Amit O, Bakst A, Ayres JG, Creemers JP, Schultze-Werninghaus G, Brombilla C et al. Cilomilast, a selective phosphodiesterase-4 inhibitor for treatment of patients with chronic obstructive pulmonary disease: a randomised, dose-ranging study. Lancet 2001; 358(9278):265–270.

175. Vignola AM. PDE4 inhibitors in COPD—a more selective approach to treatment. Respir Med 2004; 98(6):495–503.

176. Manthous CA Morgan S, Pohlman A, Hall JB. Heliox in the treatment of airflow obstruction: a critical review of the literature. Respiratory Care 1997; 42(11): 1034–1042.

177. Kass JE, Terregino CA. The effect of heliox in acute severe asthma: a randomized controlled trial. Chest 1999; 116(2):296–300.

178. Manthous CA, Hall JB, Caputo MA, Walter J, Klocksieben JM, Schmidt GA, Wood LD. Heliox improves pulsus paradoxus and peak expiratory flow in non-intubated patients with severe asthma. Am J Respir Crit Care Med 1995; 151(2 Pt 1):310–314.

179. Kass JE, Castriotta RJ. Heliox therapy in acute severe asthma. Chest 1995; 107(3):757–760.

180. Kress JP, Noth I, Gehlbach BK, Barman N, Pohlman AS, Miller A, Morgan S, Hall JB. The utility of albuterol nebulized with heliox during acute asthma exacer-bations. Am J Respir Crit Care Med 2002; 165(9):1317–1321.

181. Gerbeaux P, Gainnier M, Boussuges A, Rakotonirina J, Nelh P, Torro D, Arnal JM, Jean P. Use of heliox in patients with severe exacerbation of chronic obstructive pulmonary disease. Crit Care Med 2001; 29(12):2322–2324.

182. DeBoisblanc BP, Burch WC Jr, Buechner HA, Haponik EF. Computed tomo-graphic appearance of an oleothorax. Thorax 1988; 43(7):572–573.

183. Jaber S, Carlucci A, Boussarsar M, Fodil R, Pigeot J, Maggiore S Harf A, Isabey D, Brochard L. Helium–oxygen in the postextubation period decreases inspiratory effort. Am J Respir Crit Care Med 2001; 164(4): 633–637.

184. Jolliet P, Tassaux D, Roeseler J, Burdet L, Broccard A, D'Hoore W, Borst F, Reynaert M, Schaller MD, Cherrolet JC. Helium–oxygen versus air–oxygen non-invasive pressure support in decompensated chronic obstructive disease: A prospec-tive, multicenter study. Crit Care Med 2003; 31(3):878–884.

185. Silverman RA, Osborn H, Runge J, Gallagher EJ, Chiang W, Feldman J, Gaeta T, Freeman K, Levin B, Mancherje N, et al. IV magnesium sulfate in the treatment of

acute severe asthma: a multicenter randomized controlled trial. Chest 2002; 122(2):489–497.

186. Skorodin MS, Tenholder MF, Yetter B, Owen KA, Waller RF, Khandelwahl S, Maki K, Rohail T, D'Alfonson N. Magnesium sulfate in exacerbations of chronic obstructive pulmonary disease. Arch Intern Med 1995; 155(5):496–500.

187. Moser KM, Luchsinger PC, Adamson JS, McMahon SM, Schlueter DP, Spivack M, Weg J. Respiratory stimulation with intravenous doxapram in respiratory failure. A double-blind co-operative study. N Engl J Med 1973; 288(9):427–431.

188. Angus RM, Ahmed AA, Fenwick LJ, Peacock AJ. Comparison of the acute effects on gas exchange of nasal ventilation and doxapram in exacerbations of chronic obstructive pulmonary disease. Thorax 1996; 51(10):1048–1050.

189. Kerr HD. Doxapram in hypercapnic chronic obstructive pulmonary disease with respiratory failure. J Emerg Med 1997; 15(4):513–515.

190. Wagenaar M, Vos P, Heijdra Y, Teppema L, Folgering H. Comparison of acetazo-lamide and medroxyprogesterone as respiratory stimulants in hypercapnic patients with COPD. Chest 2003; 123(5):1450–1459.

191. McCrory DC, Brown C, Gelfand SE, Bach PB. Management of acute exacerbations of COPD: a summary and appraisal of published evidence. Chest 2001; 119(4):1190–1209.

192. Wollmer P, Ursing K, Midgren B, Eriksson L. Inefficiency of chest percussion in the physical therapy of chronic bronchitis. Eur J Respir Dis 1985; 66(4):233–239.

193. Gerrits CM, Herings RM, Leufkens HG, Lammers JW. N-acetylcysteine reduces the risk of re-hospitalisation among patients with chronic obstructive pulmonary disease. Eur Respir J 2003; 21(5):795–798.

194. Dekhuijzen PN. Antioxidant properties of N-acetylcysteine: their relevance in relation to chronic obstructive pulmonary disease. Eur Respir J 2004; 23(4):629–636.

195. Peter JV, Moran JL, Phillips-Hughes J, Warn D. Noninvasive ventilation in acute respiratory failure—a meta-analysis update. Crit Care Med 2002; 30(3): 555–562.

196. Keenan SP, Sinuff T, Cook DJ, Hill NS. Which patients with acute exacerbation of chronic obstructive pulmonary disease benefit from noninvasive positive-pressure ven-tilation? A systematic review of the literature. Ann Intern Med 2003; 138(11):861–870.

197. Liesching T, Kwok H, Hill NS. Acute applications of noninvasive positive pressure ventilation. Chest 2003; 124(2):699–713.

198. Chu CM, Chan VL, Wong IW, Leung WS, Lin AW, Cheung KF. Noninvasive ventilation in patients with acute hypercapnic exacerbation of chronic obstructive pulmonary disease who refused endotracheal intubation. Crit Care Med 2004; 32(2):372–377.

199. Tobin MJ. Respiratory muscles in disease. Clin Chest Med 1988; 9(2):263–286.

200. Rochester DF. Respiratory muscle weakness, pattern of breathing, and CO_2 retention in chronic obstructive pulmonary disease. Am Rev Respir Dis 1991; 143(5 Pt 1):901–903.

201. Pepe PE, Marini JJ. Occult positive end-expiratory pressure in mechanically venti-lated patients with airflow obstruction: the auto-PEEP effect. Am Rev Respir Dis 1982; 126(1):166–170.

202. Marini JJ, Culver BH, Kirk W. Flow resistance of exhalation valves and positive end-expiratory pressure devices used in mechanical ventilation. Am Rev Respir Dis 1985; 131(6):850–854.

203. Ninane V, Yernault JC, De Troyer A. Intrinsic PEEP in patients with chronic obstructive pulmonary disease. Role of expiratory muscles. Am Rev Respir Dis 1993; 148(4 Pt 1):1037–1042.

204. Lessard MR, Lofaso F, Brochard L. Expiratory muscle activity increases intrinsic positive end-expiratory pressure independently of dynamic hyperinflation in mechanically ventilated patients. Am J Respir Crit Care Med 1995; 151(2 Pt 1): 562–569.

205. Brown D, Pierson D. Auto-PEEP is common in mechanically ventilated patients: a study of incidence, severity, and detection. Respir Care 1986; 31(11):1069–1074.

206. Smith TC, Marini JJ. Impact of PEEP on lung mechanics and work of breathing in severe airflow obstruction. J Appl Physiol 1988; 65(4):1488–1499.

207. Marini JJ, Rodriguez RM, Lamb V. The inspiratory workload of patient-initiated mechanical ventilation. Am Rev Respir Dis 1986; 134(5):902–909.

208. Kress JP, O'Connor MF, Schmidt GA. Clinical examination reliably detects intrinsic positive end-expiratory pressure in critically ill, mechanically ventilated patients. Am J Respir Crit Care Med 1999; 159(1):290–294.

209. Rossi A, Gottfried SB, Zocchi L, Higgs BD, Lennox S, Calverley PM, Begin P, Grassino A, Mili-Emili J. Measurement of static compliance of the total respiratory system in patients with acute respiratory failure during mechanical ventilation. The effect of intrinsic positive end-expiratory pressure. Am Rev Respir Dis 1985; 131(5):672–677.

210. Leatherman JW, Ravenscraft SA. Low measured auto-positive end-expiratory pressure during mechanical ventilation of patients with severe asthma: hidden auto-positive end-expiratory pressure. Crit Care Med 1996; 24(3):541–546.

211. Maltais F, Reissmann H, Navalesi P, Hernandez P, Gursahaney A, Ranieri VM, Sovilj M, Gottfried SB. Comparison of static and dynamic measurements of intrinsic PEEP in mechanically ventilated patients. Am J Respir Crit Care Med 1994; 150(6 Pt 1):1318–1324.

212. Petrof BJ, Legare M, Goldberg P, Milic-Emili J, Gottfried SB. Continuous positive airway pressure reduces work of breathing and dyspnea during weaning from mechanical ventilation in severe chronic obstructive pulmonary disease. Am Rev Respir Dis 1990; 141(2):281–289.

213. Zakynthinos SG, Vassilakopoulos T, Zakynthinos E, Roussos C, Tzelepis GE. Correcting static intrinsic positive end-expiratory pressure for expiratory muscle contraction. Validation of a new method. Am J Respir Crit Care Med 1999; 160(3):785–790.

214. Zakynthinos SG, Vassilakopoulos T, Zakynthinos E, Mavrommatis A, Roussos C. Contribution of expiratory muscle pressure to dynamic intrinsic positive end-expiratory pressure: validation using the Campbell diagram. Am J Respir Crit Care Med 2000; 162(5):1633–1640.

215. Younes M. Dynamic intrinsic PEEP (PEEP(i),dyn): is it worth saving? Am J Respir Crit Care Med 2000; 162(5):1608–1609.

216. Tuxen DV, Lane S. The effects of ventilatory pattern on hyperinflation, airway pressures, and circulation in mechanical ventilation of patients with severe airflow obstruction. Am Rev Respir Dis 1987; 136(4):872–879.

217. Laghi F, Segal J, Choe WK, Tobin MJ. Effect of imposed inflation time on respiratory frequency and hyperinflation in patients with chronic obstructive pulmonary disease. Am J Respir Crit Care Med 2001; 163(6):1365–1370.

218. Marini JJ. Should PEEP be used in airflow obstruction? Am Rev Respir Dis 1989; 140(1):1–3.
219. Tuxen DV. Detrimental effects of positive end-expiratory pressure during controlled mechanical ventilation of patients with severe airflow obstruction. Am Rev Respir Dis 1989; 140(1):5–9.
220. Tobin MJ, Lodato RF. PEEP, auto-PEEP, and waterfalls. Chest 1989; 96(3):449–451.
221. Hoffman RA, Ershowsky P, Krieger BP. Determination of auto-PEEP during spontaneous and controlled ventilation by monitoring changes in end-expiratory thoracic gas volume. Chest 1989; 96(3):613–616.
222. Brain JD, Valberg PA. Deposition of aerosol in the respiratory tract. Am Rev Respir Dis 1979; 120(6):1325–1373.
223. Fink JB, Dhand R, Duarte AG, Jenne JW, Tobin MJ. Aerosol delivery from a metered-dose inhaler during mechanical ventilation. An in vitro model. Am J Respir Crit Care Med 1996; 154(2 Pt 1):382–387.
224. O'Doherty MJ, Thomas SH, Page CJ, Treacher DF, Nunan TO. Delivery of a nebulized aerosol to a lung model during mechanical ventilation. Effect of ventilator settings and nebulizer type, position, and volume of fill. Am Rev Respir Dis 1992; 146(2):383–388.
225. Dhand R, Tobin MJ. Inhaled bronchodilator therapy in mechanically ventilated patients. Am J Respir Crit Care Med 1997; 156(1):3–10.
226. Duarte AG, Momii K, Bidani A. Bronchodilator therapy with metered-dose inhaler and spacer versus nebulizer in mechanically ventilated patients: comparison of magnitude and duration of response. Respir Care 2000; 45(7):817–823.
227. Dhand R, Duarte AG, Jubran A, Jenne JW, Fink JB, Fahey PJ, Tobin MJ. Dose-response to bronchodilator delivered by metered-dose inhaler in ventilator-supported patients. Am J Respir Crit Care Med 1996; 154(2 Pt 1):388–393.
228. Guerin C, Chevre A, Dessirier P, Poncet T, Bacquemin MH, Dequin PF, LeGuellec C, Jacque SD, Fournier G. Inhaled fenoterol-ipratropium bromide in mechanically ventilated patients with chronic obstructive pulmonary disease. Am J Respir Crit Care Med 1999; 159(4 Pt 1):1036–1042.
229. Miller DD, Amin MM, Palmer LB, Shah AR, Smaldone GC. Aerosol delivery and modern mechanical ventilation: in vitro/in vivo evaluation. Am J Respir Crit Care Med 2003; 168(10):1205–1209.
230. Duarte AG. Inhaled bronchodilator administration during mechanical ventilation. Respir Care 2004; 49(6):623–634.
231. Smaldone GC. Aerosolized bronchodilators in the intensive care unit: much ado about nothing? Am J Respir Crit Care Med 1999; 159(4 Pt 1):1029–1030.
232. Nava S, Compagnoni ML. Controlled short-term trial of fluticasone propionate in ventilator-dependent patients with COPD. Chest 2000; 118(4):990–999.
233. Tassaux D, Jolliet P, Roeseler J, Chevrolet JC. Effects of helium–oxygen on intrinsic positive end-expiratory pressure in intubated and mechanically ventilated patients with severe chronic obstructive pulmonary disease. Crit Care Med 2000; 28(8):2721–2728.
234. Diehl JL, Mercat A, Guerot E, Aissa F, Teboul JL, Richard C, Labrousse J. Helium/oxygen mixture reduces the work of breathing at the end of the weaning process in patients with severe chronic obstructive pulmonary disease. Crit Care Med 2003; 31(5):1415–1420.

235. Manthous CA MSPAHJ. Heliox in the treatment of airflow obstruction: a critical review of the literature. Respiratory Care 1997; 42(11):1034–1042.

236. Saudny-Unterberger H, Martin JG, Gray-Donald K. Impact of nutritional support on functional status during an acute exacerbation of chronic obstructive pulmonary disease. Am J Respir Crit Care Med 1997; 156(3 Pt 1):794–799.

237. Covelli HD, Black JW, Olsen MS, Beekman JF. Respiratory failure precipitated by high carbohydrate loads. Ann Intern Med 1981; 95(5):579–581.

238. Talpers SS, Romberger DJ, Bunce SB, Pingleton SK. Nutritionally associated increased carbon dioxide production. Excess total calories vs. high proportion of carbohydrate calories. Chest 1992; 102(2):551–555.

239. Angelillo VA, Bedi S, Durfee D, Dahl J, Patterson AJ, O'Donohue WJ, Jr. Effects of low and high carbohydrate feedings in ambulatory patients with chronic obstructive pulmonary disease and chronic hypercapnia. Ann Intern Med 1985; 103(6 Pt 1):883–885.

240. Nava S, Ambrosino N, Clini E, Prato M, Orlando G, Vitacca M, Brigada P, Fracchia C, Rogini F. Noninvasive mechanical ventilation in theweaning of patients with respiratory failure due to chronic obstructive pulmonary disease. A randomized, controlled trial. Ann Intern Med 1998; 128(9):721–728.

241. Girault C, Daudenthun I, Chevron V, Tamion F, Leroy J, Bonmarchand G. Noninvasive ventilation as a systematic extubation and weaning technique in acute-on-chronic respiratory failure: a prospective, randomized controlled study. Am J Respir Crit Care Med 1999; 160(1):86–92.

242. Ferrer M, Esquinas A, Arancibia F, Bauer TT, Gonzalez G, Carrillo A, Rodrigwez-Roisin R, Torres A. Noninvasive ventilation during persistent weaning failure: a randomized controlled trial. Am J Respir Crit Care Med 2003; 168(1):70–76.

243. Keenan SP, Powers C, McCormack DG, Block G. Noninvasive positive-pressure ventilation for postextubation respiratory distress: a randomized controlled trial. J Am Med Assoc 2002; 287(24):3238–3244.

244. Esteban A, Frutos-Vivar F, Ferguson ND, Arabi Y, Apezteguia C, Gonzalez M, Epstein SK, Hill NS, Nava S, Soares MA, et al. Noninvasive positive-pressure ventilation for respiratory failure after extubation. N Engl J Med 2004; 350(24):2452–2460.

245. Laghi F, Cattapan SE, Jubran A, Parthasarathy S, Warshawsky P, Choi YS, Togin MJ. Is weaning failure caused by low-frequency fatigue of the diaphragm? Am J Respir Crit Care Med 2003; 167(2):120–127.

246. Aldrich TK, Karpel JP, Uhrlass RM, Sparapani MA, Eramo D, Ferranti R. Weaning from mechanical ventilation: adjunctive use of inspiratory muscle resistive training. Crit Care Med 1989; 17(2):143–147.

247. Martin AD, Davenport PD, Franceschi AC, Harman E. Use of inspiratory muscle strength training to facilitate ventilator weaning: a series of 10 consecutive patients. Chest 2002; 122(1):192–196.

248. Pacht ER. Emergent bullectomy in a patient with severe bullous emphysema receiving mechanical ventilatory assistance. Chest 1995; 108(5):1454–1456.

249. Pacht ER. Emergent bullectomy in a patient with severe bullous emphysema receiving mechanical ventilatory assistance. Chest 1995; 108(5):1454–1456.

250. Criner GJ, O'Brien G, Furukawa S, Cordova F, Swartz M, Fallahnejad M, D'Aconzoe. Lung volume reduction surgery in ventilator-dependent COPD patients. Chest 1996; 110(4):877–884.

251. Low DE, Trulock EP, Kaiser LR, Pasque MK, Ettinger NA, Dresler C, Cooper JD. Lung transplantation of ventilator-dependent patients. The Washington University Lung Transplantation Group. Chest 1992; 101(1):8–11.

252. Maziak W, Loukides S, Culpitt S, Sullivan P, Kharitonov SA, Barnes PJ. Exhaled nitric oxide in chronic obstructive pulmonary disease. Am J Respir Crit Care Med 1998; 157(3 Pt 1): 998–1002.

253. Kharitonov SA, Barnes PJ. Exhaled markers of pulmonary disease. Am J Respir Crit Care Med 2001; 163(7):1693–1722.

254. Biernacki WA, Kharitonov SA, Barnes PJ. Increased leukotriene B4 and 8-isoprostane in exhaled breath condensate of patients with exacerbations of COPD. Thorax 2003; 58(4):294–298.

255. Montuschi P, Kharitonov SA, Ciabattoni G, Barnes PJ. Exhaled leukotrienes and prostaglandins in COPD. Thorax 2003; 58(7):585–588.

256. Chelluri L, Im KA, Belle SH, Schulz R, Rotondi AJ, Donahoe MP, Sirio CA, Mendelsohn AB, Pinsky MR. Long-term mortality and quality of life after prolonged mechanical ventilation. Crit Care Med 2004; 32(1):61–69.

257. Bach PB, Carson SS, Leff A. Outcomes and resource utilization for patients with prolonged critical illness managed by university-based or community-based subspecialists. Am J Respir Crit Care Med 1998; 158(5 Pt 1):1410–1415.

258. Scheinhorn DJ, Chao DC, Stearn-Hassenpflug M, LaBree LD, Heltsley DJ. Post-ICU mechanical ventilation: treatment of 1,123 patients at a regional weaning center. Chest 1997; 111(6):1654–1659.

259. Scheinhorn DJ, Chao DC, Stearn-Hassenpflug M. Liberation from prolonged mechanical ventilation. Crit Care Clin 2002; 18(3):569–595.

260. Pearlman RA. Variability in physician estimates of survival for acute respiratory failure in chronic obstructive pulmonary disease. Chest 1987; 91(4): 515–521.

261. Seneff MG, Wagner DP, Wagner RP, Zimmerman JE, Knaus WA. Hospital and 1-year survival of patients admitted to intensive care units with acute exacerbation of chronic obstructive pulmonary disease. J Am Med Assoc 1995; 274(23):1852–1857.

262. Wildman MJ, O'Dea J, Kostopoulou O, Tindall M, Walia S, Khan Z. Variation in intubation decisions for patients with chronic obstructive pulmonary disease in one critical care network. QJM 2003; 96(8):583–591.

263. Pearlman RA, Inui TS, Carter WB. Variability in physician bioethical decision-making. A case study of euthanasia. Ann Intern Med 1982; 97(3):420–425.

264. Fox E, Landrum-McNiff K, Zhong Z, Dawson NV, Wu AW, Lynn J. Evaluation of prognostic criteria for determining hospice eligibility in patients with advanced lung, heart, or liver disease. SUPPORT Investigators. Study to Understand Prognoses and Preferences for Outcomes and Risks of Treatments. J Am Med Assoc 1999; 282(17):1638–1645.

265. Nishimura K, Izumi T, Tsukino M, Oga T. Dyspnea is a better predictor of 5-year survival than airway obstruction in patients with COPD. Chest 2002; 121(5):1434–1440.

266. Domingo-Salvany A, Lamarca R, Ferrer M, Garcia-Aymerich J, Alonso J, Felez M, Khalaf A, Marrades RM, Monso E, Serra-Batlleset, et al. Health-related quality of life and mortality in male patients with chronic obstructive pulmonary disease. Am J Respir Crit Care Med 2002; 166(5):680–685.
267. Hansen-Flaschen J. Chronic obstructive pulmonary disease: the last year of life. Respir Care 2004; 49(1):90–97.
268. Gore JM, Brophy CJ, Greenstone MA. How well do we care for patients with end stage chronic obstructive pulmonary disease (COPD)? A comparison of palliative care and quality of life in COPD and lung cancer. Thorax 2000; 55(12):1000–1006.
269. Wenger NS, Phillips RS, Teno JM, Oye RK, Dawson NV, Liu H, Califf R, Layde P, Hakim R, Lynn J. Physician understanding of patient resuscitation preferences: insights and clinical implications. J Am Geriatr Soc 2000; 48(suppl 5):S44–S51.
270. Dales RE, O'Connor A, Hebert P, Sullivan K, McKim D, Llewellyn-Thomas H. Intubation and mechanical ventilation for COPD: development of an instrument to elicit patient preferences. Chest 1999; 116(3):792–800.
271. McNeely PD, Hebert PC, Dales RE, O'Connor AM, Wells G, McKim D, Sullivan KE. Deciding about mechanical ventilation in end-stage chronic obstructive pulmonary disease: how respirologists perceive their role. CMAJ 1997; 156(2):177–183.
272. Sullivan KE, Hebert PC, Logan J, O'Connor AM, McNeely PD. What do physicians tell patients with end-stage COPD about intubation and mechanical ventilation? Chest 1996; 109(1):258–264.
273. Claessens MT, Lynn J, Zhong Z, Desbiens NA, Phillips RS, Wu AW, Harrell FE, Connors AF. Dying with lung cancer or chronic obstructive pulmonary disease: insights from SUPPORT. Study to Understand Prognoses and Preferences for Outcomes and Risks of Treatments. J Am Geriatr Soc 2000; 48(suppl 5):S146–S153.

4

Hemoptysis

NADER KAMANGAR

Division of Pulmonary and Critical Care
Olive View–UCLA Medical Center
Geffen School of Medicine at UCLA
Los Angeles, California, U.S.A.

HSIN-YI LEE

Department of Imaging
VA Greater Los Angeles Healthcare
    System and Geffen School of
    Medicine at UCLA
Los Angeles, California, U.S.A.

SILVERIO SANTIAGO

Pulmonary and Critical Care Section
    West Los Angeles Healthcare Center
    VA Greater Los Angeles Healthcare System
    and Geffen School of Medicine at UCLA
Los Angeles, California, U.S.A.

I. Introduction

Hemoptysis is defined as the expectoration of blood that originates from the tracheobronchial tree or the pulmonary parenchyma. It can be the presenting sign of serious pulmonary and cardiac disorders and needs to be differentiated from blood loss arising from the upper respiratory tract or the gastrointestinal tract. Blood loss from a variety of nonpulmonary sources can also be aspirated and later expectorated, thus confounding this differentiation. This is especially likely if bleeding originates from the vallecula and hypopharynx (1). If there is doubt about the source of bleeding, it should be assumed that the patient is bleeding from the tracheobronchial tree or pulmonary parenchyma.

It is usually not problematic to differentiate hemoptysis from hematemesis. Blood originating from the lungs is more likely to be bright red, mixed with sputum, and associated with cough, whereas blood originating from the gastrointestinal tract is more likely to be dark, mixed with food particles, and associated with nausea and vomiting. A history of underlying upper gastrointestinal disease or hepatic disease may also be valuable in helping elucidate a non-pulmonary origin of bleeding.

The initial step in the assessment of a patient with hemoptysis is dictated by the amount of expectorated blood. Hemoptysis can range from mild blood-streaked sputum to massive, life-threatening hemorrhage. Massive hemoptysis has been variously defined as expectoration of blood in the amount of 100 to 1000 mL during a 24-hour period. This highly variable amount is based on the fact that the anatomic dead space in most adults is 100–200 mL. Thus, it becomes apparent that even relatively small volumes of blood can lead to asphyxiation. Mortality rates as high as 75% are reported indicating the need for rapid implementation of an appropriate diagnostic and therapeutic plan (2,3). Fortunately, massive hemoptysis is rare, occurring in <5% of cases of hemoptysis (4,5).

II. Vascular Anatomy of the Lung

The lung receives its blood supply from two different circulations, the pulmonary and bronchial circulations. Since hemoptysis may occur from either circulation, it is essential to understand each of these systems.

A. Bronchial Circulation

The bronchial circulation is the source of bleeding in the majority of cases of hemoptysis, and it also represents the source of most episodes of massive hemoptysis. Unlike the pulmonary circulation, the bronchial circulation arises from the aorta and is under systemic pressure. Bronchial arteries originate directly from the descending thoracic aorta, most commonly (nearly 80%) between the levels of the T5 and T6 vertebrae (6). A number of anatomic variations have been described. Cauldwell described four classic origin variations in 1948: type 1 (40%)—two on the left and one on the right, presenting as an intercostobronchial (ICBT) trunk; type 2 (21%)—one on the left and one ICBT on the right; type 3 (20%)—two on the left and two on the right (one ICBT and one bronchial artery); and type 4 (9.7%)—one on the left and two on the right (one ICBT and one bronchial artery) (7). The right ICBT, the most consistently seen vessel at angiography, usually arises from the right posterolateral aspect of the thoracic aorta. The right and left bronchial arteries, on the other hand, typically branch from the anterolateral aspect of the aorta (8). It is important to note that the anterior medullary branch supplying the anterior spinal artery is known to arise from the right ICBT in 5% of the population. Left bronchial arteries, on the other hand, rarely supply the anterior spinal artery. Other aberrant origins of the bronchial arteries include the aortic arch, the abdominal aorta, and the subclavian, thyrocervical, internal mammary, innominate, pericardiophrenic, superior intercostal, and inferior phrenic arteries.

The bronchial arteries send branches to the esophagus, trachea, pericardium, hilar nodes, and visceral pleura. As they enter the lungs at the hilar region, they follow the branches of the bronchial tree, giving rise to small penetrating arteries that form submucosal plexi supplying the bronchial mucosa. There are anastamoses between the bronchial and pulmonary circulations at the level of both medium-sized arteries and precapillary vessels (9).

The bronchial circulation plays an important role in hemoptysis by virtue of its close association with the entire length of the tracheobronchial tree. Massive hemoptysis generally involves bleeding from the bronchial circulation or, less frequently, from a pulmonary artery that is pathologically exposed to the high pressure bronchial circulation through enlarged bronchopulmonary anastamoses.

The response of the bronchial circulation to both acute and chronic disease involves vascular proliferation. The ability to proliferate distinguishes the bronchial from the pulmonary circulation. Mechanisms by which massive hemoptysis is produced include the following (10):

1. Chronic parenchymal inflammation leading to erosion of bronchial and vascular walls, enlargement and proliferation of bronchial vessels, formation of anastamoses between bronchial and pulmonary circulation, and formation of bronchiectasis or lung abscesses.
2. Various vascular alterations, such as aneurysmal formation, vasculitis (Goodpasture's syndrome, systemic lupus erythematosus, idiopathic pulmonary hemosiderosis), and pulmonary embolism.
3. Erosion of a calcified lymph node into the tracheobronchial tree (broncholithiasis) with disruption of peribronchial and submucosal blood vessels.
4. Vascular invasion by tumor.

Hence, the bronchial circulation is the usual source of bleeding in chronic parenchymal lung infections, such as lung abscesses, mycetomas, chronic fungal infections, and pulmonary tuberculosis. It is also the source of bleeding in bronchogenic carcinoma, endobronchial metastases, congenital heart disease, and broncholithiasis.

B. Pulmonary Circulation

The pulmonary circulation is a low-pressure circuit with normal pressures of 15–20 mmHg systolic and 5–10 mmHg diastolic. However, these pressures may rise to approach systemic pressures in both pulmonary vascular and parenchymal diseases. Although the pulmonary arteries travel alongside the bronchial tree, they only interact with the airways at the level of the terminal bronchiole. It is there where they branch extensively, forming the capillary bed around the alveoli and allowing for efficient gas exchange (9).

Aneurysms and false aneurysms of the pulmonary artery, arteriovenous malformations (AVMs), and iatrogenic pulmonary artery rupture by balloon flotation pulmonary arterial catheters are common causes of bleeding arising from the pulmonary circulation. Additionally, pulmonary arterial bleeding has been observed in a variety of destructive pulmonary processes, such as tuberculosis, lung abscesses, and aspergillomas (11).

C. Non-Bronchial Systemic Collateral Circulation

Systemic arteries may cross the pleural space and neovascularize the lung in a number of disease processes associated with inflammation of the lung parenchyma and the pleura. Such vascular networks arising from systemic arteries are commonly seen in cystic fibrosis and aspergillomas. New collaterals from the bronchial arteries or adjacent intrathoracic systemic arteries may also develop (12). Nonbronchial collateral arteries commonly arise from the phrenic, intercostal, subclavian, and axillary arteries. The internal mammary, coronary, or carotid arteries represent some of the more unusual sources. Such exuberant networks of collaterals can undermine the success of bronchial artery embolization (9,12).

III. Etiology

Hemoptysis may result from a broad range of etiologies, including many systemic illnesses. Some of the most common causes are listed in Table 1. The frequency of reported causes varies with the demography of the population studied. In addition, in contrast to older studies which list tuberculosis, bronchiectasis, and lung abscesses as the most common causes, more recent studies demonstrate a different trend. For example, in one retrospective investigation of elderly males, the most common causes were pulmonary carcinoma (29%), bronchitis (23%), idiopathic (22%), and infectious causes (12%), with tuberculosis accounting for only 6% of cases (13). In another retrospective study, 37% suffered from bronchitis, 19% from bronchogenic carcinoma, 6% from infectious causes, and only 7% from mycobacterium tuberculosis (14). Similarly, a recent report from a tertiary referral hospital listed bronchiectasis in 20%, bronchogenic cancer in 19%, infectious causes in 16%, and tuberculosis in only 1.4% (15). Tuberculosis, however, continues to be a leading cause of hemoptysis in underdeveloped countries (16). Additionally, paragonomiasis continues to be a major cause of hemoptysis in Southeast Asia (17).

The quantity of blood loss cannot be used to determine the etiology of hemoptysis with certainty. However, certain causes of hemoptysis which are more likely to be associated with massive hemoptysis are listed in Table 2. As noted, tuberculosis and bronchiectasis have become less common causes of massive hemoptysis. The survival of more patients with cystic fibrosis into adulthood has made this a more common etiology of massive hemoptysis (18). Similarly, early recognition and treatment of arteriovenous malformations (AVMs) have increased the survival of patients with hereditary hemorrhagic telangiectasia (HHT), with a large number of these patients presenting with recurrent episodes of massive hemoptysis (19).

Table 1 Causes of Hemoptysis

Infection
  Necrotizing pneumonia (Staphyloccus,
    Klebsiella, Gram-negatives,
    Anaerobes, Legionella)
  Anaerobic lung abscess
  Bronchitis, acute or chronic
  Mycetoma
  Parasitic (Paragonimiasis, Echinococcus,
    Ascariasis, Amebiasis,
    Schistosomiasis, Strongyloidiasis,
    Ancylostomiasis)
  Fungal pneumonia (Aspergillosis,
    Mucormycosis, Coccidioidomycosis,
    Histoplasmosis, Blastomycosis)
  Viral pneumonia (Varicella, Influenza)
  Infected pulmonary sequestration
  Septic pulmonary emboli
Neoplastic
  Bronchogenic carcinoma
  Bronchial adenoma
  Metastatic carcinoma
Pulmonary venous hypertension
  Mitral stenosis
  Left ventricular failure
  Fibrosing mediastinitis
  Pulmonary veno-occlusive disease
  Pulmonary vein congenital stenosis
Vascular
  Arteriovenous malformation
  Pulmonary hypertension
  Aortic aneurysm
  Vascular prosthesis
Traumatic
  Aortic aneurysm
  Pulmonary contusion
  Pulmonary laceration
  Thoracic splenosis
  Ruptured bronchus
  Fat embolism
  Lightning injury
  Aorto-bronchial fistula
  Tracheal-innominate artery fistula
  Coronary artery-bronchial fistula

Systemic disease
  Goodpasture's syndrome
  Idiopathic pulmonary hemosiderosis
  Systemic lupus erythematosus
  Other pulmonary vasculitis
    (Wegener's granulomatosis,
    Henoch-Schonlein purpura,
    Churg-Strauss syndrome,
    Bechet's syndrome)
Hematologic
  Disseminated intravascular
    coagulation
  Thrombocytopenia
  Platelet dysfunction
  Coagulopathy
Pulmonary
  Bronchiectasis
  Bronchitis
  Pulmonary embolism
  Bullous emphysema
  Cystic fibrosis
Iatrogenic
  Right heart catheterization
  Bronchoscopy
  Transtracheal aspiration
  Transbronchial biopsy
  Endobronchial biopsy
Pseudohemoptysis
  Serratia marcescens pneumonia
Drugs/toxins
  Nitrofurantoin
  Aspirin
  Anticoagulants
  Cocaine
  Penicillamine
  Trimellitic anhydride
  Solvents
Miscellaneous
  Broncholithiasis
  Endometriosis (catamenial hemoptysis)
  Aspirated foreign body
  Amyloidosis
  Lymphangioleiomyomatosis
  Cryptogenic hemoptysis

Table 2   Causes of Massive Hemoptysis

Cardiovascular disorders	Broncholithiasis
Pulmonary arteriovenous fistula	Tracheobronchial trauma
Mitral stenosis	Malignancies
Arteriobronchial fistula	Bronchogenic carcinoma
Septic pulmonary emboli	Bronchial adenoma
Pulmonary infarct, emboli	Metastatic carcinoma
Ruptured thoracic aneurysm	Leukemia
Infectious disorders	Diffuse parenchymal disease
Aspergilloma	Systemic lupus erythematosus
Tuberculosis	Idiopathic pulmonary hemosiderosis
Paragonimiasis	Goodpasture's syndrome
Coccidioidomycosis	Wegener's greanulomatosis
Lung abscess, necrotizing	Polyarteritis nodosa
pneumonia	Bechet's disease
Hydatid cyst	Lymphangioleiomyomatosis
Sporotrichosis	Iatrogenic
Mucormycosis	Bronchoscopy
Atypical mycobacterial infection	Pulmonary artery rupture
Tracheobronchial disorders	Tracheo-artery fistula
Bronchitis	Malposition of chest tube
Bronchiectasis	Miscellaneous
Bronchogenic carcinoma	Anticoagulant therapy
Cystic fibrosis	Coagulopathies
Foreign body aspiration	Thrombocytopenia

A.   Infections

Infection is a common cause of hemoptysis, especially in underdeveloped countries. Although the incidence of tuberculosis, mycetomas, and lung abscesses is declining, they continue to be significant causes of massive hemoptysis.

Tuberculosis

Hemoptysis complicates the course of approximately 25% of all cases of tuberculosis (20,21). Hemoptysis in patients with tuberculosis occurs through a variety of mechanisms. The pathological lesions responsible for bleeding include:

1.   Rupture of Rasmussen's aneurysms, which represent small ectatic portions of pulmonary arteries traversing thick walled cavities of chronic tuberculosis (22). Autopsy series from the 1930s and 1940s indicate that sudden, massive hemoptysis accounted for 5–7% of deaths in patients with longstanding tuberculosis (23,24).

2. Bronchial artery erosions from parenchymal/airway necrosis and tuberculous bronchiectasis (25). Additionally, healed calcified lymph nodes can impinge on the airway and erode through bronchial arteries. This is rarely preceded by the expectoration of the broncholith itself.
3. Chronic cavitary disease predisposing to the formation of secondary infections, such as mycetomas.

The course of hemoptysis from tuberculosis is commonly unpredictable, and the ability to predict if a sentinel bleed will proceed to massive hemoptysis is quite difficult. In a recent series of patients with massive hemoptysis, only 43% of patients had a previous episode of major hemoptysis (26). Of note, only a minority of patients with a history of tuberculosis who present with hemoptysis will have active tuberculosis.

Fungal Infections

Fungal infections can lead to hemoptysis by mechanisms similar to tuberculosis. These infections are increasing in frequency, particularly in immune-compromised patients. Aspergillus can cause hemoptysis via direct parenchymal invasion or by angioinvasion with distal infarction (27). Other invasive fungal infections, such as mucormycosis, cause hemoptysis by similar mechanisms. Although chronic cavitary coccidioidomycosis commonly causes hemoptysis, it is relatively uncommon in primary coccidioidomycosis. Acute histoplasma or blastomyces pneumonitis is rarely associated with bronchial mucosal erosion and variable degrees of hemoptysis (28). Broncholithiasis is another cause of hemoptysis related to histoplasmosis. In addition, hemoptysis has been reported in over 40% of patients with fibrosing mediastinitis complicating histoplasmosis (29).

Hemoptysis occurs in 50–78% of patients with aspergillomas and may be massive (30–34). Aspergillus fungus balls begin with colonization of pre-existing lung cavities and may not cause symptoms for years. However, the accompanying intense inflammation and neovascularization not infrequently lead to the occurrence of massive hemoptysis.

Lung Abscess

Anaerobic lung abscesses can cause sudden massive hemoptysis from erosion of a bronchial vessel in a cavity wall. These cavities can also erode into major pulmonary arteries and other thoracic vessels, such as the aorta (35). Although changes in both pulmonary and bronchial circulations occur, autopsy studies reveal that hemoptysis is likely due to destruction of fairly normal vessels by overwhelming inflammation (36).

Bacterial and Viral Infections

Bacterial and viral infections are less common causes of significant hemoptysis. However, it is not uncommon to see blood-streaked or "rusty" sputum in a variety of bacterial and viral pneumonias. Tissue necrosis is usually present when significant hemoptysis occurs in infections such as staphylococcus pneumonia or actinomycosis (37,38). Klebsiella pneumoniae pneumonia can mimic reactivation tuberculosis since patients can present with cavitary lesions and hemoptysis, which often resembles currant jelly (39). Varicella pneumonia associated with vesicular rupture and pulmonary infarction has also been reported as a cause of significant hemoptysis (40–43). Of note, Serratia marcescens, a common saprophyte of soil and water, can produce a red pigment in expectorated material, resulting in "pseudohemoptysis" (44,45).

Parasitic Infections

Parasitic infection is the most common cause of hemoptysis worldwide. Paragonimiasis, prevalent in Southeast Asia, is the leading parasitic disease causing hemoptysis (46,47). A variety of other parasites, such as Amoeba, Ascaris, Echinococcus, Ancylostoma, Necator, Clonorchis, Strongyloides, and Trichinella, may cause hemoptysis when they involve the lung.

B. Chronic Airway Inflammation

Bronchiectasis

Historically, bronchiectasis, along with tuberculosis and lung abscess, was the major cause of hemoptysis (2). Bronchiectasis during the early- to mid-20th century was attributable to tuberculosis, necrotizing pneumonia, and childhood infections such as whooping cough. Presently, however, cystic fibrosis, mucociliary clearance defects, and immune deficiencies represent more common causes of bronchiectasis.

Bronchiectasis is best characterized by bronchial dilatation, persistent bacterial colonization, chronic mucosal inflammation, and airway neovascularization (48). Hemoptysis occurs in 25–50% in patients with bronchiectasis (49). It can present as a single massive episode of hemorrhage, but is more commonly heralded by intermittent blood streaking intermixed with purulent sputum. In this condition, the bronchial arteries are hypertrophied and ectatic, and accompanied by enlarged submucosal anastomotic plexi in the bronchial walls. The bleeding is commonly brisk given that it originates from the bronchial circulation. The evaluation of these patients can be difficult since the chest radiograph is either normal or opacified by alveolar hemorrhage.

Today, high resolution computerized tomography (HRCT) has been clearly identified as the most sensitive diagnostic test in patients with suspected bronchiectasis (50,51).

Cystic Fibrosis

The spectrum of disease in patients with cystic fibrosis has markedly changed during the past few decades, as more individuals are surviving into adulthood.

The majority of patients with cystic fibrosis have hemoptysis sometime in the course of their disease, with 50–70% having massive hemoptysis (52). Approximately 11% of these patients will die within 48 hours of presentation because of uncontrolled hemoptysis and asphyxiation (53). Postmortem studies reveal extensive bronchiectasis, lung abscesses, granulation tissue, and patchy bronchopneumonia. Hypervascularity due to extensive neovascularization of the bronchial circulation and engorged bronchopulmonary anastamoses are observed in areas of bronchiectasis (52). These abnormalities, in conjunction with pulmonary arterial hypertension, account for the high incidence of hemoptysis observed in these patients (53,54).

Chronic Bronchitis

Chronic bronchitis is frequently cited as a cause of hemoptysis in the presence of small amounts of bleeding from the airways. It is a relatively uncommon cause of massive hemoptysis. The pathological lesions are likely dilated, tortuous bronchial arteries just below the bronchial mucosa, with sites of both current and healing arterial rupture (55). In patients with acute exacerbations of chronic obstructive pulmonary disease (COPD), small amounts of hemoptysis are exceedingly common and usually transient.

C. Neoplastic Diseases

Bronchogenic Carcinoma

Hemoptysis is exceedingly common during the course of bronchogenic carcinoma and is a common initial manifestation (56). Approximately 7–10% of patients with bronchogenic carcinoma present with a history of blood-streaked sputum or expectoration of small clots (52).

In a large retrospective analysis of 877 patients with lung cancer, massive, terminal hemoptysis was noted in 29 (3%) (57). This report and other studies have confirmed that those who present with massive hemoptysis secondary to lung cancer typically have a centrally located cavitary squamous cell carcinoma (58).

Although rare, direct tumor invasion of the pulmonary vasculature can lead to rapid demise, especially if there is communication with the tracheobronchial tree (57).

Carcinoid Tumors

Bronchial carcinoids are a frequent cause of hemoptysis due to their endobronchial location and their abundant vascularity. Carcinoids are typically seen in younger individuals who present with a history of a chronic cough, recurrent obstructive pneumonitis, or peripheral atelectasis. The majority of these tumors arise in lobar, segmental, or proximal subsegmental bronchi, although they can also arise rarely from the lung periphery or trachea (59,60). Hemoptysis occurs in 30–50% of cases (61–63). Despite reports of increased risk of massive hemorrhage after endobronchial biopsy during rigid bronchoscopy, biopsies performed with smaller forceps using a flexible bronchoscope can be performed safely (64).

Lung Metastases and Other Malignancies

Hemoptysis due to metastatic disease is mostly due to endobronchial metastases. The most common primary sites of endobronchial metastatic tumors include breast, melanoma, colon, and kidney (52). Hemoptysis may also occur in patients with mediastinal malignancies, such as esophageal carcinoma, which may directly erode into the tracheobronchial tree and result in massive hemoptysis (65). Severe intractable hemoptysis and fatal pulmonary hemorrhage have also been reported in patients with Kaposi's sarcoma and angiosarcomas (66–68).

Hematological Malignancies

Diffuse alveolar hemorrhage is an important complication of both autologous and, less commonly, allogeneic bone marrow transplantation (BMT) (58,69). Among this group of patients, pulmonary hemorrhage is strongly associated with fungal infections, especially invasive aspergillosis. The latter is particularly common in granulocytopenic patients receiving treatment for acute leukemia (70–72).

D. Cardiovascular Disorders

Mitral stenosis associated with rheumatic heart disease is one of the most common cardiovascular abnormalities known to cause hemoptysis (73). The source of bleeding is the submucosal bronchial veins, which proliferate considerably in this disorder. Precipitating factors for hemoptysis in patients with mitral stenosis include upper respiratory tract infections, simple coughing, and pregnancy (74–76). With the advent of surgical interventions and decline in the incidence of rheumatic fever, hemoptysis secondary to mitral stenosis has become relatively uncommon (52).

A variety of other causes of pulmonary venous hypertension, including hypertensive and ischemic cardiomyopathy and mitral regurgitation, may result in hemoptysis that usually presents as expectoration of pink frothy sputum. Less common causes of pulmonary venous hypertension that may result in hemoptysis include congenital cardiac anomalies such as cor triatriatum, capillary hemangiomatosis, chronic sclerosing mediastinitis, atrial myxoma, total anomalous venous drainage, and pulmonary veno-occlusive disease (77–79).

Hemoptysis can also occur in patients with pulmonary hypertension and Eisenmenger's Syndrome and bodes a poor prognosis (80,81). Usually, the amounts of bleeding are relatively small in the absence of coagulopathy or anticoagulation.

Hemoptysis is also a common symptom in patients with congenital pulmonary AVMs and is frequently the presenting complaint (82–84). Massive hemoptysis may occur, but is rarely fatal (85). It is estimated that approximately

60% of patients with pulmonary AVMs have arteriovenous communications in the skin, mucous membranes, or other organs (86).

Bleeding from pulmonary artery aneurysms has also been reported in patients with Bechet's disease and the Hughes–Stovin syndrome, a syndrome consisting of multiple pulmonary aneurysms and peripheral venous thrombosis (87–89).

E. Pulmonary Embolism

Hemoptysis occurs in less than 30% of patients with pulmonary embolism and is rarely associated with massive hemorrhage (90–93). Hemorrhage in the setting of pulmonary embolism is commonly seen in patients with pulmonary infarction who present with acute onset dyspnea and pleuritic pain (94). With anticoagulation, thrombolytic therapy, or an underlying coagulopathy, massive hemoptysis can occur.

F. Diffuse Alveolar Hemorrhage

The differential diagnosis of diffuse alveolar hemorrhage (DAH) is quite extensive and is listed in Table 3. DAH is a common feature of many autoimmune, vasculitic, and idiopathic systemic diseases. Specific disorders mediated by immunologic mechanisms include Goodpasture's syndrome, Wegener's granulomatosis, systemic lupus erythematosus, and idiopathic pulmonary hemosiderosis (95–98). The cardinal features of alveolar hemorrhage include hemoptysis, anemia, and rapidly progressive bilateral alveolar infiltrates on chest roentgenograms. Other clinical clues that may be present include renal dysfunction and other systemic manifestations of vasculitis.

The initial approach to patients presenting with diffuse alveolar hemorrhage includes bronchoscopy in order to help confirm the diagnosis and to rule out potential infectious etiologies. Sequential bronchoalveolar lavage in patients with unexplained diffuse alveolar infiltrates on chest roentgenograms and occult alveolar hemorrhage may show a progressive hemorrhagic return and hemosiderin-laden macrophages on histological analysis (99). Serial measurements of diffusing capacity for carbon monoxide have also been suggested as a sensitive marker of bleeding in patients with recurrent alveolar hemorrhage (100,101). Although informative, this test cannot be performed in most patients with DAH due to the severity of illness.

G. Iatrogenic Hemoptysis

Iatrogenic hemoptysis is most frequently associated with bronchoscopy with biopsy, transthoracic needle biopsy, or pulmonary artery perforation induced by inflation of a pulmonary artery (PA) catheter. Hemoptysis induced during bronchoscopy may occur via brushing, endobronchial biopsy, or transbronchial biopsy, with the latter being more frequently associated with significant bleeding

Table 3 Causes of Diffuse Alveolar Hemorrhage

Immunologic	Retinoic acid
Systemic vasculitides	Nitrofurantoin
• Wegener's granulomatosis	Abciximab
• Microscopic polyangiitis	Crack cocaine
• Henoch–Schonlein purpura	Isocyanates
• Cryglobulinemia	Trimellitic anhydride
• Goodpasture's syndrome	Amiodarone
• Bechet's syndrome	Tissue plasminogen activator
• Polyarteritis nodosa	Lymphangiography contrast
• Tumor-related vasculitis	Coumadin overdose
• Endocarditis-related vasculitis	Clotting disorders
• Systemic necrotizing vasculitis	Cirrhosis
Collagen vascular disease	DIC
• Systemic lupus erythematosus	Other disorders of coagulation
• Primary antiphospholipid syndrome	Thrombotic thrombocytopenic purpura
• Polymyositis	Infections
• Rheumatoid arthritis	Necrotizing pneumonia
• Scleroderma	Infections in the immune-compromised
• Mixed connective tissue disease	host
Glomerulopathies associated with	Legionnaire's disease
multisystem diseases	Diffuse lung injury
• Membranoproliferative	ARDS—any cause
glomerulonephritis	Negative pressure pulmonary
• IgA nephropathy	hemorrhage
• Diffuse endocapillary proliferative	Cytotoxic drug toxicity
glomerulonephritis	Breath-hold diving
• Focal proliferative	Pulmonary venous hypertension
glomerulonephritis	Mitral stenosis
Transplant related	Mitral regurgitation
Bone marrow transplant	Pulmonary veno-occlusive disease
Renal transplant	Fibrosing mediastinitis
Lung transplant rejection	Pulmonary capillary hemangiomatosis
Drug or chemical related	Congenital heart disease
Propylthiouracil	Miscellaneous conditions
Phenytoin	Lymphangioleiomyomatosis
D-penicillamine	Tuberous sclerosis
Mitomycin C	Pulmonary infarction

Abbreviations: DIC, disseminated intravascular coagulation; ARDS, acute respiratory distress syndrome.

(102). The risk of hemoptysis due to transbronchial biopsy is estimated to range from 2% to 9% (103–108).

Perforation of the pulmonary artery is a catastrophic complication associated with catheterization. Catheter-induced pulmonary artery rupture is rare, with an incidence of 0.016–0.2%, but it remains the most dreaded complication, with reported mortality rates above 50% (109). Distal and prolonged balloon inflation can cause catastrophic PA dissection, pseudoaneuysm formation, or PA rupture (110–114). In addition, endovascular damage leading to the development of thrombus formation and pulmonary infarction can occur. The diagnosis of infarction is occasionally suggested by the presence of a local patchy infiltrate near the tip of a catheter. Preventive maneuvers that can be undertaken include notation of the insertion distance during placement of the catheter, full inflation of the balloon to prevent the catheter tip from projecting beyond the balloon, and routine monitoring of catheter position with daily chest roentgenograms (115). The risk factors for massive hemoptysis secondary to PA perforation include advanced age, anticoagulation, distal catheter tip position, prolonged balloon inflation, and the presence of pulmonary hypertension (116).

Treatment options for PA rupture include surgical resection of the involved lobe and angiography-guided embolization of the involved pulmonary artery (117–119). Some conservative, temporizing therapeutic alternatives with limited efficacy include re-inflation of the PA catheter balloon and high levels of positive end-expiratory pressure (PEEP) to decrease the pulmonary artery-to-bronchial pressure gradient (120,121).

H. Trauma

Chest trauma is a relatively common and potentially lethal cause of hemoptysis, requiring urgent thoracic surgery consultation and management. Injuries occurring after severe blunt trauma include puncture of a lung by a fractured rib, lung contusions, and laceration of the tracheobronchial tree. Tracheobronchial disruption should always be considered when managing patients with blunt trauma, especially when barotrauma and air leaks persist (122,123). Stab or gunshot wounds, in addition, can also lacerate the lungs or the tracheobronchial tree. Early diagnostic bronchoscopy is recommended to confirm the diagnosis of tracheobronchial tears, which are usually within a few centimeters of the carina and often involve the membranous trachea (124–126). Initial stabilization prior to surgical repair often requires placement of a double-lumen endotracheal tube or use of high-frequency jet ventilation (125,127).

I. Cryptogenic Hemoptysis

Cryptogenic or idiopathic hemoptysis refers to hemoptysis in which the cause remains unclear despite a thorough diagnostic evaluation. It is estimated that up to 30% of patients examined by bronchoscopy for hemoptysis (128,129) and about 8–15% of patients with massive hemoptysis are ultimately given the diagnosis of cryptogenic hemoptysis 26, 130–131. Several explanations have been proposed for the pathogenesis of cryptogenic hemoptysis, although few data support any single hypothesis. Acute and chronic bronchial inflammation is the most frequently implicated cause of bleeding (132–134). Other potential etiologies include isolated bronchial telangiectasias (135), occult pulmonary embolism (132–134), occult bronchiectasis (130,132,133), coagulation abnormalities related to medications (136), thrombocytopenia (137–139), and broncholithiasis associated with inactive tuberculosis (130,132,133). Carcinoma is found during follow-up in 2–6% of patients with cryptogenic hemoptysis. The prognosis of patients with cryptogenic hemoptysis is generally favorable, usually with resolution of bleeding within six months of evaluation (140).

J. Factitious Hemoptysis

A factitious cause should be considered in the differential diagnosis of hemoptysis of unclear etiology, especially when the medical history or the patient's behavior is unusual (142). This is a unique form of Munchausen syndrome that is rarely reported in the literature (142,143).

IV. Diagnostic Evaluation

A. History

The initial approach to patients with suspected hemoptysis should be directed towards determination of the site of bleeding. Characterization of the expectorated blood together with some simple tests may be sufficient to determine whether the source of bleeding is the respiratory tract or the gastrointestinal tract. Patients with hemoptysis may experience a gurgling sensation in the chest, whereas patients with hematemesis experience nausea and vomiting (144,145). Hemoptysis is usually characterized by frothy bright red blood, which may be mixed with sputum. Microscopic analysis may reveal hemosiderin-laden macrophages, and the pH should be alkaline. Hematemesis, on the other hand, is classically characterized by dark red blood, occasionally intermixed with food particles, and usually has an acidic pH. A thorough evaluation of the upper airway along with indirect examination of the posterior pharynx is indicated if there is a question as to the source of bleeding. Occasionally, both upper gastrointestinal endoscopy and bronchoscopy are required to clarify the source of bleeding (146).

In patients with massive bleeding, investigation should be initiated with speed with attention to resuscitation of the patient. Massive hemoptysis is a life-threatening event that requires intensive care unit (ICU) admission and urgent evaluation for localization of the bleeding site. Management should be individualized and requires prompt consultation with cardiothoracic surgery, pulmonary medicine, anesthesia, and interventional radiology staff. The yield of individual strategies for localization of the bleeding source varies considerably. Rarely, patients themselves can localize the source of bleeding (4).

B. Physical Examination

Although useful in assessing cause and sometimes severity of bleeding, the physical examination can be unreliable in localizing the site of bleeding. However, inspection of the thorax for signs of penetration and blunt trauma is important and can be helpful in localizing the site of bleeding (147).

C. Sputum Examination

Examination of the sputum is an adjunctive test guided by the differential diagnosis. Sputum should be examined for the presence of bacteria, acid-fast bacilli, or fungi if such infectious etiologies are suspected. Sputum for cytology can be collected if lung cancer is suspected, especially if the patient is older than 40 years of age and a smoker.

D. Chest Roentgenography

Roentgenographic examination of the thorax should be obtained routinely in all cases of hemoptysis. Frequently, a pulmonary parenchymal source of bleeding is associated with an infiltrate, cavity, mass, or atelectasis. An airway source is suggested if the chest roentgenogram is normal (148). Chest roentgenography is, however, frequently not helpful in localization since blood may be aspirated into portions of the lung distant from the source of bleeding (149). In addition, interpretation of chest roentgenograms is normal or nonlocalizing in 20–40% of patients with hemoptysis (150).

E. Radionuclide Studies

Radionuclide scanning with technetium-99m sulfur colloid or technetium-99m labeled red blood cells have localized bleeding in some patients with hemoptysis (151–153). However, this modality requires a rapid rate of bleeding in order to be diagnostic. In cases where the bleeding is significant, chest roentgenography and bronchoscopy provide a more accurate identification of the source of hemorrhage.

F. Chest Computed Tomography

The potential role of chest computed tomography (CT) in the evaluation of hemoptysis continues to evolve. In cases of hemoptysis with normal chest roentgenograms, fiberoptic bronchoscopy (FOB) has not been shown to be of significant utility. In a retrospective evaluation of 113 patients with hemoptysis who underwent FOB, a specific etiology was not found in 26 patients (0%) with normal chest roentgenograms, compared with 35 of 87 patients (40%) in whom chest roentgenograms proved localizing (154). In another study of 196 patients with normal or nonlocalizing chest roentgenograms who underwent FOB, specific causes were established in only 33 patients (17%) (155).

Lesions that may not be visible on chest roentgenograms, such as bronchiectasis, broncholithiasis, and small bronchial carcinomas, can occasionally be detected by chest CT (156–158). In a prospective study of 20 patients with unexplained hemoptysis, normal chest roentgenograms, and normal FOB, chest CT demonstrated abnormalities in 50% of patients (159). In another study of 93 patients with hemoptysis, chest CT demonstrated all 27 tumors that were detected by FOB and an additional seven tumors, five of which were beyond the visual range of bronchoscopy (160). Chest CT, however, failed to demonstrate early mucosal abnormalities, bronchitis, squamous metaplasia, and a benign papilloma, all of which were detected by FOB.

More recent studies have demonstrated a favorable role for high-resolution computed tomography (HRCT) in the assessment of patients with hemoptysis. In a prospective study, the overall diagnostic yield of HRCT was 61%, compared to 43% for FOB. In addition, a specific diagnosis was made based on the HRCT findings in 50% of cases with nondiagnostic FOB (161).

Routine use of chest CT in the evaluation of patients with submassive or massive hemoptysis is not supported, however, by the literature (51). Chest CT obtained during active hemorrhage is frequently misleading since aspirated blood may obscure a mass or incorrectly simulate a parenchymal mass. Given that approximately 20–40% of patients presenting with hemoptysis have normal chest roentgenograms, chest CT may be preferred over other modalities in the stable patient presenting with hemoptysis (162). Abnormalities that can be reliably diagnosed by chest CT include peripheral masses, alveolar consolidation, bronchiectasis, broncholithiasis, and abnormally enhancing vessels. Ultimately, however, the potential impact of FOB or HRCT on patient management will determine whether chest CT or FOB, or both, are indicated in the assessment of patients with hemoptysis (163).

G. Bronchoscopy

Bronchoscopy is an appropriate first diagnostic test in the evaluation of patients with hemoptysis and should be considered for localization and diagnosis whether the patient presents with blood-streaked sputum or massive hemoptysis. The risk of recurrent bleeding also adds urgency to bronchoscopic evaluation. However, the timing of bronchoscopy in the evaluation of hemoptysis is controversial (128). In a survey of specialists performed by Haponik and Chin, 50% of 106 respondents favored immediate bronchoscopy in massive hemoptysis, 34% advocated bronchoscopy within 24 hours, and 16% favored bronchoscopy later, after bleeding had subsided (164). The diagnostic yield for elucidating the site of bleeding is enhanced, however, if there is active bleeding at the time of bronchoscopy (165–167). If bronchoscopy is performed during active hemoptysis, the site of bleeding can be localized in 93% of patients (167). If bronchoscopy is performed after bleeding ceases entirely, the etiology is determined in no more than 52% of cases (4). Hence for patients with massive hemoptysis or those with rapid clinical deterioration, early bronchoscopy is the recommended approach (168). In addition, bronchoscopy will provide opportunities for treatment, e.g., endobronchial tamponade, and will also serve as a guide for surgical resection, if necessary (52,128,153).

Performing rigid versus flexible bronchoscopy to assess patients with massive hemoptysis is another area of controversy (169). In the survey conducted by Haponik and Chin, 41% of respondents favored FOB through an endotracheal tube, 17% favored rigid bronchoscopy, and 7% advocated FOB without an endotracheal tube (167). Theoretically, however, there are potential benefits and disadvantages to either procedure.

Rigid bronchoscopy has several potential advantages in the evaluation of patients with massive hemoptysis. These include improved suctioning capability, maintenance of airway patency, and a larger lumen for introducing packing materials to control hemorrhage (26,170–171). Rigid bronchoscopy is also safe and well tolerated under local anesthesia and conscious sedation when performed by experienced practitioners. Failure to visualize the upper lobes and peripheral lesions remains a major limitation to the use of rigid bronchoscopy. However, the fiberoptic bronchoscope can be used in conjunction with the rigid broncho-scope in order to visualize the more distal tracheobronchial tree (146).

The fiberoptic bronchoscope can reach lesions that are located distally up to the fifth and sixth bronchial orifices, which are not within reach of a rigid bronchoscope. FOB is a technique that is extremely safe and can be performed at the patient's bedside without general anesthesia. Additionally, the flexible bronchoscope allows the introduction of balloon catheters to tamponade sites of bleeding (173). Suction capability with the flexible bronchoscope is, however, limited because of the narrow suction channel (174).

Thus, in the unstable patient with hemoptysis, FOB through an endotracheal tube should be attempted first, with consideration given for rigid broncho-scopy in the event of unsuccessful localization and control of hemorrhage.

V. Management

The initial steps involved in the management of patients with hemoptysis should run concurrent with the initial diagnostic steps and should be dictated by the initial clinical presentation (175). In view of the significant mortality in patients with massive hemoptysis, initial management is mostly dependent on the rate of bleeding. Sputum containers should be left at the bedside in order to precisely quantitate the amount of bleeding. Because asphyxiation is the usual cause of death, immediate treatment goals in patients with massive hemoptysis should include maintenance of airway patency and control of hemorrhage. Subsequent goals should include determination of the site of bleeding and evaluation of the patient's candidacy for a variety of therapeutic interventions. Early consultation by pulmonary medicine, thoracic surgery, and invasive radiology is recommended.

A. Resuscitation and Supportive Measures

Due to the inability to predict which patients will accelerate their rate of hemop-tysis, it is recommended that those with hemoptysis greater than 200 mL be admitted to a setting where rapid airway support can be initiated (115). Patients' vital signs and arterial oxygen saturation should be closely monitored. Two large-bore peripheral intravenous catheters should be placed in anticipation of active volume resuscitation. Blood should be drawn for typing and crossmatching and sent for laboratory analyses, including hematocrit, coagulation parameters, blood urea nitrogen, creatinine, and arterial blood gases. Any coagulation or platelet abnormality should be aggressively corrected, along with volume and red blood cell replacement. Patients with worsening hypoxemia should be given high-flow supplemental oxygen and considered for intubation (176).

B. Antitussive Therapy

Initiation of adequate sedation and judicious use of cough suppressants to prevent vigorous coughing should be considered in patients with massive hemoptysis (52). The patient needs to remain awake, however, in order to be able to expectorate clots within the central airways (177). Most commonly, moderate doses of codeine or codeine-based antitussive agents are used, which also help reduce patient anxiety (178). The dose of the antitussive agent should be carefully titrated in order to suppress cough without affecting the patient's mental status. Overzealous use of cough suppressants may increase the risk of blood retention and worsening alveolar flooding due to inadequate airway clearance.

C. Patient Positioning

The patient should be placed in the lateral decubitus position with the involved side down to prevent spill-over into the non-involved lung. A patient with massive hemoptysis may, however, not tolerate a full lateral decubitus position without sedation. In this setting, intubation is usually required (178). The head of the bed should also be lowered to promote drainage of blood from the airway.

D. Endotracheal Intubation

Death from hemoptysis results from asphyxia produced by flooding of the airways with aspirated blood. Therefore, control of the airways is the most important aspect of initial patient management. If bleeding does not subside promptly, the patient should be electively intubated using an endotracheal tube with an internal diameter of at least 8 mm. The use of a large endotracheal tube is essential in order to permit passage of suction catheters or a flexible bronchoscope. Oral intubation is preferred over nasal intubation since this allows insertion of larger endotracheal tubes and provides sufficient endotracheal tube length for mainstem bronchial intubation.

    Selective bronchial intubation involves placement of a single lumen endotracheal tube into either the left or right mainstem bronchus in order to protect the unaffected lung from spillage of blood (144). Because of the leftward displacement of the carina, selective right bronchial intubation is easier to achieve.

However, a potential problem that may occur is right upper lobe atelectasis due to the proximity of the right upper lobe bronchus to the carina. If an effort is made not to place the cuff of the endotracheal tube directly over the right upper lobe orifice or in the bronchus intermedius, the Murphy opening on the right side of the tip of a standard endotracheal tube will allow some ventilation of the right upper lobe. This is an important consideration in performing isolated right lung ventilation in patients with limited pulmonary reserve.

Selective intubation of the left mainstem bronchus is more challenging in the absence of bronchoscopic guidance. This problem can occasionally be facilitated by placing the patient in the right lateral decubitus position, angulation of the endotracheal tube to the left, and placement over a coude catheter (115).

E. Double-Lumen Endotracheal Tubes

Double-lumen endotracheal tubes (Combitube® Esophageal/Tracheal Double-Lumen Airway, Nellcor, Pleasanton, CA, USA) have been used to allow independent isolation of each mainstem bronchus in order to protect the nonbleeding lung from blood spillage (179). A double-lumen endotracheal tube may offer advantages over standard intubation, provided that the individual lumina are large enough to allow clearance of the airways and the passage of a fiberoptic bronchoscope (180). Unfortunately, there are significant problems associated with the use of double-lumen endotracheal tubes. Misplacement and difficulty maintaining proper placement are serious problems that are frequently encountered. In a prospective study of 200 patients who had double-lumen endotracheal tubes placed blindly, initial malpositioning was clinically and bronchoscopically detected in 28 and 79 cases, respectively. Additionally, after patient positioning, double-lumen endotracheal tubes were found displaced in 93 patients, 48 of which were deemed critical (181). Consequently, due to difficulties in maintaining the position of such endotracheal tubes, higher doses of sedatives and paralytics are frequently used. In a series of 62 patients with massive hemoptysis, four of seven patients died as a direct result of intraoperative aspiration of blood due to loss of pulmonary separation while being ventilated with double-lumen endotracheal tubes (3). Furthermore, the small channels of these tubes do not allow a therapeutic bronchoscope or large suction catheter to pass through and frequently become obstructed with blood (165). Given these difficulties, the use of double-lumen endotracheal tubes is not recommended in patients with acute massive hemoptysis (177).

F. Endobronchial Tamponade

Endobronchial tamponade with fiberoptic bronchoscopy represents a potentially life-saving technique in patients who are not considered suitable candidates for bronchial artery embolization or surgery, and in patients who cannot be transferred due to logistical problems or who have rapidly deteriorated in the ICU. Endobronchial tamponade can be achieved with a 4 Fr, 80–100 cm Fogarty balloon catheter (Fogarty balloon catheter®, Edwards Lifesciences, Irvine, CA,

USA), which is introduced through the channel of the bronchoscope (173,182–184). The classic technique entails the inflation of the balloon at the distal hub of the catheter in a mainstem or lobar bronchus in order to achieve occlusion. The bronchoscope is then removed by sliding it over the Fogarty catheter after cutting off the proximal hub of the catheter. A larger Fogarty catheter can also be passed outside the endobronchial tube into the trachea, and then placed into the bleeding bronchus via the guidance of the bronchoscope. The balloon usually remains in place for 24 to 48 hours. Another technique that has been described involves the use of a pulmonary artery catheter in order to achieve occlusion of bleeding segments (185).

A double-lumen, bronchus-blocking catheter that can be introduced through the working channel of a standard fiberoptic bronchoscope has also been developed. This is a 6 Fr, 170 cm long catheter with a distal balloon that can be inflated thru a detachable valve at the proximal end. This detachable valve facilitates removal of the bronchoscope without requiring modification to the catheter. This catheter was used successfully in 26 of 27 patients with hemoptysis and was left in place for up to seven days while patients underwent other treatment modalities (186,187).

An alternative method for allowing single-lung ventilation in critically ill patients utilizes a fiberoptically directed wire-guided endobronchial blocker (Fig. 1, Arndt Endobronchial Blocker® [AEB]; Cook Critical Care, Bloomington, IN, USA) (188–190). The endobronchial blocker has a central lumen through which a wire with a looped end has been passed. The loop on the distal end is placed over a fiberoptic bronchoscope, which is then used as a guide to facilitate bronchial placement of the balloon-tipped endobronchial blocker. The AEB can be piggybacked on a small bronchoscope within a large endotracheal tube. If using a larger bronchoscope, it is preferable to pass the AEB outside the endotracheal tube using either a bronchoscope or a laryngoscope (177). Once in the trachea, the distal loop of the AEB can be guided into its final position with the aid of the bronchoscope (191).

G. Endobronchial Pharmacotherapy

Numerous hemostatic agents have been infused through the bronchoscope in patients with massive hemoptysis. There has been limited success with the use of iced saline (171,192), and although topical epinephrine has been advocated as an effective means of controlling hemorrhage, its efficacy in the management of massive hemoptysis has not been adequately assessed (193–195).

Fiberoptic bronchoscopy-based infusion of thrombin and fibrinogen-thrombin has been used with relatively good success (196). In a study by Tsukamoto and colleagues, hemostasis was achieved using this technique in 31 of 33 patients studied, and only two patients required surgical intervention following infusion. Fibrin precursors sprayed selectively into bleeding bronchi have also been used successfully in a small group of patients (197). More recently, a prospective

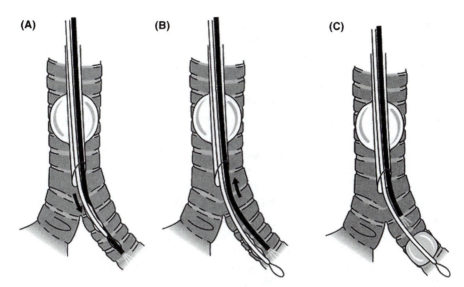

Figure 1 The AEB is an alternative method of securing the airway for unilateral tamponade. (**A**) Using an Arndt Multiport Airway Adaptor, the loop on the distal end is placed over a small FOB, which is then used as a guide to facilitate bronchial placement of the balloon-tipped endobronchial blocker. The AEB is advanced until the guide loop, which is piggybacked on the bronchoscope, is seen to exit. (**B**) The FOB is retracted to view the endobronchial blocker within the bronchial lumen. The AEB should then be advanced distally in to the right or left mainstem bronchus. (**C**) Following positioning, under direct visualization, the balloon is inflated with air using the pilot balloon assembly. The AEB should be inspected and adjusted so the inflated balloon fills the bronchial lumen without herniation into the trachea. The balloon inflation volume should also be noted. *Abbreviations*: AEB, Arndt endobronchial blocker; FOB, fiberoptic bronchoscope.

study analyzed the efficacy of endoscopic fibrinogen-thrombin instillation in 11 of 101 patients with severe hemoptysis ($>$150 mL/12 hr) in whom bronchial artery embolization was not possible or had proved ineffective (198). Immediate control of severe hemoptysis was noted in all patients who received endoscopic instillation of fibrinogen-thrombin. Additionally, the authors noted a very low rebleed rate and no attributable complications. Fibrin precursors can be injected through the bronchoscope wedged against the bleeding bronchus. The fiberoptic broncoscope is usually retained in place for about five minutes following infusion and is removed after confirming, by aspiration, that hemostasis has occurred. In the study by Tsukamoto and colleagues, 5–10 mL of a 2% fibrinogen solution and 5–10 mL of thrombin (1000 U/mL) were instilled directly through the channel used for aspiration. Most blood banks can readily provide fibrinogen for topical use in the form of cryoprecipitate. One unit of cryoprecipitate is derived from one unit of fresh frozen plasma and contains at least 150 mg of fibrinogen in a volume of 15–25 mL. Generally, a single bag of cryoprecipitate contains sufficient fibrinogen for topical use. Fibrin sealants are also commercially available (Tisseel® VH, Baxter Healthcare, Deerfield, IL, USA). Despite the encouraging results from these reports, additional controlled studies are required to confirm the efficacy of bronchoscopic infusion of coagulants.

H. Nonbronchoscopic Pharmacotherapy

Intravenous vasopressin has been used to control massive hemoptysis due to its potent vasoconstrictor effect on systemic vessels (199). Recent case reports have demonstrated successful outcomes following use of vasopressin in patients with massive hemoptysis due to cystic fibrosis and leptospirosis (200,201). The recommended dose of intravenous vasopressin for the treatment of massive hemoptysis is 0.2–0.4 units/min as a continuous infusion (202). This modality should at best be considered a temporizing measure. Additionally, bronchial artery constriction caused by vasopressin has been shown to hinder successful angiographic visualization of the bleeding source during bronchial artery embolization (203).

Systemic corticosteroids and cytotoxic agents are treatment options available to patients presenting with diffuse alveolar hemorrhage (DAH) accompanying pulmonary vasculitides (204,205). In addition, recombinant factor VIIa has been used successfully in patients with DAH following hematopoietic stem-cell transplantation (206,207).

In the management of patients with pulmonary aspergilloma and massive hemoptysis who have severe chronic respiratory insufficiency, intracavitary therapy with amphotericin B and N-acetylcysteine with or without aminocaproic acid represent treatment options (208–211).

Gonadotropin-releasing hormone analogues (GnRH), danazol, and low dose corticosteroids have also been shown to be effective in the management of patients with catamenial hemoptysis (212–215).

I. Laser Photocoagulation and Argon Plasma Coagulation

Coagulating laser phototherapy using a neodymium-yttrium-aluminum-garnet (Nd-YAG) laser through either a flexible fiberoptic bronchoscope or rigid bronchoscope has been utilized, with mixed results, to control massive hemoptysis (216–219). Laser therapy is limited to patients with hemorrhage from endobronchial lesions and is occasionally used for palliation in patients with carcinomatous bleeding after chemotherapy and radiation therapy.

More recently, Argon Plasma Coagulation (APC) has been used with good success for controlling hemoptysis in patients with endobronchial disease (220,221). APC is a simpler, lower-risk treatment modality compared to other interventional endobronchial techniques.

J. Radiation Therapy

External beam radiation therapy is used for palliation of lung cancer-related symptoms, such as hemoptysis, and those related to endobronchial obstruction. When bronchoscopy reveals bleeding from an endoscopically visible, unresectable lung cancer, external beam radiation serves as an additional treatment option (222). However, radiation therapy has no role in the acute management of patients with massive hemoptysis secondary to bronchogenic carcinoma.

External beam radiation therapy has also been utilized successfully in patients with life-threatening hemoptysis secondary to mycetomas (223,224).

K. Transcatheter Bronchial Artery Embolization

Massive hemoptysis is the principal indication for bronchial artery embolization. In patients with isolated abnormalities and adequate pulmonary reserve, surgical resection of the hemorrhagic source may be feasible. However, in patients with diffuse underlying lung disease and limited pulmonary reserve, bronchial artery embolization is the treatment of choice. In addition, there is evidence that preoperative bronchial artery embolization may reduce the risk of death following surgery (225). In 90% of the cases, the source of massive hemoptysis is the bronchial circulation (Figs. 2 and 3). The pulmonary circulation accounts for 5%, and the remainder is attributable to the aorta or other systemic arterial supply to the lungs (226–228).

When performing bronchial arteriography and embolization, special attention must be given to the arterial supply of the spinal cord, as devastating sequelae can result if its circulation is compromised. The largest anterior medullary branch supplying the anterior spinal artery (the artery of Adamkiewics), most commonly found at the T8 to L1 level, is known to arise from the right ICBT in 5% of the population (229). Left bronchial arteries and other systemic arteries rarely supply the anterior spinal artery (Fig. 4).

A descending thoracic aortogram serves as a helpful roadmap during bronchial embolization. Cobra-type curved catheters are most commonly used, but others such as Simmons-1®, Headhunter®, Mikaelsson®, or shepherd's hook are also used. A five French catheter is often used. For subselective embolization, a coaxial system with a three French catheter (i.e., a microcatheter such as a Tracker® system; Target Therapeutics, Fremont, CA, USA) may be used. This prevents occlusion of the bronchial artery by the catheter, avoiding potential spinal cord ischemia should a spinal branch originate from this vessel. For embolization, the more peripherally placed coaxial catheter may also prevent reflux of embolic material into the aorta.

Selective catheterization is performed by searching for the bronchial artery at the T5 to T6 level. The origin of the right and left bronchial arteries is found within or near the shadow of the left main bronchus in 94% of bronchial angiograms performed in patients with and without distorted thoracic anatomy (230).

When abnormal bronchial arteries are not identified, arch aortography and selective arteriography should be performed to search for anomalous bronchial

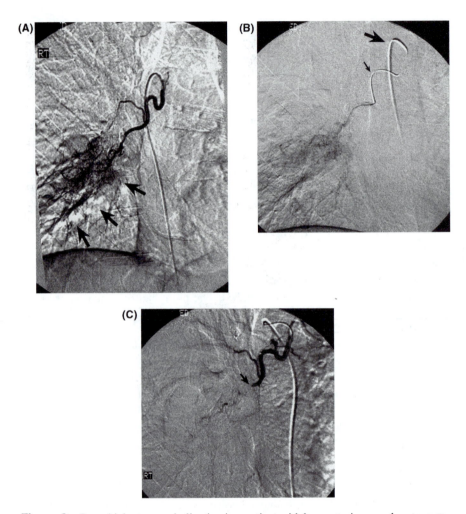

Figure 2   Bronchial artery embolization in a patient with hemoptysis secondary to metastatic renal cell carcinoma. (**A**) Initial diagnostic angiogram demonstrating a hypertrophied right bronchial artery supplying a hypervascular tumor mass (*arrows*) in the right
lung base. (**B**) Right bronchial artery embolized selectively with PVA particles using
a coaxial system with an outer 5 French Cobra catheter (*large arrow*) and an inner
3 French microcatheter (*small arrow*). (**C**) Postembolization angiogram demonstrating
cessation of flow (*arrow*) to the tumor mass as well as the distal right bronchial artery.
Abbreviation: PVA, polyvinyl alcohol.

arteries, nonbronchial systemic arterial supply, or both (Fig. 5). If lower lobe
disease is present, an abdominal aortogram and examination of the inferior
phrenic arteries should also be performed. If no systemic arterial supply is identified, selective pulmonary arteriography is performed to rule out pulmonary

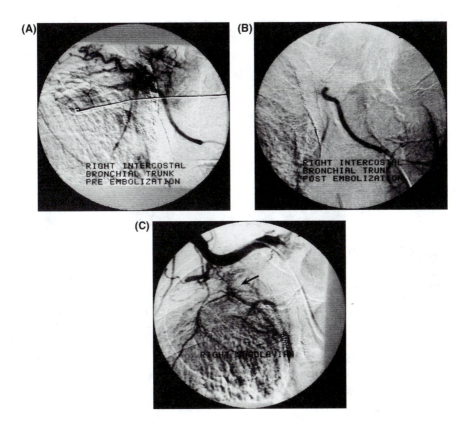

Figure 3 Bronchial artery embolization in a patient with massive hemoptysis due to tuberculosis. (**A**) Arteriography demonstrating a large right intercostobronchial trunk with multiple large, tortuous branch vessels and a capillary stain, supplying the right lung apex. (**B**) Postembolization angiogram demonstrating termination of the contrast column and cessation of blood flow after successful embolization with PVA particles. (**C**) Selective right subclavian artery injection demonstrating parasitization via systemic collaterals into the lung (*arrow*). *Abbreviation*: PVA, polyvinyl alcohol.

pseudoaneurysm or AV fistula, especially in patients with cavitary lung disease or a history of recent Swan–Ganz catheterization.

In cases of chronic inflammation, the bronchial arteries are hypertrophied and tortuous. Other signs that may be observed include bronchial or peribronchial hypervascularity, systemic-to-pulmonary artery or venous shunting, and bronchial artery aneurysms. However, the hypervascularity shown on bronchial arteriogram does not consistently predict the site of bleeding. In addition, frank contrast extravasation and aneurysm are rarely observed. Aneurysms may be observed, however, on pulmonary angiograms, e.g., Rasmussen's aneurysm in cavitary tuberculosis and mycotic aneurysms resulting from drug abuse.

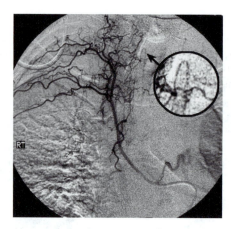

Figure 4 Injection at the origin of the right superior intercostal artery demonstrating an anterior spinal artery arising from it, with the characteristic hairpin loop appearance (*arrow*).

Bronchial artery embolization may be performed in the absence of active contrast extravasation since hemorrhage from bronchial arteries is usually intermittent and slow. Nonionic contrast should be used routinely to minimize the cough response and to lower the risk of spinal cord injury (231,232). A short acting barbiturate, amobarbital, or lidocaine solution, which temporarily produces the symptoms of spinal cord ischemia, can be injected intra-arterially as

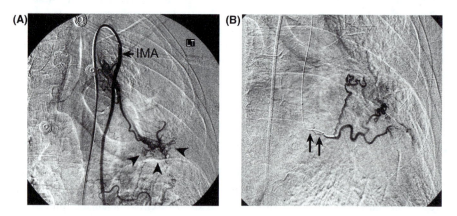

Figure 5 Embolization of abnormal feeding vessels arising from the internal mammary artery (IMA) in a patient with recurrent hemoptysis. (**A**) Abnormal feeding vessels (*arrowheads*) to the lingula arising from the left internal mammary artery. (**B**) Successful embolization with PVA particles using a coaxial system with an inner microcatheter (*arrows*). *Abbreviation*: PVA, polyvinyl alcohol.

a provocative test to detect any occult spinal artery branch before bronchial artery embolization (233,234).

The most frequently used embolic materials are gelfoams and polyvinyl alcohol (PVA) particles. Both are non-radiopaque and require mixture with contrast material during the procedure. The disadvantage of gelfoam is its resolvability leading to recanalization. PVA particles (350–500 μm in diameter), on the other hand, are permanent embolic agents. Particles with dimensions of 350 μm or greater are used to prevent tissue necrosis or neurologic damage. Smaller particles can pass through bronchial artery–pulmonary artery anastomosis to cause pulmonary infarction, or pass through bronchial artery–pulmonary vein anastomosis to cause systemic artery embolization (6,8,235,236).

Enormous bronchial arteries with high flow and large systemic-to-pulmonary shunts are sometimes encountered in cystic fibrosis and may require the use of coil embolization for safe and adequate occlusion (237,238). Such type of proximal coil occlusion should not be considered routine practice because it is important to preserve the proximal part of any abnormal vessel for future embolization access in case of recurrent bleeding. It is to be used only when other methods fail or are contraindicated, or when the patient's clinical condition demands very rapid control. Liquids such as ethanol or fine particles (gelfoam powder) produce distal embolization with occlusion of the capillary bed, leading to possible tissue infarction. They should, therefore, be avoided.

Complications of bronchial artery embolization include chest pain (24–91%) and dysphagia (0.7–18.2%), which can occur two to seven days after embolization (239–241). These symptoms usually regress. Subintimal dissection of aorta or bronchial artery can also occur, but is frequently asymptomatic. Pulmonary infarction can complicate bronchial embolization when the bronchial artery is the only source of vascular supply to the lung, as in the case of chronic proximal pulmonary artery occlusion. The most devastating complication is spinal cord ischemia following inadvertent occlusion of the anterior spinal artery. Careful analysis of the angiogram, before and during the embolization procedure, is crucial to prevent this complication. Transverse myelitis has also been reported after diagnostic bronchial arteriography with the use of - ionic hyperosmolar contrast agents (231,232). The risk of this contrast-induced neurotoxicity can be minimized with the use of a diluted non-ionic contrast medium.

Bronchial artery embolization is a very effective technique for the immediate control of hemoptysis of inflammatory origin, with a success rate in the range of 77–91% (242–245). Overall, the long-term control rate of hemoptysis is about 70–80% and is largely a function of the natural progression of the underlying disease (243). However, recurrent bleeding can also be attributed to recanalization of the embolized vessels or achievement only of partial embolization.

The presence of pleural abnormalities significantly lowers the long term effectiveness of bronchial artery embolization. Tamura and colleagues showed long term hemostasis in 70% of patients without evidence of pleural thickening, whereas the same was accomplished in only 29% of patients with significant pleural thickening (246).

In patients with cystic fibrosis, bronchial artery embolization is a valuable tool for palliation of hemoptysis. Excellent immediate control rate can be achieved (247,248). Palliation is especially crucial to these young patients awaiting lung transplantation.

Bronchial embolization is an effective tool for massive hemoptysis. More recently, its indications have been broadened to include mild and chronic hemoptysis. With careful technique, it can be performed safely and with minimum risk.

L. Surgery

Surgical therapy should be considered in the management of patients for whom hemoptysis is life-threatening or not controlled by nonsurgical interventions. Patients with lateralized, uncontrollable hemoptysis should be assessed early for candidacy for surgery in case bleeding persists and is unresponsive to other interventions. Until three decades ago, surgical therapy was considered the treatment of choice in patients with localized sites of bleeding (2,3,26,144,165,249,250). This conclusion was based on lower mortality rates among patients treated with surgery compared to patients who were treated conservatively. The surgical mortality rates from observational uncontrolled studies published between the 1960s and the 1990s range from 0–50%, compared with mortality rates as high as 80% for medically managed patients (Table 4) (2,3,26,144,145,165,249–251).

Table 4 Outcomes of Surgical Versus Medical Treatment of Massive Hemoptysis

Author, year (Ref. number)	Total number of patients	Number of patients treated medically (% mortality)	Number of patients treated surgically (% mortality)	Mortality of surgical candidates managed medically
Yeoh et al., 1967	56	43 (23%)	13 (15%)	—
Crocco et al., 1968 (2)	67	35 (54%)	32 (19%)	78%
Gourin and Garzon, 1974 (3)	62	5 (80%)	57 (18%)	—
Sehhat et al., 1978 (145)	146	40 (80%)	106 (0.9%)	85%
Yang and Berger, 1978	20	17 (17%)	3 (0%)	—
Garzon et al., 1982 (165)	24	—	24 (25%)	—
Bobrowitz et al., 1983 (149)	113	82 (22%)	31 (13%)	1.6%
Conlan et al., 1983 (192)	100	66 (32%)	34 (18%)	10%
Corey and Hla, 1987 (251)	59	55 (29%)	4 (50%)	11%
Knott-Craig et al., 1993 (26)	120	778 (11.5%)	42 (7%)	—
Chen et al., 1997	15	—	15 (6.7%)	—

Source: Ref. 169.

Appropriate interpretation of mortality rates in patients treated medically, however, requires a study of patients deemed operable who are managed medically (251). Additionally, bronchial artery embolization was not utilized in any of these reports. Today, with increasing availability of bronchial artery embolization, emergent surgical resection has become less frequent. This current trend towards non-surgical treatment is supported by the results of a large survey comparing management of life-threatening hemoptysis in 1988 and 1998 (252). This survey showed that in 1998, 50% of clinicians preferred interventional radiography to surgery, compared to 23% questioned in 1988 ($P < 0.0001$).

The evaluation of patients for surgery requires assessment of underlying cardiopulmonary reserve, precise localization of bleeding, and observation of a source amendable to resection. Spirometry has been performed safely in patients with massive hemoptysis. Frequently, however, patients are too ill to undergo pulmonary function testing; therefore, historical data are used to assess their surgical candidacy. Additional helpful information includes arterial blood gas results, dyspnea scores, and overall functional status. Surgery may be contraindicated if, historically, there is arterial hypoxemia, carbon dioxide retention, dyspnea at rest, or severe dyspnea on exertion. Additional contraindications to surgery include nonlateralized bleeding site, unresectable carcinoma, hemoptysis secondary to valvular heart disease, and diffuse alveolar hemorrhage.

Morbidity and mortality rates are significantly greater with emergent surgery compared to elective surgery in the nonbleeding patient (192). Common postoperative complications include broncho-pleural fistula, empyema, hemorrhage requiring re-exploration, respiratory insufficiency requiring prolonged ventilatory support, hemothorax and wound infection (3,165). Because the decision regarding surgery is difficult and often made without the benefit of a diagnosis, a multidisciplinary approach involving pulmonologists, thoracic surgeons, and anesthesiologists is essential.

References

1. Premachandra DJ, Prinsley PR, McRae D. Massive haemorrhage from the vallecula: a diagnostic difficulty. Case report. Eur J Surg 1991; 157:297–298.
2. Crocco JA, Rooney JJ, Frankushen DS, DiBenedetto RJ, Lyons HA. Massive hemoptysis. Arch Intern Med 1968; 121:495–498.
3. Gourin A, Garzon AA. Operative treatment of massive hemoptysis. Ann Thorac Surg 1974; 18:52–60.
4. Pursel SE, Lindskog GE. Hemoptysis: a clinical evaluation of 103 patients examined consecutively on a thoracic surgical service. Am Rev Respir Dis 1961; 84:329–336.
5. Johnston RN, Lockhart W, Richie RT. Hemoptysis. Br Med J 1960; 1:592–595.
6. Marshall TJ, Jackson JE. Vascular intervention in the thorax: bronchial artery embolization for hemoptysis. Eur Radiol 1997; 7:1221–1227.
7. Cauldwell EW, Siekert RG, Lininger RE, Anson BJ. The bronchial arteries: an anatomic study of 150 human cadavers. Surg Gynecol Obstet 1948; 86:395–412.

8. Yoon WY, Kim FK, Kim YH, Chung TW, Kang HK. Bronchial and nonbronchial systemic systemic artery embolization for life-threatening hemoptysis; a comprehensive review. Radiographics 2002; 22:1395–1409.

9. Deffebach ME, Charan NB, Lashminarayan S, Bulter J. The bronchial circulation: small, but a vital attribute of the lung. Am Rev Respir Dis 1987; 135:463–481.

10. Stenbach G, Varon J. Massive hemoptysis. Intensive Care World 1995; 12:74–79.

11. Remy J, Lemaitre L, Lafitte JJ, Vilain MO, Saint Michel J, Steenhouwer F. Massive hemoptysis of pulmonary arterial origin: diagnosis and treatment. Am J Roentgenol 1984; 143:963–969.

12. Keller FS, Rosch J, Loflin TG, Nath PH, McElvein RB. Nonbronchial systemic collateral arteries: significance in percutaneous embolotherapy for hemoptysis. Radiology 1987; 164:687–692.

13. Santiago S, Tobias J, Williams AJ. A reappraisal of the causes of hemoptysis. Arch Intern Med 1991; 151:2449–2451.

14. Johnston H, Reisz G. Changing spectrum of hemoptysis. Underlying causes in 148 patients undergoing diagnostic flexible fiberoptic bronchoscopy. Arch Intern Med 1989; 149:1666–1668.

15. Hirshberg B, Biran I, Glazer M, Kramer MR. Hemoptysis: etiology, evaluation, and outcome in a tertiary referral hospital. Chest 1997; 112:440–444.

16. Yaacob I, Harun Z, Ahmad Z. Fibreoptic bronchoscopy—a Malaysian experience. Singapore Med J 1991; 32:26–28.

17. Razaque MA, Mutum SS, Singh TS. Recurrent haemoptysis? Think of paragonimiasis. Trop Doct 1991; 2:153–155.

18. Porter DK, Van Every MJ, Anthracite RF, Mack JW Jr. Massive hemoptysis in cystic fibrosis. Arch Intern Med 1983; 143:287–290.

19. Ference BA, Shannon TM, White RI Jr, Zawin M, Burdge CM. Life-threatening pulmonary hemorrhage with pulmonary arteriovenous malformations and hereditary hemorrhagic telangiectasia. Chest 1994; 106:1387–1390.

20. Levitt N. Clinical significance of hemoptysis. J Mich State Med Soc 1951; 50:606–610.

21. Minor GR. Haemorrhage in pulmonary tuberculosis. Am Rev Tuberc 1943; 48:109–114

22. Rasmussen V. Hemoptysis, especially when fatal, in its anatomical and clinical aspects. Edinburgh Medical Journal 1868; 14:385–404.

23. Auerbach O. Pathology and pathogenesis of pulmonary arterial aneurysm in tuberculous cavities. Am Rev Tuberc 1939; 39:99–115.

24. Plessinger VA, Jolly PN. Rasmussen's aneurysms and fatal hemorrhage in pulmonary tuberculosis. Am Rev Tuberc 1949; 60:589–603.

25. Stinghe RV, Mangiulea VG. Hemoptysis of bronchial origin occurring in patients with arrested tuberculosis. Am Rev Respir Dis 1970; 101:84–89.

26. Knott-Craig CJ, Oostuizen JG, Rossouw G, Joubert JR, Barnard PM. Management and prognosis of massive hemoptysis. Recent experience with 120 patients. J Thorac Cardiovasc Surg 1993; 10:394–397.

27. Albelda SM, Talbot GH, Gerson SL, Miller WT, Cassileth PA. Pulmonary cavitation and massive hemoptysis in invasive pulmonary aspergillosis. Influence of bone marrow recovery in patients with acute leukemia. Am Rev Respir Dis 1985; 131:115–120.

28. Jerray M, Hayouni A, Benzarti M, Klabi N, Garrouche A. Blastomycosis in Africa: a new case from Tunisia. Eur Respir J 1992; 5:365–367.

29. Loyd JE, Tillman BF, Atkinson JB, Des Prez RM. Mediastinal fibrosis complicating histoplasmosis. Medicine 1988; 67:295–310.

30. Breuer R, Baigelman W, Pugatch RD. Occult mycetoma. J Comput Assist Tomogr 1982; 6:166–168.

31. Butz RO, Zvetina JR, Leininger BJ. Ten-year experience with mycetomas in patients with pulmonary tuberculosis. Chest 1985; 87:356–358.

32. Hughes CF, Waugh R, Lindsay D. Surgery for pulmonary aspergilloma: preoperative embolisation of the bronchial circulation. Thorax 1986; 41:324–325.

33. Jewkes J, Kay PH, Paneth M, Citron KM. Pulmonary aspergilloma: analysis of prognosis in relation to haemoptysis and survey of treatment. Thorax 1983; 38:572–578.

34. Uflacker R, Kaemmerer A, Neves C, Picon PD. Management of massive hemoptysis by bronchial artery embolization. Radiology 1983; 146:627–634.

35. Rogol PR. Fatal hemoptysis due to lung abscess and pulmoaortic fistula. Chest 1988; 94:441–442.

36. Thoms NW, Wilson RF, Puro HE, Arbulu A. Life-threatening hemoptysis in primary lung abscess. Ann Thorac Surg 1972; 14:347–358.

37. Silverman NA, Levitsky S, Spigos DG, Tan WS, Amiry AA. Massive hemoptysis and recurrent tricuspid infective endocarditis in a heroin addict. Successful treatment by bronchial artery embolization and valvulectomy. Chest 1982; 82:195–196.

38. Hamer DH, Schwab LE, Gray R. Massive hemoptysis from thoracic actinomycosis successfully treated by embolization. Chest 1992; 101:1442–1443.

39. Prince SE, Dominger KA, Cunha BA, Klein NC. Klebsiella pneumoniae pneumonia. Heart Lung 1997; 26:413–417.

40. De la Pena L, Izaguirre D, Aguirrebengoa K, Grande C, Montejo M. Varicella pneumonia in the adult: study of 22 cases. Enferm Infecc Microbiol Clin 2000; 18:493–495.

41. Paytubi C, Negredo E, Ferrer S, Monmany J, Barrio JL. Varicella pneumonia in the adult. Study of 9 cases. An Med Interna 2001; 18:312–316.

42. Gomez de la Torre R, Alvarez Carreno F, Rubio Barbon S, Lopez Muniz C. Multiple pulmonary nodules as a manifestation of varicella. An Med Interna 1998; 15:31–32.

43. Glick N, Levin S, Nelson K. Recurrent pulmonary infarction in adult chickenpox pneumonia. JAMA 1972; 222:173–177.

44. Gale D, Lord JD. Overgrowth of Serratia marcescens in respiratory tract, simulating hemoptysis; report of a case. J Am Med Assoc 1957; 164:1328–1330.

45. Hurtado Ayuso JE, Otero Candelera R, Lopez Casanova C. Pseudo-hemoptysis due to Serratia marcescens, an etiology to remember. Arch Bronconeumol 1999; 35:194–195.

46. Choi WY. Paragonimus westermani: pathogenesis and clinical features of infection. Arzneimittelforschung 1984; 34:1184–1185.

47. Singh NB, Singh KC. Pulmonary paragonimiasis in childhood—a cause of recurrent haemoptysis and pneumonia. Indian J Chest Dis Allied Sci 1989; 31:211–215.

48. Bone RC. Pulmonary & Critical Care Medicine. Mosby-Year Book, Inc., 1998: R19–R13.

49. Field EC. Bronchiectasis: a long term follow-up of medical and surgical cases from child hood. Arch Dis Child 1969; 44:551–561.

50. Ooi GC, Khong PL, Chan-Yeung M, Ho JC, Chan PK, Lee JC, Lam WK, Tsang KW. High-resolution CT quantification of bronchiectasis: clinical and functional correlation. Radiology 2002; 225:663–672.

51. Lee JH, Kim YK, Kwag HJ, Chang JH. Relationships between high-resolution computed tomography, lung function and bacteriology in stable bronchiectasis. J Korean Med Sci 2004; 19:62–68.

52. Cahill BC, Ingbar DH. Massive hemoptysis. Assessment and management. Clin Chest Med 1994; 15:147–167.

53. Porter DK, Van Every MJ, Anthracite RF, Mack JW Jr. Massive hemoptysis in cystic fibrosis. Arch Intern Med 1983; 143:287–290.

54. Porter DK, Van Every MJ, Mack JW Jr. Emergency lobectomy for massive hemoptysis in cystic fibrosis. J Thorac Cardiovasc Surg 1983; 86:409–411.

55. Spark RP, Sobonya RE, Armbruster RJ, Marco JD, Rotkis TC. Pathologic bronchial vasculature in a case of massive hemoptysis due to chronic bronchitis. Chest 1991; 99:504–505.

56. Levitt N. Clinical significance of hemoptysis. J Mich State Med Soc 1951; 50:606–610.

57. Miller RR, McGregor DH. Hemorrhage from carcinoma of the lung. Cancer 1980; 46:200–205.

58. Panos RJ, Barr LF, Walsh TJ, Silverman HJ. Factors associated with fatal hemoptysis in cancer patients. Chest 1988; 94:1008–1013.

59. Salyer DC, Salyer WR, Eggleston JC. Bronchial carcinoid tumors. Cancer 1975; 36:1522–1537.

60. Briselli M, Mark GJ, Grillo HC. Tracheal carcinoids. Cancer 1978; 42:2870–2879.

61. Hurt R, Bates M. Carcinoid tumours of the bronchus: a 33 year experience. Thorax 1984; 39:617–623.

62. Bower G. Bronchial adenoma. A review of twenty-eight cases. Am Rev Respir Dis 1965; 92:558–563.

63. Todd TR, Cooper JD, Weissberg D, Delarue NC, Pearson FG. Bronchial carcinoid tumors: twenty years' experience. J Thorac Cardiovasc Surg 1980; 79:532–536.

64. Warren WH, Faber LP, Gould VE. Neuroendocrine neoplasms of the lung. A clinicopathologic update. J Thorac Cardiovasc Surg 1989; 98:321–332.

65. Panos RJ, Barr LF, Walsh TJ, Silverman HJ. Factors associated with fatal hemoptysis in cancer patients. Chest 1988; 94:1008–1013.

66. Dantzig PI, Richardson D, Rayhanzadeh S, Mauro J, Shoss R. Thoracic involvement of non-African Kaposi's sarcoma. Chest 1974; 66:522–525.

67. Meduri GU, Stover DE, Lee M, Myskowski PL, Caravelli JF, Zaman MB. Pulmonary Kaposi's sarcoma in the acquired immune deficiency syndrome. Clinical, radiographic, and pathologic manifestations. Am J Med 1986; 8:11–88.

68. Palvio DH, Paulsen SM, Henneberg EW. Primary angiosarcoma of the lung presenting as intractable hemoptysis. Thorac Cardiovasc Surg 1987; 35:105–107.

69. Schmidt-Wolf I. Schwerdtfeger R, Schwella N, Gallardo J, Schmid HJ, Huhn D, Siegert W. Diffuse pulmonary alveolar hemorrhage after allogeneic bone marrow transplantation. Ann Hematol 1993; 67:139–141.

70. Gerson SL, Talbot GH, Hurwitz S, Strom BL, Lusk EJ, Cassileth PA. Prolonged granulocytopenia: the major risk factor for invasive pulmonary aspergillosis in patients with acute leukemia. Ann Intern Med 1984; 100:345–351.

71. Meyer RD, Young LS, Armstrong D, Yu B. Aspergillosis complicating neoplastic disease. Am J Med 1973; 54:6–15.

72. Muller NL, Miller RR. Diffuse pulmonary hemorrhage. Radiol Clin North Am 1991; 29:965–971.

73. Scarlat A, Bodner G, Liron M. Massive haemoptysis as the presenting symptom in mitral stenosis. Thorax 1986; 41:413–414.

74. Hodes RM. Hemoptysis in rheumatic heart disease. Trop Geogr Med 1992; 44:328–330.

75. Ferguson FC, Kobilak RE, Deitrick JE. Varices of the bronchial veins as a source of hemoptysis in mitral stenosis. Am Heart J 1944; 28:445–456.

76. Szekely P, Turner R, Snaith L. Pregnancy and the changing pattern of rheumatic heart disease. Br Heart J 1973; 35:1293–1303.

77. Hicks GL Jr. Fibrosing mediastinitis. Causing pulmonary artery and vein obstruction with hemoptysis. N Y State J Med 1983; 83:242–244.

78. Bindelglass IL, Trubowitz S. Pulmonary vein obstruction: an uncommon sequel to chronic fibrous mediastinitis. Ann Intern Med 1958; 48:876–891.

79. Cohn RC, Wong R, Spohn WA, Komer M. Death due to diffuse alveolar hemorrhage in a child with pulmonary veno-occlusive disease. Chest 1991; 100:1456–1458.

80. Granton JT. Pulmonary arterial hypertension in congenital heart disease. Cardiol Clin 2002; 20:441–457.

81. Oya H. Poor prognosis and related factors in adults with Eisenmenger syndrome. Am Heart J 2002; 143:739–744.

82. Dines DE, Seward JB, Bernatz PE. Pulmonary arteriovenous fistulas. Mayo Clin Proc 1983; 58:176–181.

83. Hodgson CH, Burchell HB, Good CA, Clagett OT. Hereditary hemorrhagic telangiectasia and pulmonary arteriovenous fistula: survey of a large family. N Engl J Med 1959; 261:625–636.

84. Sluiter-Eringa H, Orie NG, Sluiter HJ. Pulmonary arteriovenous fistula. Diagnosis and prognosis in noncomplainant patients. Am Rev Respir Dis 1969; 100:177–188.

85. Hoffman WS, Weinberg PM, Ring E, Edmunds LH Jr. Massive hemoptysis secondary to pulmonary arteriovenous fistula. Treatment by a catheterization procedure. Chest 1980; 77:697–700.

86. Dines DE, Arms RA, Bernatz PE, Gomes MR. Pulmonary arteriovenous fistulas. Mayo Clin Proc 1974; 49:460–465.

87. Erkan F, Gul A, Tasali E. Pulmonary manifestations of Behcet's disease. Thorax 2001; 56:572–578.

88. Herb S, Hetzel M, Hetzel J, Friedrich J, Weber J. An unusual case of Hughes-Stovin syndrome. Eur Respir J 1998; 11:1191–1193.

89. Riantawan P, Yodtasurodom C, Chotivatanapong T, Subhannachart P. Hughes-Stovin syndrome: a case report and review of the literature. J Med Assoc Thai 1999; 82:312–316.

90. Stein PD, Terrin ML, Hales CA, Palevsky HI, Saltzman HA, Thompson BT, Weg JG. Clinical, laboratory, roentgenographic, and electrocardiographic findings in patients with acute pulmonary embolism and no pre-existing cardiac or pulmonary disease. Chest 1991; 100:598–603.

91. Anderson FA Jr, Wheeler HB, Goldberg RJ, Hosmer DW, Patwardhan NA, Jovanovic B, Forcier A, Dalen JE. A population-based perspective of the hospital

incidence and case-fatality rates of deep vein thrombosis and pulmonary embolism. The Worcester DVT Study. Arch Intern Med 1991; 15:933–938.

92. Stein PD, Willis PW 3rd, DeMets DL. History and physical examination in acute pulmonary embolism in patients without preexisting cardiac or pulmonary disease. Am J Cardiol 1981; 47:218–223.

93. Bell WR, Simon TL, DeMets DL. The clinical features of submassive and massive pulmonary emboli. Am J Med 1977; 62:355–360.

94. Stein PD, Henry JW. Acute pulmonary embolism presenting as pulmonary hemorrhage/infarction syndrome in the elderly. Am J Geriatr Cardiol 1998; 7:36–42.

95. Briggs WA, Johnson JP, Teichman S, Yeager HC, Wilson CB. Antiglomerular basement membrane antibody-mediated glomerulonephritis and Goodpasture's syndrome. Medicine 1979; 58:348–361.

96. Haworth SJ, Savage CO, Carr D, Hughes JM, Rees AJ. Pulmonary haemorrhage complicating Wegener's granulomatosis and microscopic polyarteritis. Br Med J 1985; 290:1775–1778.

97. Gamsu G, Webb WR. Pulmonary hemorrhage in systemic lupus erythematosus. J Can Assoc Radiol 1978; 29:66–68.

98. Milman N, Pedersen FM. Idiopathic pulmonary haemosiderosis. Epidemiology, pathogenic aspects and diagnosis. Respir Med 1998; 92:902–907.

99. Drew WL, Finley TN, Golde DW. Diagnostic lavage and occult pulmonary hemorrhage in thrombocytopenic immunocompromised patients. Am Rev Respir Dis 1977; 116:215–221.

100. Ewan PW, Jones HA, Rhodes CG, Hughes JM. Detection of intrapulmonary hemorrhage with carbon monoxide uptake. Application in goodpasture's syndrome. N Engl J Med 1976; 295:1391–1396.

101. Greening AP, Hughes JM. Serial estimations of carbon monoxide diffusing capacity in intrapulmonary haemorrhage. Clin Sci 1981; 60:507–512.

102. Cordasco EM Jr, Mehta AC, Ahmad M. Bronchoscopically induced bleeding. A summary of nine years' Cleveland clinic experience and review of the literature. Chest 1991; 100:1141–1147.

103. Ahmad M, Livingston DR, Golish JA, Mehta AC, Wiedemann HP. The safety of outpatient transbronchial biopsy. Chest 1986; 90:403–405.

104. Mitchell DM, Emerson CJ, Collyer J, Collins JV. Fibreoptic bronchoscopy: ten years on. Br Med J 1980; 281:360–363.

105. Stableforth DE, Knight RK, Collins JV, Heard BE, Clarke SW. Transbronchial lung biopsy through the fibreoptic bronchoscope. Br J Dis Chest 1978; 72:108–114.

106. Miller JI, Grossman GD. Bronchoscopy in the community hospital. South Med J 1978; 71:129–130.

107. Zavala DC. Pulmonary hemorrhage in fiberoptic transbronchial biopsy. Chest; 70:584–588.

108. Mitchell DM, Emerson CJ, Collyer J, Collins JV. Fibreoptic bronchoscopy: ten years on. Br Med J 1980; 281:360–363.

109. Stancofski ED, Sardi A, Conaway GL. Recognition and management of catheter-induced pulmonary artery rupture. Ann Thorac Surg 1998; 66:1242–1245.

110. Wajon P. Avoiding pulmonary artery rupture. Anaesth Intensive Care 1997; 25:578–579.

111. Poplausky MR, Rozenblit G, Rundback JH, Crea G, Maddineni S, Leonardo R. Swan-Ganz catheter-induced pulmonary artery pseudoaneurysm formation: three case reports and a review of the literature. Chest 2001; 120:2105–2111.

112. Bowdle TA. Complications of invasive monitoring. Anesthesiol Clin North America 2002; 20:571–588.

113. Mullerworth MH, Angelopoulos P, Couyant MA, Horton AM, Robinson SM, Petring OU, Mitchell PJ, Presneill J. Recognition and management of catheter-induced pulmonary artery rupture. Ann Thorac Surg 1998; 66:1242–1245.

114. Kearney TJ, Shabot MM. Pulmonary artery rupture associated with the Swan-Ganz catheter. Chest 1995; 108:1349–1352.

115. Strange C, Sahn SA. Massive Hemoptysis. In Parrillo JE, Dellinger RP, eds. Crtical Care Medicine: Principles and Management in the Adult. 2nd ed. St. Louis: Mosby, 2001:910–929.

116. Pape LA, Haffajee CI, Markis JE, Ockene IS, Paraskos JA, Dalen JE, Alpert JS. Fatal pulmonary hemorrhage after use of the flow-directed balloon-tipped catheter. Ann Intern Med 1979; 90:344–347.

117. Mullerworth MH, Angelopoulos P, Couyant MA, Horton AM, Robinson SM, Petring OU, Mitchell PJ, Presneill JJ. Successful outcome in Swan-Ganz catheter-induced rupture of pulmonary artery. Am Surg 1998; 64:1062–1065.

118. Gottwalles Y, Wunschel-Joseph ME, Hanssen M. Coil embolization treatment in pulmonary artery branch rupture during Swan-Ganz catheterization. Cardiovasc Intervent Radiol 2000; 23:477–479.

119. Tayoro J, Dequin PF, Delhommais A, Alison D, Perrotin D. Rupture of pulmonary artery induced by Swan-Ganz catheter: success of coil embolization. Intensive Care Med 1997; 23:198–200.

120. Thomas R, Siproudhis L, Laurent JF, Bouget J, Bousser J, Camus C, Michelet C. Massive hemoptysis from iatrogenic balloon catheter rupture of pulmonary artery: successful early management by balloon tamponade. Crit Care Med 1987; 15:272–273.

121. Scuderi PE, Prough DS, Price JD, Comer PB. Cessation of pulmonary artery catheter-induced endobronchial hemorrhage associated with the use of PEEP. Anesth Analg 1983; 62:236–238.

122. Jones WS, Mavroudis C, Richardson JD, Gray LA Jr, Howe WR. Management of tracheobronchial disruption resulting from blunt trauma. Surgery 1984; 95:319–323.

123. Unger JM, Schuchmann GG, Grossman JE, Pellett JR. Tears of the trachea and main bronchi caused by blunt trauma: radiologic findings. Am J Roentgenol 1989; 153:1175–1180.

124. Chu CP, Chen PP. Tracheobronchial injury secondary to blunt chest trauma: diagnosis and management. Anaesth Intensive Care 2002; 30:145–152.

125. Kshettry VR, Bolman RM III. Chest trauma. Assessment, diagnosis, and management. Clin Chest Med 1994; 15:137–146.

126. Halttunen PE, Kostiainen SA, Meurala HG. Bronchial rupture caused by blunt chest trauma. Scand J Thorac Cardiovasc Surg 1984; 18:141–144.

127. Shimazu T, Sugimoto H, Nishide K, Terai C, Ohashi N, Yoshioka T, Sugimoto T. Tracheobronchial rupture caused by blunt chest trauma: acute respiratory management. Am J Emerg Med 1988; 6:427–434.

128. Gong H Jr, Salvatierra C. Clinical efficacy of early and delayed fiberoptic broncho-scopy in patients with hemoptysis. Am Rev Respir Dis 1981; 124:221–225.

129. Adelman M, Haponik EF, Bleecker ER, Britt EJ. Cryptogenic hemoptysis. Clinical features, bronchoscopic findings, and natural history in 67 patients. Ann Intern Med 1985; 102:829–834.

130. Barrett RJ, Tuttle WM. A study of essential hemoptysis. J Thorac Cardiovasc Surg 1960; 40:468–474.

131. Pursel SE, Lindskog GE. Hemoptysis. A clinical evaluation of 105 patients examined consecutively on a thoracic surgical service. Am Rev Respir Dis 1961; 84:329–336.

132. Wolfe JD, Simmons DH. Hemoptysis: diagnosis and management. West J Med 1977; 127:383–390.

133. Douglas BE, Carr DT. Prognosis in idiopathic hemoptysis. JAMA 1952; 150:468–473.

134. Souders CR, Smith AT. The clinical significance of hemoptysis. N Engl J Med 1952; 247:790–793.

135. Masson RG, Altose MD, Mayock RL. Isolated bronchial telangiectasia. Chest 1974; 65:450–452.

136. Winter JH. Haemoptysis and aspirin ingestion. Lancet 1983; 1:1441.

137. Smith LJ, Katzenstein AL. Pathogenesis of massive pulmonary hemorrhage in acute leukemia. Arch Intern Med 1982; 142:2149–2152.

138. Golde DW, Drew WL, Klein HZ, Finley TN, Cline MJ. Occult pulmonary haem-orrhage in leukaemia. Br Med J 1975; 2:166–168.

139. Finley TN, Aronow A, Cosentino AM, Golde DW. Occult pulmonary hemorrhage in anticoagulated patients. Am Rev Respir Dis 1975; 112:23–29.

140. Adelman M, Haponik EF, Bleecker ER, Britt EJ. Cryptogenic hemoptysis. Clinical features, bronchoscopic findings, and natural history in 67 patients. Ann Intern Med 1985; 102:829–834.

141. Baktari JB, Tashkin DP, Small GW. Factitious hemoptysis. Adding to the differen-tial diagnosis. Chest 1994; 105:943–945.

142. Saed G, Potalivo S, Panzini L, Bisetti A. Munchausen's syndrome. A case of facti-tious hemoptysis. Panminerva Med 1999; 41:62–67.

143. O'Shea B, Falvey J, Cahill M, McGennis A. Factitious hemoptysis. Arch Intern Med 1984; 144:415–419.

144. Gourin A, Garzon AA. Control of hemorrhage in emergency pulmonary resection for massive hemoptysis. Chest 1975; 68:120–121.

145. Sehhat S, Oreizie M, Moinedine K. Massive pulmonary hemorrhage: surgical approach as choice of treatment. Ann Thorac Surg 1978; 25:12–15.

146. Winter SM, Ingbar DH. Massive hemoptysis: pathogenesis and management. J Inten Care Med 1988; 3:171–188.

147. Corder R. Hemoptysis. Emerg Med Clin North Am 2003; 21:421–435.

148. Israel RH, Poe RH. Hemoptysis. Clin Chest Med 1987; 8:197–205.

149. Bobrowitz ID, Ramakrishna S, Shim YS. Comparison of medical v surgical treat-ment of major hemoptysis. Arch Intern Med 1983; 143:1343–1346.

150. Marshall TJ, Flower CD, Jackson JE. The role of radiology in the investigation and management of patients with haemoptysis. Clin Radiol 1996; 51:391–400.

151. Haponik EF, Rothfeld B, Britt EJ, Bleecker ER. Radionuclide localization of massive pulmonary hemorrhage. Chest 1984; 86:208–212.

152. Coel MN, Druger G. Radionuclide detection of the site of hemoptysis. Chest 1982; 81:242–243.
153. Winzelberg GG, Wholey MH, Jarmolowski CA, Sachs M, Weinberg JH. Patients with hemoptysis examined by Tc-99 m sulfur colloid and Tc-99 m-labeled red blood cells: a preliminary appraisal. Radiology 1984; 153:523–526.
154. Peters J, McClung HC, Teague RB. Evaluation of hemoptysis in patients with a normal chest roentgenogram. West J Med 1984; 141:624–626.
155. Poe RH, Israel RH, Marin MG, Ortiz CR, Dale RC, Wahl GW, Kallay MC, Greenblatt DG. Utility of fiberoptic bronchoscopy in patients with hemoptysis and a nonlocalizing chest roentgenogram. Chest 1988; 93:70–75.
156. Stanford W, Galvin JR. The diagnosis of bronchiectasis. Clin Chest Med 1988; 9:691–699.
157. Shin MS, Ho KJ. Broncholithiasis: its detection by computed tomography in patients with recurrent hemoptysis of unknown etiology. J Comput Tomogr 1983; 7:189–193.
158. Haponik EF, Britt EJ, Smith PL, Bleecker ER. Computed chest tomography in the evaluation of hemoptysis. Impact on diagnosis and treatment. Chest 1987; 91:80–85.
159. Millar AB, Boothroyd AE, Edwards D, Hetzel MR. The role of computed tomography (CT) in the investigation of unexplained haemoptysis. Respir Med 1992; 86:39–44.
160. Set PA, Flower CD, Smith IE, Chan AP, Twentyman OP, Shneerson JM. Hemoptysis: comparative study of the role of CT and fiberoptic bronchoscopy. Radiology 1993; 89:677–680.
161. McGuinness G, Beacher JR, Harkin TJ, Garay SM, Rom WN, Naidich DP. Hemoptysis: prospective high-resolution CT/bronchoscopic correlation. Chest 1994; 105:1155–1162.
162. Jackson CV, Savage PJ, Quinn DL. Role of fiberoptic bronchoscopy in patients with hemoptysis and a normal chest roentgenogram. Chest 1985; 87:142–144.
163. Muller NL. Hemoptysis: high-resolution CT vs bronchoscopy. Chest 1994; 105:982–983.
164. Haponik EF, Chin R. Hemoptysis: clinicians' perspectives. Chest 1990; 97:469–475.
165. Garzon AA, Cerruti MM, Golding ME. Exsanguinating hemoptysis. J Thorac Cardiovasc Surg 1982; 84:829–833.
166. Weaver LJ, Solliday N, Cugell DW. Selection of patients with hemoptysis for fiberoptic bronchoscopy. Chest 1979; 76:7–10.
167. Smiddy JF, Elliott RC. The evaluation of hemoptysis with fiberoptic bronchoscopy. Chest 1973; 64:158–162.
168. Fishman AP. Pulmonary Disease and Disorders. 2nd ed. New York: McGraw Hill, 1988:436–467.
169. Dweik RA, Stoller JK. Role of bronchoscopy in massive hemoptysis. Clin Chest Med 1999; 20:89–105.
170. Helmers RA, Sanderson DR. Rigid bronchoscopy. The forgotten art. Clin Chest Med 1995; 16:393–399.
171. Conlan AA, Hurwitz SS. Management of massive haemoptysis with the rigid bronchoscope and cold saline lavage. Thorax 1980; 35:901–904.
172. Goldman JM. Hemoptysis: emergency assessment and management. Emerg Med Clin North Am 1989; 7:325–338.

173. Hiebert CA. Balloon catheter control of life-threatening hemoptysis. Chest 1974; 66:308–309.

174. Williams MH Jr. Life-threatening haemoptysis. Lancet 1987; 1:1354–1356.

175. Thompson AB, Teschler H, Rennard SI. Pathogenesis, evaluation, and therapy for massive hemoptysis. Clin Chest Med 1992; 13:69–82.

176. Jean-Baptiste E. Clinical assessment and management of massive hemoptysis. Crit Care Med 2000; 28:1642–1647.

177. Susanto I. Managing a patient with hemoptysis. J Bronchology 2002; 9:40–45.

178. Szekely SM, Vickers MD. A comparison of the effects of codeine and tramadol on laryngeal reactivity. Eur J Anaesthesiol 1992; 9:111–120.

179. Strange C. Double lumen endotracheal tubes. Clin Chest Med 1991; 12:497–506.

180. Shivaram U, Finch P, Nowak P. Plastic endobronchial tubes in the management of life-threatening hemoptysis. Chest 1987; 92:1108–1110.

181. Klein U, Karzai W, Bloos F, Wohlfarth M, Gottschall R, Fritz H, Gugel M, Seifert A. Role of fiberoptic bronchoscopy in conjunction with the use of double-lumen tubes for thoracic anesthesia: a prospective study. Anesthesiology 1998; 88:346–350.

182. Saw EC, Gottlieb LS, Yokoyama T, Lee BC. Flexible fiberoptic bronchoscopy and endobronchial tamponade in the management of massive hemoptysis. Chest 1976; 70:589–591.

183. Gottlieb LS, Hillberg R. Endobronchial tamponade therapy for intractable hemoptysis. Chest 1975; 67:482–483.

184. Swersky RB, Chang JB, Wisoff BG, Gorvoy J. Endobronchial balloon tamponade of hemoptysis in patients with cystic fibrosis. Ann Thorac Surg 1979; 27:262–264.

185. Jolliet P, Soccal P, Chevrolet JC. Control of massive hemoptysis by endobronchial tamponade with a pulmonary artery balloon catheter. Crit Care Med 1992; 20:1730–1732.

186. Freitag L. Development of a new balloon catheter for management of hemoptysis with bronchofiberscopes. Chest 1993; 103:593.

187. Freitag L, Tekolf E, Stamatis G, Montag M, Greschuchna D. Three years experience with a new balloon catheter for the management of haemoptysis. Eur Respir J 1994; 7:2033–2037.

188. Arndt GA, Kranner PW, Lorenz D. Co-axial placement of endobronchial blocker. Can J Anaesth 1994; 41:1126–1127.

189. Arndt GA, DeLessio ST, Kranner PW, Orzepowski W, Ceranski B, Valtysson B. One-lung ventilation when intubation is difficult—presentation of a new endobronchial blocker. Acta Anaesthesiol Scand 1999; 43:356–358.

190. Arndt GA, Kranner PW, Rusy DA, Love R. Single-lung ventilation in a critically ill patient using a fiberoptically directed wire-guided endobronchial blocker. Anesthesiology 1999; 90:1484–1486.

191. Campos JH. An update on bronchial blockers during lung separation techniques in adults. Anesth Analg 2003; 97:1266–1274.

192. Conlan AA, Hurwitz SS, Krige L, Nicolaou N, Pool R. Massive hemoptysis. Review of 123 cases. J Thorac Cardiovasc Surg 1983; 85:120–124.

193. Dupree HJ, Lewejohann JC, Gleiss J, Muhl E, Bruch HP. Role of bronchoscopy in massive hemoptysis. Chest Surg Clin N Am 2001; 11:873–906.

194. Dupree HJ, Lewejohann JC, Gleiss J, Muhl E, Bruch HP. Fiberoptic bronchoscopy of intubated patients with life-threatening hemoptysis. World J Surg 2001; 25:104–107.

195. Sidman JD, Wheeler WB, Cabalka AK, Soumekh B, Brown CA, Wright GB. Management of acute pulmonary hemorrhage in children. Laryngoscope 2001; 111:33–35.

196. Tsukamoto T, Sasaki H, Nakamura H. Treatment of hemoptysis by thrombin and fibrinogen-thrombin infusion therapy using a fiberoptic bronchoscope. Chest 1988; 96:473–476.

197. Bense L. Intrabronchial selective coagulative treatment of hemoptysis. Report of three cases. Chest 1990; 97:990–996.

198. de Gracia J, de la Rosa D, Catalan E, Alvarez A, Bravo C, Morell F. Use of endoscopic fibrinogen-thrombin in the treatment of severe hemoptysis. Respir Med 2003; 97:790–795.

199. Magee G, Williams MH Jr. Treatment of massive hemoptysis with intravenous pitressin. Lung 1982; 160:165–169.

200. Bilton D, Webb AK, Foster H, Mulvenna P, Dodd M. Life threatening haemoptysis in cystic fibrosis: an alternative therapeutic approach. Thorax 1990; 45:975–976.

201. Pea L, Roda L, Boussaud V, Lonjon B. Desmopressin therapy for massive hemoptysis associated with severe leptospirosis. Am J Respir Crit Care Med 2003; 167:726–728.

202. Stoller JK. Diagnosis and management of massive hemoptysis: a review. Respir Care 1992; 37:564–581.

203. Remy J, Arnaud A, Fardou H, Giraud R, Voisin C. Treatment of hemoptysis by embolization of bronchial arteries. Radiology 1977; 122:33–37.

204. Green RJ, Ruoss SJ, Kraft SA, Duncan SR, Berry GJ, Raffin TA. Pulmonary capillaritis and alveolar hemorrhage. Update on diagnosis and management. Chest 1996; 110:1305–1316.

205. Leatherman JW, Davies SF, Hoidal JR. Alveolar hemorrhage syndromes: diffuse microvascular lung hemorrhage in immune and idiopathic disorders. Medicine 1984; 63:343–361.

206. Pastores SM, Papadopoulos E, Voigt L, Halpern NA. Diffuse alveolar hemorrhage after allogeneic hematopoietic stem-cell transplantation: treatment with recombinant factor VIIa. Chest 2003; 124:2400–2403.

207. Henke D, Falk RJ, Gabriel DA. Successful treatment of diffuse alveolar hemorrhage with activated factor VII. Ann Intern Med 2004; 140:493–494.

208. Hargis JL, Bone RC, Stewart J, Rector N, Hiller FC. Intracavitary amphotereicin B in the treatment of symptomatic pulmonary aspergillomas. Am J Med 1980; 68:389–394.

209. Glimp RA, Bayer AS. Pulmonary aspergilloma. Diagnostic and therapeutic considerations. Arch Intern Med 1983; 143:303–308.

210. Jewkes J, Kay PH, Paneth M, Citron KM. Pulmonary aspergilloma: analysis of prognosis in relation to haemoptysis and survey of treatment. Thorax 1983; 38:572–578.

211. Shapiro MJ, Albelda SM, Mayock RL, McLean GK. Severe hemoptysis associated with pulmonary aspergilloma. Percutaneous intracavitary treatment. Chest 1988; 94:1225–1231.

212. Rosenberg SM, Riddick DH. Successful treatment of catamenial hemoptysis with danazol. Obstet Gynecol 1981; 57:130–132.

213. Elliot DL, Barker AF, Dixon LM. Catamenial hemoptysis. New methods of diagnosis and therapy. Chest 1985; 87:687–688.

214. Di Palo S, Mari G, Castoldi R, Staudacher C, Taccagni G, Di Carlo V. Endometriosis of the lung. Respir Med 1989; 83:255–258.

215. Espaulella J, Armengol J, Bella F, Lain JM, Calaf J. Pulmonary endometriosis: conservative treatment with GnRH agonists. Obstet Gynecol 1991; 78:535–537.

216. Lang N, Maners A, Broadwater J, Shewmake K, Chu D, Westbrook K. Management of airway problems in lung cancer patients using the neodymium-yttrium-aluminum-garnet (Nd-YAG) laser and endobronchial radiotherapy. Am J Surg 1988; 156:463–465.

217. Edmondstone WM, Nanson EM, Woodcock AA, Millard FJ, Hetzel MR. Life threatening haemoptysis controlled by laser photocoagulation. Thorax 1983; 38:788–789.

218. Hetzel MR, Nixon C, Edmondstone WM, Mitchell DM, Millard FJ, Nanson EM, Woodcock AA, Bridges CE, Humberstone AM. Laser therapy in 100 tracheobronchial tumours. Thorax 1985; 40:341–345.

219. Shankar S, George PJ, Hetzel MR, Goldstraw P. Elective resection of tumours of the trachea and main carina after endoscopic laser therapy. Thorax 1990; 45:493–495.

220. Morice RC, Ece T, Ece F, Keus L. Endobronchial argon plasma coagulation for treatment of hemoptysis and neoplastic airway obstruction. Chest 2001; 119:781–787.

221. Keller CA, Hinerman R, Singh A, Alvarez F. The use of endoscopic argon plasma coagulation in airway complications after solid organ transplantation. Chest 2001; 119:1968–1975.

222. Hoegler D. Radiotherapy for palliation of symptoms in incurable cancer. Curr Probl Cancer 1997; 21:129–183.

223. Falkson C, Sur R, Pacella J. External beam radiotherapy: a treatment option for massive haemoptysis caused by mycetoma. Clin Oncol 2002; 14:233–235.

224. Shneerson JM, Emerson PA, Phillips RH. Radiotherapy for massive haemoptysis from an aspergilloma. Thorax 1980; 35:953–954.

225. Fernando HC, Stein M, Benfield JR, Link DP. Role of bronchial artery embolization in the management of hemoptysis. Arch Surg 1998; 133:862–866.

226. MacIntosh EL, Parrott JCW, Unrhu HW. Fistulas between the aorta and tracheobronchial tree. Ann Thorac Surg 1991; 51:515–519.

227. Hakanson E, Konstantinov IE, Fransson SG. Management of life-threatening haemoptysis. Br J Anaesth 2001; 88:291–295.

228. Pearse IO, Bryan AJ. Massive hemoptysis 27 years after surgery for coarctation of the aorta. J R Soc Med 2001; 94:640–641.

229. Mauro MA, Jaques PF. Transcatheter bronchial artery embolization for inflammation (hemoptysis). In: Baum S, Pentecost MJ, eds. Abrams' Angiography: International Radiology. Vol. 3. Boston: Little, Brown and Company, 1997; 819–828.

230. Tanomkiat W, Tanisaro K. Radiographic relationship of the origin of the bronchial arteries to the left main bronchus. J Thorac Imaging 2003; 18:27–33.

231. Kardjiev V, Symeonov A, Chankov I. Etiology, pathogenesis, and prevention of spinal cord lesions in selective angiography of the bronchial and intercostals arteries. Radiology 1974; 112:81–83.

232. Feigelson HH, Ravin HA. Transverse myelitis following selective bronchial arteriography. Radiology 1965; 85:663–665.

233. Lois JF, Gomes AS, Smith DC, Laks H. Systemic-to-pulmonary collateral vessels and shunts: treatment with embolization. Radiology 1988; 169:671–676.

234. Doppman JL, Girton M, Oldfield EH. Spinal WADA test. Radiology 1986; 161:319–321.

235. White RI Jr. Bronchial artery embolotherapy for control of acute hemoptysis: analysis of outcome. Chest 1999; 115:912–915.

236. Pump K. Distribution of bronchial arteries in human lung. Chest 1972; 62:447–451.

237. Boushy SF, Helgason AH, North LB. Occlusion of the bronchial arteries by glass microspheres. Am Rev Respir Dis 1971; 103:249–263.

238. Fuhrman BP, Bass JL, Castaneda-Zuniga W, Fuhrman BP, Rashkind WJ, Lucas RV Jr. Coil embolization of congenital thoracic vascular anomalies in infants and children. Circulation 1984; 70:285–289.

239. Ramakantan R, Bandekar VG, Gandhi MS, Aulakh BG, Deshmukh HL. Massive hemoptysis due to pulmonary tuberculosis: control with bronchial artery embolization. Radiology 1996; 200:691–694.

240. Cohen AM, Doershuk CF, Stern RC. Bronchial artery embolization to control hemoptysis in cystic fibrosis. Radiology 1990; 175:401–405.

241. Tonkin IL, Hanissian AS, Boulden TF, Baum SL, Gavant ML, Gold RE, George P, Green WJ. Bronchial arteriography and embolotherapy for hemoptysis in patients with cystic fibrosis. Cardiovasc Intervent Radiol 1991; 14:241–246.

242. Remy J, Arnaud A, Fardou H, Giroud R, Voisin C. Treatment of hemoptysis by embolization of bronchial arteries. Radiology 1977; 122:33–37.

243. Hayakawa K, Tanaka F, Torizuka T, Mitsumori M, Okuno Y, Matsui A, Satoh Y, Fujiwara K, Misaki T. Bronchial artery embolization for hemoptysis: immediate and long-term results. Cardiovasc Intervent Radiol 1992; 15:154–159.

244. Uflacker R, Kaemmerer A, Picon PD, Rizzon CF, Neves CM, Oliveira ES, Oliveira ME, Azevedo SN, Ossanai R. Bronchial artery embolization in the management of hemoptysis: technical aspects and long-term results. Radiology 1985; 157:637–644.

245. Rabkin JE, Astafjev VI, Gothman LN, Grigorjev YG. Transcatheter embolization in the management of pulmonary hemorrhage. Radiology 1987; 163:361–365.

246. Tamura S, Kodama T, Otsuka N, Kihara Y, Nisikawa K, Yuki Y, Samejima M, Uwada O, Watanabe K, Minoda S. Embolotherapy for persistent hemoptysis: the significance of pleural thickening. Cardiovasc Intervent Radiol 1993; 16:85–88.

247. Cohen AM, Doershuk CF, Stern RC. Bronchial artery embolization to control hemoptysis in cystic fibrosis. Radiology 1990; 175:401–405.

248. Fellows KE, Khaw KT, Schuster S, Shwachman H. Bronchial artery embolization in cystic fibrosis: technique and long-term results. J Pediatr 1979; 95:959–963.

249. Garzon AA, Gourin A. Surgical management of massive hemoptysis. A ten-year experience. Ann Surg 1978; 187:267–271.
250. Garzon AA, Cerruti M, Gourin A, Karlson KE. Pulmonary resection for massive hemoptysis. Surgery 1970; 67:633–638.
251. Corey R, Hla KM. Major and massive hemoptysis: reassessment of conservative management. Am J Med Sci 1987; 294:301–309.
252. Haponik EF, Fein A, Chin R. Managing life-threatening hemoptysis:has anything really changed? Chest 2000; 118:1431–1435.

5

Pneumonia in the ICU

RICHARD G. WUNDERINK

Division of Pulmonary and Critical Care, Northwestern University
   Feinberg School of Medicine
Chicago, Illinois, U.S.A.

I. Introduction

Pneumonia is one of the most common clinical problems presenting to critical care physicians. The pneumonia can present as four main syndromes—severe community-acquired pneumonia (SCAP), hospital-acquired pneumonia (HAP), pneumonia in the immunocompromised patient, and intensive care unit (ICU)-acquired pneumonia, which is principally ventilator-associated pneumonia (VAP). The first three are primarily causes for ICU admission while the latter is one of the most common complications of ICU care. This review will focus predominantly on SCAP and VAP. Pneumonia in the immunocompromised patient is in many ways just a more severe manifestation of SCAP, while VAP represents the severe end of the spectrum of HAP. Where differences between these overlapping syndromes may occur will be commented upon briefly.

II. Ventilator-Associated Pneumonia

While few intensive care physicians doubt the clinical importance of VAP, little agreement exists about any other aspect of VAP. This is unfortunate since VAP is such an important clinical problem.

A. Diagnosis

The key controversy in VAP management is the uncertainty regarding diagnosis. This diagnostic dilemma revolves around three important issues: (1) the

167

nonspecificity of clinical signs and symptoms, (2) association of inappropriate initial antibiotic therapy with excess mortality, and (3) the increased mortality and selection for antibiotic-resistant micro-organisms caused by excessive antibiotic therapy.

The cardinal signs and symptoms of VAP are similar to that of SCAP—fever, purulent sputum, leukocytosis, hypoxemia, and radiographic infiltrates. However, what is a very accurate set of diagnostic criteria in community-acquired pneumonia (CAP) patients is extremely compromised for VAP diagnosis. Critically ill patients, especially when ventilated, have multiple other potential sources for fever and leukocytosis (1). Increased or purulent sputum production and radiographic infiltrates are the principal means of localizing the source of infection to the lung. Unfortunately, both are inaccurate in the ventilated patient.

Tracheal colonization by pathogenic microorganisms occurs in a large (>30%) proportion of ventilated patients. This colonization occurs early in the course of ventilation and tends to increase in proportion to the duration of mechanical ventilation, such that by the end of three to four weeks on a ventilator, most patients have at least transiently harbored pathogenic micro-organisms in their lower airways. Therefore, the presence of pathogenic micro-organisms alone is insufficient evidence of the presence of VAP. Hospitalized but nonintubated patients also are frequently colonized with pathogenic bacteria, but to a much lower degree than intubated patients. An increased volume of secretions also can occur for noninfectious reasons, such as fluid overload or a decrease in the endotracheal tube cuff pressure. Both increased volume of secretions and purulence increase the probability of VAP but remain very nonspecific.

A new or worsening radiographic infiltrate is felt to be required for the diagnosis of VAP. An absolutely normal chest X-ray (CXR) is fairly strong evidence against pneumonia. However, chest computerized tomography (CT) scans can pick up basilar infiltrates in up to 20% of patients whose plain CXRs are considered normal (2). The more common problem is that ventilated patients often have abnormal CXRs before developing other symptoms suggestive of VAP. Detecting a new infiltrate may be nearly impossible, such as in patients with ARDS. New infiltrates or changes in existing infiltrates can also occur from multiple other common clinical problems in the ICU (3). The most common are pulmonary edema (ARDS, fluid overload, or cardiogenic), atelectasis, and pleural effusions, but pulmonary hemorrhage, infarction, and chemical pneumonitis from aspiration are also not uncommon.

The net result is that VAP is significantly overdiagnosed by the usual clinical criteria. This knowledge has led to intense research on improving the accuracy of the diagnosis of VAP. This research has revolved around obtaining more peripheral samples of respiratory secretions to culture and the use of quantitative cultures of secretions to separate colonization from infection.

Despite ongoing controversy regarding which strategy is best, these studies have led to several important areas of consensus. The first is that, when sought aggressively, other sources of fever and causes of radiographic infiltrates will be identified in patients whose suspicion of VAP has not been confirmed (1,4). A second is that a diagnostic strategy that leads to more antibiotic use is consistently associated with an increased mortality (4,5). The important philosophical implication is that antibiotics are not benign, and careful consideration of the risk benefit ratio is needed their use. The third is that no gold standard exists to which diagnostic techniques can be compared in order to know the "truth" about sensitivity or specificity. Even interpretation of lung histology has been shown to vary between pathologists (6). Understanding of this latter fact has led to an appropriate shift in focus from studies of the sensitivity and specificity of diagnostic tests to studies of clinical outcome based on different diagnostic strategies.

A general misconception is that only two diagnostic strategies for VAP exist—the invasive (usually bronchoscopic) and the noninvasive (usually based on nonquantitative cultures of endotracheal aspirates). Multiple options at specific decision points are possible (Table 1). The main decision points are when VAP is initially suspected, when results of initial cultures return, and when the patient appears to not respond clinically. Unfortunately, most of the clinical trials force patients to all be managed with the same strategy, while clinicians often use the pretest probability of VAP to individualize management strategy. If the pretest probability of VAP is low, many physicians are comfortable with waiting on culture results, while this approach as a general strategy would probably not be acceptable.

The best-studied strategy is to test, screen, start empiric antibiotics based on a positive screening test, and modify antibiotics when culture results return. This strategy was used in both arms of the randomized controlled trial of invasive versus noninvasive diagnosis (4). A bronchoalveolar lavage (BAL) or endotracheal aspirate (ETA) Gram stain was the screening test used. No antibiotics were started in either arm if no organisms were seen. The number of subsequent positive cultures was very low and the mortality of patients in whom antibiotics were withheld in either group was low, especially for a group of patients in whom VAP is suspected. This outcome confirms previous data that suggests that the probability of VAP is <5% when a ETA has <1 micro-organism per high power field (7). Screening by Gram stain also led to one of the lowest incidence rates of inappropriate initial antibiotic therapy in *both* groups reported in the literature. A carefully done Gram stain of ETA therefore appears to be adequate to exclude VAP, guide initial empiric therapy, and possibly to screen for patients who may need a more definitive positive diagnosis via invasive quantitative cultures. The practical clinical limitation of this strategy is the inability of many microbiology laboratories to provide this accurately and in a timely manner.

This study of Fagon et al. (4) is presently the largest and only multicenter randomized trial of diagnostic strategy in the VAP literature. The invasive strategy resulted in a lower 14-day mortality rate (the primary endpoint) and a severity-adjusted 28-day mortality. The 9.6% absolute mortality risk reduction at 14 days (number needed to treat to avoid one death of <11) compares favorably with

Table 1 Management Strategies for VAP and Appropriateness of Strategy Based on Pretest Probability of VAP

Strategy	Initial	Subsequent	Example (Ref.)
1	Quantitative culture (QC)	Treat only positive	
2	QC, screen, empiric treatment of positive	Stop or modify based on culture	Fagon (4)
3	QC, start empiric	Stop or modify based on culture	Singh (5)
4	QC, start empiric	Modify only based on culture	Ruiz (10),
			Sanchez-Nieto (12)
5	Start empiric, QC culture	Modify only based on culture	
6	Non-QC culture, start empiric	Stop or modify based on culture	
7	Non-QC culture, start empiric	Modify based on culture,	Ioanas (14)
		QC only if not responding	
8	Non-QC culture	Modify based on culture	
9	Empiric	Empiric change if not responding	

other critical care interventions (8). The invasive strategy also clearly led to fewer antibiotic days and less use of every antibiotic class except carbapenems. This study is one of those that demonstrate an association between lower mortality and a diagnostic strategy that leads to fewer antibiotics. The temptation is to suggest that this is cause and effect, most likely through less antibiotic pressure to select for highly resistant bacteria. However, a lower incidence of subsequent infections with resistant microorganisms was not found, possibly because the invasive strategy was not applied to all patients in each ICU and cross infection may have occurred. An alternative explanation for the lower mortality is that more extrapulmonary infections were documented in the invasive group, which may also have resulted in lower mortality via more effective treatment of these infections.

Another diagnostic/treatment strategy is to test, start empiric therapy, and either stop or modify antibiotics when cultures return. This strategy was used by Singh et al. (5) to focus on patients with a low modified clinical pulmonary infection score (CPIS). The original CPIS score suggested that VAP was unlikely with a CPIS <6, but required results of ETA cultures (9). Since these are not routinely available at the time that VAP is first suspected, a modified CPIS score used (Table 2). Patients with an initial CPIS score of <6 were randomized to three

Table 2 Modified Clinical Pulmonary Infection Score (CPIS)

Factor	Points
Temperature ($^{\circ}$C)	
$\geq 38.5^{\circ}$ and $< 38.9^{\circ}$	1
$\geq 39.0^{\circ}$ or $< 38.5^{\circ}$	2
Blood leukocytes (mm^3)	
< 4000 or $> 11,000$	1
Above plus bands $\geq 50\%$	2
Tracheal secretions	
Present but nonpurulent	1
Purulence	2
Oxygenation (P_aO_2/F_IO_2, mmHg)	
< 240 and no ARDS	2
Chest radiograph	
Diffuse or patchy infiltrate	1
Localized infiltrate	2
[a]Progression of chest radiograph	
Progression (but no CHF or ARDS)	2
[a]Culture of tracheal aspirate	
Pathogenic bacteria in moderate or heavy growth	1
Above, plus same pathogenic species seen on Gram stain	2

[a]Criteria only assessed on day 3 of diagnosis.
Abbreviations: ARDS, acute respiratory distress syndrome; CHF, congestive heart failure.
Source: From Ref. 5.

days of ciprofloxacin or standard antibiotic therapy. After three days, if the CPIS score (which now included results of the ETA culture) remained <6, antibiotics were stopped in the ciprofloxacin arm or modified based on culture and continued if the CPIS score now rose above six. Results of the study demonstrated that the short course therapy group had fewer superinfections, less development of resistance, and a trend toward lower mortality, again confirming the association between less antibiotic therapy and lower mortality. This study confirms that even if antibiotics are started empirically for suspected VAP, discontinuation after only a few doses if the clinical suspicion is not confirmed is not only safe, but will have beneficial outcomes.

A fourth strategy is to test, start empiric therapy, and only modify therapy based on culture results. This is the strategy used by the other three randomized controlled trials of diagnostic strategies (10–12). Narrowing of the antibiotic spectrum was significantly more common in the one study that compared quantitative cultures to nonquantitative ETA cultures (11). This study included mainly patients with early onset VAP and a low baseline mortality. The other two studies compared quantitative ETA cultures to quantitative bronchoscopy cultures (10,12). The main differences between groups in the latter two studies probably reflected differences based on randomization in a relatively small population, that is, more Pseudomonas VAP in the invasive group, than any differences resulting from the diagnostic strategy. In none of these studies were antibiotics discontinued based on a negative culture. Correspondingly, no statistically significant differences in mortality were found between the groups in any study. While this may reflect the smaller numbers and a possible beta-error, the pattern also fits the positive association between antibiotic use and death. The Singh et al. study noted above (5) and multiple other observational studies of BAL and PSB quantitative cultures suggest that continuing antibiotics with negative cultures should be discouraged. The one exception is if the patient has developed hemodynamic instability or significantly worsening respiratory failure. However, the assumption in these cases is that if cultures for pneumonia are negative, a different source of infection that needs antibiotic therapy is present.

The two studies that compared quantitative ETA cultures to bronchoscopy cultures (10,12) suggest that, from a practical standpoint, either type of quantitative culture can be used to manage patients with a strategy to minimize antibiotic therapy. A study of 400 patients was required to demonstrate a survival difference between invasive quantitative cultures and nonquantitative ETA cultures. A significantly larger population would be needed to demonstrate a difference between two quantitative culture strategies. Choice of technique must take into account the probabilities of a false positive. The consistent pattern is that the number of positive cultures and the number of organisms cultured (and therefore potentially needing treatment) ranks, from greatest to least, as nonquantitative ETA > quantitative ETA (10^5 colony forming units [cfu]/mL) > nonbronchoscopic BAL (10^4 cfu/mL) > bronchoscopic BAL (10^4 cfu/mL) > bronchoscopic PSB (10^3 cfu/mL).

The last strategy is to culture only if empiric therapy appears to be failing. While generally not recommended, this is in fact a not uncommon situation, especially in hospitals that do not have in-house physicians. Nursing priorities are for starting antibiotics, and cultures may be delayed or not obtained. The rapid response of many micro-organisms to appropriate antibiotic therapy makes quantitative cultures in this setting difficult to interpret. Because of these complexities, cultures are often reserved till the time that suspicion of failure is raised. In this setting, invasive quantitative cultures probably are most helpful, although lowering the threshold for a positive culture may be required.

Unfortunately, failure of even "appropriate" therapy is being recognized with greater frequency. Clinical response should track closely with the parameters in the CPIS score, especially oxygenation (13). If these are not improving by day 3 of therapy, concern regarding failure of therapy should be raised. In this setting, bronchoscopy with quantitative cultures is the most reliable method to diagnose local failure (14). Persistance of positive ETA cultures is unreliable, especially this early in the course of treatment. A search for alternative sites of infection is mandatory, as is consideration of complications of therapy, such as drug fever, or of the original infection, such as empyema, secondary intravascular catheter infections, and so on.

B. Treatment

One of the other consistent findings in the VAP literature is the relationship between inappropriate initial antibiotic therapy and increased mortality. Most studies document an inappropriate initial therapy rate of 25–50% (10,12,15,16). It is unclear that correction of inappropriate therapy once cultures return improves mortality (10,12). Therefore, emphasis has been directed at broad-spectrum initial therapy, particularly for late onset VAP or patients who have received prior antibiotic therapy. In essence, empiric therapy must be directed at the multidrug resistant microorganisms such as methicillin-resistant *Staphylococcus aureus* (MRSA), *Pseudomonas aeruginosa*, *Acinetobacter* species, and Enterobacteriaceae with extended spectrum beta-lactamases (ESBLs) (15,17). Frequencies of the latter two will vary greatly from institution to institution (18), and even between ICUs in the same institution. For appropriate initial empiric therapy, knowledge of the local frequencies of etiologies and resistance patterns is therefore critical.

For most institutions, appropriate empiric therapy will require a three-drug regimen with dual gram negative coverage and coverage for MRSA (15,17). Ibrahim et al. found that routine use of a combination of imipenem, ciprofloxacin, and vancomycin reduced their inappropriate initial therapy from approximately 50% to approximately 5% (15). An important aspect of this strategy is de-escalating therapy. In the Ibrahim et al. study (15), the three-drug regimen was only required for the whole course of treatment in 2% of cases. One-third could have one drug stopped and nearly two-thirds required only monotherapy.

As noted above, the ability to de-escalate therapy will be very dependent on the diagnostic culture used.

A second important concept to the use of broad-spectrum empiric therapy is to shorten the overall course of therapy. Ibrahim et al. included this in their protocol, and one of the results is a significantly lower incidence of subsequent multidrug resistant isolates (15). Recently, a randomized controlled trial demonstrated that an 8-day course of antibiotics was just as effective as a 15-day course (19). A small trend toward more recurrent Pseudomonas VAP was found in the shorter course therapy group. However, given the marked propensity for *P. aeruginosa* to develop resistance while on therapy (20), longer courses of the same antibiotic regimen are less likely to improve cure, so choosing an alternative regimen may be necessary if longer therapy is felt to be needed.

A distinction has been made in the past between early-onset and late-onset VAP, with a cut-off ranging from five to seven days of mechanical ventilation. Unfortunately, this concept has not been demonstrated to discriminate between patients at high risk of multidrug-resistant (MDR) microorganisms and those who were not. It also does not address the other types of healthcare-related pneumonias. Therefore, new antibiotic treatment guidelines will discriminate only between patients at risk for MDR microorganisms and those who are not. The major risk factors for MDR microorganisms are prior hospitalization and prior antibiotic use, especially broad-spectrum. Other risk factors are listed in Table 3. Recommendations for treatment are outlined in Table 4.

Another important concept in management of VAP is antibiotic prescription heterogeneity. Consistent use of the same antibiotic regimen is likely to result in selection of a resistant clone or species of bacteria because of selective pressure. The most immediate priority is to not use the same antibiotic repeatedly in the same patient (21). Clinicians should avoid empirically starting a specific antibiotic or even the same class of agent if previously used during the same hospitalization, at least until culture and sensitivity results are available. Even repeated use of the same antibiotic(s) for multiple patients in the same unit

Table 3   Risk Factors for Multidrug Resistant Microorganisms

---

Prior antimicrobial therapy in preceding 90 days
Current hospitalization of ≥ 5 days
High frequency of antibiotic resistance in the community or in the specific hospital unit
Presence of other risk factors:
    Hospitalization for ≥ 2 days in the preceding 90 days
    Residence in a nursing home or extended care facility
    Home infusion therapy (including antibiotics)
    Chronic dialysis within 30 days
    Home wound care
    Family member with multidrug-resistant pathogen
Immunosuppressive disease and/or therapy

Source: From Ref. 59.

Table 4 Recommended Therapy for Ventilator-Associated or ICU Nosocomial Pneumonia

No MDR pathogen risk factors	MDR pathogen risk factors present
CHOICE of:	COMBINATION of:
Beta-lactam	*Beta-lactam*
Ceftriaxone	Cephalosporin (cefipime or ceftazidime)
Ampicillin/sulbactam	Carbapenem (imipenem or meropenem)
Ertapenem	Piperacillin/tazobactam
OR	AND
Quinolone	*Second gram-negative agent*
Ciprofloxacin, levofloxacin,	Quinolone (ciprofloxacin, levofloxacin)
moxifloxacin	Aminoglycoside (gentamicin,
	tobramycin, amikacin)
	AND
	MRSA coverage
	Linezolid
	Vancomycin

Abbreviation: MDR, Multidrug-resistant.
Source: Ref. 59.

may result in increased antibiotic resistance, with a resultant increase in inappropriate initial empiric therapy. In these situations, conscious rotation of the usual empiric antibiotic choice will result in a lower rate of resistant isolates (22).

Unfortunately, simply decreasing the incidence of inappropriate initial empiric therapy will not necessarily lead to lower VAP mortality (15). Increasing attention is being directed to ineffective subsequent antibiotic therapy. The microorganisms associated with a high frequency of inappropriate initial empiric therapy are also the ones associated with ineffective therapy, especially MRSA and Pseudomonas. Treatment of *P. aeruginosa* VAP fails in almost 50% of cases, despite use of potent single agents or combinations (20,23). Treatment of MRSA VAP with vancomycin has a consistent 40% clinical failure rate (24,25). New strategies are needed for these serious causes of VAP. Use of linezolid has demonstrated both lower mortality and greater clinical response than vancomycin but still has a failure rate (24). Other drugs or more effective delivery of antibiotics to the site of infection may be needed for better cure rates.

C. Prevention

Given the significant morbidity, mortality, and difficulties in diagnostic and treatment decisions, prevention of VAP would appear to be a prudent priority. Unfortunately, years of attempts have only yielded minor gains in the understanding of prevention.

By far the most effective prevention strategy is avoidance of intubation. Use of noninvasive ventilation to treat exacerbations of chronic obstructive lung disease or CAP has demonstrated a corresponding decrease in HAP rates

(26–28). Shortening the duration of ventilation is also an important strategy. Use of weaning protocols (29) and daily sedation holidays (30,31) can shorten the duration of ventilation and lead to a lower incidence of VAP.

Airway management that decreases the incidence of microaspiration around the endotracheal tube is also an appropriate direction. The easiest to apply technique is simply to position the patient in the semi-upright position as much as possible (32). Use of specialized endotracheal tubes, which allow aspiration of subglottic secretions, can prevent some early-onset pneumonias and delay the onset to initial VAP (33), potentially allowing extubation in the interval. Early tracheostomy, especially via the percutaneous technique, in patients with anticipated prolonged ventilation decreases mortality, possibly by decreasing VAP rates (34).

The most effective strategy to avoid colonization with more virulent and antibiotic-resistant isolates is to avoid the use of antibiotics. This may be the main benefit of the invasive VAP diagnostic strategy (4). Attention to hand washing and other infection control practices may prevent cross contamination between patients. The data on other strategies remains inconclusive.

III. Severe Community-Acquired Pneumonia

Severe community-acquired pneumonia is one of the most common causes for admission to a medical ICU, therefore representing an important specific clinical entity. Nevertheless, the mortality of SCAP remains unacceptably high. Despite the common idea that death from pneumonia is the culmination of progressive underlying medical illness and is the "old man's friend," the mortality in patients without endstage comorbid illnesses remains high. For example, more than 50% of the deaths from bacteremic pneumococcal pneumonia occur to patients age 18–65 years (35).

A. Definition

One of the potential influences on SCAP mortality is inappropriate initial placement of the patient on a regular ward rather then in the ICU. Delayed transfer to the ICU is associated with an increased risk of death compared to patients initially admitted to the higher acuity unit. The recent data on early aggressive resuscitation (36) and early provision of antibiotic therapy (37) suggests that early intervention may be helpful.

A variety of definitions of SCAP have been used in the literature. Most studies use the very practical definition of any patient admitted to the ICU. However, characteristics of patients admitted to the ICU vary from institution to institution and physician to physician. The corresponding mortality rates therefore also vary, as does the frequency of subsequent transfer from the general floors to the ICU. Some of the variability is due to limited availability of ICU beds, but this is not the sole cause.

A better characterization of SCAP in order to define which patients warrant ICU admission appears desirable. Patients with septic shock requiring vasopressor therapy or immediate need for endotracheal intubation obviously require ICU admission. The real need is for criteria to define appropriate candidates for the ICU without these overt reasons. Unfortunately, determination of the operating characteristics of the criteria for ICU admission recommended by professional society guidelines has included these patients, resulting in an overestimation of their accuracy in patients with more subtle indications for ICU care. Despite this, none of the standard criteria correlate well with which patients are actually admitted to the ICU (38).

Table 5 lists clinical factors associated with increased mortality in SCAP. Presence of several of these adverse risk factors should suggest the need for ICU monitoring. The exact number needed to define SCAP is still unclear, especially since several of the important risk factors occur in clusters. A good example is the common occurrence of leukopenia and alcoholism, often with bilateral infiltrates (39). A particularly insidious problem is the occurrence of an increased anion gap in patients with underlying COPD and a chronic respiratory acidosis.

B. Microbiologic Etiology and Diagnosis

Once the decision to admit a patient to an ICU bed has been made, the next critical decision is appropriate therapy. Unfortunately, therapeutic choices are not so simple in SCAP as they are in CAP patients admitted to the floor or treated as outpatients. The main reason is that the spectrum of etiologies shifts toward microorganisms that are not covered by the usual empiric antibiotics.

Table 5   Clinical Factors Associated with Increased Mortality in SCAP

Respiratory	Neurologic
Need for intubation	Confusion or altered mental status
Noninvasive ventilation	Delerium tremens
$P_aO_2/F_IO_2 < 250$	Metabolic
Respiratory rate >30	Hypoglycemia (especially in absence
Multilobar infiltrates	of hypoglycemic agents)
Cardiovascular	Hyponatremia
Hypotension requiring pressors	Hypothermia
Hypotension requiring massive	Predisposing diseases
volume infusion	Cirrhosis
Lactic acidosis	Active alcohol ingestion
Renal	Postsplenectomy
Blood urea nitrogen >20 mg/dl	Chemotherapy-induced neutropenia
Hematologic	Sickle cell disease
Thrombocytopenia	Leukemia/lymphoma
Neutropenia	

The pneumococcus remains the most common etiology in SCAP. However, the next most common causes vary from nonsevere cases of CAP. In some centers, *Legionella*, especially *L. pneumophilia*, is the next most common cause of SCAP. However, the frequency will vary from year to year even within the same institution and when sought for by the same or more accurate diagnostic tools (40,41). *Legionella* SCAP is also a geographic disease, with some centers never seeing a case or seeing species other than *L. pneumophilia*. In some ICUs, *S. aureus* is the second most common documented etiology (16). Recent reports of community-acquired MRSA pneumonia also make antibiotic choices more complicated. Gram-negative bacilli, such as *Pseudomonas* and *Klebsiella pneumoniae*, are also more common in SCAP (40). In contrast, *Mycoplasma, Chlamydia pneumoniae*, and even *Hemophilus pneumoniae* are less common than in non-SCAP patients. However, when they do occur in SCAP, the reason for ICU admission is more often the exacerbation of the patient's underlying cardiopulmonary disease, rather than because of the severity of the pneumonia. Because of this shift in causative etiologies, diagnostic testing takes a greater priority in SCAP than in non-ICU patients.

Thankfully, diagnostic testing is more often helpful in SCAP patients. Metersky et al. determined risk factors for bacteremia in CAP patients (42). Presence of two or more risk factors, especially in the absence of prior antibiotic therapy, was associated with a significantly greater probability of positive blood cultures. The risk factors for bacteremia in their study included most of the mortality risk factors listed in Table 5. Of the true positive blood cultures, >20% of positive cultures in this elderly population had gram-negative pathogens.

Tracheal aspirates from intubated SCAP patients have a higher diagnostic yield than expectorated sputum (43,44). A major reason is that tracheal aspirates avoid many of the issues that make expectorated sputum diagnosis problematic. The samples clearly come from the lower respiratory tract, are not contaminated by oropharyngeal flora, and are accessible even if the patient is uncooperative or too weak to cough. In addition, a single dose of antibiotic prior to culturing is less likely to result in a negative culture with the SCAP pathogens other than the pneumococcus. For all these reasons, a tracheal aspirate should be obtained in all intubated SCAP patients. The diagnostic yield of expectorated sputum in patients with SCAP may also be slightly higher than for non-SCAP patients, mainly because of the difference in pathogens, many of which are associated with an increased amount of purulent sputum.

The real hope is for improved diagnostic techniques, such as polymerase chain reaction or other molecular techniques. A dipstick bedside test for pneumococcal and Legionella urinary antigens are already available (45,46). Wider use may lead to a higher percentage of patients with a specific CAP diagnosis. Whether this leads to changes in antibiotic treatment will need to be demonstrated.

C. Treatment

Just as in VAP, antibiotic therapy should never be discussed outside the context of diagnostic testing in SCAP. However, the situation in SCAP is very different than for VAP. Despite aggressive attempts at diagnosis, many patients will still not have a microbial etiology established. Guidelines for empiric therapy are therefore more important (47,48), since the ability to modify therapy after culture results return is less common. In addition, the higher incidence of less common micro-organisms discussed above makes an efficient regimen that does not include four to five drugs for all the possible etiologies nearly impossible. Therefore, most recommendations include coverage of the most common etiologies and rely on diagnostic testing to detect less common micro-organisms, with subsequent modifications.

The standard antibiotic recommendation for SCAP is combination therapy with a beta-lactam antibiotic and either a macrolide or a fluoroquinolone. Despite very adequate in vitro activity against the pneumococcus, *Legionella*, *Hemophilus*, and other common CAP pathogens, neither the American Thoracic Society (ATS) (48) nor the Infectious Disease Society of America (IDSA) guidelines (47) recommended monotherapy with a fluoroquinolone. Retrospective studies in elderly patients with CAP have demonstrated that a fluoroquinolone was superior to monotherapy with a cephalosporin and equivalent to a cephalosporin/macrolide combination (49). These studies did not specifically include SCAP patients and were limited to the elderly. The benefit of the macrolide or use of a quinolone was suggested to be the coverage of micro-organisms such as *Legionella*, *Mycoplasma*, and *Chlamydia*. This was particularly important in SCAP where some studies suggested that Legionella was the second most common cause after the pneumococcus (41).

Recent studies have suggested an alternative benefit of combination antibiotics: lower mortality for bacteremic pneumococcal pneumonia. This finding has been seen in one prospective observational study (50) and in three retrospective analyses (51–53), including single site, single area, and international collections of patients. Multivariate analysis has suggested that this effect is most apparent in the more severely ill (51,53), and therefore most pertinent to SCAP patients. All but one study has only compared the outcome of cephalosporin monotherapy versus a combination with a macrolide. However, Waterer et al. did show that combination therapy was better than a quinolone monotherapy, although numbers are small (51). In their study, the worst outcome was from the use of the penicillin class of antibiotics, despite only analyzing penicillin- sensitive strains. While the explanation for this consistent finding is unclear, combination therapy with a cephalosporin and either a macrolide or a quinolone is presently the standard.

Empiric coverage for all the other potential causes of SCAP is extremely difficult. The best strategy may be use of one of the standard combinations with an aggressive search for evidence of a less common pathogen. The retrospective study of Gleason et al. (49) suggested that use of aminoglycosides was associated with an increase in mortality. Many have suggested that this finding indicates that aminoglycoside use is poor practice. However, the indication for aminoglycosides would be a suspicion of gram-negative CAP, which is known to be associated with higher mortality (40). Therefore, while not needed in the overwhelming majority of SCAP patients, appropriate suspicion of gram-negative SCAP based on tracheal aspirate gram stain or clinical epidemiologic risk factors is an appropriate indication for aminoglycosides, carbapenems, and several other drugs not usually in the armamentarium of SCAP treatment. A similar argument can be made for *S. aureus* coverage with either oxacillin or linezolid, depending on the incidence of community-acquired MRSA pneumonia in the area. The latter has been shown to be superior to vancomycin in HAP (24), and community-acquired MRSA pneumonia is unlikely to be significantly different.

D. Immunomodulatory Treatment

The mortality of CAP has not changed significantly in the United States since penicillin became readily available. Therefore, newer, more potent antibiotics are unlikely to significantly improve mortality, as the historical trend documents. Immunomodulatory therapy therefore offers the best hope of improving mortality in CAP. Immunomodulatory therapy can occur in two forms—prevention and active treatment once infection occurs.

The release of drotrecogin alfa activated (Xigris®) represents the first successful immunomodulatory therapy for severe sepsis and septic shock (8). CAP patients made up 35% of the trial and the survival advantage to active treatment was statistically significant in the SCAP subgroup, with an 8.8% absolute risk reduction (ARR) at 28 days overall and a 17.3% ARR in the group with APACHE II score >25 (54). Pneumococcal SCAP was present in 159 patients and had an ARR of 12.9% with drotrecogin alfa activated. The coagulation system activation may be particularly important in SCAP since other interventions in the coagulation system, such tissue factor pathway inhibitor and antithrombin III, also appear to be disproportionately beneficial in CAP. If aggressive resuscitation does not restore blood pressure, SCAP patients should be considered for this immunomodulatory therapy.

Other forms of immunomodulation to consider in SCAP include the use of corticosteroids. Recent data has suggested a high frequency of occult or relative adrenal insufficiency in patients with sepsis (55). Since many of the underlying diseases predisposing to SCAP, such as COPD, are treated intermittently with corticosteroids, adrenal insufficiency should be considered in these patients. Clearly, chemotherapy-induced neutropenic patients should receive filgrastim or sargmostatin in order to increase circulating neutrophils counts. However, filgrastim also increases activation of neutrophils and may potentiate their antimicrobial capacity. The benefit in non-neutropenic patients is unclear but is more likely to benefit patients who do not present with SCAP than those with severe sepsis secondary to SCAP (56,57).

E. Prevention

Given the persistent mortality of SCAP unresponsive to new antibiotics, prevention appears to be warranted. Generally, prevention is thought of in terms of immunization, both pneumococcal and influenza. However, a consistent pattern is that active smoking is associated with an increased risk of developing CAP and an increased risk bacteremia. Therefore, encouragement of smoking cessation represents an important primary and secondary prevention strategy. Hospitalization for CAP is once again an optimal time to reiterate the benefits of smoking cessation. Simple physician advice and referral for assistance can significantly increase long-term quit rates in similar circumstances.

One of the more exciting developments in CAP prevention is the success of the new conjugate vaccine in children (58). The interesting information is that by immunizing at-risk children, invasive pneumococcal disease has also decreased in adults, including the elderly. This most likely represents prevention of colonization in the child's caregivers, which increasingly includes grandparents in our society. More widespread use of the vaccine may finally lead to lower CAP mortality, not just in children (still a high risk group) but also in their adult caregivers.

IV. Conclusion

VAP and SCAP are important entities in the critical care unit. Any active ICU will see many patients with pneumonia and ICU practitioners should be well versed in their diagnosis and management. Significant further research is needed to improve the persistent unacceptably high mortality of both entities.

References

1. Meduri GU, Mauldin GL, Wunderink RG, Leeper KV, Jones CB, Tolley E, et al. Causes of fever and pulmonary densities in patients with clinical manifestations of ventilator-associated pneumonia. Chest 1994; 106:221–225.
2. Beydon L, Saada M, Liu N, Becquemin JP, Harf A, Bonnet F, et al. Can portable chest X-ray examination accurately diagnose lung consolidation after major abdominal surgery? A comparison with computed tomography scan. Chest 1992; 102:1698–1703.
3. Wunderink RG, Woldenberg LS, Zeiss J, Day CM, Ciemons J, Lacher DA. Radiologic diagnosis of autopsy-proven ventilator-associated pneumonia. Chest 1992; 101:458–463.

4.   Fagon JY, Chastre J, Wolff M, Gervais C, Parer-Aubas S, Stephan F, et al. Invasive
     and noninvasive strategies for management of suspected ventilator-associated pneu-
     monia. A randomized trial. Ann Intern Med 2000; 132:621–630.
5.   Singh N, Rogers P, Atwood CW, Wagener MM, Yu VL. Short-course empiric
     antibiotic therapy for patients with pulmonary infiltrates in the intensive care unit.
     A proposed solution for indiscriminate antibiotic prescription. Am J Respir Crit
     Care Med 2000; 162:505–511.
6.   Corley DE, Kirtland SH, Winterbauer RH, Hammar SP, Dail DH, Bauermeister DE,
     et al. Reproducibility of the histologic diagnosis of pneumonia among a panel of four
     pathologists: analysis of a gold standard. Chest 1997; 112:458–465.
7.   Salata RA, Lederman MM, Shlaes DM, Jacobs MR, Eckstein E, Tweardy D, et al.
     Diagnosis of nosocomial pneumonia in intubated, intensive care unit patients. Am
     Rev Respir Dis 1987; 135:426–432.
8.   Bernard GR, Vincent JL, Laterre PF, LaRosa SP, Dhainaut JF, Lopez-Rodriguez A,
     et al. Efficacy and safety of recombinant human activated protein C for severe sepsis.
     N Engl J Med 2001; 344:699–709.
9.   Pugin J, Auckenthaler R, Mili N, Janssens JP, Lew PD, Suter PM. Diagnosis of
     ventilator-associated pneumonia by bacteriologic analysis of bronchoscopic and
     nonbronchoscopic "blind" bronchoalveolar lavage fluid. Am Rev Respir Dis 1991;
     143:1121–1129.
10. Ruiz M, Torres A, Ewig S, Marcos MA, Alcon A, Lledo R, et al. Noninvasive versus
     invasive microbial investigation in ventilator-associated pneumonia: evaluation of
     outcome. Am J Respir Crit Care Med 2000; 162:119–125.
11. Sole VJ, Fernandez JA, Benitez AB, Cardenosa Cendrero JA, Rodriguez DC. Impact
     of quantitative invasive diagnostic techniques in the management and outcome of
     mechanically ventilated patients with suspected pneumonia. Crit Care Med 2000;
     28:2737–2741.
12. Sanchez-Nieto JM, Torres A, Garcia-Cordoba F, El Ebiary M, Carrillo A, Ruiz J,
     et al. Impact of invasive and noninvasive quantitative culture sampling on
     outcome of ventilator-associated pneumonia: a pilot study. Am J Respir Crit Care
     Med 1998; 157:371–376.
13. Luna CM, Blanzaco D, Niederman MS, Matarucco W, Baredes NC, Desmery P,
     et al. Resolution of ventilator-associated pneumonia: prospective evaluation of the
     clinical pulmonary infection score as an early clinical predictor of outcome. Crit
     Care Med 2003; 31:676–682.
14. Ioanas M, Ferrer M, Cavalcanti M, Ferrer R, Ewig S, Filella X, et al. Causes and
     predictors of nonresponse to treatment of intensive care unit-acquired pneumonia.
     Crit Care Med 2004; 32:938–945.
15. Ibrahim EH, Ward S, Sherman G, Schaiff R, Fraser VJ, Kollef MH. Experience with
     a clinical guideline for the treatment of ventilator-associated pneumonia. Crit Care
     Med 2001; 29:1109–1115.
16. Kollef MH, Sherman G, Ward S, Fraser VJ. Inadequate antimicrobial treatment of
     infections: a risk factor for hospital mortality among critically ill patients. Chest
     1999; 115:462–474.
17. Trouillet J-L, Chastre J, Vuagnat A, Joly-Guillou M-L, Combaux D, Dombret M-C,
     et al. Ventilator-associated pneumonia caused by potentially drug-resistant bacteria.
     Am J Respir Crit Care Med 1998; 157:531–539.

18. Rello J, Sa-Borges M, Correa H, Leal SR, Baraibar J. Variations in etiology of ventilator-associated pneumonia across four treatment sites: implications for antimicrobial prescribing practices. Am J Respir Crit Care Med 1999; 160:608–613.

19. Chastre J, Wolff M, Fagon JY, Chevret S, Thomas F, Wermert D, et al. Comparison of 8 vs 15 days of antibiotic therapy for ventilator-associated pneumonia in adults: a randomized trial. J Am Med Assoc 2003; 290:2588–2598.

20. Fink MP, Snydman DR, Niederman MS, Leeper KV Jr, Johnson RH, Heard SO, et al. Treatment of severe pneumonia in hospitalized patients: results of a multicenter, randomized, double-blind trial comparing intravenous ciprofloxacin with imipenem-cilastatin. The Severe Pneumonia Study Group. Antimicrob Agents Chemother 1994; 38:547–557.

21. Trouillet JL, Vuagnat A, Combes A, Kassis N, Chastre J, Gibert C. Pseudomonas aeruginosa ventilator-associated pneumonia: comparison of episodes due to piperacillin-resistant versus piperacillin-susceptible organisms. Clin Infect Dis 2002; 34:1047–1054.

22. Kollef MH, Vlasnik J, Sharpless L, Pasque C, Murphy D, Fraser V. Scheduled change of antibiotic classes: a strategy to decrease the incidence of ventilator-associated pneumonia. Am J Respir Crit Care Med 1997; 156:1040–1048.

23. Brun-Buisson C, Sollet JP, Schweich H, Briere S, Petit C. Treatment of ventilator-associated pneumonia with piperacillin-tazobactam/amikacin versus ceftazidime/amikacin: a multicenter, randomized controlled trial. VAP Study Group. Clin Infect Dis 1998; 26:346–354.

24. Wunderink RG, Rello J, Cammarata SK, Croos-Dabrera RV, Kollef MH. Linezolid vs vancomycin: analysis of two double-blind studies of patients with methicillin-resistant Staphylococcus aureus nosocomial pneumonia. Chest 2003; 124:1789–1797.

25. Fagon J, Patrick H, Haas DW, Torres A, Gibert C, Cheadle WG, et al. Treatment of gram-positive nosocomial pneumonia. Prospective randomized comparison of quinupristin/dalfopristin versus vancomycin. Nosocomial Pneumonia Group. Am J Respir Crit Care Med 2000; 161:753–762.

26. Brochard L, Mancebo J, Wysocki M, Lofaso F, Conti G, Rauss A, et al. Noninvasive ventilation for acute exacerbations of chronic obstructive pulmonary disease. N Engl J Med 1995; 333:817–822.

27. Guerin C, Girard R, Chemorin C, De Varax R, Fournier G. Facial mask noninvasive mechanical ventilation reduces the incidence of nosocomial pneumonia. A prospective epidemiological survey from a single ICU. Intensive Care Med 1997; 23:1024–1032.

28. Confalonieri M, Potena A, Carbone G, Porta RD, Tolley EA, Umberto MG. Acute respiratory failure in patients with severe community-acquired pneumonia. A prospective randomized evaluation of noninvasive ventilation. Am J Respir Crit Care Med 1999; 160:1585–1591.

29. Ely EW, Baker AM, Dunagan DP, Burke HL, Smith AC, Kelly PT, et al. Effect on the duration of mechanical ventilation of identifying patients capable of breathing spontaneously. N Engl J Med 1996; 335:1864–1869.

30. Kress JP, Pohlman AS, O'Connor MF, Hall JB. Daily interruption of sedative infusions in critically ill patients undergoing mechanical ventilation. N Engl J Med 2000; 342:1471–1477.

31. Schweickert WD, Gehlbach BK, Pohlman AS, Hall JB, Kress JP. Daily interruption of sedative infusions and complications of critical illness in mechanically ventilated patients. Crit Care Med 2004; 32:1272–1276.

32. Drakulovic MB, Torres A, Bauer TT, Nicolas JM, Nogue S, Ferrer M. Supine body position as a risk factor for nosocomial pneumonia in mechanically ventilated patients: a randomised trial. Lancet 1999; 354:1851–1858.

33. Rello J, Sonora R, Jubert P, Artigas A, Rue M, Valles J. Pneumonia in intubated patietns: Role of respiratory airway care. Am J Respir Crit Care Med 1996; 154:111–115.

34. Rumbak MJ, Newton M, Truncale T, Schwartz SW, Adams JW, Hazard PB. A prospective, randomized, study comparing early percutaneous dilational tracheotomy to prolonged translaryngeal intubation (delayed tracheotomy) in critically ill medical patients. Crit Care Med 2004; 32:1689–1694.

35. Feikin DR, Schuchat A, Kolczak M, Barrett NL, Harrison LH, Lefkowitz L, et al. Mortality from invasive pneumococcal pneumonia in the era of antibiotic resistance, 1995–1997. Am J Public Health 2000; 90:223–229.

36. Rivers E, Nguyen B, Havstad S, Ressler J, Muzzin A, Knoblich B, et al. Early goal-directed therapy in the treatment of severe sepsis and septic shock. N Engl J Med 2001; 345:1368–1377.

37. Houck PM, Bratzler DW, Nsa W, Ma A, Bartlett JG. Timing of antibiotic administration and outcomes for Medicare patients hospitalized with community-acquired pneumonia. Arch Intern Med 2004; 164:637–644.

38. Angus DC, Marrie TJ, Obrosky DS, Clermont G, Dremsizov TT, Coley C, et al. Severe community-acquired pneumonia: use of intensive care services and evaluation of American and British Thoracic Society Diagnostic criteria. Am J Respir Crit Care Med 2002; 166:717–723.

39. Perlino CA, Rimland D. Alcoholism, leukopenia and pneumococcal sepsis. Am Rev Respir Dis 1985; 132:757–760.

40. Ruiz M, Ewig S, Torres A, Arancibia F, Marco F, Mensa J, et al. Severe community-acquired pneumonia. Am J Respir Crit Care Med 1999; 160:923–929.

41. Torres A, Serra-Batlles J, Ferrer A, Jimenez P, Celis R, Cobo E, et al. Severe community-acquired pneumonia: epidemiology and prognostic factors. Am Rev Respir Dis 1991; 144:312–318.

42. Metersky ML, Ma A, Bratzler DW, Houck PM. Predicting bacteremia in patients with community-acquired pneumonia. Am J Respir Crit Care Med 2004; 169:342–347.

43. Sanyal S, Smith PR, Saha AC, Gupta S, Berkowitz L, Homel P. Initial microbiologic studies did not affect outcome in adults hospitalized with community-acquired pneumonia. Am J Respir Crit Care Med 1999; 160:346–348.

44. Garcia-Vazquez E, Marcos MA, Mensa J, de Roux A, Puig J, Font C, et al. Assessment of the usefulness of sputum culture for diagnosis of community-acquired pneumonia using the PORT predictive scoring system. Arch Intern Med 2004; 164:1807–1811.

45. Benson RF, Tang PW, Fields BS. Evaluation of the binax and biotest urinary antigen kits for detection of legionnaires' disease due to multiple serogroups and species of Legionella. J Clin Microbiol 2000; 38:2763–2765.

46. Dominguez J, Blanco S, Rodrigo C, Azuara M, Gali N, Mainou A, et al. Usefulness of urinary antigen detection by an immunochromatographic test for diagnosis of Pneumococcal pneumonia in children. J Clin Microbiol 2003; 41:2161.

47. Mandell LA, Bartlett JG, Dowell SF, File TM Jr, Musher DM, Whitney C. Update of practice guidelines for the management of community-acquired pneumonia in immunocompetent adults. Clin Infect Dis 2003; 37:1405–1433.

48. Niederman MS, Mandell LA, Anzueto A, Bass JB, Broughton WA, Campbell GD, et al. Guidelines for the management of adults with community-acquired pneumonia. Diagnosis, assessment of severity, antimicrobial therapy, and prevention. Am J Respir Crit Care Med 2001; 163:1730–1754.

49. Gleason PP, Meehan TP, Fine JM, Galusha DH, Fine MJ. Associations between initial antimicrobial therapy and medical outcomes for hospitalized elderly patients with pneumonia. Arch Intern Med 1999; 159:2562–2572.

50. Mufson MA, Stanek RJ. Bacteremic pneumococcal pneumonia in one American city: a 20-year longitudinal study, 1978–1997. Am J Med 1999; 107:34S–43S.

51. Waterer GW, Somes GW, Wunderink RG. Monotherapy may be suboptimal for severe bacteremic pneumococcal pneumonia. Arch Intern Med 2001; 161:1837–1842.

52. Baddour LM, Yu VL, Klugman KP, Feldman C, Ortqvist A, Rello J, et al. Combination antibiotic therapy lowers mortality among severely ill patients with pneumococcal bacteremia. Am J Respir Crit Care Med 2004; 170:440–444.

53. Martinez JA, Horcajada JP, Almela M, Marco F, Soriano A, Garcia E, et al. Addition of a macrolide to a beta-lactam-based empirical antibiotic regimen is associated with lower in-hospital mortality for patients with bacteremic pneumococcal pneumonia. Clin Infect Dis 2003; 36:389–395.

54. Laterre PF, Garber G, Levy H, Wunderink, R, Kinasewitz GT, Sollet JP, Maki DG, Bates B, Sau CBY, Dhainaut JF. Severe community-acquired pneumonia as a cause of severe sepsis: data from the PROWESS trial. Crit Care Med 2004.

55. Annane D, Sebille V, Charpentier C, Bollaert PE, Francois B, Korach JM, et al. Effect of treatment with low doses of hydrocortisone and fludrocortisone on mortality in patients with septic shock. J Am Med Assoc 2002; 288:862–871.

56. Root RK, Lodato RF, Patrick W, Cade JF, Fotheringham N, Milwee S, et al. Multicenter, double-blind, placebo-controlled study of the use of filgrastim in patients hospitalized with pneumonia and severe sepsis. Crit Care Med 2003; 31:367–373.

57. Nelson S, Heyder AM, Stone J, Bergeron MG, Daugherty S, Peterson G, et al. A randomized controlled trial of filgrastim for the treatment of hospitalized patients with multilobar pneumonia. J Infect Dis 2000; 182:970–973.

58. Whitney CG, Farley MM, Hadler J, Harrison LH, Bennett NM, Lynfield R, et al. Decline in invasive pneumococcal disease after the introduction of protein-polysaccharide conjugate vaccine. N Engl J Med 2003; 348:1737–1746.

59. American Thoracic Society; Infectious Diseases Society of America. Guidelines for the management of adults with hospital-acquired, ventilator-associated, and healthcare-associated pneumonia. Am J Respir Crit Care Med. 2005 Feb 15; 171:388–416.

6

Pulmonary Embolism

TIMOTHY L. WILLIAMSON

Division of Pulmonary and Critical
Care Medicine, University of
Kansas Medical Center,
Kansas City, Kansas, U.S.A.

PETER F. FEDULLO

Division of Pulmonary and Critical
Care Medicine, University of
California San Diego,
La Jolla, California, U.S.A.

I. Introduction

The 19th-century German pathologist Rudolf Virchow was one of the first physicians to characterize pulmonary embolism (PE), christening the phenomenon "Embolia" (1). Since that time, tens of thousands of publications have addressed the spectrum of venous thromboembolic disease, yet more controversy and question surrounds this particular ailment than perhaps any other disease process in medicine.

What is not controversial, however, is the considerable impact of pulmonary embolism in terms of morbidity and mortality. In the United States alone, the annual incidence of embolism is in excess of 600,000 cases per year; it is the primary cause of death in over a 100,000 patients each year, and likely contributes to 100,000 more deaths in individuals with serious comorbidities, such as heart disease or malignancy (2). The true impact of embolism, however, may be underestimated, as the incidence of the disease as a finding at autopsy has remained relatively constant over the past 40 years (3–5).

II. Epidemiology and Risk Factors

Nearly 150 years ago, Virchow postulated that thrombosis was caused by changes in the flow of blood, the vessel wall, or the composition of blood (6). Abundant clinical data support this proposition. Although thromboembolism can occur without a definable risk factor (idiopathic thrombosis), the overwhelming majority of patients experiencing a venous thromboembolic event are placed at risk by one or more predisposing clinical factors that result in endothelial injury, venous stasis, or hypercoagulability (7).

187

The identification of congenital predispositions to venous thromboembolism, commonly referred to as thrombophilias, provided additional insight into the pathogenesis and natural history of the disease (8). The earliest of these to be described was antithrombin III deficiency in 1965, followed by the description of Protein C deficiency in 1981 and that of Protein S deficiency in 1984 (9–11). These abnormalities, however, were identified in less than 10% of patients with venous thrombosis (12).

In 1993, Dahlbeck and associates described a single point mutation on the factor V gene resulting in factor V_a with diminished sensitivity to activated Protein C (13). Designated Factor V Leiden, this mutation is present in approximately five percent of Caucasians in Europe and North America; lower rates of carrier frequency have been reported among Native-American, African, and Asian populations. Although initially detected in as many as 60% of selected patients with venous thromboembolism, subsequent studies have detected the mutation in 10–20% of unselected patients. The heterozygous state carries a 5- to 10-fold increase in lifetime risk for venous thromboembolism, while the risk among patients homozygous for this mutation may be increased 80-fold.

A sequence variation in the prothrombin gene (20210G > A) was described in 1996 and is estimated to occur in approximately 2–4% of the population (14). This mutation results in an overproduction of prothrombin, which is otherwise normal. It is associated with a 3–4-fold increased risk of lower extremity venous thrombosis and appears to act in a synergistic manner with other forms of thrombophilia in increasing both the initial and recurrent thrombosis risk (15).

The identification of these inherited risk factors has proven useful in providing insight into the etiologic basis for thromboembolism in the majority of patients with idiopathic disease. However, most patients who develop venous thromboembolism do so as the consequence of some clinical predisposition. Even in those with an identified thrombophilic predisposition, interaction with a defined clinical state is necessary to shift the normal hemostatic balance towards thrombosis (6). Major risk factors include pelvic or lower extremity fractures, hip and knee surgery, spinal injury, major traumatic injury, and major surgery including, but not limited to, open prostatectomy and abdominal or pelvic surgery for malignant disease. Other factors that enhance risk include a past history of venous thromboembolism, acute paralytic stroke, advancing age, congestive heart failure, pregnancy, the post-partum period, the use of estrogen-containing compounds, malignancy, the presence of a lupus anticoagulant or antiphospholipid antibody, and prolonged immobilization.

III. Natural History

A. Deep Venous Thrombosis

Thrombi originate in the deep venous system either near venous valve cusps, an area of altered blood flow, or at sites of intimal injury. Thrombus propagation is associated with a concurrent local fibrinolytic state, resulting in a "dynamic process" wherein these two forces compete. The outcome may result in total dissolution of the thrombus, partial resolution with variable degrees of intimal and valvular damage, progressive proximal propagation, or embolization (16). By noninvasive measures, roughly half of patients with proximal venous thrombosis will have an incompletely compressible vein on ultrasound at one year following treatment (17–20). Invasive venographic studies performed six months after an acute deep venous thrombosis (DVT) in treated patients with femoral or distal DVTs will demonstrate complete lysis in 38%, partial lysis in just over half, and evidence of thrombus extension in 7% (21).

Embolism occurs in the overwhelming majority of patients as a consequence of dislodgment of thrombus from the deep venous system of the lower legs (22). Calf veins are rarely the source of embolism (23). If left untreated, though, roughly a quarter of patients with untreated calf vein thrombosis will have extension to involve proximal vessels with subsequent risk for embolism, typically within a week of presentation (24,25). Approximately 50% of these patients may go on to develop associate pulmonary embolism, the mortality of which varies depending on embolus size and underlying cardiopulmonary reserve. PE can also result as a consequence of thrombus formation in the axillary or subclavian veins, either spontaneously, as a consequence of congenital abnormalities, or as a consequence of foreign bodies such as central lines, pulmonary artery catheters, or transvenous pacemaker wires (26).

B. Pulmonary Embolism

Not surprisingly, the natural history of PE parallels that of DVT, with potential for resolution, partial resolution, or propagation. In most patients there is significant resolution during the first week of therapy, which continues for four to eight weeks (27,28). Residual defects on lung scintigraphy are common, and complete resolution is unusual (29). Patients with PE who receive anticoagulation but no thrombolytic therapy have, on angiography and scintigraphy, essentially no resolution at two hours, approximately 10% at 24 hours, 40% at a week, and 50% at two to four weeks. Complete resolution occurs in about two-thirds of patients with partial resolution in the remainder (30–32).

Resolution occurs as a result of fibrinolysis, re-organization, and recannalization. It may be that emboli resolve faster than similar thrombi in the deep venous systems. It has been postulated that higher flow rates in the pulmonary arterial system may expose the thrombi to more plasminogen, and that the thrombolytic capacity of the pulmonary artery is greater than that of peripheral veins (33). These postulates remain largely unproven, however.

Most patients who initially manifest elevated pulmonary artery pressures with acute embolism will reach a stable pulmonary artery pressure within six weeks from the event (34). A small number of patients will not have normalization of their pulmonary artery pressures, and will go on to develop chronic thromboembolic pulmonary hypertension (CTEPH). The true percentage of patients who experience acute embolism and subsequently develop pulmonary hypertension is unknown but has been estimated to be as high as 5%. Mean pulmonary artery pressures exceeding 50 mmHg at presentation and an age greater than 70 years have been independently associated with persistent pulmonary hypertension (34).

IV. Physiologic Consequences of PE

A. Pulmonary

Roughly half of patients with acute PE will develop increased pulmonary artery pressures during the acute phase of their disease, but with endogenous thrombolysis and reversal of hypoxic vasoconstriction, pulmonary arterial pressures will drop progressively with treatment. Most patients will normalize pulmonary hemodynamics by one month post event (27,34).

Arterial hypoxemia often accompanies acute pulmonary embolism, the reasons for which are manifold (35). The major mechanisms involved in the hypoxemia associated with embolism appear to be a redistribution of perfusion to low ventilation areas, resulting in ventilation–perfusion mismatch, and a decrease in cardiac output resulting in a lower mixed venous oxygen content, thereby magnifying the effect of the normal venous admixture (36,37). Shunting may also occur at either an intrapulmonary or intracardiac level (38). If right atrial pressure is substantially elevated, right to left shunting may occur through a patent foramen ovale. Finally, acute embolism can be associated with loss of pulmonary surfactant (39). This loss of surfactant takes approximately 24 hours following complete occlusion to occur, and can result in atelectasis or edema.

B. Cardiovascular

The physiological impact upon the cardiovascular system is dependent largely on three determining conditions: the magnitude of decrease in the cross-sectional area of the pulmonary vascular bed, the pre-existing status of the cardiopulmonary system, and the effect of hypoxic and neurohumorally mediated vasoconstriction (40–44). In the absence of prior cardiopulmonary disease, embolic obstruction of 20% or less of the vascular bed results in recruitment and distention of pulmonary vessels to maintain normal or near normal pulmonary hemodynamics. Right ventricular stroke volume and heart rate increase modestly to preserve cardiac output. With vascular obstruction ranging from 30% to 40%, PA pressures begin to increase, accompanied by a modest increase in right atrial pressure. As obstruction exceeds 50% of the pulmonary vascular bed, compensatory mechanisms are overcome, right atrial pressure increases, and cardiac output decreases. Further obstruction leads to right ventricular dilation, increases in right ventricular wall tension, and the potential for right ventricular ischemia. As cardiac output falls, systemic hypotension ensues. In general, the highest mean pulmonary artery pressure thought able to be generated by a previously normal right ventricle is

40 mmHg, which approximates a pulmonary artery systolic pressure of approximately 70 mmHg as measured by echocardiogram (45). In the absence of preexisting cardiopulmonary disease, there is a general relationship between the extent of vascular obstruction and level of PA pressure elevation.

In patients with prior cardiopulmonary disease, however, the severity of pulmonary hypertension is disproportionate to the magnitude of obstruction. Relatively small decreases in pulmonary vascular cross-sectional area may result in severe pulmonary hypertension. Indeed, the right ventricle is often hypertrophied instead of dilated (reflecting the chronicity of increase in PA pressures), and is able to generate mean PA pressures that exceed 40 mmHg (42).

V. Clinical Presentation

A. DVT

Pulmonary embolism is not a separate disease entity, but rather a complication of deep venous thrombosis. Consequently, the presentation of embolism cannot be fully discussed without also discussing the presentation of DVT. Clinically apparent venous thrombosis often presents as edema of one or both lower extremities, sometimes accompanied by erythema or warmth. Homan's sign (calf pain with flexion of the knee and dorsiflexion of the ankle), Moses' sign (pain associated with calf compression against the tibia), and a palpable venous cord are all variably present and nonspecific for the diagnosis of DVT.

The clinical diagnosis of deep venous thrombosis can be quite difficult to establish (22,46–48). The vast majority of patients with clinical symptoms suggestive of the disease do not have evidence of such by objective testing. Alternatively, the majority of high risk patients who are serially monitored and who develop DVT do not manifest clinical signs or symptoms of the disease (49).

B. PE

The symptoms of pulmonary embolism are non-specific and common to a multitude of cardiopulmonary disorders. Although the diagnosis of embolism cannot be excluded solely on clinical findings, clinical suspicion is important, as it is the first step in each of the many potential diagnostic algorithms (50–53).

PE may present as one of three recognized clinical syndromes: isolated dyspnea, pulmonary infarct or hemorrhage, or circulatory collapse. One of the most common symptoms associated with embolism by clinicians is dyspnea, and indeed, the sudden onset of unexplained dyspnea is one of the most common presenting symptoms of an acute embolic event (52–54). The syndrome of isolated dyspnea, however, occurs in only 25% of patients with angiographically proven embolism (53). This dyspnea is variable in intensity and duration, often lasting only a few minutes, and results from the sudden appearance of alveolar dead space and the perception of altered pulmonary compliance related to the embolism. With more extensive embolization, the sensation of dyspnea tends to be striking and persistent. It is important to emphasize, however, that dyspnea is not present in approximately 25% of patients with the disease (53). The differential diagnosis of dyspnea, particularly in the hospitalized patient, is diverse and includes anemia, congestive heart failure, chronic lung disease, postoperative atelectasis, pneumonia, pneumothorax, and diaphragmatic dysfunction.

Steell first described the constellation of findings comprising the pulmonary infarction/hemorrhage syndrome in 1906—hemoptysis, pleuritic chest pain, a pleural friction rub, evidence of lung consolidation, and small pleural effusions (55). The majority of patients with embolism will present with some variation of this syndrome (56–59). Pulmonary infarction typically results from submassive obstruction of segmental branches of the pulmonary artery, not massive central obstruction. In fact, ligation of the main right pulmonary artery does not lead to pulmonary infarction. Given the dual circulation of the lungs from pulmonary and bronchial arterial sources, infarction in patients without pre-existing cardiopulmonary disease is rare. In patients without congestive heart failure, the syndrome may present with hemoptysis and a chest radiograph demonstrating a pleural-based infiltrate that clears over two to four days. Pathologically, these patients have evidence of intra-alveolar hemorrhage but no evidence of alveolar wall necrosis. Patients with underlying congestive heart failure, however, may progress to complete infarction associated with persistent radiographic scarring (56–59).

The remaining 10–15% of patients with embolism present with circulatory collapse (54,60,61). This represents the most dramatic of possible presentations in which mortality is high, and many patients may not survive the first hour following clinical onset.

The signs associated with PE are nonspecific and common to a variety of cardiopulmonary processes. Although tachypnea is frequent, it is not noted in roughly 30% of patients with PE. Other physical finding in patients without pre-existing cardiac or pulmonary disease included rales (51%), tachycardia (30%), a fourth heart sound (24%), and an increased pulmonic component of the second heart sound (23%) (53). Fever may be present but rarely exceeds 38.3°C. Additional findings associated with massive pulmonary embolism include a sense of impending doom, anginal type chest pain secondary to right ventricular ischemia, syncope or near syncope, or clinical evidence of right ventricular failure. The presentation of PE may or may not be accompanied by findings suggestive of DVT. In the PIOPED trial, for example, just over a quarter of patients with PE had lower extremity edema or pain at presentation (53).

It should be re-emphasized that patients without pre-existing cardiopulmonary disease and small to moderate emboli can exhibit few if any signs or symptoms. In prospective surveillance studies of high risk patients, for example, 40% or more of patients with proximal DVT and no pulmonary symptoms were found to have lung scans consistent with the presence of embolism (50,62). In patients with pre-existing cardiopulmonary disease, symptoms may be more common or more severe, but may be mistaken as manifestations of the underlying disease process.

VI. Diagnostic Approach to PE

The diagnostic approach to patients with suspected PE has undergone a fundamental transition over the past decade. Once dependent almost exclusively on the results of ventilation/perfusion scanning and pulmonary angiography, the diagnosis of PE can now be reliably confirmed or excluded in the majority of patients through a risk stratification approach combined with one or more noninvasive techniques that includes D-dimer determination, lower extremity ultrasonography, and computerized tomography (CT). As a result, ventilation/ perfusion scanning, although serving adequately in its diagnostic role for more than three decades, has assumed a secondary role in embolism diagnostic strategies. This transition was based on the realization that lung scanning was nondiagnostic (neither normal nor high-probability) in 60–70% of patients with suspected embolism (53). Figures 1 and 2 demonstrate the appearance of a normal and a high-probability scan.

It was also based on investigations supporting a Bayesian approach to embolism diagnosis, thereby optimizing the positive and negative predictive values of noninvasive diagnostic tests; on the development and validation of rapid, highly-sensitive D-dimer assays capable of excluding embolism in those with a low or intermediate clinical likelihood of embolism; and on advances in CT technology that allow higher resolution, dramatically faster scanning times,

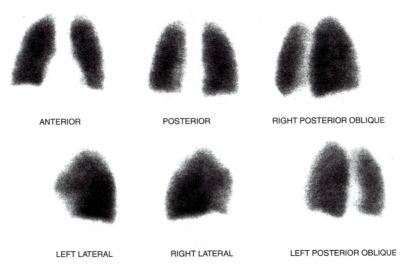

Figure 1 Normal 6-view ventilation-perfusion scan.

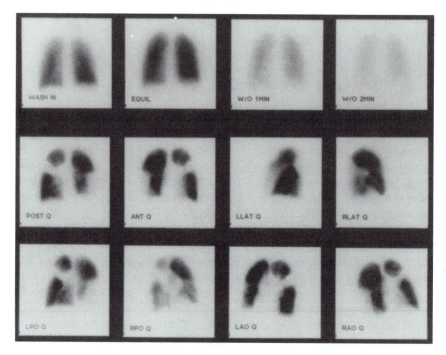

Figure 2 High-probability ventilation–perfusion scan. Note multiple segmental perfusion defects in the presence of normal ventilation.

more peripheral visualization, and less motion artifact than that provided by earlier generation scanners (63–65).

Multiple studies have demonstrated that clinical evidence in isolation, although capable of raising a suspicion of pulmonary embolism, cannot be relied on to confirm or exclude the diagnosis. In the PIOPED trial, for example, presenting symptoms and signs proved incapable of differentiating those patients who had pulmonary embolism from those who did not. Likewise, chest radiography, electrocardiography, and arterial blood gas analysis, although often providing useful clinical information, do not have the discriminatory power to confirm or exclude the diagnosis of embolism (52).

A major advance in the diagnostic approach to embolism, as it has been in the diagnostic approach to venous thrombosis, has been the derivation and validation of clinical prediction rules, such as the Wells Prediction Rule (Table 1), and their introduction into clinical practice. Standardized prediction rules range from those that are simple, involving information that can be easily acquired even in an outpatient setting, to those that are more complex, involving an increased number of clinical variables requiring expert interpretation (66,67). Objective rules have not been demonstrated to be superior to empiric assessment but can help avoid variance among practitioners with different levels of

Table 1 Wells Clinical Model for Predicting the Pretest Probability of Pulmonary Embolism

Variable	Points assigned
Clinical signs and symptoms of deep venous thrombosis	3.0
An alternative diagnosis is less likely than pulmonary embolism	3.0
Heart rate >100	1.5
Immobilization or surgery in the previous four weeks	1.5
Previous deep vein thrombosis or pulmonary embolism	1.5
Hemoptysis	1.0
Malignancy (on treatment, treated in the last six months, or palliative)	1.0
Score	Clinical assessment probability
<2 points	Low-probability
2–6 points	Intermediate-probability
>6 points	High-probability

Source: From Ref. 149.

experience and training (66). Prediction rules in isolation are incapable of confirming or excluding the likelihood of pulmonary embolism with a clinically acceptable degree of certainty but have proven capable of stratifying patients into probability categories. By combining this derived clinical probability with the results of a noninvasive diagnostic technique, diagnostic accuracy in terms of both the confirmation and exclusion of embolism can be increased well beyond that achieved by either the use of clinical probability or the noninvasive diagnostic technique alone, and can substantially limit the number of patients who require pulmonary angiography.

The development of an accurate blood test capable of diagnosing venous thromboembolism has been the focus of considerable investigative interest. Studies suggested as potential screening techniques for PE have included the measurement of plasma DNA levels as well as the measurement of factors involved in hemostasis such as platelets, fibrinogen, thrombin–antithrombin III complexes, and various products of fibrin metabolism (68–70). The potential of D-dimer testing as an exclusionary technique for pulmonary embolism has been recognized for almost 20 years (71). D-dimer testing has proven to be highly sensitive but not specific; that is, elevated levels are present in nearly all patients with embolism but also occur in a wide range of disorders including advancing age, trauma, the postoperative period, pregnancy, inflammatory states, and malignancy (72). Problems limiting the widespread application of D-dimer testing to embolism diagnosis included the wide array of available techniques, variations in sensitivity and specificity among assays, a range of discriminate values for positivity, lack of standardization, and uncertainty among clinicians regarding the sensitivity of the assay they are utilizing. Recent outcome studies utilizing validated techniques have demonstrated that treatment may be safely withheld in patients presenting with suspected embolism who have a low clinical probability of embolism and a negative sensitive D-dimer assay (e.g., SimpliRED) and in patients with a low or intermediate clinical probability using selected highly sensitive assays (e.g., Vidas ELISA) (73). A negative D-dimer test should not be utilized as the sole exclusionary technique in patients with a high pretest probability of disease. Multiple D-dimer assays are available; selection of assays appears to be largely institution specific. These assays have been reviewed in greater detail elsewhere (148).

Because the majority of pulmonary emboli arise from the deep veins of the lower extremities, the detection of lower extremity, proximal-vein thrombosis in a patient suspected of embolism, although not confirming that embolism has occurred, is strongly suggestive of that diagnosis and has an equivalent therapeutic implication. Ultrasonography has been reported to be positive in approximately 10–20% of patients with suspected embolism and in 50% of patients with proven embolism (74). A negative ultrasound finding, therefore, cannot exclude the diagnosis. A positive ultrasound finding in an embolic suspect, particularly one with a low probability of disease and without symptoms or signs referable to the lower extremities, should be interpreted judiciously and supported by additional diagnostic data given the possibility this may represent a false positive study (75). CT venography as an adjunct to helical CT scanning has been investigated, and preliminary results suggest that it is capable of detecting femoropopliteal thrombosis with the same accuracy as duplex ultrasonography while also detecting pelvic and abdominal thrombosis (76).

CT has represented a major advance in embolism diagnosis (65). Unlike ventilation–perfusion scanning, it provides the ability to directly visualize emboli as well as to detect parenchymal abnormalities that may support the diagnosis of embolism or provide an alternative basis for the patient's complaints. The reported sensitivity of helical CT scanning for embolism has ranged from 57–100%, with a specificity ranging from 78–100%. Factors responsible for this wide divergence relate to the proximal extent of vascular obstruction that can be detected and, in part, to advances in CT technology. Sensitivity and specificity of CT scanning for emboli involving the main and lobar pulmonary arteries exceeds 95%. Figure 3 illustrates characteristic findings seen on a diagnostic CT pulmonary angiogram. Vascular involvement confined to segmental or subsegmental pulmonary vessels is associated with a decline in both sensitivity and specificity. These findings suggest that filling defects consistent with embolism involving the main or lobar pulmonary arteries can be considered diagnostic of embolism. Defects involving the segmental and subsegmental arteries can be considered suggestive of embolism but should be supported by additional objective data. The absence of detectable filling defects reduces the likelihood of

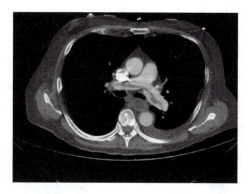

Figure 3 CT pulmonary angiogram of a patient with a serpentine thrombus obstructing the right pulmonary artery extending across the pulmonary bifurcation into the left pulmonary artery.

embolism but appears incapable of excluding the possibility with the same degree of certainty as a negative ventilation–perfusion scan. Outcome studies have demonstrated, however, that withholding anticoagulant therapy in patients with a negative CT scan, coupled with a negative lower extremity ultrasound study, is a safe strategy except in those patients who present with a high-clinical likelihood of embolism (77,78).

The out-patient approach to the diagnosis of suspected embolism, therefore, should be initiated with a clinical probability assessment, either objective or empiric. For institutions using a sensitive D-dimer assay, a negative result can exclude the diagnosis of embolism in patients with a low probability of disease; for institutions using a highly sensitive assay, a negative result can exclude the diagnosis in patients with both a low or intermediate probability of disease. In patients with a positive D-dimer assay or a high clinical probability of disease, lower-extremity ultrasonography should then be performed. A positive study in patients with an intermediate or high clinical probability of disease would confirm the diagnosis. In patients with negative lower extremity ultrasonography, a helical CT scan should be performed. A negative study would exclude the diagnosis in patients with a low or intermediate probability of disease. Pulmonary angiography should be considered in that small subset of patients with a high pretest probability of disease but negative D-dimer testing, negative lower extremity ultrasonography, and negative helical CT scan, especially those patients with pre-existing cardiopulmonary disease in whom a missed diagnosis might have catastrophic consequences. By utilizing this approach, angiography would be required in less than 1% of patients presenting with suspected embolism (79). Sometimes alternative diagnoses become evident and this is demonstrated in the pulmonary angiograms presented in Figures 4 and 5.

In patients with a relative or absolute contraindication to CT scanning (e.g., dye allergy, renal insufficiency, pregnancy), ventilation/perfusion scanning can

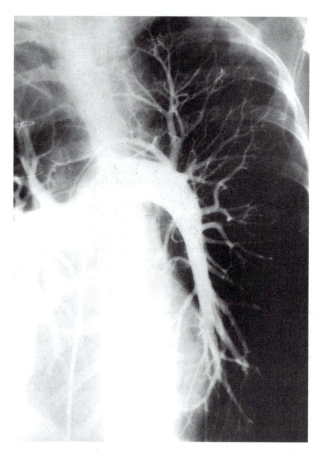

Figure 4   Left-sided contrast pulmonary angiogram in a patient with idiopathic pulmonary arterial hypertension. Note absence of intraluminal defects with paucity and peripheral tapering of pulmonary vessels.

be substituted for CT scanning in this diagnostic algorithm. A normal ventilation/perfusion scan would exclude the diagnosis, while a high probability scan in patients with a high pretest probability of disease would confirm it (53). Because patients with indeterminate scan results and a moderate or high clinical probability of disease would require additional testing, such an approach would require a substantial increase in the number of pulmonary angiograms performed. This approach is summarized in Figure 6.

The diagnostic approach to PE in inpatients has been studied less comprehensively than in outpatients. D-dimer testing has limited value given its low specificity (10–20%) and its consequentially high frequency of positive results in an inpatient population (80,81). In terms of the use of prediction rules, care

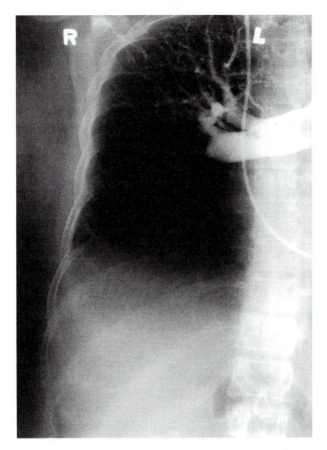

Figure 5 Right-sided contrast pulmonary angiogram in a patient with chronic thromboembolic pulmonary hypertension. A "pouch" defect is present in the proximal interlobar artery immediately below the right upper lobe vessels with complete absence of flow to the right middle and lower lobes.

must be taken in applying an objective probability assessment tool derived in outpatients to an inpatient population with confounding medical problems. Regardless of these complexities, however, the combination of a negative helical CT scan in conjunction with a negative lower ultrasound exam appears capable of excluding embolism in inpatients with a low or intermediate probability of disease. However, pending the results of future investigations, strong consideration should be given to performing conventional pulmonary angiography in inpatients with a high pretest probability of disease, even in the setting of a negative helical CT scan and lower extremity ultrasound (78). A suggested approach to these patients is presented in Figure 7.

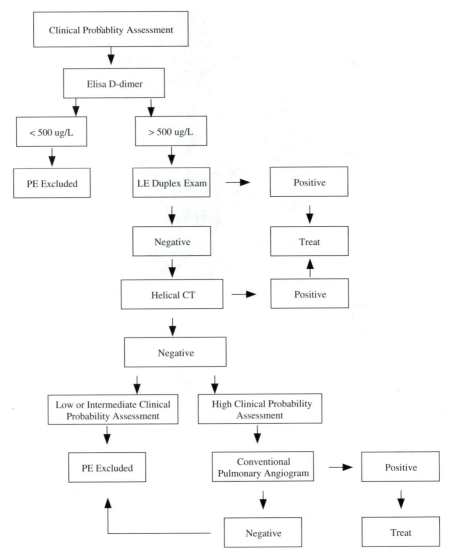

Figure 6   Algorithmic approach to suspected pulmonary embolism in outpatients.

VII.   Treatment of Acute PE

The goals of therapy in pulmonary embolism include interventions to compensate for the cardiac and pulmonary consequences of the disease and to prevent thrombus propagation or recurrence. Anticoagulation remains the mainstay of therapy in venous thromboembolic disease by preventing further thrombus extension,

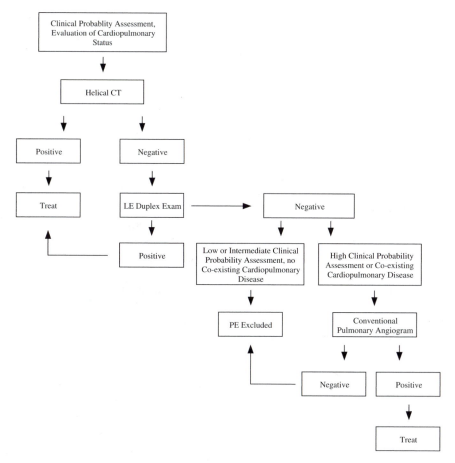

Figure 7 Algorithmic approach to suspected pulmonary embolism in inpatients.

thereby allowing established thrombi to undergo endogenous lysis, and by reducing the risk of recurrent thrombosis.

A. Unfractionated Heparin

Heparin, discovered by Howell and Holt in 1918, is the anticoagulant with which we have the most experience (82). In an era that champions the virtue of evidence-based medicine, it is ironic that a drug as widely utilized as heparin has been subjected to only one randomized placebo controlled trial comprising 35 patients with pulmonary embolism, and no such trials in patients with deep venous thrombosis (61,83). In the study that enrolled patients with embolism, the diagnosis was entirely clinically-based, but the difference in mortality amongst treatment and placebo groups was striking. Although there are those who have suggested that the effects of heparin on the morbidity and mortality from PE are not known, numerous studies have clearly demonstrated that the risk of embolic recurrence is significantly reduced by adequate heparin therapy.

Given that failure to achieve therapeutic levels of anticoagulation within the first 24 hours appears to be associated with an increased recurrence rate, it seems reasonable to attempt to ensure adequate anticoagulation within this time frame (84). One commonly employed dosing regimen utilizing an initial intravenous bolus of 80 units of heparin per kilogram followed by a continuous infusion initiated at 18 units per kilogram per hour has been demonstrated to reach therapeutic thresholds more quickly than regimens utilizing fixed dosing (85). The heparin drip is adjusted based on activated partial thromboplastin time (aPTT) monitoring, drawn six hours after the initial bolus dose, and then six hours after each dose adjustment. The therapeutic range of aPTT may vary substantially depending on the sensitivity of the reagent utilized and among coagulometers. Therefore, unless internal validation has been performed, a target aPTT ratio of 2.0 to 3.5 should be attained. A subtherapeutic level of anticoagulation may be associated with increased risk for thromboembolic occurrence, but a supratherapeutic level does not appear to be associated with increased risk of clinically important bleeding complications (86).

Rare patients may demonstrate significant heparin resistance, requiring 40,000 or more units per day. In this population, monitoring of anticoagulation with antifactor Xa assays is a safe and effective alternative to monitoring patients with aPTT levels, and may subsequently result in less escalation of heparin dosing (87).

B.   Low-Molecular Weight Heparin

Low-molecular weight heparin (LMWH) preparations have been demonstrated safe and effective in the treatment of DVT, and their allure for the treatment of submassive PE is fairly intuitive.

LMWH preparations have increased bioavailability, a predictable dose response curve, and a longer half life, all of which permit once or twice daily subcutaneous dosing without any need for aPTT monitoring. Additionally, they are associated with a decreased incidence of heparin-induced thrombocytopenia (HIT) and have been proven cost-effective when compared with regimens utilizing unfractionated heparin preparations. Nonetheless, LMWH preparations are not without shortcomings: dosing is problematic at extremes of body weight, necessitating dose adjustment, and monitoring with anti-Xa levels may be required in renal insufficiency because the drug is renally excreted, reversal of anticoagulant effect with protamine is imprecise, and the anticoagulant effect is not easily monitored. Furthermore, in patients with an increased risk of hemorrhage, the increased half-life of LMWH may be undesirable.

Several studies and meta-analyses have compared the subcutaneous administration of a number of LMWH preparations with the administration of intravenous unfractionated heparin in acute, submassive PE (88–91). No statistically significant difference in recurrent venous thromboembolic phenomenon, major bleeding, or mortality has been demonstrated. No single LMWH preparation has been demonstrated superior to any other in regards to safety or efficacy (88).

Most patients with acute DVT can be safely managed on an outpatient basis with LMWH, reducing total medical expenditures and decreasing length of stay parameters (92). A similar therapeutic paradigm for treating acute PE would, of course, be attractive for analogous reasons. Kovacs and colleagues looked at treating acute PE as an outpatient with dalteparin (93), including patients treated wholly as outpatients, as well as those treated initially as inpatients and transitioned after several days to the outpatient arena. Their study enrolled 158 patients, 81 of whom were treated exclusively as outpatients. Their conclusion was that outpatient management utilizing LMWH was safe and feasible for the majority of patients.

A significant number of patients, however, may not be candidates for outpatient therapy as a result of hemorrhagic risk, compliance issues, renal insufficiency, significant comorbidity, inadequate cardiopulmonary reserve, or poor likelihood of obtaining post-discharge care. There is promise, however, for the subset of patients who have suffered a submassive embolic event associated with preserved right ventricular function and whose care is not complicated by one of the above concerns to be treated on an outpatient basis with LMWH. Further prospective studies are required, however, to more completely evaluate the safety and efficacy of this management strategy.

C. Novel Agents

Fondaparinux is a synthetic anti-thrombotic agent possessing specific anti-factor Xa activity. Subcutaneous administration of fondaparinux has been compared to intravenous unfractionated heparin in an open-label, noninferiority study enrolling 2200 patients with acute symptomatic embolism, approximately 15% of whom received at least part of their therapy as an outpatient (94). There was no statistically significant difference in major bleeding episodes, recurrent venous thromboembolic disease, or mortality.

Ximelagatran is a novel oral direct thrombin inhibitor that has been investigated in a small trial of 12 patients with PE (95). It was found to be safe and efficacious without need for monitoring of anticoagulation parameters. Both drugs hold promise for use in the treatment of embolism, but recommendations regarding their use should be held pending further investigation.

D. Long Term Oral Anticoagulation

Warfarin

The birth of oral anticoagulation was heralded by the discovery of dicumarol in spoiled sweet clover, which was responsible for a fatal hemorrhagic disorder in livestock (96). It was subsequently synthesized by Stahmann in 1940 (97). Since that time it has remained the backbone of oral anticoagulation for outpatient therapy.

Coumarins are antagonists of vitamin K and affect anticoagulation by interfering with the cyclic interconversion of vitamin K, and its vitamin K epoxide, consequently affecting vitamin K-dependent factors II, VII, IX, and X (98). There may be, however, a concurrent inhibition of carboxylation of anticoagulant proteins C and S, with a resultant potential for an initial procoagulant effect. The half-life of warfarin is 36 to 42 hours, and the drug is protein bound in plasma, largely to albumin. Therapeutic response to warfarin is gauged by monitoring the prothrombin time, which reflects activity of coagulation factors II, VII, and X. The dose-response of warfarin varies with a number of factors, including genetic factors, environmental factors, disease states, concurrent medication utilization, and dietary issues (98). As a result of the considerable variability in the sensitivity of commercially available thromboplastins, a reliance on the absolute prothrombin time or the prothrombin time ratio may lead to either excessive or inadequate anticoagulation. These concerns have resulted in adoption of the international normalized ratio (INR), which corrects for the thromboplastin sensitivity, as a means of reporting warfarin effect.

The duration of oral therapy with vitamin K antagonists following an initial venous thromboembolic episode is controversial. The goal is to balance the risks of extended anticoagulation with the risk of recurrent thromboembolic phenomenon. The risk of having a recurrent PE after an initial episode diminishes over time, but appears to stabilize after approximately nine months, regardless of the duration of initial therapy with warfarin (99). It is widely accepted that duration of therapy is individualized to each patient and is dependent on whether the thrombosis is idiopathic, associated with ongoing risk factors such as malignancy or thrombophilia, or is secondary to a reversible underlying process. In general, patients should receive a longer duration of therapy if the thrombotic event is idiopathic, originates in a proximal lower extremity vessel versus distal, or is a recurrent event. Consideration should be given to indefinite anticoagulation if a persistent risk factor exists. Current recommendations from the Sixth American College of Chest Physicians (ACCP) Consensus Conference on Anti-Thrombotic Therapy are that patients with proximal venous thrombosis should receive a minimum of three months of anticoagulation, patients with pulmonary embolism associated with proximal venous thrombosis or recurrent venous thrombosis should receive six months, and patients with symptomatic calf vein thrombosis should receive six weeks to three months of therapy (98). Patients recommended to receive anticoagulation for an indefinite period of time include patients with greater than one episode of idiopathic proximal vein thrombosis or pulmonary embolism, those with malignancy, or those with idiopathic venous thromboembolism associated with the following procoagulant states: homozygous factor V Leiden genotype, heterozygous Factor V Leiden genotype combined with heterozygous prothrombin mutation, antiphospholipid antibody syndrome, or protein C or S deficiency (98).

Hemorrhage is the most notable adverse effect associated with warfarin, and appears proportional to the degree of anticoagulation. A targeted INR of 2.0 to 3.0 confers less risk of bleeding than that associated with an INR of 3.0 to 4.5 (100–103). A recent large randomized trial, however, demonstrated no significant difference in the risk of bleeding for patients with a targeted INR of 2.0 to 3.0 versus those with a lower targeted INR of 1.5 to 1.9, but did exhibit a significantly higher incidence of recurrent PE in the patients receiving lower levels of anti-coagulation (104). The official recommendation of the Sixth ACCP Consensus Conference on Anti-Thrombotic Therapy is that warfarin should be dosed to target an INR of 2.0 to 3.0 in most patients, although patients with the antiphospholipid antibody syndrome may require a higher INR range (98).

Certain medications administered concurrently with warfarin will increase bleeding risk. Aspirin, nonsteroidal anti-inflammatory agents, and high doses of penicillin all increase this risk through their associated inhibition of platelet function (105–107). Skin necrosis is the other adverse effect most associated with warfarin usage. It is uncommon, but when it does occur it tends to do so between the third and eighth days following the initiation of therapy. Necrosis results from extensive thrombosis of venules and capillaries within subcutaneous fat and may be associated with deficiencies of protein C. Treatment is problematic, but the mainstay is future avoidance of warfarin (108,109).

Ximelagatran

As mentioned previously, ximelagatran is a novel oral direct thrombin inhibitor demonstrated to be safe and efficacious in a small pilot study (95). A recent larger randomized double-blind multicenter trial investigated the role of ximelagatran in over 1200 patients who had received six months of conventional anticoagulation following venous thromboembolism (VTE) (110). Patients were treated for a total of 18 additional months with ximelagatran or placebo. The primary end point of symptomatic recurrent VTE was met in 12 of 612 patients receiving ximelagatran and 71 of 611 patients receiving placebo, with no associated differences in mortality or bleeding events.

Given the difficulties maintaining rigid therapeutic levels with warfarin and the associated need for frequent laboratory monitoring, a drug without such need for monitoring is highly desirable. The results of studies such as these are encouraging, but further studies are needed prior to the routine use of ximelagatran for the secondary prevention of VTE.

E. Inferior Vena Cava Filters

Interruption of the inferior vena cava (IVC) to prevent PE as a consequence of DVT is not a new concept. Trousseau suggested in 1868 that a barrier might be able to be placed in the IVC for such a purpose (111). The first surgical ligation of the IVC was performed in 1893, and percutaneous filters eventually became available in the 1960s (111,112). By the early 1990s, 30,000 to 40,000 IVC filters were placed every year in the United States alone, despite a limited evidence base for their efficacy (111,113,114). Data suggest, however, that IVC filters do lessen the incidence of early thromboembolic recurrence, but may be accompanied by an increased long term risk of recurrent DVT. There is no significant impact on survival (111).

Generally accepted criteria for IVC filter placement include an absolute contraindication to anticoagulation, complications of anticoagulation, failure of anticoagulation, massive embolism with residual DVT, free floating ilio-femoral or IVC thrombus, severe cardiopulmonary disease and concurrent DVT, or poor compliance with anticoagulation medicines. Additionally, place-ment may be considered in select patients with severe trauma without documen-ted VTE, particularly those with closed head injuries, spinal cord injuries, or multiple long bone or pelvic fractures (115). Relative contraindications to percu-taneous IVC placement include uncorrectable severe coagulopathy and patients with bacteremia or untreated infection. The long-term durability of these devices is unknown; placement in children and young adults should require careful consideration (115).

In experienced centers, percutaneous placement of IVC filters is safe, with a mortality of approximately 0.1%. Other reported complications include IVC occlusion (2–30%), filter embolization (2–5%), IVC penetration (0–41%), filter migration (0–18%), and filter fracture (2–10%) (115). Even given its rela-tive safety, IVC filter placement should not be considered sole therapy unless absolute contraindications to anticoagulation exist. Although filter placement may help protect the pulmonary vascular bed from embolic material, it does nothing to retard extension of existing venous thrombi and does not affect the sys-temic prothrombotic state. Small thrombi may pass through the IVC filter or through well-developed venous collaterals, and thrombus can extend through the filter. Given these issues, long-term anticoagulation should be provided con-currently with the filter if no contraindications exist or if contraindications later resolve.

VIII. Special Situations

A. Massive Pulmonary Embolism

The diagnosis of massive pulmonary embolism should be based upon the pre-sence of hemodynamic compromise, and not on the anatomical extent of occlusion of the pulmonary vasculature. Not all anatomically massive pul-monary emboli lead to hemodynamic compromise, and smaller emboli can lead to circulatory collapse in a patient with compromised cardiopulmonary reserve.

The pathophysiological changes that accompany massive pulmonary embolism have already been discussed. Therapy is directed at countering the physiologic consequences of vascular obstruction. Supportive care should be provided in a closely monitored environment in which critical care expertise is readily available. As with any critical illness, attention to basics such as airway, breathing, and circulation are paramount. Oxygen administration is nearly universal, and may improve hypoxic pulmonary vasoconstriction. In some patients, endotracheal intubation and mechanical ventilation may be required to improve oxygenation and decrease metabolic demands. Some degree of volume resuscitation may be necessary to support systemic blood pressure, but excessive preload may further distend an already dilated right ventricle with resultant increase in right ventricular wall tension and subsequent decreased right coronary perfusion. This may lead to right ventricular ischemia. Inotropic agents may improve systemic blood pressure, preserve right coronary artery perfusion, and support right ventricular function (116). The use of central hemodynamic monitoring in this setting is tempting given the potential hemodynamic complexities. Placement of a pulmonary artery catheter from a femoral approach, however, can dislodge residual thrombotic material, and balloon flotation from an internal jugular or subclavian approach may be associated with a theoretical risk of dislodging embolic material in transit in the right sided chambers of the heart.

Given the success of thrombolytic agents for myocardial infarction, it was anticipated that similar success would be achieved with their application to pulmonary embolic disease. Since the first use of streptokinase in 1964 in four patients with massive PE (all four patients survived), a number of clinical trials and meta-analyses have evaluated the role of thrombolysis in such patients (60,117–123). Although thrombolytics lead to increased resolution in the first 24 hours when compared to heparin therapy, no significant positive impact has been demonstrated on mortality or recurrence rates. What is clear from these studies, however, is that thrombolysis is associated with an increase in major hemorrhagic complications, including an incidence of intracranial bleeding of 0.5–2.0%, nearly all of which are fatal (124).

Given the increased bleeding risk and lack of impact on mortality, the role of thrombolytic therapy in pulmonary embolism remains undefined. It seems reasonable to limit the use of such therapy to circumstances in which an accelerated rate of thrombolysis has the potential to be life-saving. Specifically, consideration should be given for its use in patients with hemodynamic compromise or in patients with intra-cavitary right heart thrombi (125,126). The use of intravenous and intrapulmonary thrombolytics appears to be equivalent (127), as does the choice of thrombolytic. Thrombolysis does not obviate the need for anticoagulation, which should be initiated in a manner similar to that of other patients with thromboembolic disease.

The role of thrombolytic therapy in hemodynamically stable patients with echocardiographic evidence of right ventricular function remains controversial (128). There is no compelling evidence that thrombolytics affect survival in these patients in the absence of subsequent hemodynamic decline (129). Given the bleeding risk associated with thrombolytic therapy, routine use of these agents in this population cannot be advocated.

Embolectomy for acute massive pulmonary embolism was first proposed by Trendelenberg in 1908, though all three patients initially treated with this procedure died (61). The first successful embolectomy was subsequently performed by Kirschner in 1924. Not surprisingly, randomized trials examining the safety and efficacy of embolectomy in patients with acute, hemodynamically-massive embolism have not been undertaken. The procedure should be reserved for patients with hemodynamically massive PE who have absolute contraindications to anticoagulation or thrombolysis, those in whom the most aggressive medical therapy has failed, and those who have suffered a cardiac arrest, although the mortality in this latter group exceeds 80% (130,131). Percutaneous devices for catheter embolectomy have been investigated (132). Catheter embolectomy has been demonstrated to reverse systemic hypotension, improve pulmonary artery hemodynamics, and improve cardiac output, but with a mortality rate roughly similar to that of surgical embolectomy (133,134).

B. PE in Pregnancy

A number of physiologic perturbations occur in pregnancy that places the gravid patient at increased risk for venous thromboembolism. These include an increase in clotting factors I, VII, VIII, and IX, a decrease in protein S, decreased fibrinolytic activity, increased venous stasis, increased platelet activity, and resistance to activated protein C (135). Even given these changes that may predispose to clotting, VTE in this population is less common than previously thought. In a retrospective review of nearly 270,000 deliveries, there were only 165 (0.06%) episodes of VTE, or approximately one in every 1627 births (136). Of these 165 episodes, 127 patients suffered DVT, while 38 had pulmonary embolism. The majority of cases of venous thrombosis occurred ante partum, while most episodes of embolism occurred post partum and were strongly associated with delivery by cesarean section.

The diagnosis of pulmonary embolism in pregnancy is complicated by the significant overlap between the symptoms of that disease and the dyspnea and lower extremity edema that may accompany normal pregnancy. A natural concern regarding the evaluation of suspected embolism in pregnant patients is the potential radiation exposure of the fetus. This concern is largely unfounded, and the workup of pregnant patients with suspected embolism should not differ substantially from that of nongravid patients, as the well-being of the fetus is ultimately dependent on the welfare of the mother.

The treatment of PE in pregnancy differs substantially from that of nonpregnant patients in that warfarin is contraindicated secondary to its teratogenic effects on the fetus. Warfarin, which crosses the placental barrier, may cause a skeletal embryopathy with stippled epiphyses, as well as nasal and limb hypoplasia when given between six and 12 weeks gestation. Mid-trimester exposures may lead to optic atrophy, microcephaly, and developmental delay, and fetal hemorrhage may occur at any time during the pregnancy, resulting in a high fetal loss rate (137).

Heparin is currently the treatment of choice in pregnancy for both the acute treatment of venous thromboembolic disease as well as long term prevention of recurrence. Neither low-molecular weight heparin or unfractionated heparin cross the placenta, so both are safe for the fetus (138,139). Heparin requirements are amplified in pregnancy given increases in heparin-binding proteins, plasma volume, renal clearance, and heparin degradation by the placenta, all of which reduce heparin bioavailability (140). Long-term use of heparin may also affect bone density, with an average bone loss of approximately 5%, with one-third of patients experiencing a 10% or more decrease in bone density (140,141).

C. Chronic Thromboembolic Pulmonary Hypertension

Chronic thromboembolic pulmonary hypertension (CTEPH) represents a rare sequelae of acute pulmonary embolism. Dexter laboratories assessed 60 consecutive patients with angiographically proven embolism one to seven years after their initial embolic event (30). Complete resolution was noted in 39 patients, partial resolution in 16 patients, and no resolution in five, though only one had chronic cor pulmonale. Although 19 patients in this series died during the study period, only one death could be attributed to chronic thromboembolic disease. Others have estimated that CTEPH of sufficient severity to warrant surgical intervention afflicts approximately 500–2500 patients annually in the United States, or approximately 0.1–0.5% of patients who survive their initial embolic event (142,143). It is essential to identify patients with symptomatic CTEPH, as a potentially curative surgery exists for these patients.

Inadequate thromboembolic resolution following one or more embolic events, regardless of whether those events are clinically symptomatic, appears to represent the predisposing condition in the majority of patients who develop the disease (144). The extent of residual pulmonary vascular obstruction appears to be a major determinant of disease initiation, with involvement of greater than 30–40% of the pulmonary vascular bed present in most patients. If the obstruction is of sufficient magnitude to substantially increase right ventricular afterload, pulmonary hypertension, right ventricular failure, or death may ensue.

Symptoms of CTEPH, like those of other forms of pulmonary hypertension, are fairly protean and difficult to discern from other cardiopulmonary disorders. This explains, in part, the average delay of two to three years between symptom onset and correct diagnosis in this disorder (145). Contributing to the diagnostic delay is a failure to consider disorders of the pulmonary vascular bed in patients presenting with unexplained dyspnea. Dyspnea and impaired exercise tolerance are the most common manifestations, but fatigue, weakness, cough, chest pain or discomfort, and syncope or near-syncope are also reported (146).

Physical exam findings in CTEPH are quite similar to those in other variants of pulmonary hypertension and are dependent on the degree of pulmonary hypertension present when the patient is evaluated. With mild pulmonary hypertension, physical examination findings may be subtle, limited to an accentuation of the pulmonic component of the second heart sound. With the development of right heart failure, additional findings may ensue, such as jugular venous distention, hepatomegaly, ascites, lower extremity edema, and cyanosis.

Once the diagnosis of pulmonary hypertension has been confirmed, ventilation–perfusion lung scanning represents a simple, noninvasive means of differentiating disorders of the peripheral pulmonary vascular bed from those of the central. In chronic thromboembolic disease, at least one (and more commonly, several) segmental or larger mismatched perfusion defects are present. In disorders of the distal pulmonary vascular bed, perfusion scans are either normal or exhibit a "mottled" appearance characterized by subsegmental defects.

Right heart catheterization with pulmonary angiography remains the diagnostic "gold standard" for the disease. An absolute criterion for surgery is the presence of accessible chronic thrombi. Current surgical techniques allow removal of organized thrombi whose proximal extent is in the main and lobar arteries and, depending on surgical skill and experience, those involving the proximal segmental arteries. The presence of comorbid conditions that may adversely affect perioperative mortality or morbidity as well as long term survival must also be considered prior to surgical referral. In patients deemed to be operative candidates, the mainstay of therapy for CTEPH is pulmonary thromboendarterectomy (PTE). The majority of patients who undergo this intervention exhibit a pulmonary vascular resistance greater than $300 \, \text{dynes/sec/cm}^{-5}$. At centers reporting their experience with thromboendarterectomy surgery, preoperative pulmonary vascular resistance is typically in the range of 700–$1100 \, \text{dynes/sec/cm}^{-5}$. In experienced, larger-volume programs, mortality rates associated with the procedure approximate 4–7%. The major causes of death, beyond those associated with other open-heart cardiac procedures, result from reperfusion pulmonary edema and residual pulmonary hypertension.

For the majority of survivors, both the short-term and long-term hemodynamic outcomes are favorable. The pulmonary artery pressure and pulmonary vascular resistance are dramatically reduced and at times normalized. In published series, the mean reduction in pulmonary vascular resistance has approximated 70%, and a PVR in the range of $200–350 \, \text{dynes/sec/cm}^{-5}$ can be achieved. A corresponding improvement in right ventricular function determined by echocardiography, gas exchange, exercise capacity, and quality of life has also been reported. Most patients initially in New York Heart Association (NYHA) Functional Class III or IV preoperatively return postoperatively to NYHA Class I or II and are able to resume normal activities.

Approximately 10–15% of patients have significant residual persistent pulmonary hypertension (147). Treatment options for patients not considered operative candidates and for those with persistent pulmonary hypertension following thromboendarterectomy include medical therapies such as prostaglandin analogues or endothelin antagonists, or lung transplantation.

References

1. Virchow RLK. Cellular Pathology. 1859 special edition. London, UK: John Churchill, 1978.
2. Dalen JE, Alpert JS. Natural history of pulmonary embolism. Prog Cardiovasc Dis 1975; 17:259–270.
3. Nordstrom M, Lindblad B. Autopsy-verified venous thromboembolism within a defined urban population—the city of Malmo, Sweden. Apmis 1998; 106(3): 378–384.
4. Coon WW, Coller FA. Clinicopathologic correlation in thromboembolism. Surg Gynecol Obstet 1959; 109:259–269.
5. Morrell MT, Dunnill MS. The post-mortem incidence of pulmonary embolism in a hospital population. Br J Surg 1968; 55:347–352.
6. Anderson FA Jr, Spencer FA. Risk factors for venous thromboembolism. Circulation 2003; 107(23 suppl 1):I9–I16.
7. Anderson FA, Wheeler HB. Physician practices in the management of venous thromboembolism: a community-wide survey. J Vasc Surg 1992; 16:707–714.
8. Matei D, Brenner B, Marder VJ. Acquired thrombophilic syndromes. Blood Rev 2001; 15:31–48.
9. Egeberg O. Inherited antithrombin deficiency causing thrombophilia. Thromb Diath Haemorrh 1965; 13:516.
10. Griffin JH, Evatt B, Zimmerman TS, et al. Deficiency of protein C in congenital thrombotic disease. J Clin Invest 1981; 68:1370–1373.
11. Comp P, Esmon C. Recurrent venous thromboembolism in patients with a partial deficiency of protein S. N Eng J Med 1984; 311:1525–1528.
12. Heijboer H, et al. Deficiencies of coagulation-inhibiting and fibrinolytic proteins in outpatients with deep vein thrombosis. N Eng J Med 1990; 323:1512–1516.
13. Dahlback B, Carlsson M, Svensson PJ. Familial thrombophilia due to a previously unrecognized mechanism characterized by poor anticoagulant response to activated protein C: prediction of a cofactor to activated protein C. Pro Natl Acad Sci USA 1993; 90:1004–1008.
14. Poort SR, Rosendaal FR, Reitsma PH, Bertina RM. A common genetic variation in the 3′-untranslated region of the prothrombin gene is associated with elevated plasma prothrombin levels and an increase in venous thrombosis. Blood 1996; 88:3698–3703.
15. De Stefano V, Martinelli I, Mannucci PM, et al. The risk of recurrent deep venous thrombosis among heterozygous carriers of both factors V Leiden and the G20210A prothrombin mutation. N Eng J Med 1999; 341:801–806.
16. Kearon C. Natural history of venous thromboembolism. Circulation 2003; 107(23 suppl 1):I22–I30.
17. Heijboer H, Jongbloets LMM, Buller HR. Clinical utility of real-time compression ultrasonography for diagnostic management of patients with recurrent venous thrombosis. Acta Radiol 1992; 33:297–300.

18. Prandoni P, Cogo A, Bernardi E. A simple ultrasound approach for detection of recurrent proximal vein thrombosis. Circulation 1993; 88:1730–1735.

19. Piovella F, Crippa L, Barone M. Normalization rates of compression ultrasonography in patients with a first episode of deep vein thrombosis of the lower limbs: association with recurrence and new thrombosis. Haematologica 2002; 87:515–522.

20. Prandoni P, Lensing AW, Prins MH. Residual venous thrombosis as a predictive factor of reurrent venous thromboembolism. Ann Intern Med 2002; 2002:137.

21. Holmstrom M, Lindmarker P, Granqvist S. A 6-month venographic follow-up in 164 patients with acute deep vein thrombosis. Thromb Haemost 1997; 78:803–807.

22. Sevitt S, Gallagher N. Venous thrombosis and pulmonary embolism: a clinico-pathological study in injured and burned patients. Br J Surg 1961; 48:475–489.

23. Moser KM, LeMoine JR. Is embolic risk conditioned by location of deep venous thrombosis? Ann Intern Med 1981; 94(4 Pt 1):439–444.

24. Kearon C, Julian JA, Newman TE. Non-invasive diagnosis of deep vein thrombosis. Ann Intern Med 1998; 128:663–677.

25. Lagerstedt CI, Olsson CG, Fagher BO. Need for long-term anticoagulant treatment in symptomatic calf-vein thrombosis. Lancet 1985; 2:515–518.

26. Haire D. Arm vein thrombosis. Clin Chest Med 16(2):341–352.

27. Dalen JE, Banas JS, Brooks HL. Resolution rate of acute pulmonary embolism in man. N Engl J Med 1969; 280:1194–1199.

28. Tow DE, Wagner HN Jr. Recovery of pulmonary arterial blood flow in patients with pulmonary embolism. N Engl J Med 1967; 275:1053–1059.

29. Wartski M, Collignon MA. Incomplete recovery of lung perfusion after 3 months in patients with acute pulmonary embolism treated with antithrombotic agents. THESEE Study Group. Tinzaparin ou Heparin Standard: Evaluation dans l'Embolie Pulmonaire Study. J Nucl Med 2000; 41(6):1043–1048.

30. Paraskos JA, Adelstein SJ, Smith RE, et al. Late prognosis of acute pulmonary embolism. N Engl J Med 1973; 289:55–58.

31. Hall RJC, Sutton GC, Kerr IH. Long-term prognosis of treated acute massive pulmonary embolism. Br Heart J 1977; 39:1128–1134.

32. Riedel M, Stanek V, Widimsky J, Prerovsky I. Longterm follow-up of patients with pulmonary thromboembolism. Late prognosis and evolution of hemodynamic and respiratory data. Chest 1982; 81(2):151–158.

33. Rosenberg RD, Aird WC. Vascular-bed-specific hemostasis and hypercoagulable states. N Engl J Med 1999; 340:1555–1564.

34. Ribeiro A, Lindmarker P, Johnsson H, Juhlin-Dannfelt A, Jorfeldt L. Pulmonary embolism: one-year follow-up with echocardiography doppler and five-year survival analysis. Circulation 1999; 99(10):1325–1330.

35. Sergysels R. Pulmonary gas exchange abnormalities in pulmonary embolism. In: Morpurgo M, ed. Pulmonary Embolism Lung Biology in Health and Disease. New York: Marcel Dekker, 1994:89–96.

36. Manier G, Castaing Y, Guenard H. Determinants of hypoxemia during the acute phase of pulmonary embolism in humans. Am Rev Respir Dis 1985; 132(2):332–338.

37. Huet Y, Lemaire F, Brun-Buisson C, et al. Hypoxemia in acute pulmonary embolism. Chest 1985; 88(6):829–836.

38. D'Alonzo GE, Bower JS, DeHart P, Dantzker DR. The mechanisms of abnormal gas exchange in acute massive pulmonary embolism. Am Rev Respir Dis 1983; 128(1):170–172.

39. Cherniak V, Hodson WA, Greenfield LJ. Effect of chonic pulmonary artery ligation on pulmonary mechanics and surfactant. J Appl Physiol 1966; 21:1315–1319.

40. Wood KE. Major pulmonary embolism: review of a pathophysiologic approach to the golden hour of hemodynamically significant pulmonary embolism. Chest 2002; 121(3):877–905.

41. McIntyre KM, Sasahara AA. The hemodynamic response to pulmonary embolism in patients without prior cardiopulmonary disease. Am J Cardiol 1971; 17:288–294.

42. McIntyre KM, Sasahara AA. Hemodynamic and ventricular response to pulmonary embolism. Prog Cardiovasc Dis 1974; 17:175–190.

43. Elliott CG. Pulmonary physiology during pulmonary embolism. Chest 1992; 101(4 suppl):163S–171S.

44. Smulders YM. Pathophysiology and treatment of haemodynamic instability in acute pulmonary embolism: the pivotal role of pulmonary vasoconstriction. Cardiovasc Res 2000; 48(1):23–33.

45. Azarian R, Wartski M, Collignon MA, et al. Lung perfusion scans and hemodynamics in acute and chronic pulmonary embolism. J Nucl Med 1997; 38(6):980–983.

46. Haeger K. Problems of acute deep venous thrombosis, I: the interpretation of signs and symptoms. Angiology 1969; 20:219–223.

47. Cranley JJ, Canos AJ, Sull WJ. The diagnosis of deep venous thrombosis: fallibility of clinical symptoms and signs. Arch Surg 1976; 111:34–36.

48. Anand S, Wells PS, Hunt D, et al. Does this patient have deep venous thrombosis? JAMA 1998; 279:1998.

49. Wells PS, Lensing AW, Davidson BL. Accuracy of ultrasound for the diagnosis of deep venous thrombosis in asymptomatic patients after orthopedic surgery: a meta-analysis. Ann Intern Med 1995; 122:47–53.

50. Ryu JH, Olson EJ, Pellikka PA. Clinical recognition of pulmonary embolism: problem of unrecognized and asymptomatic cases. Mayo Clin Proc 1998; 73(9):873–879.

51. Goldhaber SZ, Hennekens CH, Evans DA, Newton EC, Godleski JJ. Factors associated with correct antemortem diagnosis of major pulmonary embolism. Am J Med 1982; 73(6):822–826.

52. Stein PD, Terrin M, Hales CA, et al. Clinical, laboratory, roentgenographic, and electrocardiographic findings in patients with acute pulmonary embolism and no pre-existing cardiac or pulmonary disease. Chest 1991; 100:698–603.

53. Value of the ventilation/perfusion scan in acute pulmonary embolism. Results of the prospective investigation of pulmonary embolism diagnosis (PIOPED). The PIOPED Investigators. J Am Med Assoc 1990; 263(20):2753–2759.

54. Stein PD, Henry JW. Clinical characteristics of patients with acute pulmonary embolism stratified according to their presenting syndromes. Chest 1997; 112(4):974–979.

55. Steell G. Text book on diseases of the heart. Special ed. Manchester, UK: University Press, 1906.

56. Karsner HT, Ash JE. Studies in infarctions: I. Experimental bland infarction of the lung. J Med Res 1912–1913; 27:205–211.

57. Chapman DW, Gugle LJ, Wheeler PW. Experimental pulmonary infarction: abnormal pulmonary circulation's a prerequisite for pulmonary infarction following an embolus. Arch Intern Med 1949; 83:158–163.

58. Hampton AO, Castleman B. Correlation of postmortem chest teleroentgenograms with autopsy findings. Am J Roentgenol Radium Ther 1940; 43:305–326.

59. Dalen JE, Haffajee CI, Alpert JS, et al. Pulmonary embolism, pulmonary hemorrhage and pulmonary infarction. N Engl J Med 1977; 296:1431–1440.

60. Urokinase-Streptokinase Embolism Trial: phase 2 results. JAMA 1974; 229: 1606–1613.

61. Dalen JE. Pulmonary embolism: what have we learned since Virchow? Treatment and prevention. Chest 2002; 122(5):1801–1817.

62. Monreal M, Ruiz J, Olazabal A, Arias A, Roca J. Deep venous thrombosis and the risk of pulmonary embolism. A systematic study. Chest 1992; 102(3):677–681.

63. Kelly J, Hunt BJ. The utility of pretest probability assessment in patients with clinically suspected venous thromboembolism. J Thromb Haemost 2003; 1(9):1888–1896.

64. Kelly J, Hunt BJ. A clinical probability assessment and D-dimer measurement should be the initial step in the investigation of suspected venous thromboembolism. Chest 2003; 124(3):1116–1119.

65. Schoepf UJ, Costello P. CT Angiography for diagnosis of pulmonary embolism: state of the art. Radiology 2004; 230:329–337.

66. Chagnon I, Bounameaux H, Aujesky D, et al. Comparison of two clinical prediction rules and implicit assessment among patients with suspected pulmonary embolism. Am J Med 2002; 113(4):269–275.

67. Miniati M, Monti S, Bottai M. A structured clinical model for predicting the probability of pulmonary embolism. Am J Med 2003; 114(3):173–179.

68. Bynum LJ, Crotty CM, Wilson JE 3rd. Diagnostic value of tests of fibrin metabolism in patients predisposed to pulmonary embolism. Arch Intern Med 1979; 139(3):283–285.

69. Klotz TA, Cohn LS, Zipser RD. Urinary excretion of thromboxane B2 in patients with venous thromboembolic disease. Chest 1984; 85(3):329–335.

70. Bounameaux H, Slosman D, de Moerloose P, Reber G. Laboratory diagnosis of pulmonary embolism: value of increased levels of plasma D-dimer and thrombin—antithrombin III complexes. Biomed Pharmacother 1989; 43(5): 385–388.

71. Goldhaber SZ, Vaughan DE, Tumeh SS, Loscalzo J. Utility of cross-linked fibrin degradation products in the diagnosis of pulmonary embolism. Am Heart J 1988; 116(2 Pt 1):505–508.

72. Kelly J, Rudd A, Lewis RR, Hunt BJ. Plasma D-dimers in the diagnosis of venous thromboembolism. Arch Intern Med 2002; 162(7):747–756.

73. Kruip MJ, Leclercq MG, van der Heul C, Prins MH, Buller HR. Diagnostic strategies for excluding pulmonary embolism in clinical outcome studies. A systematic review. Ann Intern Med 2003; 138(12):941–951.

74. Perrier A. Diagnosis of acute pulmonary embolism: an update. Schweiz Med Wochenschr 2000; 130(8):264–271.

75. Turkstra F, Kuijer PM, van Beek EJ, Brandjes DP, ten Cate JW, Buller HR. Diagnostic utility of ultrasonography of leg veins in patients suspected of having pulmonary embolism. Ann Intern Med 1997; 126(10):775–781.

76. Loud PA, Katz DS, Bruce DA, Klippenstein DL, Grossman ZD. Accuracy of combined CT venography and pulmonary angiography for lower extremity DVT. Radiology 2001; 219:498–502.
77. van Strijen MJ, de Monye W, Schiereck J, et al. Single-detector helical computed tomography as the primary diagnostic test in suspected pulmonary embolism: a multicenter clinical management study of 510 patients. Ann Intern Med 2003; 138(4):307–314.
78. Musset D, Parent F, Meyer G, et al. Diagnostic strategy for patients with suspected pulmonary embolism: a prospective multicentre outcome study. Lancet 2002; 360(9349):1914–1920.
79. Perrier A, Roy PM, Aujesky D, et al. Diagnosing pulmonary embolism in outpatients with clinical assessment, D-Dimer measurement, venous ultrasound, and helical computed tomography: a multicenter management study. Am J Med 2004; 116:291–299.
80. Schrecengost JE, LeGallo RD, Boyd JC, et al. Comparison of diagnostic accuracies in outpatients and hospitalized patients of D-dimer testing for the evaluation of suspected pulmonary embolism. Clin Chem 2003; 49(9):1483–1490.
81. Rathbun SW, Whitsett TL, Vesely SK, Raskob GE. Clinical utility of D-dimer in patients with suspected pulmonary embolism and nondiagnostic lung scans or negative CT findings. Chest 2004; 125:807–809.
82. Howell WH, Holt E. Two new factors in blood coagulation—heparin and proantithrombin. Am J Physiol 1918; 427:328–333.
83. Barritt DW, Jordan SC. Anticoagulant drugs in treatment of pulmonary embolism: controlled trial. Lancet 1960; 1:1309–1312.
84. Hull RD, Raskob G, Brant RF, et al. The importance of initial heparin treatment on long-term clinical outcomes of antithrombotic therapy. The emerging theme of delayed recurrence. Arch Intern Med 1997; 157:2317–2321.
85. Raschke RA, Reilly BM, Guidry JR, et al. The weight based heparin dosing nomogram compared with a "standard care" nomogram: a randomized controlled study. Ann Intern Med 1993; 119:874–881.
86. Hull RD, Raskob G, Rosenbloom DR, et al. Optimal therapeutic level of heparin therapy in patients with venous thromboembolism. Arch Intern Med 1992; 152:1589–1595.
87. Levine MN, Hirsh J, Gent M, et al. A randomized trial comparing activated thromboplastin time with heparin assay in patients with acute venous thromboembolism requiring large daily doses of heparin. Arch Intern Med 1994; 154(1):49–56.
88. Quinlan DJ, McQuillan A, Eikelboom JW. Low-molecular weight heparin compared with intravenous unfractionated heparin for treatment of pulmonary embolism. Ann Intern Med 2004; 140:175–183.
89. Low-molecular-weight heparin in the treatment of patients with venous thromboembolism. The Columbus Investigators. N Engl J Med 1997; 337(10):657–662.
90. Simonneau G, Sors H, Charbonnier B, et al. A comparison of low-molecular-weight heparin with unfractionated heparin for acute pulmonary embolism. The THESEE Study Group. Tinzaparine ou Heparine Standard: Evaluations dans l'Embolie Pulmonaire. N Engl J Med 1997; 337(10):663–669.
91. Findik S, Erkan ML, Selcuk MB, Albayrak S, Atici AG, Doru F. Low-molecular-weight heparin versus unfractionated heparin in the treatment of patients with acute pulmonary thromboembolism. Respiration 2002; 69(5):440–444.

92.   Segal JB, Bolger DT, Jenckes MW, et al. Outpatient therapy with low molecular weight heparin for the treatment of venous thromboembolism: a review of efficacy, safety, and costs. Am J Med 2003; 115:298–308.

93.   Kovacs MJ, Anderson D, Morrow B, Gray L, Touchie D, Wells PS. Outpatient treatment of pulmonary embolism with dalteparin. Thromb Haemost 2000; 83(2):209–211.

94.   Investigators TM. Subcutaneous fondaparinux versus intravenous unfractionated heparin in the initial treatment of pulmonary embolism. N Engl J Med 2003; 349(18):1695–1702.

95.   Wahlander K, Lapidus L, Olsson CG, et al. Pharmacokinetics, pharmacodynamics and clinical effects of the oral direct thrombin inhibitor ximelagatran in acute treatment of patients with pulmonary embolism and deep vein thrombosis. Thromb Res 2002; 107(3–4):93–99.

96.   Link KP. The discovery of dicumarol and its sequels. Circulation 1959; 19:97–107.

97.   Stahmann MA, Huebner CH, Link KP. Studies on the hemorrhagic sweet clover disease v. identification and synthesis of the hemorrhagic agent. J Biol Chem 1941; 138:513–527.

98.   Hirsh J, Dalen JE, Anderson DR, et al. Oral anticoagulants: Mechanism of action, clinical effectiveness, and optimal therapeutic range. Chest 2001; 119:8s–21s.

99.   van Dongen CJ, Vink R, Hutten BA, Buller HR, Prins MH. The incidence of recurrent venous thromboembolism after treatment with vitamin K antagonists in relation to time since first event: a meta-analysis. Arch Intern Med 2003; 163(11):1285–1293.

100. Hull R, Hirsh J, Jay R, et al. Different intensities of oral anticoagulant therapy in the treatment of proximal-vein thrombosis. N Engl J Med 1982; 307:1676–1681.

101. Turpie AGG, Gunstensen J, Hirsh J, et al. Randomized comparison of two intensities of oral anticoagulant therapy after tissue heart valve replacement. Lancet 1988; 1:1242–1245.

102. Saour JN, Sieck JO, Mamo LAR, et al. Trial of different intensities of anticoagulation in patients with prosthetic heart valves. N Engl J Med 1990; 322:428–432.

103. Altman R, Rouvier J, Gurfinkel E, Comparison of two levels of anticoagulant therapy in patients with substitute heart valves. J Thorac Cardiovasc Surg 1991; 101:427–431.

104. Kearon C, Ginsberg JS, Kovacs MJ, et al. Comparison of low-intensity warfarin therapy with conventional-intensity warfarin therapy for long-term prevention of recurrent venous thromboembolism. N Engl J Med 2003; 349(7):631–639.

105. Dale J, Myhre E, Loew D. Bleeding during acetysalicylic acid and anticoagulant therapy in patients with reduced platelet reactivity after aortic valve replacement. Am Heart J 1980; 99:746–751.

106. Schulman S, Henriksson K. Interaction of ibuprofen and warfarin on primary hemostasis. Br J Rheumatol 1989; 38:46–49.

107. Casenave J-P, Packham MA, Guccione MA, et al. Effects of penicillin G on platelet aggregation, release and adherence to collagen. Proc Soc Exp 1973; 142:159–166.

108. Verhagen H. Local hemorrhage and necrosis of the skin and underlying tissues at starting therapy with dicumarol or dicumacyl. Acta Med Scand 1954; 148:455–467.

109. Weinberg AC, Lieskovsky G, McGehee WG, et al. Warfarin necrosis of the skin and subcutaneous tissue of the male genitalia. J Urol 1983; 130:352–354.

110. Schulman S, Wahlander K, Lundstrom T, Blason SB, Eriksson H. Secondary prevention of venous thromboembolism with the oral direct thrombin inhibitor ximelagatran. N Engl J Med 2003; 349:1713–1721.

111. Decousus H, Leizorovicz A, Parent F, et al. A clinical trial of vena caval filters in the prevention of pulmonary embolism in patients with proximal deep-vein thrombosis. Prevention du Risque d'Embolie Pulmonaire par Interruption Cave Study Group. N Engl J Med 1998; 338(7):409–415.

112. Becker DM, Philbrick JT, Selby JB. Inferior vena cava filters. Indications, safety, effectiveness. Arch Intern Med 1992; 152(10):1985–1994.

113. Magnant JG, Walsh DB, Juravsky LI, Cronenwett JL. Current use of inferior vena cava filters. J Vasc Surg 1992; 16(5):701–706.

114. Streiff MB. Vena caval filters: a comprehensive review. Blood 2000; 95(12): 3669–3677.

115. Grassi CJ, Swan TL, Cardella JF, et al. Quality improvement guidelines for percutaneous permanent inferior vena cava filter placement for the prevention of pulmonary embolism. SCVIR Standards of Practice Committee. J Vasc Interv Radiol 2001; 12(2):137–141.

116. Layish DT, Tapson VF. Pharmacologic hemodynamic support in massive pulmonary embolism. Chest 1997; 111:218–224.

117. Browse NL, James DCO. Streptokinase and pulmonary embolism. Lancet 1964; 2:1039–1043.

118. Bounameaux H, Vermylen J, Collen D. Thrombolytic treatment with recombinant tissue-type plasminogen activator in a patient with massive pulmonary embolism. Ann Intern Med 1985; 103(1):64–65.

119. Levine M, Hirsh J, Weitz J, et al. A randomized trial of a single bolus dosage regimen of recombinant tissue plasminogen activator in patients with acute pulmonary embolism. Chest 1990; 98(6):1473–1479.

120. Tissue plasminogen activator for the treatment of acute pulmonary embolism. A collaborative study by the PIOPED Investigators. Chest 1990; 97(3):528–533.

121. Dalla-Volta S, Palla A, Santolicandro A, et al. PAIMS 2: alteplase combined with heparin versus heparin in the treatment of acute pulmonary embolism. Plasminogen activator Italian multicenter study 2. J Am Coll Cardiol 1992; 20(3):520–526.

122. Goldhaber SZ, Haire WD, Feldstein ML, et al. Alteplase versus heparin in acute pulmonary embolism: randomised trial assessing right-ventricular function and pulmonary perfusion. Lancet 1993; 341(8844):507–511.

123. Thabut G, Thabut D, Myers RP, et al. Thrombolytic therapy of pulmonary embolism: a meta-analysis. J Am Coll Cardiol 2002; 40(9):1660–1667.

124. Dalen JE, Alpert JS, Hirsch J. Thrombolytic therapy for pulmonary embolism: is it effective? Is it safe? When is it indicated? Arch Intern Med 1997; 157(22):2550–2556.

125. Rose PS, Punjabi NM, Pearse DB. Treatment of right heart thromboemboli. Chest 2002; 121(3):806–814.

126. Chartier L, Bera J, Delomez M, et al. Free-floating thrombi in the right heart: diagnosis, management, and prognostic indexes in 38 consecutive patients. Circulation 1999; 99(21):2779–2783.

127. Verstraete M, Miller GA, Bounameaux H, et al. Intravenous and intrapulmonary recombinant tissue-type plasminogen activator in the treatment of acute massive pulmonary embolism. Circulation 1988; 77(2):353–360.

128. Konstantinides S, Geibel A, Heusel G, Heinrich F, Kasper W. Heparin plus alteplase compared with heparin alone in patients with submassive pulmonary embolism. N Engl J Med 2002; 347(15):1143–1150.

129. Hamel E, Pacouret G, Vincentelli D, et al. Thrombolysis or heparin therapy in massive pulmonary embolism with right ventricular dilation: results from a 128-patient monocenter registry. Chest 2001; 120(1):120–125.

130. Gray HH, Miller GA, Paneth M. Pulmonary embolectomy: its place in the management of pulmonary embolism. Lancet 1988; 1(8600):1441–1445.

131. Doerge HC, Schoendube FA, Loeser H, Walter M, Messmer BJ. Pulmonary embolectomy: review of a 15-year experience and role in the age of thrombolytic therapy. Eur J Cardiothorac Surg 1996; 10(11):952–957.

132. Uflacker R. Interventional therapy for pulmonary embolism. J Vasc Interv Radiol 2001; 12(2):147–164.

133. Greenfield LJ, Proctor MC, Williams DM, Wakefield TW. Long-term experience with transvenous catheter pulmonary embolectomy. J Vasc Surg 1993; 18(3): 450–457; discussion 7–8.

134. Timsit JF, Reynaud P, Meyer G, Sors H. Pulmonary embolectomy by catheter device in massive pulmonary embolism. Chest 1991; 100(3):655–658.

135. Barbour LA. ACOG practice bulletin. Thrombembolism in pregnancy. Int J Gynaecol Obstet 2001; 75(2):203–212.

136. Gherman RB, Goodwin TM, Leung B, Byrne JD, Hethumumi R, Montoro M. Incidence, clinical characteristics, and timing of objectively diagnosed venous thromboembolism during pregnancy. Obstet Gynecol 1999; 94(5 Pt 1):730–734.

137. Hall JG, Pauli RM, Wilson KM. Maternal and fetal sequelae of anticoagulation during pregnancy. Am J Med 1980; 68:122–140.

138. Forestier F, Sole Y, Aiach M, Alhenc GM, Daffos F. Absence of transplacental fragmin (Kabi) during second and third trimesters of pregnancy. Thromb Haemost 1992; 67:180–181.

139. Omri A, Delaloye JF, Andersen H, Bachmann F. Low molecular weight hepain Novo (LHN-1) does not cross the placenta during the second trimester of pregnancy. Thromb Haemost 1989; 61:55–56.

140. Barbour LA, Smith JM, Marlar RA. Heparin levels to guide thromboembolism prophylaxis during pregnancy. Am J Obstet Gynecol 1995; 173:1869–1873.

141. Dahlman TC, Sjoberg HE, Ringertz H. Bone mineral density during long-term prophylaxis with heparin in pregnancy. Am J Obstet Gynecol 1994; 170:1315–1320.

142. Moser KM, Auger WR, Fedullo PF. Chronic major-vessel thromboembolic pulmonary hypertension. Circulation 1990; 81(6):1735–1743.

143. Jamieson SW, Kapelanski DP. Pulmonary endarterectomy. Curr Probl Surg 2000; 37(3):165–252.

144. Daily PO, Dembitsky WP, Jamieson SW. The evolution and the current state of the art of pulmonary thromboendarterectomy. Semin Thorac Cardiovasc Surg 1999; 11:152–163.

145. Simonneau G, Azarian R, Brenot F, Dartevelle PG, Musset D, Duroux P. Surgical management of unresolved pulmonary embolism. A personal series of 72 patients. Chest 1995; 107(1 suppl):52S–55S.

146. D'Alonzo GE, Bower JS, Dantzker DR. Differentiation of patients with primary and thromboembolic pulmonary hypertension. Chest 1984; 85(4):457–461.

147. Fedullo PF, Auger WR, Channick RN, Kerr KM, Rubin LJ. Chronic thromboembolic pulmonary hypertension. Clin Chest Med 2001; 22(3):561–581.

148. Kelly J, Rudd A, Lewis RR, Hunt BJ. Plasma D-dimers in the diagnosis of venous thromboembolism. Arch Intern Med 2002; 162:747–756.

149. Wells PS, Anderson DR, Rodger M, Stiell I, Dreyer JF, Barnes D, Forgie M, Kovacs G, Ward J, Kovacs MJ. Excluding pulmonary embolism at the bedside without diagnostic imaging: management of patients with suspected pulmonary embolism presenting to the emergency department by using a simple clinical model and d-dimer. Ann Intern Med 2001; 135:98–107.

7

Neuromuscular Respiratory Failure

SUNIT D. MISTRY and MICHAEL I. LEWIS

Division of Pulmonary and Critical Care Medicine, Cedars–Sinai Medical Center
Geffen School of Medicine at UCLA
Los Angeles, California, U.S.A.

I. Introduction: Applied Respiratory Muscle Physiology

The respiratory muscles operate as a vital "air pump" promoting effective ventilation both at rest as well as under conditions of increased demand. Dysfunction or weakness may thus compromise ventilatory ability and capacity. In this chapter, we will focus on neuromuscular conditions involving the respiratory muscles that may be managed in the intensive care unit (ICU) arena. However, in order to fully appreciate the pathophysiology of the specific conditions, key common principles governing functional anatomy, physiology, and functional assessment of the respiratory muscles will first be introduced.

A. Respiratory Muscles: Functional Anatomy (1,2)

Primary inspiratory muscles are those which are phasically recruited under resting conditions with each ventilatory effort. In humans, the diaphragm, parasternal intercostals, and scalene muscles are considered primary. The diaphragm is responsible for expanding the lower chest cage. Geometric configuration affects diaphragm function. For example, with hyperinflation, the diaphragm becomes flatter and shorter, reducing its force-generating potential. The diaphragm is innervated by the right and left phrenic nerves, which arise from cervical roots 3, 4, and 5. The parasternal intercostals are the interchondral portion of the internal intercostals and produce cranial motion of the ribs and an increased anteroposterior dimension of the upper rib cage. They are innervated by the intercostal nerves. The scalene neck muscles increase the anteroposterior and

transverse diameters of the upper rib cage and elevate the sternum. They are innervated by cervical nerves C4–C8. Accessory respiratory muscles are those
recruited under conditions of increased demand (load, chemical drive, exercise,
etc.). These include the external intercostals and levator costae, which generally
function as reserve inspiratory muscle groups, the sternocleidomastoids (inspiratory, innervated by the X1 cranial nerves), and the internal interosseous intercostals, which generally subserve an expiratory function. The abdominal
muscles are silent at rest, but exert phasic expiratory influences on the chest
cage under conditions of increased ventilatory demand. In addition, they subserve
an important functional role in the act of coughing. They are innervated by
branches of T7 to T12.

B. Respiratory Muscles: Motor Units and Fiber Types

Motor units are comprised of a motor neuron (e.g., phrenic motor neuron in the
case of the diaphragm), its axon, and the motor fibers it innervates, as depicted in
Figure 1 (3). Slow (type S) motor units produce the lowest levels of force, but are
the most fatigue resistant. By contrast, types FR, F int, and FF produce progressive increments in force, respectively, but at the cost of increased fatigability
(Fig. 1). Recruitment of motor units generally follows an orderly progression
(i.e., S → FR → F int → FF). Thus, for the diaphragm, resting ventilation can
be accomplished by the recruitment of mainly type S and some FR motor units
at low frequencies (e.g., 8–16 Hz) (4). With increased ventilatory demand,
recruitment of fast motor units and/or an increase in firing frequency occur.
While force generation increases, this cannot be sustained for long periods
because of the fatigable nature of the fast motor units producing high levels of
force (4). In general, type S motor units are composed of type 1 fiber types,
and FR, F int, and FF of types IIa, IIx, and IIb, respectively. In humans, type
IIb fibers are not noted in the diaphragm (5). Muscle fibers may be classified
histochemically based on pH lability of myofibrillar ATPase staining or
immunohistochemically using monoclonal antibodies to important contractile
proteins, myosin heavy chains (HC; slow, 2A, 2B, and 2X). The specific
myosin heavy chain (MHC) content of muscle fibers influences specific force
(6). Co-expression of different MHC isoforms can occur within single muscle
fibers, especially under pathologic conditions. The latter would be expected to
alter contractile properties.

C. Respiratory Muscles: Weakness and Fatigue

Respiratory muscle weakness is defined as "a condition in which the capacity of a
rested muscle to generate force is impaired" (7). By contrast, respiratory muscle
fatigue is defined as "a condition in which there is a loss in the capacity for developing force and/or velocity of a muscle, resulting from muscle activity under
load and which is reversible by rest" (7). Clinically, the latter translates into
the impaired ability of the respiratory muscles to generate pressure and/or

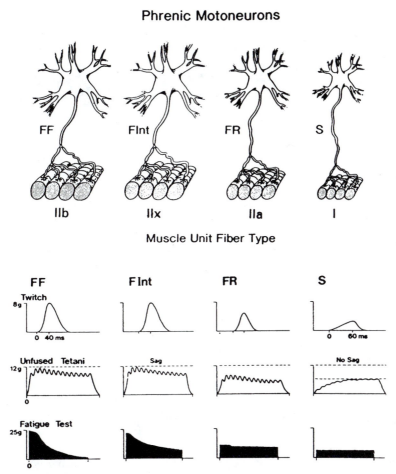

Figure 1 Diaphragm motor units comprising the phrenic motoneuron and the muscle fibers innervated. Twitch force, presence or absence of "sag" during unfused teatany, and a fatigue test are used to distinguish the different motor unit types. Muscle unit fibers can be subclassified histochemically as types I, IIa, IIb, and IIx. *Source*: From Ref. 3.

airflow due to increased contractile activity of the respiratory muscles relative to strength and/or a decrease in energy supply. A weak muscle under load is, thus, highly susceptible to fatigue. Task failure is another term worth emphasizing. This is defined as the point at which the required force (or pressure) needed to subserve a physiologic function can no longer be maintained. For the respiratory muscles, task failure is represented by ventilatory insufficiency and failure (7) (Fig. 2). Respiratory muscle fatigue may be classified as peripheral (contractile

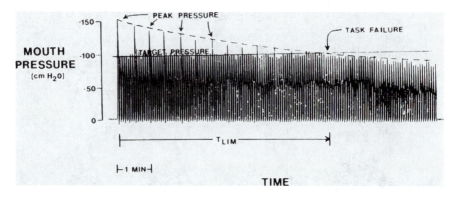

Figure 2 Changes in the capacity to generate pressure during a submaximal endurance run at a target pressure of 67% of peak pressure, measured prior to the endurance challenge. Note that peak pressure measured every 30 sec falls progressively during the endurance run, indicating that a "fatiguing process" is under way. The point of task failure is defined in this endurance run as the inability to generate the target pressure (i.e., maximum efforts now fall below the target pressure). *Source*: From Ref. 8.

fatigue; neurotransmission fatigue) and central fatigue (8–12). Contractile fatigue relates to impaired contractile function of the muscle, despite increased drive, due to sarcolemmal dysfunction or injury, cellular metabolic aberrations, cellular chemical factors (e.g., effects of reactive oxygen species, peroxynitrites, etc.), critical substrate depletion, alterations in excitation–contraction coupling, and injury or dysfunction of cellular constituents/organelles (12,13). Clinically, contractile fatigue may be relatively long-lasting (14). Neurotransmission fatigue refers to reduced amplitude of action potentials due to axonal branch point conduction failure or impaired release, binding, or re-uptake of the neurotransmitter at the neuromuscular junction. Central fatigue refers to a diminution in force generation because of reduced central neural drive, which may be overcome by nerve stimulation (nonmotivational) or voluntary super-effort (motivational). Central fatigue has been viewed as a "protective mechanism" to offset muscle fiber injury to which the term "central wisdom" has been applied. The mechanisms underlying central fatigue are complex, ill-understood, and variable between subjects. Central fatigue of the respiratory muscles, however, likely contributes to or influences the development of task failure to an extent greater than is generally appreciated clinically (15). A number of clinical signs may indicate a loading response of the respiratory muscles without implying the presence of overt fatigue. These include: rapid shallow breathing (16), respiratory alternans (17), paradoxical abdominal or rib cage motion (18), and accessory and/or abdominal muscle recruitment (19).

D. Respiratory Muscles: Assessment of Function in the ICU

The recent American Thoracic Society/European Respiratory Society joint statement on respiratory muscle testing is an excellent resource (20).

Pulmonary Function Tests

While the vital capacity (VC) may be influenced by inspiratory and ± expiratory muscle strength, other factors such as compliance of the lungs and/or chest wall and airway closure may also contribute (21,22). The VC may, thus, exhibit poor specificity in the diagnosis of respiratory muscle weakness. In addition, it is generally considered less sensitive than maximum mouth pressures in the presence of mild respiratory muscle weakness (23). Serial measurements in the ICU offer more reliable data and trends.

Arterial Blood Gases

Awake arterial blood gases are relatively insensitive indices of respiratory muscle weakness until late and severe impairment of respiratory muscles is present. In patients with chronic myopathics and no associated lung disease per se, Braun et al. reported that daytime awake hypercapnia was unlikely, until respiratory muscle strength was reduced to <40% of predicted and VC to <50% (45). Incipient hypercapnia may rapidly change to overt respiratory failure when even mild changes in load or ventilatory drive ensue.

Measures of Respiratory Muscle Strength

The maximum inspiratory mouth pressure (PI_{max}) is a global test of inspiratory muscle strength and reflects the pressure generated by the inspiratory muscles (P mus) plus the passive elastic recoil pressure of the respiratory system (lung and chest wall; Prs). At functional residual capacity (FRC), Prs = 0, while at residual volume (RV), Prs can be considerable (e.g., −30 cmH$_2$O). In the ICU, therefore, it makes more sense to measure PI_{max} at FRC rather than at RV. Normal values are depicted in Table 1. The major disadvantage in measuring PI_{max} is that the test is effort-dependent and requires patient motivation, cooperation, and coordination, all of which may be difficult to obtain in critically ill patients where variances within patients can be wide (24). Further, in the presence of intrinsic positive end-expiratory pressure (PEEP), the pressure generated by the inspiratory muscles will be underestimated. Maximum expiratory mouth pressure (PE_{max}) is measured at total lung capacity (TLC) and is a global measure of expiratory muscle strength. (*Note*: At TLC, Prs can be as high as +40 cmH$_2$O.) In general, multiple efforts may be required to ensure three maximal values with less than 20% variance are obtained. This is difficult to achieve in critically ill patients who may exhibit marginal, if any, reserve and does not ensure that maximal efforts have indeed been produced (25).

Table 1   Normal Values for Tests of Respiratory Muscle Performance

Test		Male	Female	Reference
PI^a_{max}	(tube MP)	-123 ± 21	-87 ± 15	b
(cmH$_2$O)	(flanged MP)	-106 ± 30	-73 ± 21	c
PE^a_{max}	(tube MP)	232 ± 427	152 ± 56	b
(cmH$_2$O)	(flanged MP)	148 ± 34	93 ± 16	c
Sniff Pes		-105 ± 25	-89 ± 21	31
(cmH$_2$O)				
Sniff Pdi		145 ± 24	121 ± 25	31
(cmH$_2$O)				
Maximum static Pdi		108 ± 30	65 ± 31	31
(Mueller) (cmH$_2$O)				
Pdi (combined		180 ± 14		30
Mueller/expulsive				
technique)				
(cmH$_2$O)				
UMS-Tw-Pdi		16 ± 3		34, 36
(cmH$_2$O)		(left; <10 abnormal)		
		12 ± 4		34, 36
		(right; <6 abnormal)		
BAMPS-Tw-Pdi		27.6 ± 1.6		35, 36
(cmH$_2$O)		(male and female;		
		<20 abnormal)		

Note: Phrenic nerve stimulation in intubated patients or with tracheostomy requires occlusion of the artificial airway at end expiration just prior to stimulation.

[a]Normal values in the elderly are available: Enright PL, Kronmal RA, Monolio TA, Schenker MB, Hyatt RF. Respiratory muscle strength in the elderly. Am J Respir Crit Care Med 1994; 149:430–438.

[b]Black LF, Hyatt RE. Maximal respiratory pressures: normal values and relationship to age and sex. Am Rev Respir Dis 1969; 99:698–702.

[c]Wilson SH, Cooke NT, Edwards NT, Edwards RH, Spiro SG. Predicted normal values for maximum respiratory pressures in Caucasian adults and children. *Thorax* 1984; 39:535–538.

Abbreviations: UMS-Tw-Pdi, unilateral magnetic stimulation twitch Pdi; BAMPS, bilateral anterior magnetic phrenic stimulation.

Less variances may be evident by measuring maximal esophageal pressures (Pes), but this requires the insertion of an esophageal balloon catheter. In nonintubated patients, measuring Pes following a maximum sniff may be easier to perform (26). Nasal sniff pressures (Pnas, sn), using a catheter wedged in one nostril, may represent a relatively noninvasive measure mirroring Pes measurements (27). However, Pnas, sn tends to underestimate Pes, sn in patients with lung disease [e.g., chronic obstructive pulmonary disease (COPD)] (28). PI$_{max}$ values greater than -80 cmH$_2$O and Pes (or Pnas) greater than -70 cmH$_2$O (males) or -60 cmH$_2$O (females) are not likely associated with significant respiratory muscle weakness.

Transdiaphragmatic pressure (Pdi) measured as the difference between gastric pressure (Pga) and Pes (i.e., Pdi = Pga − Pes) is a measure of diaphragm strength. Maximal Pdi (Pdi_{max}) may be achieved using different techniques, which include a maximal static inspiratory effort (Mueller maneuver) (29), a Mueller maneuver combined with an abdominal expulsive effort (30), and a maximal sniff (sniff Pdi) (31). Such efforts require patient motivation, cooperation, and coordination, which may be difficult to achieve in critically ill patients (see Table 1 for normal values). Phrenic nerve stimulation at FRC provides an objective, reproducible nonvolitional test. This can be achieved using either electrical stimulation (surface or needle electrodes) (32) or magnetic stimulation, in which rapidly changing magnetic fields produce brief electric fields within conducting tissues. While cervical magnetic stimulation produces bilateral phrenic stimulation, it requires the stimulating coil to be positioned behind the neck, making this technically challenging in ICU patients who are commonly supine (33). Unilateral or bilateral anterior magnetic stimulation approaches to stimulate the phrenic nerves are better suited to the ICU environment (Fig. 3) (34–36). As critically ill patients are most often supine, a greater volume of air may need to be placed in the esophageal balloon. Electrical or magnetic phrenic nerve stimulation uses single supramaximal stimuli to produce a twitch (Tw) Pdi. In general, bilateral phrenic nerve Tw Pdi's are about a quarter of the Pdi_{max} achieved by maximum voluntary effort (37) (Table 1).

In patients in whom it is not feasible to insert balloon catheters into esophagus and stomach and/or who are intubated on mechanical ventilation, endotracheal tube pressure change (TwPet) during magnetic stimulation of the phrenic nerves may be performed. This is closely correlated with TwPes, but not TwPdi (38,39). Thus, this provides another nonvolitional test of respiratory muscle strength (40).

1. *Impaired cough* may be common in patients with neuromuscular disorders and contribute to pulmonary morbidity (infections, retained secretions, atelectasis). Cough strength can be assessed by measuring Pga with a maximal cough (lower limit of normal for adults: 160 cmH_2O (males), 120 cmH_2O (females) (44).

2. *Electrophysiology.* Phrenic nerve conduction time (PNCT) may also be measured following unilateral phrenic nerve stimulation (normal in adults: 6–8 ms) (41). In general, marked prolongation of PNCT suggests a demyelinating process, whereas preserved PNCT coupled with reduced amplitude of the compound action potential suggests axonal damage (41). While surface and needle electrodes have been utilized, the recent use of esophageal electrodes offers precise and reproducible measurement of PNCT and amplitude of the diaphragm compound action potential (42,43).

E. Respiratory Muscles: Functional Force Reserve

The concepts underlying sustainable levels of force (or load) by the respiratory muscles are useful in approaching the factors governing endurance capacity and

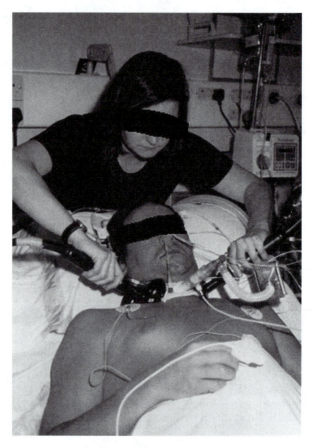

Figure 3 Bilateral anterior magnetic stimulation of phrenic nerves. *Source*: From Polkey MI, Moxham J. Clinical aspects of respiratory muscle dysfunction in the critically ill. Chest 2001; 119:926–939.

functional force reserve of the respiratory pump. Skeletal muscles can sustain repetitive loads or forces for prolonged periods or indefinitely, provided the forces generated are below a critical (threshold) percentage of the maximum force generating capacity. In the case of the diaphragm, fatigue ensued in normal subjects when breathing against inspiratory resistive loads when the ratio of Pdi with each inspiratory to Pdi_{max} exceeded 40% (46). With resting ventilation, the ratio is generally $\leq 5\%$, highlighting considerable reserve capacity. The ratio may approach or exceed the critical threshold if Pdi_{max} is reduced, Pdi breath is increased, or with a combination of the two. The tension time index of the diaphragm (TTdi) is the product of Pdi/Pdi_{max} and the duty cycle (inspiratory time/total respiratory time) and is about 0.02 in normal subjects under resting conditions. A TTdi of 0.15–0.18 proved to be a fatiguing threshold, beyond which respiratory

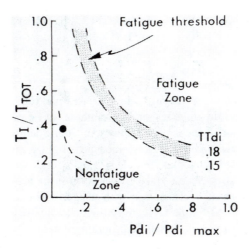

Figure 4 Relationship between duty cycle (Ti/Ttot) and mean spontaneous Pdi expressed as a percentage of Pdi_{max}. The fatigue threshold and fatigue zone are depicted in the figure; endurance capacity of the ventilatory pump may also be influenced independently by either lung volume or flow rate. *Source*: From Ref. 47.

muscle fatigue ensues (Fig. 4) (47). The TTdi is strongly related to endurance, blood flow, and oxygen consumption of the diaphragm (47–49).

II. Specific Neuromuscular Disorders

A. Guillain-Barré Syndrome

Introduction

Of the reversible neuromuscular disorders encountered in the ICU, Guillain-Barré (GBS) syndrome is probably the most common and well known. It is classically defined as an idiopathic acute demyelinating polyneuropathy characterized by progressive muscle weakness and areflexia, and associated with spontaneous remission as a rule. However, forms of the GBS exhibiting predominantly axonal degeneration have been described, accounting for up to 20% of cases. These include an acute motor-sensory axonal neuropathy (50,51) associated with severe Wallerian degeneration in peripheral nerves and a poor prognosis, and an acute motor axonal neuropathy (52) with more rapid recovery and better long-term prognosis. The Miller Fisher syndrome is an unusual variant of the GBS associated with opthalmoplegia, ataxia, and areflexia with minimal weakness (53). GBS is now the most common cause of acute flaccid paralysis and is associated with significant morbidity and, rarely, mortality (2.4–6.4%). Indeed, respiratory failure requiring mechanical ventilation and ICU care occurs in up to 30% of cases (54–56). Mortality in patients requiring mechanical ventilation is higher (15–30% reported) (57,58).

Demographics

The annual incidence ranges from 0.6 to 2.4 cases per 100,000 people per year (56,59). Cases occur in all ages and throughout the world, but there does appear to be a bimodal peak in incidences in young adults and between the fifth and eighth decades. Furthermore, men are slightly more likely to suffer this disease than women (male:female = 1.5:1), and whites slightly more likely than blacks (60). Also, a seasonal variation in incidence has been noted, likely due to the disease's association with triggering infections (and possible vaccines). The reported temporal increase in incidence of GBS in 1976 with the U.S. swine influenza vaccination program remains a controversial issue (61,62).

Pathogenesis

Pathology studies reveal an inflammatory peripheral neuropathy with lymphocytes and macrophages surrounding endoneural vessels, together with demyelination (or axonal degeneration) (63). A predilection for nerve roots is evident. There is evidence for both humoral and cell-mediated neuronal injury. Humoral antibodies are thought to be directed against peripheral nerve tissue. This is supported by the fact that serum from Guillain-Barre' patients has been found to damage Schwann cells in vitro; furthermore, antibodies to *Campylobacter jejuni* have also been noted to cross-react with neuronal gangliosides. Humoral factors can disturb electrical nerve conduction. However, cell-mediated immune response is also involved, evidenced by the invasion of macrophages and lymphocytes leading to splitting of myelin and demyelination. Inflammation can lead to primary or secondary axonal injury in a proportion of cases (64–66).

Associated Conditions or Factors

Two-thirds of patients have a history of upper respiratory infection or gastroenteritis (two to four weeks prior to onset) (56). Infectious associations include *Campylobacter jejuni*, mycoplasma, Lyme disease, *H. influenza*, Epstein–Barr virus, cytomegalovirus, herpes simplex virus, and recent HIV sero-conversion, or HIV with relatively preserved immune function (67–69). Of these, Campylobacter, Cytomegalovirus, and Epstein–Barr virus infections are the most common (70). Campylobacter infection precedes 26% of Guillain-Barre' cases (range: 14–38%) (71,72) and is associated with worse prognosis, slower recovery, acute axonal degeneration and, thus, severe disease, and a greater degree of chronic neurologic residual defects (71).

The association is likely the result of molecular mimicry whereby peripheral nerves share epitopes with the organism, culminating in antibodies misdirected against nerve tissue. With campylobacter-associated GBS, cross-reacting antibodies to GM-I ganglioside (a component of myelin) is present (73). Further, unusual campylobactor serotypes are associated with the GBS. These include 0:19 (most common in the U.S.), 0:41, and four other unusual serotypes (74,75).

Other associations preceding GBS include: Hodgkin's lymphoma (and rarely other malignancies), sarcoidosis, systemic lupus erythematosis, and a variety of drugs (e.g., streptokinase, penicillamine, heroin, epidural anesthesia) (56,68).

Clinical Manifestations and Diagnosis

Initial symptoms include parasthesiae in fingers and toes due to spontaneous discharges in demyelinated sensory nerves. This is followed by lower extremity weakness, which progresses in an ascending fashion to involve the upper extremities. Cranial nerve involvement (facial, bulbar), autonomic dysfunction, and respiratory muscle involvement can ensue. Pain in limb muscles, flank, and back is common. Weakness and other neurologic signs tend to be symmetrical, and areflexia is prominent. There is minimal evidence of sensory loss despite prominent symptoms of parasthesias. Most signs and symptoms peak in severity in two to four weeks, followed by a plateau phase of variable time, with recovery of function returning slowly over weeks to months (76–79).

Table 2 reports the frequency of clinical features at disease onset and with the fully developed illness (nadir in function). Table 3 highlights diagnostic criteria supporting the diagnosis of GBS compared to features which cast doubt on the diagnosis or exclude it.

Diagnostic Studies

Electrophysiology

Electrophysiologic Studies are the most sensitive and specific, with findings reflecting type and extent of nerve injury. These include reduced nerve conduction velocities, partial motor conduction block, or prolonged distal latencies. Roper and coworkers (80) evaluated electrodiagnostic abnormalities in a large consecutive cohort of patients with GBS. The most common abnormalities were proximal conduction block (27%), proximal conduction block associated with a distal lesion (increased duration of compound action potential on distal stimulation $\pm$ increased distal latency) (27%), and generalized slowing in 22%. Evidence of axonal damage or absent response was evident in a minority of patients (80). Moreover, electrophysiologic studies may help in the prognosis of the disease in that action potentials reduced to less than 20% of the lower limit of normal suggest a poorer outcome (81).

Table 2 Frequency of Features of Acute Guillain-Barré Syndrome

Condition	Frequency	
	Initially (%)	In fully developed illness (%)
Features of syndrome		
Parasthesias	70	85
Weakness		
Arms	20	90
Legs	60	95
Face	35	60
Oropharynx	25	50
Ophthalmoparesis	5	15
Sphincter dysfunction	15	5
Ataxia	10	15
Areflexia	75	90
Pain	25	30
Sensory loss	40	75
Respiratory failure	10	30
CSF protein >0.55 g/L	50	90
Abnormal electrophysiologic findings	95	99

Source: From Ref. 68.

Cerebrospinal Fluid (CSF) Analysis

Early in the disease, CSF studies may be essentially normal, but after one week of symptoms, the CSF typically shows normal opening pressures, elevated protein concentrations of greater than 50 mg/dL, and few cells (mononuclear; <10). A pleocytosis of >50 cells suggests another process such as HIV, Lyme disease, malignancy, or sarcoidosis. A protein level >250 mg/dL suggests spinal cord compression (77,68).

Respiratory and ICU Considerations

Respiratory Failure

Twenty-five to 30% of patients will progress to respiratory failure. The factors involved include inspiratory pump weakness, expiratory muscle weakness giving rise to poor cough and clearance of secretions, and bulbar weakness predisposing to aspiration (75,82).

Ideally, one would want to intervene preemptively, prior to late stages of the disease and florid respiratory failure in which risk of respiratory arrest is high. As there can be discordance between limb muscle, bulbar, and respiratory muscle weakness, serial measurements of respiratory muscle function are essential (see Introduction).

Table 3   Diagnostic Criteria for Typical Guillain-Barré Syndrome

---

Features required for diagnosis
   Progressive weakness in both arms and both legs
   Areflexia

Features strongly supporting the diagnosis
   Progression of symptoms over days to 4 wk
   Relative symmetry of symptoms
   Mild sensory symptoms or signs
   Cranial-nerve involvement, especially bilateral weakness of facial muscles
   Recovery beginning two to four weeks after progression ceases
   Autonomic dysfunction
   Absence of fever at the onset
   Elevated concentration of protein in cerebrospinal fluid, with fewer than 10 cells/mm^3
   Typical electrodiagnostic features

Features making the diagnosis doubtful
   Sensory level
   Marked, persistent asymmetry of symptoms or signs
   Severe and persistent bladder or bowel dysfunction
   More than 50 cells/mm^3 in cerebrospinal fluid

Features excluding the diagnosis
   Diagnosis of botulism, myasthenia, poliomyelitis, or toxic neuropathy
   Abnormal porphyrin metabolism
   Recent diphtheria
   Purely sensory syndrome, without weakness

Source: From Ref. 68.

Traditionally, VC and mouth pressures have been measured. As these require volitional effort and can be inaccurate because of poor mouth seal (e.g., bilateral facial weakness), newer objective measures are superior, but not readily available (see Introduction). Chevrolet and Deleamont (83) reported significant reductions in VC 48 hours prior to intubation, with the average VC being 15.2 ± 3.7 mL/kg, while in stable patients, VC exceeded 40 mL/kg on serial measures. Early predictors of mechanical ventilation were recently reported by the French Cooperative Group on Plasma Exchange in GBS in a large cohort of patients (84). Multivariate analysis revealed a number of predictors which included: time from onset of condition to admission <7 days (odds ratio [OR], 5.0), inability to lift head (OR, 5.0), and VC < 60 predicted (OR, 2.86). In a separate analysis, excluding VC, inability to cough had an OR of 9.09. In the presence of these predictors, mechanical ventilation was required in >85% (84). It should be noted that hypercapnia is a very late sign and portends respiratory arrest. Therefore, serial reliance on PCO_2 is not recommended. This is because hypercapnia occurs only with severe inspiratory muscle weakness (85), and hypocapnia or normocapnia on blood gas analysis can rapidly transition to overt respiratory failure. Hypoxemia may be secondary to alveolar hypoventilation, microatelectasis, mucous plug obstruction, aspiration, pneumonia, and so on. Table 4 provides practical considerations in determining the need for intubation and/or mechanical ventilation. In general, multiple such factors are taken into consideration. Elective intubation is preferred, as recent reports highlight that emergent intubation was associated with a weaning time that was prolonged two-fold (86).

Special considerations regarding intubation involve the hemodynamic instability of many of these patients due to autonomic dysfunction. This may complicate the act of intubation, in which sedatives are often given that can reduce the blood pressure of a patient with already labile hemodynamics. Moreover, the act of intubation itself may promote arrhythmias in a patient already predisposed, further complicating airway control. Therefore, intubation should be performed in the most controlled of settings by one highly skilled in the act of airway management (78,86,87).

Ventilatory Support

While intubation and conventional ventilation is the traditional approach, noninvasive positive pressure ventilation (NIPPV) is an alternative to invasive

Table 4 Factors Mitigating Towards Need for Intubation and/or Mechanical Ventilation in Guillain-Barré Syndrome

---

Clinical: general
  Inability to lift head
  Time from onset to admission <7 days
  Restlessness and anxiety

Clinical: respiratory
  Inability to cough
  Inability to clear secretions (bulbar)
  Staccato speech
  Inability to count to 20 in one breath
  Use of accessory muscles
  Paradoxic respirations
  Rapid shallow respirations
  Dyspnea

Measures
  VC <20 mL/kg
  MIP < -30 cmH$_2$O
  MEP $< +40$ cmH$_2$O
  Hypoxemia
  Respiratory acidosis (late)

---

ventilation that may be considered in a subset of patients with milder abnormalities, completely intact bulbar function, or in those in whom intubation criteria are "on the fence" (borderline). Clearly, this requires a patient who is cooperative with the NIPPV, has intact upper airway function to maintain patency of the airways and prevent aspiration, minimal secretions, and hemodynamic stability. NIPPV, if used, is not a long-term solution due to pressure necrosis by a tight-fitting mask and/or disease progression. Further, as patients may take up to four weeks to peak in severity and several weeks to months thereafter to recover, consideration for early tracheostomy in mechanically ventilated patients is reasonable in anticipation of prolonged respiratory and/or bulbar compromise and to facilitate comfort, bronchial toilet, and weaning (88,89).

Liberation from mechanical ventilation depends, in large part, on improvement in respiratory muscle function. While a threshold of $VC \geq 18$ mL/kg was necessary for successful liberation in one study (83), this has not been confirmed in other studies (90). Borel and colleagues (90) found that the level of Pdi_{max} and maximum inspiratory pressure (MIP) correlated with duration of unsupported respiration, with threshold values for Pdi_{max} and MIP being 31 cmH$_2$O and -30 cmH$_2$O, respectively. Even in patients who were successfully weaned, Pdi_{max} and MIP were still markedly reduced. Improvement in Pdi_{max} was the best predictor of recovery (90). While it may be possible to liberate patients from mechanical ventilation, extubation may be prolonged to ongoing bulbar dysfunction.

Autonomic Dysfunction

Autonomic neuropathy affecting sympathetic and parasympathetic function is common in GBS, occurring in up to 69% clinically and in the majority of patients at the peak of illness with special testing (91). Manifestations include tachycardia, bradycardia and arrhythmias, labile blood pressure and orthostasis, sweating disturbance, pupillary changes, urinary retention, and gastrointestinal dysfunction (92,93). The incidence of dysautonomia is highest in patients requiring mechanical ventilation (91).

Other issues include pneumonias (aspiration or nosocomial/ventilator-associated), pulmonary embolism/deep venous thrombosis from prolonged immobility, decubitus ulcers, and impaired nutrition from poor enteral intake or gastrointestinal autonomic dysfunction (58,93).

Treatment

Current treatment for GBS involves either plasma exchange or intravenous immune globulin (IVIG).

Plasma Exchange

This involves the selective removal of plasma from circulation to eliminate or dilute circulating pathogenic factors and replacement with albumin. Large multicenter trials have demonstrated efficacy as evinced by increased muscle strength, shorter time on mechanical ventilation, and more rapid overall improvement. Furthermore, a meta-analysis of six trials involving a total of 649 patients found plasma exchange to be superior to supportive care, even in mild disease (94). This therapy is most effective when started within 7 to 14 days of symptoms, and albumin has been found as effective as fresh frozen plasma as a replacement fluid. Because of the risks of hypotension and hemodynamic instability, as well as the cost and discomfort to the patient, plasmaphoresis is recommended for patients with gait instability, worsening respiratory muscle function, or bulbar weakness. It is less indicated in ambulatory patients with mild disease or with no further progression after three weeks. Plasma exchange generally involves alternate day exchanges (50 mL/kg) for four to five exchanges. Relapse in signs and symptoms can be treated with a second course of therapy with similar efficacy (95–99).

Intravenous Immune Globulin

Intravenous immune globulin (IVIG) has been found to be as efficacious as plasma exchange when given in the first two weeks of the disease (400 mg/kg daily for five to six days). One study showed no difference when compared to plasma exchange with respect to disability scale or duration of mechanical ventilation (100). Also, no further added benefit of combined plasmaphoresis and IVIG was found over single modality therapy (101). IVIG is considered to be generally safer than plasmaphoresis but with higher cost and variable supply. IVIG is regarded as superior to plasma exchange in campylobacter-associated GBS with antibodies against GM-1 and GM-1b gangliosides (102). The immunomodulating effects of IVIG may be related to cytokine suppression, down regulation of antibody production, interference with Fc receptors, complement inhibition, and suppression of NK cells (103). Side effects include hyperviscocity and thromboembolism, aseptic meningitis, skin rashes, renal dysfunction, and migraine (103). IVIG is associated with a volume load and may be complicated by anaphylaxis in patients with IgA deficiency, which is a contraindication to its use. Relapses are not more common with IVIG (104), and a second course in select cases may have efficacy (105). The use of corticosteroids, once considered the mainstay of therapy for GBS, is now controversial. Both recent multicenter trials and meta-analyses have confirmed no benefit to their use as single modality therapy. However, there may be questionable benefit when combined with plasma exchange (54,102).

Prognosis

The overall outcome of GBS is generally favorable, with 65% progressing to complete recovery within 12 months, and 15% left with only minor deficits that do not interfere with activities of daily life. However, 20% of patients will be left with significant disabilities, including weakness, imbalance, or sensory loss. Moreover, mortality rates can vary from 2.4 to as high as 6.4%, despite aggressive ICU and supportive care, with patients often succumbing to complications such as nosocomial pneumonia, ARDS, sepsis, pulmonary embolism, and cardiac arrhythmias (104). Furthermore, if complete or near-complete recovery does not occur early after the onset of the disease, recovery tends to be slow or minimal after 1.5 to 2 years, and 3% will have one or more acute relapses over their lifetime. Factors that portend a poorer outcome include old age, severe or rapidly progressing disease, axonal degeneration, prolonged ventilation (greater than one month), persistent abnormalities on EMG, and preexisting pulmonary disease (107–109).

B. Myasthenia Gravis

Introduction

Myasthenia gravis (MG) is an acquired disorder of the neuromuscular junction, producing neurotransmission fatigue (110). The clinical manifestations are consequences of muscle fatigability and weakness. The disease is of special interest in the critical care arena in that it may affect respiratory muscles out of proportion to other muscle groups, with progressive and/or sudden deterioration ensuing, leading to respiratory failure and even unexpected respiratory arrest (111–113).

Demographics

MG is not a rare disease. Its prevalence is approximately 20 cases per 100,000 individuals, with an annual incidence of 1.3 new cases per 100,000 individuals per year. Overall, in the year 2000 (114), 53,000–59,900 people were estimated to be affected in the United States alone. All races are affected equally. A bimodel incidence exists, with females twice as likely as males to be affected during the second and third decades of life, while mostly men are affected during a second peak in the sixth and seventh decades (115). More recent epidemiologic studies highlight an increased prevalence in older individuals and likely underdiagnosis in the elderly (116,117).

Pathogenesis

MG is an autoimmune disorder most often caused by autoantibodies to postsynaptic nicotinic acetylcholine receptors. This leads to a reduction in acetylcholine receptors along with the morphologic changes at the neuromuscular junction (simplified synaptic folds; widened synaptic space) (Fig. 5). Antibodies to acetylcholine receptors may reduce their number by several mechanisms, including accelerated degradation, complement-mediated injury, and functional blockade with down regulation (118–120). This culminates in reduced amplitude of end-plate potentials and progressive inefficiency of neuromuscular synaptic transmission, leading to muscle weakness with inability to sustain muscle force.

The initiating events leading to autoimmune dysfunction are unknown. Possible links to the thymus as an inducer of the immune response in MG have been postulated and explored, particularly as thymic abnormalities are present in about 75% of patients with the disorder. In particular, thymic myoid cells which express surface acetylcholine receptors have been implicated (121). Molecular

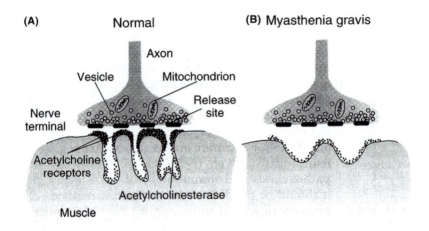

Figure 5 Normal (**A**) and abnormal neuromuscular junction as might be seen in myasthenia gravis (**B**). *Source*: From Ref. 110.

mimicry has also been proposed, as some infectious agents express peptide sequences homologous to the α subunit of the acetylcholine receptor (122). The role of T-lymphocytes and genetic factors have also been explored (123,124).

Diagnosis

Apart from clinical suspicion, a useful order of testing would be use of a short-acting anticholinergic inhibitor (edrophonium [Tensilon®]), antibody assays, and finally electrodiagnostic studies (125).

Edrophonium (Tensilon)

This agent, which potentiates muscurinic effects of acetylcholine at the receptor, lasts for only 10 minutes. A test dose of 1 mg is given to assess for cholinergic excess, followed by the remaining 9 mg over one to two minutes. Atropine is available if necessary. Objective end points need to be measured. These include VC and MIP (as indices of respiratory muscle function), evidence of sustained upward gaze, and limb muscle tests including hand-grip strength before and after. False-negative and positive results can occur.

Antibody Assays

Antibodies to the acetylcholine receptor are seen in ~80–90% of MG patients (110,126). In seronegative patients, as many as 70% have antibodies directed against the muscle-specific kinase (MuSK) (127,128). These patients often have severe bulbar disease and are resistant to treatment (127,128). In patients with MG exhibiting myopathic features, antititin antibodies have recently been reported (129).

Electrodiagnostic Studies

Repetitive nerve stimulation, at two to five pulses per second with a 10% or greater decrease in the amplitude of the compound action potential from the first to fourth or fifth waveform, has been considered valid for diagnosis of MG in a systematic review of the literature (130). Single fiber electromyography (EMG) is considered more sensitive than conventional EMG but is not specific nor readily available (130,131). Repetitive phrenic nerve stimulation is a promising new tool to assess MG involvement of diaphragm (132).

Clinical Manifestations

The cardinal feature of MG is muscle weakness and fatigability, which is aggravated by muscle recruitment/exercise. In ∼15%, MG is limited to the eyes (ocular MG), with the remaining patients exhibiting generalized disease (110,126,132). It has recently been highlighted, however, that more than 50% of patients with ocular MG will progress to generalized disease, with immunosuppressive therapy markedly reducing this progression (133). Ophthalmic features include ptosis and diplopia (extraocular muscle involvement) with sparing of pupils. Bulbar and facial muscle involvement produces a "snarly" smile, nasal speech, difficulty chewing, dysphagia, and choking (aspiration). Weakness of bulbar and upper airway muscles can result in upper airway obstruction (134,135). Limb muscle weakness is most often proximal in distribution. Neck extensor weakness may be prominent. Respiratory muscle involvement produces inspiratory muscle weakness with reduced pump capacity and expiratory muscle involvement with impaired cough and clearance of secretions (111) (see ICU considerations in the preceeding text). A clinical staging (grading) classification is presented in Table 5.

Associated Clinical Conditions

About 75% of patients with MG have thymic abnormalities (136). Of these, 85% are thymic hyperplasia and 15% thymomas (benign and malignant). By contrast, in patients with thymomas, ∼35% have MG (137). Thymic carcinoma, Hodgkin's lymphoma, and small cell lung cancer have also been associated

Table 5 Clinical Staging of Myasthenia Gravis

Stage I: Ocular (only)

Stage IIA: Mild generalized with slow progression (no crisis, drug responsive)

Stage IIB: Moderate generalized (severe skeletal and bulbar involvement, no crisis, less drug responsive)

Stage III: Acute fulminating (rapid progression of severe symptoms including respiratory compromise and poor drug response; high incidence of thymoma)

Stage IV: Late severe (severe symptoms with respiratory compromise, but longer progression from stage I or II)

with MG (138,139). Systemic lupus erythematosis and rheumatoid arthritis have likewise been associated with MG, and Graves disease and MG may co-exist or have overlapping features (140). While a number of drugs have been reported to impair neurotransmission and aggravate MG, penicillamine has been implicated in producing a form of MG (141,142).

Life-threatening crises associated with MG include myasthenic crisis, in which marked deterioration of the condition culminates in respiratory muscle pump failure and/or bulbar paralysis, with imminent or overt respiratory failure, and the less common cholinergic crisis, in which overmedication with anticholinesterase drugs leads to depolarization and weakness (143,144).

Myasthenic Crisis

Myasthenic crisis occurs in ~5–20%, with an annual incidence of 2.5% per year (145). Crises occurred more commonly in women, with the mean age $43 + 18$ years and median age 55 (range 70–82) years in two recent series (144,145). The time interval between onset of MG and a crisis is variable, but generally short on average (<3 years) (144,145). The most common precipitating cause is infection (upper or lower respiratory), occurring in ~30–40% (144,145). No obvious cause is found in close to a third (144). Thymectomy has been associated with a crisis post-op in 11–17% (145,146). (Prognostic factors—preoperative bulbar symptoms, high antibody levels, and prior crisis) (146).

Corticosteroid administration or withdrawal, underdosing or discontinuation of anticholinesterase medications, and use of agents affecting the neuromuscular junction have also been implicated (141,144,145), as have pregnancy, emotional distress, and other surgeries.

Respiratory failure usually ensues rapidly (within three days) with onset of crisis. The median duration of the crisis was 13 days in a large series (144). Independent risk factors for prolonged intubation included: (1) peak VC post-intubation in the first six days <25 mL/kg, (2) age >30, and three serum bicarbonate >30 mEq/L. The likelihood of intubation for periods >2 weeks was related to the number of risk factors present (144). Of note, limb muscle weakness was absent in 20% of patients (144). Early intubation and mechanical ventilation are key. While objective measures (VC, MIP, etc.) can be followed as with GBS, trends are more likely to be useful, especially in view of discordance between respiratory, bulbar, and limb muscle weakness. Following blood gas trends are not useful, as rapid deterioration can develop. Thus, hypercapnia is a very late sign. In select cases, NIPPV can be utilized, offsetting the need for intubation (147). The most common complication with prolonged ventilation is atelectasis (with risk of pneumonia), and aggressive pulmonary toilet, including bronchoscopic removal of secretions if necessary, is key (144,145,148). Other general supportive measures employed in ventilated patients should be used, including attention to nutrition. Successful weaning criteria reported by Thomas, et al. (144) included VC > 25 mL/kg, MIP > −40 cmH$_2$O, and MEP > 50 cmH$_2$O. Where available, measurement of Pdi (volitional or stimulated) may provide more specific data (132,149). See below for summary of specific treatment measures in myasthenic crisis. Overall, functional morbidity after a crisis is closely linked to prolonged ventilation (144). Mortality with myasthenic crisis is between 4–12%, with the majority attributable to comorbidities or cardiac arrhythmias (144,145).

Cholinergic Crisis

This is an unusual problem, accounting for <5% of cases of MG presenting in crisis (145). Overdosage of anticholinesterase drugs leads to muscarinic effects (increased pulmonary secretions, wheezes, abdominal discomfort, diarrhea, miosis, etc.) and a depolarizing block at the neuromuscular junction. While edrophonium was previously used to distinguish myasthenic from cholinergic crises, the common practice of withdrawing anticholinergic medications acutely with crises makes this unnecessary.

Anesthesia

Patients exhibit an unpredictable response to succinylcholine and a marked sensitivity to nondepolarizing blockers (141). Thus, some anesthesiologists avoid neuromuscular blocking agents and depend on deep inhalational anesthesia (150). A balanced approach using anesthetic agents in combination with short or intermediate acting agents may cautiously be titrated (mivacurium, vercuronium, *cis*-atracurium) (141,150).

Pregnancy

Pregnancy can offer unique challenges in patients with MG. The intrapartum period can produce muscle fatigue and precipitate a myasthenic crisis (151). In a large series, 17% exhibited myasthenic exacerbation with labor, while a further 15% and 16% deteriorated during pregnancy or in the early postpartum period, respectively (152). Epidural anesthesia is key to reducing pain and muscular fatigue. While Cesarean section is avoided if possible, it may be necessary in a minority of cases (152).

Treatment

Treatment modalities for MG may encompass four objectives: (1) enhancement of neuromuscular transmission, (2) suppression of the immunologic attack, (3) elimination of "antigenic cells," and (4) depletion of circulating antibodies.

Anticholinesterases

Cholinesterase inhibitors, which enhance neuromuscular transmission by preventing the breakdown of acetylcholine from the neuromuscular junction and thus saturating receptors and improving function, are the mainstay of treatment. Pyridostigmine (Mestinon®) is the oral agent of choice. A starting dose of 30–60 mg every six hours is commonly employed. The dosage and interval need to be tailored to each patient and generally should not exceed 120 mg every three hours. A long-acting preparation is available (Mestinon Timespans 180 mg) to cover sleeping hours. While benefit is noted in most patients, it tends to be incomplete and decreases after several weeks or months (110). This provides the rationale for other therapies, including immunosuppressive agents and thymectomy (110,126,153–155).

Steroids

Corticosteroids can induce remission in 30% of patients and significant benefit in a further 45% (156). Steroids can transiently worsen MG. Therefore, initially small doses of prednisone (15–25 mg/day) should be used with slow increments to a target of 60 mg/day (over two to three weeks) for two to three months. This is followed by an alternate day regimen and continued for a year, prior to progressive tapering of dose. While improvement may be noted two to four weeks after start of therapy, maximum benefit may be delayed for six to twelve months or longer (110). Few patients are tapered off completely. Pulsed IV methylprednisolone has also been used in resistant cases (157).

Immunosuppressive Agents

Azathioprine (158,159) and cyclosporine (160) have generally been used in conjunction with prednisone as steroid-sparing agents. Used alone, these agents exhibit a longer time to onset of effect and maximum response compared to prednisone (110). Mycophenolate mofetil has been used with improvement in 73%, including patients refractory to steroids or other immunosuppressive agents (161).

Thymectomy

Given that 75% of MG patients have thymic abnormalities and that the acetylcholine receptors on thymic myoid cells are thought to serve as an antigenic source, thymectomy theoretically works by removing the antigen source or reducing the reservoir of immune cells or thymic antibodies (162). Remission is seen in 35% of patients, and overall improvement is seen in 50–80% (even patients without thymomas), although the improvement may be delayed over months to years. Of note, thymectomy is not useful in the treatment of acute severe disease. In general, given the overall improvement with thymectomy, it should be strongly considered in all patients with generalized MG between the ages of puberty and 60 years (163,164).

Thymectomy may be associated with worsening of MG and/or myasthenic crisis (146). Thus, perioperative plasmapheresis may be employed to offset this. While median sternotomy has been a classic surgical approach, newer experience with thoracoscopic procedures have been reported (165).

Treatment of Myasthenic Crisis

Figure 6 provides an algorithm for management of myasthenic crisis (166). Because crises may occur in the presence of anticholinesterase therapy and risk inducing cholinergic excess including arrhythmias, a common practice is to discontinue cholinesterase inhibitors during the acute phase, with

Algorithm for management of patients in myasthenic crisis

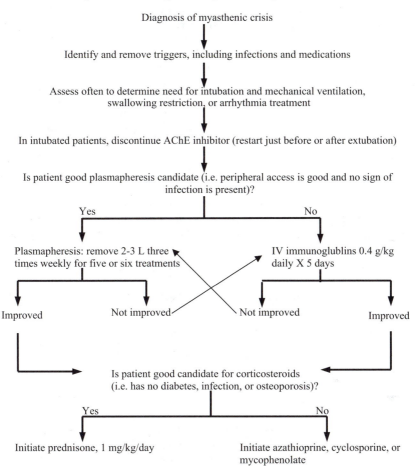

Diagnosis of myasthenic crisis

Identify and remove triggers, including infections and medications

Assess often to determine need for intubation and mechanical ventilation, swallowing restriction, or arrhythmia treatment

In intubated patients, discontinue AChE inhibitor (restart just before or after extubation)

Is patient good plasmapheresis candidate (i.e. peripheral access is good and no sign of infection is present)?

Yes — No

Plasmapheresis: remove 2-3 L three times weekly for five or six treatments

IV immunoglublins 0.4 g/kg daily X 5 days

Improved — Not improved — Not improved — Improved

Is patient good candidate for corticosteroids (i.e. has no diabetes, infection, or osteoporosis)?

Yes — No

Initiate prednisone, 1 mg/kg/day

Initiate azathioprine, cyclosporine, or mycophenolate

Figure 6 Management algorithm for myasthenic crisis. *Abbreviation*: AchE-acetyl-cholinesterase. *Source*: From Ref. 166.

reintroduction once the crisis has been adequately treated and stabilization achieved (166). However, regimens using pyridostigminal alone or in conjunction with corticosteroids or plasmapheresis had equal efficacy in patients with myasthenic crisis (145). Thus, there is no established approach.

Plasmapheresis

This modality removes antibodies to the acetylcholine receptor and can be associated with rapid improvement in ~75% of patients, often within days

(167,168). Usually, 3-L exchanges are used, three times a week for two weeks. Plasmaphoresis with an immunoabsorbent column may improve antibody clearance over conventional plasmaphoresis (169).

IVIG

This also produces rapid clinical improvement and is effective in 75% (170). The dose is 400 mg/kg daily for five days. Some reserve this therapy for patients in whom plasmaphoresis is clinically problematic (166). Cochrane data base systematic reviews of either plasma exchange (171) or IVIG (172) in MG, highlighting the paucity of randomized controlled trials. The benefits from both modalities are relatively short-lived.

Prognosis

The overall prognosis of MG has improved over recent years. Most patients will show improvement within two weeks of initiation of therapy. Equal severity and long-term outcome has been reported in both thymoma and nonthymoma MG (173). However, the presence of antiryanodine receptor antibodies in thymoma-MG and antititin/ryanodine receptor antibodies in nonthymoma MG portend a less favorable prognosis (173). Similarly a worse outcome may be noted in patients exhibiting anti-MuSK antibodies (127).

Differential Diagnosis

A number of conditions may mimic generalized MG. Three such conditions will be briefly discussed.

Lambert–Eaton Syndrome

This syndrome may be associated with small cell lung cancer (174). Pelvic girdle weakness usually exceeds shoulder girdle. Ptosis is common but diplopia rare. Respiratory muscle involvement and respiratory failure has been reported (175). Repetitive nerve stimulation typically produces augmentation of the amplitude of compound action potentials. Antibodies directed against voltage gated calcium channels on presynaptic nerve terminals occur in 95% (176). Plasma exchange and 3,4,diaminopyridine (which releases acetylcholine from nerve terminals) have been used therapeutically.

Botulism

Botulin toxins (A–G) are produced by clostridium botulinum. They impair neurotransmission by preventing presynaptic acetylcholine containing vesicles from fusing with the presynaptic membrane (177). Botulism produces a descending flaccid paralysis, bulbar dysfunction, and prominent eye signs (pupillary paralysis) (197). Respiratory muscle involvement and ventilatory failure occur in 19–75% early in the disease process (178). Prolonged mechanical ventilation may be required and recovery delayed over many months. Repetitive nerve studies produce similar findings to that noted with Lambert–Eaton. Treatment is mainly supportive with antitoxin, effective if given early (within 24 hours of symptom onset).

Tick Paralysis

Neurotoxins produced by the wood, dog, and marsupial ticks can impair ion flux at nerve terminals or the presynaptic release of acetylcholine and may simulate MG. An acute ascending flaccid paralysis with bulbar and respiratory muscle involvement can ensue (179,180). Treatment is supportive and the efficacy of an antitoxin is unclear.

C. Neuromuscular Disorders of Critical Illness

Introduction

Neurological manifestations of critical illness, particularly in the setting of sepsis, have recently been highlighted and may be construed as the neurological components of multiple organ dysfunction. These include: (1) critical illness polyneuropathy, (2) delayed reversal of neuromuscular blockade, (3) the spectrum of critical illness myopathies, and (4) septic encephalopathy. These entities can co-exist or manifest as isolated conditions.

Critical Illness Polyneuropathy

Critical illness polyneuropathy (CIP), an acute sensory-motor distal axonal polyneuropathy complicating critical illness, was first described in 1984 (181). Recent studies suggest early development of the disease process following the onset of critical illness (two to five days) (182,183). The incidence of CIP is high, with incidence reports in 10 prospective studies ranging from 25–100% (62 ± 23%) (184,185).

Clinical Features

Clinical signs of sensorimotor polyneuropathy include limb muscle weakness and atrophy, reduced or absent deep tendon reflexes, loss of sensation to light touch or pin-prick, and relatively preserved cranial nerve function. In less severe cases, weakness is greater distally. In severe cases, a flaccid quadriplegia may be evident. Preserved deep tendon reflexes do not necessarily exclude the diagnosis of CIP. For example, Zifko et al. (186) reported preserved upper limb reflexes in 28% and preserved knee jerks in 17% of patients with CIP. The respiratory muscles can also be involved (diaphragm, chest wall), leading to difficulty in weaning patients from mechanical ventilation. Electrodiagnostic studies have shown evidence of diaphragm denervation in 54–60% of patients with CIP, which was associated with prolonged duration of mechanical ventilation (twofold) compared to patients with no evidence of CIP (187–189).

Associations

Most studies have shown a strong association with the systemic inflammatory response syndrome (SIRS) and sepsis (190), including prolonged vasopressor support and need for renal replacement therapy. While increased muscle levels of anti- and pro-inflammatory cytokines have been reported in both CIP and critical illness myopathy (191), the exact pathogenetic mechanisms are as yet unknown. Of interest, strict glycemic control in patients with sepsis was reported to significantly reduce the incidence of CIP by 44% (192).

Diagnosis

The diagnosis may be clouded by confounding factors in the critically ill patient, including metabolic abnormalities, multiorgan dysfunction, and pharmacologic influences (e.g., sedatives, analgesics, etc.). Electrophysiologic studies can suggest motor and sensory axonal polyneuropathy (reduced amplitude of motor and/or sensory compound action potentials together with preserved latencies). EMG may show evidence of muscle denervation (fibrillations, positive sharp waves) (186). It should be highlighted, however, that critical illness myopathy can coexist with CIP, and, furthermore, conventional electrodiagnostic studies may fail to distinguish between the two (185). Direct muscle stimulation studies may assist in differentiating neuropathy and myopathy (193).

Treatment

This is mainly supportive with aggressive management of sepsis or the associated critical illness, including strict glycemic control. Attention should be directed at the prevention of decubitus ulcers, physical therapy, and optimal nutrition.

Outcome

Mortality may be increased two- to three-fold in patients with CIP compared to a similar cohort of patients without CIP (194). Much of the attributable mortality is due to the need for prolonged ventilation and associated complications. While most survivors show some improvement within three months, a high percentage of severe cases remain with significant residual weakness at two years (42%), including quadraparesis (195). Survivors with mild to moderate nerve injury generally recover muscle strength slowly over weeks to months. However, electrophysiologic studies may show residual nerve dysfunction for years (187,196).

Delayed Reversal of Neuromuscular Blockade

The use of aminosteroid nondepolarizing neuromuscular blocking agents, such as pancuronium and vecuronium, can lead to prolonged neuromuscular blockade, particularly in the setting of renal dysfunction (197,198). These agents act as paralytics by reversibly binding to acetylcholine receptors on the motor end plates of neuromuscular junctions, thus inhibiting neuromuscular transmission. Normally these agents are cleared from the circulation within several hours, mostly via hepatic metabolism. However, active 3-hydroxy metabolites of these drugs require renal clearance and may accumulate in patients with impaired renal function (creatinine clearance of <30 mL/min). Neuromuscular blockade may persist for up to a week after the drug has been discontinued (197). The diagnosis is supported by the persistent suppression of train-of-four twitch responses to ulnar nerve stimulation (199). The diagnosis can be further evinced by transient improvement in muscle strength after the administration of an anticholinesterase-reversing agent.

Patients with renal failure may be better served by using benzylisoquinoline agents such as atracurium and its relatives (cisatracurium and others), which are metabolized via ester hydrolysis and Hofmann elimination to inactive metabolites and are thus not affected by renal or liver dysfunction.

Critical Illness Myopathy

This form of neuromuscular disorder is similar clinically to CIP and may also be associated with sepsis and multiorgan dysfunction. Although three distinct clinical entities have been reported (critical illness myopathy, thick filament myopathy, and acute necrotizing myopathy), pathogenetic mechanisms and associations likely overlap (190,200,201). A number of associations have been highlighted. These include the impact of sepsis, associated with cytokine-induced skeletal muscle proteolysis, the catabolic influences of endogenous and exogenously administered corticosteroids, neuromuscular blocking agents, and severe metabolic derangements (190,202–204). A combination of high dose corticosteroids and prolonged infusion of nondepolarizing neuromuscular blocking agents has been strongly associated, possibly due to the upregulation of steroid receptors in the presence of functional denervation (205). Recent reports also suggest an association with the combined use of corticosteroids and propofol (206). The incidence of critical illness myopathy is not well defined. However, one retrospective study conducted over a 10-year period in Vancouver showed that, of patients treated with a combination of corticosteroids and either pancuronium or vecuronium, 30% developed myopathy. Moreover, the duration of pharmacologic neuromuscular blockade was found to be an independent predictor for the development of myopathy (207).

Varying pathology has been reported in muscle biopsies. This ranges from atrophy of type 2 muscle fibers, as described for steroid myopathy (see general section on Myopathy in the preceeding text), to progressive necrosis of muscle fibers. Electron micrographs of muscle biopsies have shown selective loss of thick myosin filaments, particularly in patients treated with the combination of steroids and neuromuscular blocking agents (205). Helliwell et al. performed muscle biopsies on 31 patients with sepsis-related multiorgan failure and an ICU-stay >1 week. Twelve biopsies showed muscle atrophy, while 15 biopsies revealed muscle necrosis. Twelve patients underwent serial biopsies, with five showing progression of muscle necrosis (208).

As mentioned above, electrodiagnostic testing is not specific for myopathy in the setting of critical illness, and direct muscle testing may assist differentiation from CIP (193). However, small polyphasic motor unit potentials with a good interference suggest a myopathic process. CPK levels peak early and are frequently normal when the diagnosis is entertained. With severe necrosis, however, high levels of CPK and myoglobinuria may be found. Muscle biospy can be diagnostic (200).

Critical illness myopathy can be associated with severe skeletal muscle weakness, including the respiratory muscles, thus leading to the respiratory failure and/or prolonged mechanical ventilation. The mean recovery time to ambulation with critical illness myopathy tends to be shorter than reported for CIP. No specific treatment modalities are available in established disease.

Septic Encephalopathy

Septic encephalopathy presents early with impaired concentration, orientation, and a delusional state. It may progress to impaired levels of consciousness, coma, and seizures. The EEG shows nonfocal diffuse slowing of brain activity. Imaging studies (CT scan and MRI) are unremarkable and nonfocal (209,210).

D. Multiple Sclerosis

Introduction

Multiple sclerosis (MS) is generally classified as an inflammatory demyelinating disease of the central nervous system with a predilection for periventricular white matter, optic nerves, brainstem, and cervical spinal cord. Acute relapses may result in life-threatening respiratory compromise necessitating active management in the ICU. A subset of patients may also progress to chronic neuromuscular respiratory failure (211).

Demographics

MS is a disease of young adults. The mean age at onset is 30 years, with a female predominance (M:F = 1:2) (212). In the United States, the prevalence is ~100 per 100,000. Prevalence is greatest in Caucasian populations, particularly of Northern European origin.

Pathogenesis

MS is thought to be a Th1-cell-mediated autoimmune disease whereby myelin-reactive T cells cross the blood brain barrier and react to myelin antigens on microglia, astrocytes, and macrophages (213). This culminates in inflammation, release of inflammatory mediators, and damage to oligodendrocyte myelin sheaths and underlying axons. Trafficking of myelin-relative T cells to the CNS may be related to upregulation of chemokines (214,215). Genetic and environmental factors, including infection-induced immune stimuli, may play a role (216). Pathologic hallmarks include inflammation, demyelination, axon loss, and gliosis. Neuroaxonal damage and gliosis predominate in chronic progressive disease states (217).

Classification

MS is likely a series of distinct disease syndromes with both unique and overlapping clinical and pathological features (218). It is generally classified as: (1) relapsing-remitting (80–85% at onset), (2) primary progressive, (3) secondary progressive, and (4) progressive relapsing (219).

Clinical Features: General

Acute relapses produce signs and symptoms lasting at least 24 hours separated from subsequent attacks by at least 30 days. Clinical features are protean in nature. Sensory limb symptoms (secondary to posterior column, spinothalamic tract and dorsal root lesions) occur in a quarter to a third of presentation (212,220,221). Visual symptoms (eye pain, loss of visual acuity secondary to optic neuritis) and subacute motor signs (weakness, spasticity of lower limbs > arms), are also important presenting features. Other symptoms and signs include: diplopia, gait disturbances, trigeminal neuralgia, dysarthria, vertigo, Lhermitte's sign (shock-like pains with neck flexion), bowel, bladder, and sexual dysfunction, seizures, and neuropsychiatric disturbances. Accompanying signs may include: optic disc edema or atrophy, nystagmus, internuclear opthalmoplegia, spasticity, weakness, cerebellar signs and truncal ataxia, and impaired propnoception and vibration sense (212,220,221).

Clinical Features: Respiratory Disease

While respiratory complications contribute significantly to morbidity and/or mortality in the advanced stages of MS, serious respiratory compromise may complicate acute attacks (222). Of note, heat sensitivity, whereby small increases in body temperature can induce conduction block, results in exacerbation of existing signs and symptoms and may precipitate ventilatory compromise (223). Inspiratory muscle weakness, including bilateral diaphragm paralysis, may complicate lesions in the upper cervical cord. Such patients may also present with quadriparesis. It is important to note, however, that spirometry may be a relatively insensitive marker of inspiratory muscle weakness, particularly in the absence of profound clinical motor signs (224). Discordance between weakness of respiratory, bulbar, and peripheral muscles can occur. Expiratory muscle weakness is also of importance and may contribute to poor cough and clearance of secretions (resulting in pneumonia and/or atelectasis). Inspiratory muscle endurance has been reported to be significantly reduced in patients with MS able to perform exercise ergometry (225). Such patients may be vulnerable to task (ventilatory) failure with increased loads. Bulbar weakness may result in aspiration culminating in pneumonia or acute lung injury. Brain stem involvement can affect respiratory center nuclei, resulting in abnormalities of ventilatory control.

In a cohort of MS patients exhibiting respiratory abnormalities, Howard (222) reported respiratory muscle weakness in 74%, bulbar dysfunction in

47%, abnormalities of respiratory control in 32%, paroxysmal hyperventilation in 16%, and an anecdotal case of obstructive sleep apnea. Mechanical ventilation was required in 63% of the patients. In 25% of patients, noninvasive devices were used. Overall mortality for all patients was 37% and 58% in those requiring assisted ventilation (222).

Diagnostic Tests

Imaging. Magnetic resonance imaging (MRI) is the imaging test of choice. Plaques appear hyperdense on T2-weighted images and hypodense on T1. MRI detects more lesions than computerized tomography (CT) (226). Contrast enhancement (gadolinium) on T1-weighted images correlates with new active plaques (227). Depending on criteria used, MRI-sensitivity is 87–90% and specificity 71–74%.

Cerebrospinal Fluid. The total white cell count is usually normal and exceeds 15/mL in <5%. While cerebrospinal fluid (CSF) protein is normal, increased CSF immunoglobulin levels (predominantly IgG) are evident (sensitivity 90%) (228). Oligoclonal bands are found in 85–90% (229).

Evoked Potentials. Abnormal evoked visual, somatosensory, and auditory potentials are noted in 85, 77, and 67% of patients (230).

Treatment (231,232)

Acute Relapses. High-dose corticosteroids are employed short-term in high doses (0.5–1 g) of IV methyl prednisolone daily for three to seven days ± tapering schedule of oral Prednisone (1 mg/kg) over 10 days (233–235).

Disease Modifying Agents. These are used to decrease the frequency of acute attacks. Five FDA-approved medications are available. A systematic review of available interferons suggested a modest impact by one year (236). The interferons include: interferon-beta-1b (Betaseron®), interferon-beta-1a (Avonex®, given IM, and Rebif®, given SC). All the interferons are associated with prominent flu-syndrome side effects (see Refs. [231] and [232] for dosages and other details). Glatiramer acetate (Copaxone®) is a mixture of synthetic polypeptide chains originally developed as an analogue, to myelin basic protein. It is administered by daily SC injection and may decrease relapse rate (237). Side effects include dyspnea, chest pain, palpitations, and anxiety. Long-term use of mitoxantrone, an anthracycline analogue, is limited by cardiotoxicity (238). Intravenous immune globulin, plasma exchange, and a variety of immunosuppressive therapies have also been used with relapses unresponsive to steroids ± first line disease modifiers (231,232,239,240).

Differential Diagnosis

Misdiagnosis occurs in 5–10%. The following conditions may simulate MS: spinal disease (degenerative, vascular, cervical disc), collagen vascular and vasculitic disorders, infections (Lyme disease, syphilis, HTLV-1, herpes zoster, multifocal leukoencephalopathy, postinfectious encephalopathies), sarcoidosis, CNS, lymphoma, mitochondrial disorders, and other genetic disorders (241).

E. Diaphragm Paralysis

Paralysis or severe weakness of the diaphragm (unilateral or bilateral) can occur as an isolated phenomenon or as part of a more generalized neuromuscular disorder. The impact on ventilatory function depends on the degree of weakness, the extent of muscle involvement (bilateral > unilateral), the rapidity of onset, the extent of other inspiratory muscle weakness, and comorbidities (particularly cardiac, pulmonary, or chest wall abnormalities) (242).

Clinical Features

Orthopnea (occurring rapidly with supine posture) is a classic symptom of bilateral diaphragm paralysis (243). Exertional dyspnea may be seen in patients with both bilateral and unilateral paralysis (244–246), culminating in reduced exercise tolerance (247). Imersion dyspnea in water is another symptom of bilateral diaphragm paralysis (248,249). Abdominal paradox (inward inspiratory motion of the abdomen) while supine is a key sign of bilateral diaphragm paralysis (250). The sign is less evident with lesser degrees of weakness and may be absent with $Pdi_{max} > 30$ cmH_2O (251). Abdominal paradox may also be noted with unilateral diaphragm paralysis (252). In general, inspiratory muscle strength of patients with hemidiaphragm paralysis is most decreased in those with associated cardiopulmonary disease (252). Sleep-disordered breathing and nocturnal hypoventilation may occur with diaphragm paralysis, but usually in patients in whom weakness of other inspiratory muscles is present (244). Arm elevation may result in increased metabolic and ventilatory cost, producing dyspnea (253).

Diagnostic Tests

Imaging. Chest x-ray may show elevated hemidiaphragm or the appearance of small lung volumes and basilar subsegmental atelectasis which can be misinterpreted as "poor inspiratory effort." Fluoroscopy, demonstrating paradoxical motion of a hemidiaphragm when supine following a vigorous sniff, is useful with unilateral paralysis (254). However, with bilateral paralysis, the patient is unable to lie supine and the test lacks sensitivity. Expiratory muscle recruitment elevates the flaccid diaphragm, which descends passively in the upright position at the onset of inspiration with abdominal muscle relaxation. Ultrasound can also be used to assess diaphragm motion (255,256). Ultrasound has also been used to determine diaphragm atrophy with paralysis (thickness at zone of opposition with chest wall at FRC <2 mm and <20% increase in thickness during inspiration) (257).

Pulmonary Function Studies. An exaggerated fall in VC when supine is a useful test. Table 6 depicts pulmonary functions in patients with bilateral (244) and recent unilateral diaphragm weakness/paralysis (246).

Table 6 Pulmonary Function with Diaphragm Paralysis

	VC (L) (% pred)	Supine fall in VC (%)	TLC (% pred)	RV (% pred)
(A) Bilateral[a]	2.1 ± 0.7 (48)	37 ± 9	67 ± 11	104 ± 23
(B) Unilateral[b]	2.9 ± 0.9 (76)	11.8 ± 8.1	88 ± 17	108 ± 23

Note: Values are means ± SD.
[a]Ref. 244.
[b]Ref. 246.
Abbreviations: VC, vital capacity; TLC, total lung capacity; RV, residual volume; L, liters.

Maximum Respiratory Muscle Pressures. A detailed discussion is presented in the Introductory section of this chapter. Table 7 summarizes mean respiratory pressures generated in patients with bilateral severe diaphragm weakness/paralysis (244) or hemidiaphragm paralysis (246).

Typical tracings of pressure deflections for Pdi and its components (gastric and esophageal pressures) following a sniff maneuver in a patient with bilateral diaphragm weakness and a control subject are depicted in Figure 7 (257).

The ratio of Δ Pga to Δ Pes is normally < -1. With diaphragm paralysis, other chest and neck inspiratory muscles are recruited such that the ratio approaches $+1$. This index, which correlates with Pdi_{max}, may, thus, be a useful index of diaphragm weakness (258).

Nerve Conduction and Electrophysiology. See Introductory section.

Causes of Diaphragm Paralysis

A comprehensive classification of diaphragm paralysis is provided in Table 8. References for individual causes may be found in review papers and newer references cited here or in other sections of this chapter (259–266).

Table 7 Respiratory Muscle Pressures with Diaphragm Paralysis

	PI_{max} (% pred)	PE_{max} (% pred)	Pdi_{max} (Mueller)	Pdi_{max} (Sniff)	TwPdi
(A) Bilateral	4.0 ± 18 (43)	135 ± 51 (98)	11 ± 8	13 ± 6	0.8 ± 2
(B) Unilateral	49 ± 9 (62)	112 ± 53 (95)	[a]	62 ± 13	1.2 ± 1.6 (affected) 11.1 ± 3.5 (normal)

Note: Values are means ± SD.
[a]Maximum static values variable and depend on gender.
Abbreviations: PI_{max} = maximum inspiratory mouth pressure; PE_{max} = maximum expiratory mouth pressure; Pdi = transdiaphragmatic pressure; Tw = twitch.
Source: From Refs. 244 and 246.

PATIENT WITH DIAPHRAGM PARALYSIS

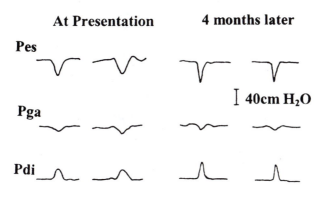

At Presentation   **4 months later**

Pes

Pga

Pdi

I 40cm H_2O

NORMAL

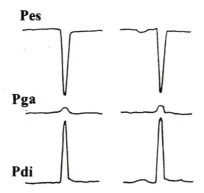

Pes

Pga

Pdi

Figure 7   Serial measurement of maximum transdiaphragmatic pressures (Pdi) in a patient with severe diaphragm weakness compared to a normal subject. *Source*: From Spireri MA, Mier AK, Pantin CF, Green M. Bilateral diaphragm weakness. Thorax 1985; 40:631–631.

Specific Conditions

Phrenic Nerve Injury Postcardiac Surgery.   Phrenic nerve injury can occur with cardiac surgery because of phrenic nerve cooling during cardioplegia. Complete phrenic nerve conduction block has been well-documented with cooling in dogs (267), and more recently, changes in the evoked EMG response of the diaphragm have been demonstrated in patients undergoing cardiac surgery using bilateral magnetic phrenic stimulation (268). Of interest, the latter occurred with mild degrees of hypothermia (31°C) (268). Internal mammary harvesting

Table 8 Etiology of Diaphragm Paralysis

(A) Spinal cord	Collagen vascular and vasculitic
High cervical cord trans-section/injury	Systemic lupus erythematosis
Multiple sclerosis	Wegener's granulomatosis
(B) Motor neurons	Radiation injury
Amyotrophic lateral sclerosis	Neuralgic amyotrophy
Post-polio syndrome	Idiopathic
Spinal muscular atrophy	(E) Diaphragm Myopathy
(C) Cervical nerve roots	Dystrophy
Cervical spondylosis	Limble girdle
Complication of spinal surgery	Collagen vascular disorders
Chiropractic manipulation	Systemic lupus erythematosis
(D) Phrenic nerves	Dermatomyositis
Trauma	Systemic sclerosis
Blunt; sharp	Mixed connective tissue disease
Surgical	Endocrine
Cooling (cardiac surgery)	Hypothyroidism
Infective	Hyperthyroidism
Herpes zoster	Gluccocorticoid excess
Lyme disease	(Cushings, iatrogenic administration)
Neoplastic	Critical illness
Tumor compression	Critical illness myopathy
Paraneoplastic	Nutrition/metabolic
Polyneuropathy	Anorexia nervosa
Gullain-Barre and associated conditions	Electrolyte deficiency
Chronic inflammatory polyneuropathy	Periodic paralysis
Critical illness polyneuropathy	Acid Maltase deficiency
Charcot Marie Tooth	Amyloidosis
Acute porphyna	Idiopathic

may also increase the risk of phrenic injury (269). Traction and vascular compromise of the phrenic nerve may contribute to injury.

Since first described, the incidence of phrenic injury following cardiac surgery has decreased with the introduction of preventive measures, including insulation. Depending on the methodologies used to define abnormalities, the incidence of abnormalities varies currently between 10–36% (270–273). However, Diehl and co-workers (274) reported the prevalence of clinically significant diaphragm dysfunction to be 2.1% (ice slush) and 0.5% (with insulation). In general, bilateral diaphragm paralysis is rare (<5% of cases with phrenic injury) (275). Of note, phrenic dysfunction has also been described after heart-lung and lung transplantation (276).

The clinical presentation of diaphragm paralysis may be acute or subacute and may contribute to significant morbidity and/or mortality (274,277) (see clinical features earlier). The natural history is such that the majority of affected patients recover function. With injury limited to the myelin sheath, recovery by

12 weeks is expected (278). With accompanying axonal damage, recovery is further delayed, and full recovery can take one to two years (272,278). About 30% of patients fail to fully recover diaphragm function (279). Supportive ventilatory measures may be required in the acute or subacute setting, including the use of noninvasive methods of support (271). In patients with prolonged chronic dysfunction which is symptomatic, diaphragm plication (either unilateral or bilateral) is a therapeutic option (see treatment of diaphragm paralysis in the preceeding text).

Neuralgic Amyotrophy. Neuralgic amyotrophy is an idiopathic inflammatory condition affecting the bronchial plexus that may lead to unilateral or bilateral diaphragm paralysis (280,281). Patients may present with dyspnea (particularly with exercise or with immersion) after a prodromal flu-like illness in which neck and shoulder pain is prominent (282). Nocturnal desaturation and obstructive sleep apnea have been described (280). The latter may be related to involvement of upper airway muscles as contributing factors (283). Upper limb weakness/paralysis recovers within three years in most cases (282). Long-term recovery of diaphragm strength was delayed and generally took greater than three years (284). No specific therapy is available for treatment of neuralgic amyotrophy. In patients with delayed recovery ($>2-3$ years), diaphragm plication can be considered (284).

Systemic Lupus Erythematosus. The mechanisms responsible for producing the "shrinking lung syndrome" in patients with systemic lupus erythematosus (SLE) are not well understood, and studies have produced conflicting results. Pathogenic mechanisms include: (1) demyelinating phrenic neuropathy, which may be responsive to corticosteroid therapy (285), (2) diaphragm myopathy (286), and (3) chest wall restriction rather than diaphragm weakness per se (287). The finding of diaphragm fiber atrophy and fibrosis in an autopsy study, however, conflicts with the latter findings and conclusions (288).

Treatment of Diaphragm Paralysis

Diaphragm Plication. Surgical plication of the diaphragm is a technique whereby sutures are placed in the paralyzed hemidiaphragm in order to render it taut, thus preventing it from being pulled up into the thorax with inspiration (289). While mostly performed in patients with symptomatic unilateral diaphragm paralysis (289,290), bilateral diaphragm plication has been used in selected cases with good long-term success (291). The procedure can be performed using a video-assisted thorascopic approach (292), conventional posterolateral thoracotomy (290), or via a laparoscopic approach (293). Diaphragm plication has been associated with improved gas exchange, chest mechanics (including supine VC), respiratory muscle function (including Pdi_{max}), exercise performance, as well as symptoms and social well-being (290,291,294–296). In children, diaphragm plication may also facilitate weaning from mechanical ventilation (294,297). Sustained long-term effects (up to 10 years) have been reported (290,295).

Diaphragm Pacing.   Diaphragm pacing may be considered in patients with high cervical spinal cord injuries (above C3), that is, high quadriplegia (298,299). This may result in independence from mechanical ventilation, the ability to speak, normalized gas exchange, reduced infections, and improved quality of life. Prerequisites for pacing include documented intact lower phrenic motor neurons, normal cognitive function, and absence of recovery of diaphragm function after a period of at least four months. Indeed, Oo and co-workers (261) reported that 21% of patients with high cervical cord injury were able to breathe independently after four to 14 months. Diaphragm pacing electrodes can be inserted around phrenic nerve trunks in the neck (cervical approach) or in the chest (standard thoracotomy or thoracoscopic approach) (300). There is also limited experience with intramuscular implantation of pacing electrodes into the diaphragm laparoscopically (301). Once electrodes are inserted, conditioning regimens of gradually increasing periods of diaphragm pacing is required for up to nine months prior to full uninterrupted pacing (302). Long-term favorable results have been reported in patients with quadriplegia, fully paced for a mean period of 14.8 years (303).

Ventilatory Support.   Acute bilateral diaphragm paralysis with or without associated pulmonary complications or other inspiratory muscle involvement may require intubation and full mechanical ventilation. Prolonged continuous or intermittent mechanical ventilatory requirements necessitate tracheostomy and positive pressure ventilation. Symptomatic patients with isolated bilateral diaphragm paralysis may be managed with nocturnal $\pm$ intermittent daytime noninvasive positive pressure ventilatory support (304). Other noninvasive devices used have included the pneumobelt, rocking bed, and negative pressure devices (Cuirass, pneumo-wrap) (259).

F.   Amyotrophic Lateral Sclerosis

Amyotrophic Lateral Sclerosis (ALS) is the most common of the progressive neurodegenerative motor neuron diseases, with an incidence of $1-3/100,000$. The mean age at onset is $\sim$56 years with a male predominance (M:F = 2:1). Familial ALS (autosomal dominant) occurs in 5–10% of cases (305–307).

Pathobiology

ALS is characterized by degeneration of upper and lower motor neurons. Lower motor neurons include anterior horn cells in the spinal cord and brainstem neuronal homologues of cranial nerves innervating bulbar muscles. Upper motor neurons include neurons in the motor cortex and their descending corticospinal tracts, which synapse on lower motor neurons. The term *amyotrophy* refers to muscle fiber atrophy and wasting secondary to denervation, and *lateral sclerosis* refers to gliosis and hardening of the lateral columns of the spinal cord with corticospinal tract degeneration (305–307). Variants of the condition include spinal muscular atrophy (progressive muscular atrophy), bulbar palsy (lower motor neuron involvement only), primary lateral sclerosis and pseudo-bulbar palsy (upper motor neuron involvement only). The cause of ALS is unknown. A number of multifactorial possibilities have been identified (305–307). Neuronal cell injury may be induced by glutamate, an excitotoxic neurotransmitter, due possibly to diminished uptake of glutamate by a specific glutamate transporter (EAAT2). Oxidant stress has also been highlighted with neuronal accumulation of reactive oxygen species important in neuronal injury. In a subset of familial cases of ALS, mutations in the cytosolic enzyme, superoxide dismutase (SOD1), important in defense against superoxide anions, have been reported. Abnormal neurofilament metabolism, autoimmunity, and abnormal responses to various growth factors have also been proposed.

Clinical Features (305–308)

The onset of the disease is often insidious with the development of asymmetric muscle weakness and cramping in a limb. Eventually, progressive muscle involvement ensues with widespread symmetric distribution. Bulbar involvement may present with difficulty chewing, swallowing, or with dysarthria. Pseudo-bulbar disease may be associated with emotional lability. Lower motor neuron signs include muscle weakness, wasting, fasciculations, and areflexia. Upper motor neuron involvement is characterized by spasticity and increased reflexes. Sensory function is normal, as is bowel and bladder function. Patients exhibit normal cognitive ability.

Respiratory Involvement (309)

Patients with ALS invariably progress to develop worsening respiratory muscle weakness and eventual ventilatory failure (310). Alveolar hypoventilation is further diminished during sleep. In patients with inspiratory muscle weakness, acute respiratory failure may also occur following the development of hypostatic or aspiration pneumonia, particularly in patients with weak cough and/or bulbar involvement. Occasionally patients with ALS can present in respiratory failure as their presenting feature (311,312).

Diagnosis

A modification of the World Federation of Neurology criteria for the diagnosis of ALS include the following (313): (1) lower motor neuron involvement in at least two limbs, (2) EMG findings and fibrillation potentials required for evidence of lower motor neuron involvement, (3) upper motor neuron involvement in at least one region (bulbar, cervical, lumbosacral), and (4) exclusion of other conditions that mimic ALS. Important conditions that may mimic ALS include: cervical cord compression, tumors at the cervicomedullary junction, multifocal motor neuropathy (axonal neuropathy), Lyme disease (axonal neuropathy), and chronic lead poisoning. Using the above criteria, the diagnosis of ALS was made an average of 9.7 months from the start of symptoms (313).

Treatment

Specific. Riluzole, a glutamate antagonist, is the only FDA-approved agent for ALS, prolonging survival by three to six months (314,315). Starting riluzole early may delay progression (316). Insulin-like growth factor-1 was shown to slow the progression of functional impairment in one placebo-controlled randomized multicenter trial (317) while no impact was observed in another study (318). The use of other neurotropic factors, antioxidants, or immunomodulators has demonstrated no efficacy (305,319).

Supportive Care. Treatment of respiratory impairment includes use of mechanical assisted coughing devices, noninvasive ventilation and tracheostomy, and mechanical ventilation, all of which have shown improvements in quality of life, reduced respiratory complications, and prolonged survival (320–322). Other issues of importance include nutritional support (nutritional depletion in 16–50%) (321,323), physical and speech therapy rehabilitative aids, management of depression and appropriate and compassionate counseling regarding end-of-life issues, and advanced directives (324).

G. Post-Polio Syndrome

While first described in 1875 (325), the syndrome has only recently been well characterized and understood (326,327). The post-polio syndrome refers to new slowly-progressive neurological symptoms and signs in polio survivors which manifest on average 28.8 years after the acute episode, with a range of 15–54 years (328–330). As it is estimated that there are 1.6 million polio survivors in the U.S.A. alone, the condition is important, and respiratory complications are likely to be encountered that require ICU care (330,331).

Pathogenesis

With acute poliomyelitis, adaptation to spinal cord motor neuron damage and denervation is the process of oversprouting of distal axons producing reinnervation of affected motor unit fibers. Post-polio syndrome occurs when the motor neurons can no longer support these reinnervating nerve sprouts, resulting in increasing denervation of motor unit fibers (328). Whether this relates to "overwork," immune dysregulation, or latent virus reactivation is unclear.

Clinical Manifestations

Protean manifestations are described (327,329–334). These include weakness and atrophy, particularly in muscles previously involved. Bulbar involvement may present with dysphonia, dysphagia, and aspiration (335). Respiratory muscle weakness can be progressive and culminate in chronic ventilatory failure and impaired secretion clearance with atelectasis and/or pneumonia (331). The latter coupled with thoracic/spinal restrictive abnormalities (see preceeding text) can result in acute respiratory decompensation and difficulty in weaning from mechanical ventilation. Further, a weak respiratory pump together with bulbar disease contributes to sleep disordered breathing and sleep apnea in these patients (336). Autonomic dysfunction together with decreased muscle bulk for heat generation produces, cold intolerance. Musculoskeletal complications (330,337) include scoliosis and spondylosis, myalgia (39–86%), and arthralgia

(51–79%). Prominent symptoms of general fatigue and lassitude are common. Patients may become deconditioned.

Diagnosis

The diagnostic criteria include (338): (1) prior episode of paralytic poliomyelitis confirmed on history, clinical findings, and compatible EMG abnormalities; (2) history of partial neurologic recovery with a substantial period (years) of clinical functional stability; (3) new complaints (gradual or overt in onset) such as muscle weakness ± atrophy which is progressive in nature, symptoms of bulbar dysfunction, myalgia, arthralgia, fatigue, and reduced endurance capacity; and (4) exclusion of other conditions. EMG shows evidence of chronic and new progressive denervation and can exclude neuropathy. Other tests, including muscle biopsy are not diagnostic.

Treatment

There are no pharmacologic or other measures that can arrest the process of progressive denervation. Treatment measures are thus supportive in nature (329) and include noninvasive positive pressure ventilatory support together with manual and/or mechanical-assisted cough and secretion clearance. This may avoid conventional mechanical ventilation and/or tracheostomy, other than when required in the management of acute complications (331). With bulbar involvement, swallowing and voice therapy or aids may be of value. Management of sleep-disordered breathing should not be overlooked. Nonfatiguing strength and endurance conditioning, pacing of activity, energy conservation, orthopedic assists, and weight loss (in the case of obesity) are of value (339,340).

H. Myopathic Disorders

Respiratory muscle involvement can complicate the course of several congenital and acquired primary muscle disorders, culminating in ventilatory failure (341). Acute or acute-on-chronic ventilatory compromise may necessitate intensive care intervention. An abbreviated classification of those myopathic disorders that may affect the respiratory muscles is presented in the Table 9.

Specific Conditions: Brief Overview

Duchenne and Becker Muscular Dystrophy

These are *x*-linked disorders associated with mutations in the dystrophin gene which codes for dystrophin, a protein component of the dystrophin–glycoprotein cytoskeletal complex, which is responsible for structural integrity of muscle fibers (342,343). Duchenne muscular dystrophy (MD) occurs in one in 3500 live male births, while Becker MD (which has a less severe clinical course) occurs in one in 30,000 live male births (344,345). In Duchenne MD, progressive proximal muscle weakness results in children being wheelchair-bound by age 12 (346). Progressive reduction in mouth pressures and vital

Table 9 Myopathic Disorders Affecting Respiratory Muscles

(A) Inherited

Muscular dystrophy (MD)
  Duchenne and Becker type MD
  Myotonic dystrophy
  Fascioscapulohumeral MD
  Limble girdle MD

Congenital myopathy
  Nemaline myopathy
  Multicore myopathy

Metabolic myopathy
  Glycolytic/glycogenolytic disorders (e.g., acid maltase deficiency)
  Disorders of lipid metabolism (defects in B oxidation enzymes, carnitine deficiency
    disorders, fatty acid transport defects)
  Mitochrondial myopathies

Periodic paralysis

(B) Acquired

Inflammatory myopathy
  Polymyositis/dermatomyositis
  Inclusion body myositis
  Infections (including HIV)

Collagen vascular disorders
  Systemic lupus erythematosus
  Other

Drugs
  Corticosteroids
  Statins
  Zidovudine
  Chloroquine
  D-penicillamine

Toxins
  Cocaine, amphetamine, alcohol

Endocrine
  Hypo- and hyperthyroidism
  Cushing's disease

Source: From Table 1 in Lynn DJ, et al. Respiratory dysfunction in muscular dystrophy and other myopathies. Clinics in Chest Medicine 1994; 15:661–674.

capacity occurs due to respiratory muscle involvement culminating in respiratory failure and death by age 20–23 (347,348). Progressive scoliosis and cardiomyopathy (associated with conduction abnormalities) also contribute to cardiopulmonary morbidity and/or mortality. Treatment measures are chiefly supportive (physical therapy and physical aids, measures to prevent or reduce progressive scoliosis, noninvasive and conventional mechanical ventilation and psychological support). Corticosteroid therapy has been shown to improve muscle strength by unexplained mechanisms (349,350), while inspiratory muscle training may offer some short-term benefits (351). Patients with Becker MD are commonly ambulatory until age 15 or later and survive into the fourth or fifth decades of life (345).

Myotonic Dystrophy (Type 1)

Myotonic dystrophy is an autosomal dominant condition in which myotonia (i.e., delayed muscle relaxation) and progressive muscle weakness and wasting is evident (352). Respiratory muscle weakness can occur early, with distinct discordance with the degree of limb muscle weakness. Early expiratory muscle weakness results in impaired cough and propensity to infection (353). Progressive weakness of the diaphragm and intercostal muscles ensues, with hypercapnia resulting when overt proximal limb muscle weakness is clinically evident (353,354). Abnormal ventilatory control and sleep disordered breathing have been described (355). While respiratory failure is the dominant cause of mortality, cardiac involvement, producing conduction defects, may contribute to morbidity and/or mortality (356).

Fascioscapulonumeral and Limb Girdle Dystrophies

Both of these autosomal dominant conditions can result in respiratory muscle weakness and failure (357). The onset of muscle weakness is in the second or third decades.

Congential Myopathies

Nemaline rod is the congenital myopathy most commonly associated with respiratory muscle weakness and failure (358). It is characterized by rod-like structure accumulation in muscle fibers. Childhood and adult-onset variants are described. Case studies of respiratory failure as a presenting feature in multicore myopathy have been reported (359).

Metabolic Myopathy: Acid Maltase Deficiency

A discussion of the metabolic myopathies is beyond the scope of this chapter. The reader is referred to comprehensive recent review articles on the subject (360–362). Acid maltase (alpha-1, 4-glucosidase) deficiency is a glycogen storage disease with both childhood and adult forms (363). The latter usually presents in the third or fourth decade as a progressive myopathy. Of interest, respiratory muscle involvement is common, and respiratory failure may be a presenting feature of the disease (364,365). Further, sleep disordered breathing is common (~50% in one series), which correlated with respiratory muscle weakness (366). Creatinine kinase is elevated in patients with acid maltase deficiency (367). Muscle biopsy shows typical vacuolar myopathy with glycogen-filled lysosomes. Deficient acid alpha-glucosidase activity may be demonstrated in muscle tissue or leukocytes (367). Muscle magnetic resonance imaging may show fatty infiltration of select muscle groups (368). Recently, enzyme replacement therapy (lysosomal alpha-glucosidase) offers new therapeutic potential (363,369) apart from supportive measures (370).

Periodic Paralysis

Of the familial periodic paralyses (autosomal dominant), hypokalemic paralysis is the most severe, characterized by attacks of severe systemic flaccid muscle weakness, including the respiratory muscles (371,372). The disorder is due to gene mutations producing abnormal sodium ion channel proteins, culminating in reduced excitability of the muscle membrane (373). While most cases of hypokalemic paralysis are familial, sporadic cases are associated with hyperthyroidism, renal disorders, potassium losing states (gastrointestinal), and mineralocorticoid excess states (371,374,375). Acute management includes potassium replacement, possible use of mannitol, and supportive care including mechanical ventilation. Preventive measures include use of oral potassium supplements, acetazolimide, and dietary modifications (low carbohydrate, low sodium) (376). Hyperkalemic paralysis is due to different mutations to the muscle membrane sodium channels (373).

Inflammatory Myopathies

While there are many similarities between polymyositis (PM) and dermatomyositis (DM), there are distinct differences in dermatologic manifestations (e.g., heliotrope rash with DM), incidence of malignancy (increased with DM), and immune pathogenesis between the two (377,378). The peak age incidence is in the fifth decade, with a female predominance (F:M = 2:1). The most common presenting feature is muscle pain and weakness of a gradually progressive nature, which is proximal and symmetric in location. An abrupt onset occasionally occurs. Respiratory muscle involvement may result in pump failure (379,380). Respiratory failure may also ensue due to aspiration (oropharyngeal dysphagia/dysfunction) or the presence of interstitial lung disease superimposed on limited functional force reserve of the respiratory muscles. Muscle enzymes, including creatinine kinase and aldolase, are elevated with correlations noted between the severity of weakness and enzyme levels (381). Myositis-specific antibodies are present in the minority. Anti-Jo-1 antibodies (20%) correlate with interstitial lung disease and anti-Mi-2 (7–30% correlates with high likelihood of complete remission with therapy) (382). Initial therapy is with prednisone (0.5–1.5 mg/day) (383). Response is monitored clinically together with the aim of normalizing muscle enzyme levels. A tapering schedule of prednisone, with or without the addition of steroid-sparing agents (e.g., azothiaprine or methotrexate), is employed (384–386). In steroid-resistant cases, intravenous immune globulin and other immunosuppresive agents have been used with some success (387,388).

The differential diagnosis includes inclusion body myositis in which muscle weakness is mainly distal (389). Respiratory failure has rarely been described (390). Generally the condition is resistant to treatment. Myositis can be observed in other collagen vascular disorders, including the overlap syndrome.

Respiratory Steroid Myopathy

Corticosteroids impair muscle protein synthesis (391) and enhance muscle protein degradation, in large part via the ubiquitin-proteasome pathways (392,393). In animal studies, atrophy of particularly type IIx diaphragm fibers was observed following corticosteroid administration, which was significantly greater than that observed in pair-weighted (diet-manipulated) controls (394). Reduced muscle mass, together with reduced force generation per unit area of muscle (specific force) markedly reduces diaphragm force generating capacity (395,396). In patients with steroid myopathy, muscle biopsies revealed necrotic and atrophic fibers (397).

Histopathology may, however, depend on the acuteness of the presentation, with necrosis of fibers noted with abrupt onset. In patients with COPD, corticosteroid myopathy of respiratory muscles has been well documented (397–400). In patients with autoimmune disorders, an average of 61 mg per day of prednisone over eight weeks reduced inspiratory muscle strength and endurance, an effect that was not completely reversible with cessation of steroid usage (401). Low dose prednisone (≤ 20 mg/day), short- (two weeks) or long-term (7.9 years), did not affect respiratory muscle strength (402,403). By contrast, Decramer and coworkers (404) reported positive correlations between average steroid dose in the prior six months (which was low) and inspiratory and quadriceps muscle strength. In general, doses of prednisone ≥ 40 mg per day for $\geq 4-6$ weeks have the potential to produce muscle wasting. However, wide variances in individual patient response and/or other contributing factors (e.g., sepsis, neuromuscular blockade, etc.) make dose–duration-response predictions difficult. Further, fluorinated steroid agents (e.g., triamcinolone) also produce greater muscle atrophy and dysfunction compared with nonfluorinated preparations. With steroid myopathy, muscle enzyme levels are generally normal (see earlier text for details on critical illness myopathy).

References

1. De Troyer Estenne M. Functional anatomy of the respiratory muscles. Clin Chest Med 1988; 9:175–193.
2. De Troyer A, Loring SH. Actions of the respiratory muscles. In: Roussos C, ed., The Thorax, 2nd ed. New York: Marcel Dekker, 1995:535–563.
3. Sieck GC. Organization and recruitment of diaphragm motor units. In: Roussos C, ed, The Thorax, 2nd ed. New York: Marcel Dekker, 1995:783–820.
4. Fournier M, Sieck GC. Mechanical properties of muscle units in the cat diaphragm. J Neurophysiol 1988; 59:1055–1066.

5. Levine S, Gregory C, Nguyen T, Shrager J, Kaiser L, Rubinstein N, Dudley G. Bioenergetic adaptation of individual human diaphragmatic myofibers to severe COPD. J Appl Physiol 2002; 92:1205–1213.

6. Geiger PC, Cody MJ, Macken RL, Sieck GC. Maximum specific force depends on myosin heavy chain content in rat diaphragm muscle fibers. J Appl Physiol 2000; 89:695–703.

7. NHLBI Workshop. Respiratory muscle fatigue: report of the respiratory muscle fatigue workshop group. Am Rev Respir Dis 1990; 142:474–480.

8. Grassino A, Clanton T. Respiratory muscle fatigue. Semin Resp Med 1991; 12:305–321.

9. Aldrich TK. Central and transmission fatigue. Semin Resp Med 1991; 12:322–330.

10. Moxham J. Respiratory muscle fatigue: mechanisms, evaluation and therapy. Br J Anesthesiol 1990; 65:43–53.

11. Roussos C, Bellmare F, Moxham J. Respiratory muscle fatigue. In: Roussos C, ed., The Thorax, 2nd ed. New York: Marcel Dekker, 1995:1405–1461.

12. Fitts RH. Cellular mechanisms of muscle fatigue. Physiol Rev 1994; 74:49–94.

13. Reid WD, Clarke TJ, Wallace AM. Respiratory muscle injury: evidence to date and potential mechanisms. Can J Appl Physiol 2001; 26:356–387.

14. Laghi F, D'Alfonso N, Tobin J. Pattern of recovery from diaphragmatic fatigue over four hours. J Appl Physiol 1995; 79:539–546.

15. Guleria R, Lyall R, Hart N, Harris ML, Hamnegard CH, Green M, Moxham J, Polkey MI. Central fatigue of the diaphragm and quadriceps during incremental loading. Lung 2002; 180:1–13.

16. Tobin MJ, Perez W, Guenther SM, Semmes BJ, Mador MJ, Allen SJ, Lodado RF, Dantzker DR. The pattern of breathing during successful and unsuccessful trials of weaning from mechanical ventilation. Am Rev Respir Dis 1986; 134:1111–1118.

17. Cohen C, Zagelbaum G, Gross D, Roussos C, Macklem PT. Clinical manifestations of inspiratory muscle fatigue. Am J Med 1982; 73:308–316.

18. Tobin JM, Perez W, Guenther SM, Lodado RF, Dantzker D. Does ribcage abdominal paradox signify respiratory muscle fatigue? J Appl Physiol 1987; 63:851–860.

19. Brochard L, Haarf A, Lorino H, Lemaire F. Inspiratory pressure support prevents diaphragmatic fatigue during weaning from mechanical ventilation. Am Rev Respir Dis 1989; 139:513–521.

20. ATS/ER Statement on respiratory muscle testing. Am J Respir Crit Care Med 2002; 166:518–624.

21. Gibson GJ, Pride NB, Newsom Davis J, Loh C. Pulmonary mechanics in patients with respiratory muscle weakness. Am Rev Respir Dis 1977; 115:389–395.

22. Estenne M, Heilporn A, Delhez L, Yernault J-C, De Troyer A. Chest wall stiffness in patients with chronic respiratory muscle weakness. Am Rev Respir Dis 1983; 128:1002–1007.

23. Black LF, Hyatt RE. Maximal static respiratory pressures in generalized neuromuscular disease. Am Rev Respir Dis 1971; 103:641–650.

24. Multz A, Aldrich TK, Prezant DJ, Karpel JP, Hendler JM. Maximal inspiratory pressure is not a reliable test of inspiratory muscle strength in mechanically ventilated patients. Am Rev Respir Dis 1990; 142:529–532.

25. Aldrich TK, Spiro P. Maximal inspiratory pressure: does reproducibility indicate full effort? Thorax 1995; 50:40–43.

26. Laroche CM, Mier AK, Moxham J, Green M. Measurement of sniff esophageal pressures to assess global inspiratory muscle strength. Am Rev Respir Dis 1988; 138:598–603.
27. Heritier F, Rahm F, Pasche P, Fitting JW. Sniff nasal pressure: a non-invasive assessment of inspiratory muscle strength. Am J Respir Crit Care Med 1994; 150:1678–1683.
28. Uldry C, Janssens JP, de Meralt B, Fitting JW. Sniff nasal inspiratory pressure in patients with chronic obstructive pulmonary disease. Eur Respir J 1997; 10:1292–1296.
29. De Troyer A, Estenne M. Limitations of measurement of transdiaphragmatic pressure in detecting diaphragm weakness. Thorax 1981; 36:169–174.
30. Laporta D, Grassino A. Assessment of transdiaphragmatic pressure in humans. J Appl Physiol 1985; 58:1469–1476.
31. Miller JM, Moxham J, Green M. The maximal sniff in the assessment of diaphragm function in man. Clin Sci 1985; 69:91–96.
32. Bellemare F, Bigland-Ritchie B. Assessment of human diaphragm strength and activation using phrenic nerve stimulation. Respir Physiol 1984; 58:263–277.
33. Simolowski T, Fleury B, Launois S, Cathala HP, Bouche P, Derenne J. Cervical magnetic stimulation: a painless method for bilateral phrenic nerve stimulation in conscious humans. J Appl Physiol 1989; 67:1311–1318.
34. Mills GH, Kyroussis D, Hamnegard C-H, Wraggs, Moxham J, Green M. Unilateral magnetic stimulation of the phrenic nerve. Thorax 1995; 50:1162–1172.
35. Mills GH, Kyroussis D, Hamnegard C-H, Polkey MI, Green M, Moxham J. Bilateral magnetic stimulation of the phrenic nerves from an anterolateral approach. Am J Respir Crit Care Med 1996; 154:1099–1105.
36. Polkey MI, Moxham J. Clinical aspects of respiratory muscle dysfunction in the critically ill. Chest 2001; 119:926–939.
37. Polkey MI, Hamnegard C-H, Hughes PD, et al. Influence of acute lung volume change on contractile properties of the human diaphragm. J Appl Physiol 1998; 85:1322–1328.
38. Watson AC, Hughes PD, Louise Harris M, Hart N, Ware RJ, Wendon J, Green M, Moxham J. Measurement of twitch transdiaphragmatic, esophageal, and endotracheal tube pressure with bilateral anterolateral magnetic phrenic nerve stimulation in patients in the intensive care unit. Crit Care Med 2001; 29:1325–1331.
39. Mills GH, Ponte J, Hamnegard CH, Kyroussis D, Polkey MI, Moxham J, Green M. Tracheal tube pressure change during magnetic stimulation of the phrenic nerves as an indicator of diaphragm strength on the intensive care unit. British Journal of Anesthesia 2001; 87:876–884.
40. Cattapan SE, Laghi F, Tobin MJ. Can diaphragmatic contractility be assessed by airway twitch pressure in mechanically ventilated patients? Thorax 2003; 58:58–62.
41. Electrophysiologic techniques for the assessment of respiratory muscle function. In: ATS/ERS Statement on Respiratory Muscle Testing. Am J Respir Crit Care Med 2002; 166:548–558.
42. Luo YM, Lyall RA, Harris ML, Rafferty GF, Polkey MI, Moxham J. Quantification of the esophageal diaphragm EMG with magnetic phrenic nerve stimulation. Am J Respir Crit Care Med 1999; 160:1629–1634.

43. Luo YM, Johnson LC, Polkey MI, Harris ML, Lyall RA, Green M, Moxham J. Diaphragm electromyogram measured with unilateral magnetic stimulation. Eur Respir J 1999; 13:385–390.

44. Kyroussis D, Polkey MI, Hughes PD, Fleming TA, Wood CN, Mills GH, Hamnegard C-H, Green M, Moxham J. Abdominal muscle strength measured by gastric pressure during maximal cough. Thorax 1996; 51(suppl 3):A45.

45. Braun NMT, Arora NS, Rochester DF. Respiratory muscle and pulmonary function in polymyositis and other proximal myopathies. Thorax 1983; 38:616–623.

46. Roussos C, Macklem PT. Diaphragmatic fatigue in man. J Appl Physiol 1977; 43:189–197.

47. Bellemare F, Grassino A. Effect of pressure and timing of contraction on human diaphragm fatigue. J Appl Physiol 1982; 53:1190–1195.

48. Bellemare F, Wright D, Levine CM, Grassino A. Effect of tension and timing of contraction on the blood flow of the diaphragm. J Appl Physiol 1983; 54:1597–1606.

49. Field S, Sanci S, Grassino A. Respiratory oxygen consumption estimated by the diaphragm pressure-time index. J Appl Physiol 1984; 57:44–51.

50. Feasby TE, Gilbert JJ, Brown WF, Bolton CF, Hahn AF, Koopman WJ, Zochod. An acute axonal form of Guillain-Barre' polyneuropathy. Brain 1986; 109:1115–1126.

51. Griffin JW, Li CY, Ho TW, Hsieh S, Xue P, Mishu B, Comblath D, McKhann G, Asbury AK. Pathology of the motor-sensory axonal Guillain-Barre' syndrome. Ann Neurol 1996; 39:17–28.

52. Hafer-Macko C, Hsieh S-T, Li CY, Ho TW, Sheikh K, Comblath D, McKhann G, Asbury AK, Griffin JW. Acute motor axonal neuropathy: an antibody-mediated attack on axolemma. Ann Neurol 1996; 40:635–644.

53. Fisher M. An unusual variant of acute idiopathic polyneuritis (syndrome of ophthalmoplegia, ataxia and areflexia). N Engl J Med 1956; 255:57–65.

54. Hughes RAC. Ineffectiveness of high-dose intravenous methylprednisolone in Guillain-Barre' syndrome. Lancet 1991; 338:1142.

55. Teitelbaum JS, Borel CO. Respiratory dysfunction in Guillain-Barre' syndrome. Clinics in Chest Medicine 1994; 15:705.

56. Hahn AF, Guillain-Barre' syndrome. Lancet 1998; 352:635–641.

57. Rees JH, Thompson RD, Smeeton NC, Hughes RA. Epidemiological study of Guillain-Barre syndrome in south east England. J Neurol Neurosurg Psychiatry 1998; 64:74–77.

58. Henderson RD, Lawn ND, Fletcher DD, McClelland RL, Wijdicks EF. The morbidity of Guillain-Barre syndrome admitted to the intensive care unit. Neurology 2003; 60:17–21.

59. Beghi E, Kurland LT, Mulder DW, Wiederholt WC. Guillain-Barre syndrome. Clinicoepidemiologic features and effect of influenza vaccine. Arch Neurol 1985; 42:1053–1057.

60. Kennedy RH, Danielson MA, Mulder DW, Kurland LT. Guillain-Barre syndrome: a 42-year epidemiologic and clinical study. Mayo Clin Proc 1978; 53:93–99.

61. Lasky T, Terracciano GJ, Magder L, Koski CL, Ballesteros M, Nash D, Clark S, Haber P, Stolley PD, Schonberger LB, Chen RT. The Guillain-Barre syndrome and the 1992–1993 and 1993–1994 influenza vaccines. N Engl J Med 1998; 339:1797–1802.

62. Kurland LT, Wiederholt WC, Kirkpatrick JW, Potter HG, Armstrong P. Swine influenza vaccine and Guillain-Barre' syndrome: epidemic or artifact? Arch Neurol 1985; 42:1089–1090.

63. Asbury AK, Arnason BG, Adams RD. The inflammatory lesion in idiopathic polyneuritis: its role in pathogenesis. Medicine (Baltimore) 1969; 48:173–215.

64. Hartung HP, Heininger K, Schafer B, Fierz W, Toyka KV. Immune mechanisms in inflammatory polyneuropathy. Ann N Y Acad Sci 1988; 540:122–161.

65. Harrison BM, Hansen LA, Pollard JD, McLeod JG. Demyelination induced by serum from patients with Guillain-Barre syndrome. Ann Neurol 1984; 15:163–170.

66. Cook SD, Dowling PC. The role of autoantibody and immune complexes in the pathogenesis of Guillain-Barre syndrome. Ann Neurol 1981; 9(suppl):70–79.

67. Schleicher GK, Black A, Mochan A, Richards GA. Effect of human immuno-deficiency virus on intensive care unit outcome of patients with Guillain-Barre syndrome. Crit Care Med 2003; 31:1848–1850.

68. Ropper AH. The Guillain-Barre' syndrome. N Engl J Med 1992; 326:1130–1136.

69. Mori M, Kuwabara S, Miyake M, et al. Haemophilus influenzae infection and Guillain-Barre' syndrome. Brain 2000; 123:2171.

70. Jacobs BC, Rothbarth PH, van der Meche FG, Herbrink P, Schmitz P, deklerk MA, vanDoor PA. The spectrum of antecedent infections in Guillain-Barre' syndrome: a case-control study. Neurology 1998; 51:1110.

71. Rees JH, Soudain SE, Gregson NA, Hughes RAC. Campylobacter jejuni infection and Guillain-Barre' syndrome. N Engl J Med 1995; 333:1374–1379.

72. McCarthy N, Giesecke J. Incidence of Guillain-Barre syndrome following infection with Campylobacter jejuni. Am J Epidemiol 2001; 153:610–614.

73. Yuki N, Handa S, Tai T, Takahashi M, Saito K, Tsujino Y, Miyatake T. Ganglioside-like epitopes of lipopolysaccharides from Campylobacter jejuni (PEN 19) in three isolates from patients with Guillain-Barre' syndrome. J Neurol Sci 1995; 130:112–116.

74. Allos BM. Campylobacter jejuni infection as a cause of the Guillain-Barre' syndrome. Infectious Disease Clinics of North America 1998; 12:173–184.

75. Goddard EA, Lastovica AJ, Argent AC. Campylobacter O:41 isolation in Guillain-Barre' syndrome. Arch Dis Child 1997; 76:526.

76. McKhann GM. Guillain-Barre syndrome: clinical and therapeutic observations. Ann Neurol 1990; 27(suppl):S13–S16.

77. Asbury AK, Cornblath DR. Assessment of current diagnostic criteria for Guillain-Barre syndrome. Ann Neurol 1990; 27(suppl):S21–S24.

78. Zochodne DW. Autonomic involvement in Guillain-Barre syndrome: a review. Muscle Nerve 1994; 17:1145–1155.

79. Ho TW, Li CY, Cornblath DR, Gao CY, Asbury AK, Griffin JW, McKhann GM. Patterns of recovery in the Guillain-Barre syndromes. Neurology 1997; 48:695–700.

80. Ropper AH, Wijdicks EFM, Shahani BT. Electrodiagnostic abnormalities in 113 consecutive patients with Guillain-Barre' syndrome. Arch Neurol 1990; 47:881–887.

81. Gordon PH, Wilbourn AJ. Early electrodiagnostic findings in Guillain-Barre syndrome. Arch Neurol 2001; 58:913–917.

82. Gracey DR, McMichan JC, Divertie MB, Howard FM Jr. Respiratory failure in Guillain-Barre syndrome: a 6-year experience. Mayo Clin Proc 1982; 57:742–746.

83. Chevrolet J-C, Deleamont P. Repeated vital capacity measurements as predictive parameters for mechanical ventilation need and weaning success in Guillain-Barre' syndrome. Am Rev Respir Dis 1991; 144:814–818.

84. Sharshar T, Chevret S, Bourdain F, Raphael JC. French Cooperative Group on Plasma Exchange in Guillain-Barre' syndrome. Crit Care Med 2003; 31:278–283.

85. Braun NMT, Arora NS, Rochester DF. Respiratory muscle and pulmonary function in polymyositis and other proximal myopathies. Thorax 1983; 38:616–623.

86. Wijdicks EF, Henderson RD, McClelland RL. Emergency intubation for respiratory failure in Guillain-Barré syndrome. Arch Neurol 2003; 60:947–948.

87. Wijdicks EF, Borel CO. Respiratory management in acute neurologic illness. Neurology 1998; 50:11–20.

88. Unterborn JN, Hill NS. Options for mechanical ventilation in neuromuscular diseases. Clin Chest Med 1994; 15:765–781.

89. Heffner JE. Timing of tracheotomy in mechanically ventilated patients. Am Rev Respir Dis 1993; 147:768–771.

90. Borel CO, Tilford C, Nichols DG, Hanley DF, Traystman RJ. Diaphragmatic performance during recovery from acute ventilatory failure in Guillain-Barré syndrome and myasthenia gravis. Chest 1991; 99:444–451.

91. Flachenecker P, Wermuth P, Hartung H-P, Reiners K. Quantitative assessment of cardiovascular autonomic function in Guillain-Barré syndrome. Ann Neurol 1997; 42:171–179.

92. Zochodne DW. Autonomic involvement in Guillain-Barré syndrome: a review. Muscle Nerve 1994; 17:1145–1155.

93. Hund EF, Borel CO, Cornblath DR, et al. Intensive management and treatment of severe Guillain-Barré syndrome. Crit Care Med 1993; 21:433–446.

94. Raphael JC, Chevret S, Hughes RA, Annane D. Plasma exchange for Guillain-Barré syndrome. Cochrane Database Syst Rev 2002; 2:CD001798.

95. Ropper AE, Albert JW, Addison R. Limited relapse in Guillain-Barré syndrome after plasma exchange. Arch Neurol 1988; 45:314–315.

96. Dyck PJ, Daube J, O'Brien P, Pineda A, Low PA, Windebank AJ, Swanson C. Plasma exchange in chronic inflammatory demyelinating polyradiculoneuropathy. N Engl J Med 1986; 314:461–465.

97. The Guillain-Barre Syndrome Study Group. Plasmapheresis and acute GBS. Neurology 1985; 35:1096–1104.

98. The French Cooperative Group on Plasma Exchange in Guillain-Barré Syndrome. Appropriate number of plasma exchanges in Guillain-Barre syndrome. Ann Neurol 1997; 41:298–306.

99. French Cooperative Group on Plasma Exchange in Guillain-Barré syndrome. Efficiency of plasma exchange in Guillain-Barre syndrome: role of replacement fluids. Ann Neurol 1987; 22:753–761.

100. van der Meche FG, Schmitz PI. A randomized trial comparing intravenous immune globulin and plasma exchange in Guillain-Barre syndrome. Dutch Guillain-Barré Study Group. N Engl J Med 1992; 326:1123–1129.

101. Plasma Exchange/Sandoglobulin Guillain-Barre Syndrome Trial Group. Randomised trial of plasma exchange, intravenous immunoglobulin, and combined treatments in Guillain-Barré syndrome. Lancet 1997; 349:225–230.

102. Yuki N, Ang CW, Koga M, Jacobs BC, van Doorn PA, Hirata K, van der Meche FG. Clinical features and response to treatment in Guillain-Barré syndrome associated with antibodies to GM_{1b} ganglioside. Ann Neurol 2000; 47:314–321.

103. Dalakas MC. Intravenous immune globulin therapy for neurologic diseases. Ann Intern Med 1997; 126:721–730.

104. Romano JG, Rotta FT, Potter P, Rosenfeld V, Santibanez R, Rocha B, Bradley WG. Relapses in the Guillain-Barré syndrome after treatment with intravenous immune globulin or plasma exchange. Muscle Nerve 1998; 21:1327–1330.

105. Nagappan R, Barker J. Second response to immunoglobulin in recurrent Guillain-Barré syndrome. N Z Med J 1998; 111:433–434.

106. Hughes RA, van Der Meche FG. Corticosteroids for treating Guillain-Barré syndrome. Cochrane Database Syst Rev 2000; 3:CD001446.

107. The Italian Guillain-Barré Study Group. The prognosis and main prognostic indicators of Guillain-Barre' syndrome: a multicentre prospective study of 297 patients. Brain 1996; 119:2053–2061.

108. Chio A, Cocito D, Leone M, Giordana MT, Mora G, Mutani R, Piemonte and Valle d'Aosta Register for Guillain-Barré Syndrome. Guillain-Barre syndrome: a prospective, population-based incidence and outcome survey. Neurology 2003; 60:1146–1150.

109. Fletcher DD, Lawn ND, Wolter TD, Wijdicks EF. Long-term outcome in patients with Guillain-Barré syndrome requiring mechanical ventilation. Neurology 2000; 54:2311–2315.

110. Drachman DB. Myasthenia gravis. N Engl J Med 1994; 330:1797–1810.

111. Zulueta JJ, Fanburg BL. Respiratory dysfunction in myasthenia gravis. Clinics in Chest Medicine 1994; 15:683–690.

112. Mier A, Laroche C, Green M. Unsuspected myasthenia gravis presenting as respiratory failure. Thorax 1990; 45:422–423.

113. Dushay KM, Zibrak JD, Jensen WA. Myasthenia gravis presenting as isolated respiratory failure. Chest 1990; 97:232–234.

114. Phillips LH 2nd. The epidemiology of myasthenia gravis. Ann N Y Acad Sci 2003; 998:407–412.

115. Simpson JA. Myasthenia gravis and related syndromes. Disorders of Voluntary Muscle. London: Churchill Livingstone, 1988:628–665.

116. Vincent A, Clover L, Buckley C, Grimley Evans J, Rothwell PM. UK Myasthenia Gravis Survey. J Neurol Neurosurg Psychiatry 2003; 74:1105–1108.

117. Aragones JM, Bolibar I, Bonfill X, Bufill E, Mummany A, Alonso F, Illa I. Myasthenia gravis: a higher than expected incidence in the elderly. Neurology 2003; 25:1024–1026.

118. Drachman DB, Angus CW, Adams RN, Michelson JD, Hoffman GJ. Myasthenic antibodies cross-link acetylcholine receptors to accelerate degradation. N Engl J Med 1978; 298:1116–1122.

119. Engel AG, Arahata K. The membrane attack complex of complement at the endplate in myasthenia gravis. Ann N Y Acad Sci 1987; 505:326–332.

120. Drachman DB, Adams RN, Josifek LF, Self SG. Functional activities of autoanti-
      bodies to acetylcholine receptors and the clinical severity of myasthenia gravis.
      N Engl J Med 1982; 307:769–775.
121. Kao I, Drachman DB. Thymic muscle cells bear acetylcholine receptors: possible
      relation to myasthenia gravis. Science 1977; 195:74–75.
122. Schwimmbeck PL, Dyrberg T, Drachman DB, Oldstone MBA. Molecular mimicry
      and myasthenia gravis: an autoantigenic site of the acetylcholine receptor α-subunit
      that has biologic activity and reacts immunochemically with herpes simplex virus.
      J Clin Invest 1989; 84:1174–1180.
123. Link H, Olsson O, Sun J, Wang W, Andersson G, Ekre H, Brenn, Abramsky O,
      Olsson T. Acetylcholine receptor-reactive T and B cells in myasthenia gravis and
      controls. J Clin Invest 1991; 87:2191–2195.
124. Carlsson B, Wallin J, Pirskanen R, Matell G, Smith CIE. Different HLA DR-DQ
      associations in subgroups of idiopathic myasthenia gravis. Immunogenetics 1990;
      31:285–290.
125. Phillips LH 2nd, Melnick PA. Diagnosis of myasthenia gravis in the 1990's. Semin
      Neurol 1990; 10:62–69.
126. Vincent A, Drachman DB. Myasthenia gravis. Adv Neurol 2002; 88:159–188.
127. Evoli A, Tonali PA, Padua L, Monaco ML, Scuderi F, Batochhi AP, Marino M,
      Bartoccioni E. Clinical correlates with anti-MuSK antibodies in generalized sero-
      negative myasthenia gravis. Brain 2003; 126:2304–2311.
128. Vincent A, McConville J, Farrugia ME, Bowen J, Plested P, Tang T, Evoli A,
      Matthews I, Sims G, Dalton P, Jacobson L, Polizzi A, Blaes F, Lang B,
      Beeson D, Willcox N, Newsom-Davis J, Hoch W. Antibodies in myasthenia
      gravis and related disorders. Ann N Y Acad Sci 2003; 998:324–335.
129. Somnier FE, Skeie GO, Aarli JA, Trojaborg W. EMG evidence of myopathy and
      the occurrence of titin autoantibodies in patients with myasthenia gravis. Eur J
      Neurol 1999; 6:555–563.
130. AAEM Quality Assurance Committee. American Association of Electrodiagnostic
      Medicine. Literature review of the usefulness of repetitive nerve stimulation and
      single fiber EMG in the electrodiagnostic evaluation of patients with suspected
      myasthenia gravis or Lambert-Eaton myasthenic syndrome. Muscle Nerve 2001;
      24:1239–1247.
131. Tanhehco JL. Single-fiber electromyography. Phys Med Rehabil Clin N AM 2003;
      24:207–229.
132. Zifko UA, Nicolle MW, Grisold W, Bolton CF. Repetitive phrenic nerve stimu-
      lation in myasthenia gravis. Neurology 1999; 53:1083–1087.
133. Barton JJ, Fouladvand M. Ocular aspects of myasthenia gravis. Semin Neurol 2000;
      20:7–20.
134. Putman MT, Wise RA. Myasthenia gravis and upper airway obstruction. Chest
      1996; 109:400–404.
135. Teramoto K, Kuwabara M, Matsubara Y. Respiratory failure due to vocal cord
      paresis in myasthenia gravis. Respiration 2002; 69:280–282.
136. Castleman B. The pathology of the thymus gland in myasthenia gravis. Ann N Y
      Acad Sci 1966; 135:496–505.
137. Leblanc J, Wood D. Diagnosis of mediastinal masses. In: Wood DE, Thomas CR
      Jr, eds. Mediastinal Tumors: Update 1995, Medical Radiology-Diagnostic

Imaging and Radiation Oncology. Heidelberg, Germany: Springer-Verlag, 1995:1–10.

138. Fujita J, Yamadori I, Yamaji Y, Yamagishi Y, Takigawa K, Takahara. Myasthenia gravis associated with small-cell carcinoma of the lung. Chest 1994; 105:624.

139. Abrey LE. Association of myasthenia gravis with extrathymic Hodgkin's lymphoma: complete resolution of myasthenic symptoms following antineoplastic therapy. Neurology 1995; 45:1019.

140. Tanwani LK, Lohano V, Ewart R, Broadstone VL, Mokshagundam SP. Myasthenia gravis in conjunction with Graves' disease: a diagnostic challenge. Endocr Pract 2001; 7:275–278.

141. Wittbrodt ET. Drugs and myasthenia gravis. Arch Intern Med 1997; 157:399–408.

142. Albers JW, Hodach RJ, Kimmel DW, Treacy WL. Penicillamine-associated myasthenia gravis. Neurology 1980; 30:1246–1250.

143. Kirmani JF, Yahia AM, Qureshi AI. Myasthenic crisis. Curr Treat Options Neurol 2004; 6:3–15.

144. Thomas CE, Mayer SA, Gungor Y, Swarup R, Webster EA, Chang I, Brannagan TH, Fink ME, Rowland LP. Myasthenic crisis: clinical features, mortality, complications, and risk factors for prolonged intubation. Neurology 1997; 48:1253–1260.

145. Berrouschot J, Baumann I, Kalischewski P, Sterker M, Schneider D. Therapy of myasthenic crisis. Crit Care Med 1997; 25:1228–1235.

146. Watanabe A, Watanabe T, Obama T, Mawatari T, Ohsawa H, Ichimiya Y, Takahashi N, Kusajima K, Abe T. Prognostic factors for myasthenic crisis after transsternal thymectomy in patients with myasthenia gravis. J Thorac Cardiovasc Surg 2004; 127:868–876.

147. Rabinstein A, Wijdicks EF. BiPAP in acute respiratory failure due to myasthenic crisis may prevent intubation. Neurology 2002; 59:1647–1649.

148. Varelas PN, Chua HC, Natterman J, Barmadia L, Zimmerman P, Yahia A, Ulatowski J, Bhardwaj A, Williams MA, Hanley DF. Ventilatory care in myasthenia gravis crisis: assessing the baseline adverse event rate. Crit Care Med 2002; 30:2663–2668.

149. Mier-Jedrzejowicz AK, Brophy C, Green M. Respiratory muscle function in myasthenia gravis. Am Rev Respir Dis 1988; 138:867–873.

150. Baraka A. Anesthesia and critical care of thymectomy for myasthenia gravis. Chest Surg Clin N Am 2001; 11:337–361.

151. Burke ME. Myasthenia gravis and pregnancy. J Perinat Neonatal Nurs 1993; 7:11–21.

152. Djelmis J, Sostarko M, Mayer D, Ivanisevic M. Myasthenia gravis in pregnancy: report on 69 cases. Eur J Obstet Gynecol Reprod Biol 2002; 104:21–25.

153. Osterman PO. Current treatment of myasthenia gravis. Prog Brain Res 1990; 84:151–161.

154. Saltis LM, Martin BR, Traeger SM, Bonfiglio MF. Continuous infusion of pyridostigmine in the management of myasthenic crisis. Crit Care Med 1993; 21:938–940.

155. Berrouschot J, Baumann I, Kalischewski P, Sterker M, Schneider D. Therapy of myasthenic crisis. Crit Care Med 1997; 25:1228–1235.

156. Mann JD, Johns TR, Campa TF. Long-term administration of corticosteroids in myasthenia gravis. Neurology 1976; 26:729.

157. Lindberg LC, Anderson O, Lefvert AK. Treatment of myasthenia gravis with methylprednisolone pulse: a double blind study. Acta Neurol Scand 1998; 97:370.

158. Richman DP, Agius MA. Treatment of autoimmune myasthenia gravis. Neurology 2003 61:1652–1661.

159. Matell G. Immunosuppressive drugs: azathioprine in the treatment of myasthenia gravis. Ann N Y Acad Sci 1987; 505:589–594.

160. Tindall RSA, Phillips JT, Rollins JA, Wells L, Hall K. A clinical therapeutic trial of cyclosporine in myasthenia gravis. Ann N Y Acad Sci 1993; 681:539.

161. Meriggioli MN, Ciafaloni E, Al-Hayk KA, Rowin J, Tucker-Lipscomb B, Massey J, Sanders D. Mycophenolate mofetil for myasthenia gravis: An analysis of efficacy, safety, and tolerability. Neurology 2003; 61:1438.

162. Gronseth GS, Barohn RJ. Practice parameter: thymectomy for autoimmune myasthenia gravis (an evidence-based review). Report of the Quality Standards Subcommittee of the American Academy of Neurology. Neurology 2000; 55:7.

163. Drachman DB. Present and future treatment of myasthenia gravis. N Engl J Med 1987; 316:743–745.

164. Fischer JE, Grinvalski HT, Nussbaum MS, Sayers HJ, Cole RE, Samaha FJ. Aggressive surgical approach for drug-free remission from myasthenia gravis. Ann Surg 1987; 205:496–503.

165. Mineo TC, Pompeo E, Lerut TE, Bernardi G, Coosemars W, Nofronti J. Thoraco-scopic thymectomy in autoimmune myasthesia: results of left-sided approach. Ann Thorac Surg 2000; 69:1537.

166. Bedlack RS, Sanders DB. How to handle myasthenic crisis. Essential steps in patient care. Postgrad Med 2000; 107:211–222.

167. Gajdos P, Chevret S, Clair B, Tranchant C, Chastang C. Clinical trial of plasma exchange and high-dose intravenous immunoglobulin in myasthenia gravis. Myasthenia Gravis Clinical Study Group. Ann Neurol 1997; 41:789.

168. Qureshi AI, Choudhry MA, Akbar MS, Mohammed Y, Chua H, Ulatowski-Krendel D, Leshner RT. Plasma exchange versus intravenous immunoglobulin treatment in myasthenic crisis. Neurology 1999; 52:629.

169. Benny WB, Sutton DM, Oger J, Bril V, McAteer M, Rock G. Clinical evaluation of a staphylococcal protein A immunosorbent system in the treatment of myasthenia gravis patients. Transfusion 1999; 39:682.

170. Arsura E. Experience with intravenous immunoglobulin in myasthenia gravis. Clin Immunol Immunopathol 1989; 53:S170.

171. Gajdos P, Chevret S, Toyka K. Plasma exchange for myasthenia gravis. Cochrane Database Syst Rev 2002; 4:CD002275.

172. Gajdos P, Chevret S, Toyka K. Intravenous immunoglobulin for myasthenia gravis. Cochrane Database Syst Rev 2003; 2:CD002277.

173. Romi F, Gilhus NE, Varhaug JE, Myking A, Aarli JA. Disease severity and outcome in thymoma myasthenia gravis: a long-term observation study. European J of Neurology 2003; 10:701–706.

174. Matell G. Immunosuppressive drugs: azathioprine in the treatment of myasthenia gravis. Ann N Y Acad Sci 1987; 505:589.

175. Smith AG, Wald J. Acute ventilatory failure in Lambert-Eaton myasthenic syndrome and its response to 3,4-diaminopyridine. Neurology 1996; 46:1143–1145.

176. Palace J, Newsom-Davis J, Lecky B, and the Myasthenia Gravis Study Group. A randomized double-blind trial of prednisolone alone or with azathioprine in myasthenia gravis. Neurology 1998; 50:1778.

177. Arnon SS, Schechter R, Inglesby TV, Henderson DA, Bartlett JG, Ascher MS, Eitzen E, Fine AD, Hauer J, Layton M, et al. Botulinum toxin as a biological weapon: Medical and public health management. J Am Med Assoc 2001; 285:1059–1070.

178. Schmidt-Nowara WW, Samet JM, Rosario PA. Early and late pulmonary complications of botulism. Arch Intern Med 1983; 143:451–456.

179. MMWR. Tick paralysis—Washington, 1005. MMWR 1996; 45:325–326.

180. Grattan-Smith PJ, Morris JG, Johnston HM, Yiannikas C, Malik R, Russell R, Ouvrier RA. Clinical and neurophysiological features of tick paralysis. Brain 1997; 120:1975–1987.

181. Bolton C, Gilbert J, Hahn A, Sibbald W. Polyneuropathy in critically ill patients. J Neurol Neurosurg Psych 1984; 47:1223–1231.

182. Tepper M, Rakic S, Haas JA, Woittiez AJ. Incidence and onset of critical illness polyneuropathy in patients with septic shock. Neth J Med 2000; 56:211–214.

183. Tennila A, Salmi T, Pettila V, Roine RO, Varpula T, Takkunen O. Early signs of critical illness polyneuropathy in ICU patients with systemic inflammatory response syndrome or sepsis. Intensive Care Med 2000; 26:1360–1363.

184. De Jonghe B, Sharshar T, Lefaucheur JP, Authier FJ, Durand-Zaleski I, Boussarsar M, Cerf C, Renaud E, Mesrati F, Carlet J, Raphael JC, Outin H, Bastuji-Garin S; Groupe de Reflexion et d'Etude des Neuromyopathies en Reanimation. Paresis acquired in the intensive care unit: a prospective multicenter study. J Am Med Assoc 2002; 288:2859–2867.

185. van Mook W, Hulsewe-Evers R. Critical illness polyneuropathy. Current Opinions Crit Care 2002; 8:302–310.

186. Zifko UA, Zipko HT, Bolton CF. Clinical and electrophysiologic findings in critical illness polyneuropathy. J Neurol Sci 1998; 159:186–193.

187. Hund EF, Fogel W, Krieger D, DeGeorgia M, Hacke W. Critical illness polyneuropathy: clinical findings and outcomes of frequent cause of neuromuscular weaning failure. Crit Care Med 1996; 24:1328–1333.

188. Maher J, Rutledge F, Remtulla H, Parkes A, Bernardi L, Bolton CF. Neuromuscular disorders associated with failure to wean from the ventilator. Intensive Care Med 1995; 21:737–743.

189. Sander HW, Saadeh PB, Chandswang N, Greenbaum D, Chokroverty S. Diaphragmatic denervation in intensive care unit patients. Electromyogr Clin Neurophysiol 1999; 39:3–5.

190. Bolton CF. Sepsis and the systemic inflammatory response syndrome: neuromuscular manifestations. Crit Care Med 1996; 24:1408–1416.

191. De Letter MA, van Doorn PA, Savelkoul HF, Laman JD, Schmitz PI, Op de Coul AA, Visser LH, Kros JM, Teepen JL, van der Meche FG. Critical illness polyneuropathy and myopathy (CIPNM): evidence for local immune activation by cytokine-expression in the muscle tissue. J Neuroimmunol 2000; 106:206–213.

192. van den Berghe G, Wouters P, Weekers F, Verwaest C, Bruyninckx F, Schetz M, Vlasselaers D, Ferdinande P, Lauwers P, Bouillon R. Intensive insulin therapy in critically ill patients. N Engl J Med 2001; 345:1359–1367.

193. Rich MM, Bird SJ, Raps EC, McCluskey LF, Teener JW. Direct muscle stimulation in acute quadriplegic myopathy. Muscle Nerve 1997; 20:665–673.

194. Leijten FS, De Weerd AW, Poortvliet DC, De Ridder VA, Ulrich C, Harink-De Weerd JE. Critical illness polyneuropathy in multiple organ dysfunction syndrome and weaning from the ventilator. Intensive Care Med 1996, 22:856–861.

195. de Seze M, Petit H, Wiart L, Cardinaud JP, Gaujard E, Joseph PA, Mazaux JM, Barat M. Critical illnss polyneuropathy: a 2-year follow-up study in 19 severe cases. Eur Neurol 2000; 43:61–69.

196. Zifko UA. Long-term outcome of critical illness polyneuropathy. MuscleNerve 2000; 52(suppl 9):49–52.

197. Segredo V, Caldwell JE, Matthay MA, Sharma ML, Gruenke LD, Miller RD. Persistent paralysis in critically ill patients after long-term administration of vecuronium. N Engl J Med 1992; 327:524–528.

198. Agoston S, Vandenbrom RH, Wierda JM. Clinical pharmacokinetics of neuro-muscular blocking drugs. Clin Pharmacokinet 1992; 22:94–115.

199. Barnette RE, Fish DJ. Monitoring neuromuscular blockade in the critically ill. Crit Care Med 1995; 23:1790–1791.

200. Hund E. Myopathy in critically ill patients. Crit Care Med 1999; 27:2544–2547.

201. Gutmann L, Gutmann L. Critical illness neuropathy and myopathy. Arch Neurol 1999; 56:527–528.

202. Hansen-Flaschen J, Cowen J, Raps EC. Neuromuscular blockade in the intensive care unit: more than we bargained for. Am Rev Respir Dis 1993; 147:234–236.

203. Sladen RN. Neuromuscular blocking agents in the intesive care unit: a two-edged sword. Crit Care Med 1995; 23:423–428.

204. Hirano M, Ott BR, Raps EC, Minetti C, Lennihan L, Libbey NP, Bonilla E, Hays AP. Acute quadriplegic myopathy: a complication of treatment with steroids, nondepolarizing drugs, or both. Neurology 1992; 42:2082–2087.

205. Larsson L, Li X, Edstrom L, Eriksson LI, Zackrisson H, Argentini C, Schiaffino S. Acute quadriplegia and loss of muscle myosin in patients treated with non-depolarizing neuromuscular blocking agents and corticosteroids: mechanisms at the cellular and molecular levels. Crit Care Med 2000; 28:34–45.

206. Hanson P, Dive A, Brucher JM, Bisteau M, Dangoisse M, Deltombe T. Acute corticosteroid myopathy in intensive care patients. Muscle Nerve 1997; 20:1371–1380.

207. Behbehani NA, Al-Mane F, D'yachkova Y, Pare P, FitzGerald JM. Myopathy fol-lowing mechanical ventilation for acute severe asthma: the role of muscle relaxants and corticosteroids. Chest 1999; 115:1627–1631.

208. Helliwell TR, Coakley JH, Wagenmakers AJ, Griffiths RD, Campbell IT, Green CJ, McClelland P, Bone JM. Necrotizing myopathy in critically ill patients. J Pathol 1991; 164:307–314.

209. Young GB, Bolton CF, Austin TW, Archibald YM, Gonder J, Wells GA. The encephalopathy associated with septic illness. Clin Invest Med 1990; 13:297–304.

210. Young GB, Bolton CF, Archibald YM, Austin TW, Wells GA. The electro-encephalogram in sepsis-associated encephalopathy. J Clin Neurophysiol 1991; 9:145–152.

211. Carter JL, Noseworthy JH. Ventilatory dysfunction in multiple sclerosis. Clinics in Chest Medicine 1994; 15:693–703.

212. Noseworthy JH, Lucchinetti C, Rodriguez M. Weinshenker BG. Multiple sclerosis. N Engl J Med 2000; 343:938–952.
213. Weiner HL, Selkoe DJ. Inflammation and therapeutic vaccination in CNS diseases. Nature 2002; 420:879–884.
214. Sorensen TL, Tani M, Jensen J, Pierce V, Lucchinetti C, Folcik VA, Qin S, Rottman J, Sellebjerg F, Strieter RM, Frederiksen JL, Ransohoff RM. Expression of specific chemokines and chemokine receptors in the central nervous system of multiple sclerosis patients. J Clin Invest 1999; 103:807–815.
215. Simpson JE, Newcombe J, Cuzner ML, Woodroofe MN. Expression of the interferon-gamma-inducible chemokines IP-10 and Mig and their receptor, CXCR3, in multiple sclerosis lesions. Neuropathol Appl Neurobiol 2000; 26:133–142.
216. Levin LI, Munger KL, Rubertone MV, Peck CA, Lennette E, Spiegelman D, Ascherio A. Multiple sclerosis and Epstein-barr virus. J Am Med Assoc 2003; 289:1533–1536.
217. Bruck W, Stadelmann C. Inflammation and degeneration in multiple sclerosis. Neurol Sci 2003; S265–267.
218. Weinshenker BG. The natural history of multiple sclerosis: update 1998. Semin Neurol 1998; 301–307.
219. Lublin FD, Reingold SC. Defining the clinical course of multiple sclerosis: results of an international survey, National Multiple Sclerosis Society IUSA) Advisory Committee on Clinical Trials of New Agents in Multiple Sclerosis. Neurology 1996; 46:907.
220. Poser CM, Paty DW, Scheinberg L, McDonald W, Davis F, Ebers G, Johnson K, Sibley W, Silberberg DH, Tourtellotte WW. New diagnostic criteria for multiple sclerosis: guidelines for research protocols. Ann Neurol 1983; 13:227.
221. McDonald WI, Compston A, Edan G, et al. Recommended diagnostic criteria for multiple sclerosis: guidelines from the International Panel on the diagnosis of multiple sclerosis. Ann Neurol 2001; 50:121.
222. Howard RS, Wiles CM, Hirsch NP, Loh L, Spencer GT, Newsom-Davis J. Respiratory involvement in multiple sclerosis. Brain 1992; 115:479–494.
223. Berger JR, Sheremata WA. Persistent neurological deficit precipitated by hot bath test in multiple sclerosis. J Am Med Assoc 1983; 249:1751–1753.
224. Gosselink R, Kovacs L, Decramer M. Respiratory muscle involvement in multiple sclerosis. Eur Respir J 1999; 13:449–454.
225. Foglio K, Clini E, Facchetti D, Vitacca M, Marangoni S, Bonomelli M, Ambrosino N. Respiratory muscle function and exercise capacity in multiple sclerosis. Eur Respir J 1994; 7:23–28.
226. Offenbacher H, Fazekas F, Schmidt R, Friedl W, Flooh E, Payer F, Lechner H. Assessment of MRI criteria for a diagnosis of MS. Neurology 1993; 43:905.
227. Tortorella C, Codella M, Rocca MA, Gasperini C, Capra R, Bastianello S, Filippi M. Disease activity in multiple sclerosis studied by weekly triple-dose magnetic resonance imaging. J Neurol 1999; 246:689.
228. McLean BN, Luxton RW, Thompson EJ. A study of immunoglobulin G in the cerebrospinal fluid of 1007 patients with suspected neurological disease using isoelectric focusing and the Log IgG-Index. A comparison and diagnostic applications. Brain 1990; 113:1269.

229. Rudick RA, Whitaker JN. Cerebrospinal fluid tests for multiple sclerosis. In: Scheinberg P, ed. Neurology/Neurosurgery Update Series. Vol. 7, Princeton, NJ: CPEC, 1987:1.

230. Gronseth GS, Ashman EJ. Practice parameter: the usefulness of evoked potentials in identifying clinically silent lesions in patients with suspected multiple sclerosis (an evidence-based review). Report of the Quality Standards Subcommittee of the American Academy of Neurology. Neurology 2000; 54:1720.

231. Samkoff LM. Multiple sclerosis: update on treatment. Hospital Physician 2002; 21–27.

232. Rudick RA, Cohen JA, Weinstock-Guttman B, Kinkel RP, Ransohoff RM. Management of multiple sclerosis. N Engl J Med 1997; 337:1604–1611.

233. Kupersmith MJ, Kaufman D, Paty DW, Ebers G, McFarland H, Johnson K, Reingold S, Whiterker J. Megadose corticosteroids in multiple sclerosis (editorial). Neurology 1994; 44:1.

234. Sellebjerg F, Frederiksen JL, Nielsen PM, Olesen J. Double-blind, randomized, placebo-controlled study of oral, high-dose methylprednisolone in attacks of MS. Neurology 1998; 51:529.

235. Barnes D, Hughes RA, Morris RW, Wade-Jones O, Brown P, Britton T, Francis D, Perkin G, Rudge P, Swash N. Randomised trial of oral and intravenous methylprednisolone in acute relapses of multiple sclerosis. Lancet 1997; 349:902–906.

236. Filippini G, Munari L, Incorvaia B, Ebers G, Polman C, Amico R, Rice G. Interferons in relapsing remitting multiple sclerosis: a systematic review. Lancet 2003; 361:545.

237. Johnson KP, Brooks BR, Cohen JA, Ford C, Goldstein J, Lisak P, Myers L, Rose J, Schiffer R. Copolymer 1 reduces relapse rate and improves disability in relapsing-remitting multiple sclerosis: results of a phase III multicenter, double-blind placebo-controlled trial. The Copolymer 1 Multiple Sclerosis Study Group. Neurology 1995; 45:1268.

238. Hartung HP, Gonsette R, Konig N, Kwiecinski H, Guseo A, Morrissey S, Krapf H, Zwingers T. Mitoxantrone in progressive multiple sclerosis: a placebo-controlled, double-blind, randomised, multicentre trial. Lancet 2002; 360:2018.

239. Fazekas F, Deisenhammer F, Strasser-Fuchs S, Nahler G, Mamoli P, Randomised placebo-controlled trial of monthly intravenous immunoglobulin therapy in relapsing-remitting multiple sclerosis. Austrian Immunoglobulin in Multiple Sclerosis Study Group. Lancet 1997; 349:589.

240. Weinshenker BG, O'Brien PC, Petterson TM, Noseworthy J, Lucchinetti C, Dodick D, Pineda A, Stevens L, Rodrigues M. A randomized trial of plasma exchange in acute central nervous system inflammatory demyelinating disease. Ann Neurol 1999; 46:878.

241. Trojano M, Paolicelli D. The differential diagnosis of multiple sclerosis: classification and clinical features of relapsing and progressive neurological syndromes. Neurol Sci 2001; 22:S98–S102.

242. Newsom Davis J, Goldman M, Loh L, Casson M. Diaphragm function and alveolar hypoventilation. Q J Med 1976; 45:87–100.

243. Sandham J, Shaw D, Guenter C. Acute supine respiratory failure due to bilateral diaphragmatic paralysis. Chest 1977; 72:96.

244. Laroche CM, Carroll N, Moxham J, Green M. Clinical significance of severe isolated diaphragm weakness. Am Rev Respir Dis 1988; 138:862–866.

245. Mills GH, Kyroussis D, Hamnegard CH, Wragg S, Polkey MI, Moxham J, Green M. Cervical magnetic stimulation of the phrenic nerves in bilateral diaphragm paralysis. Am J Respir Crit Care Med 1977; 155:1565–1569.

246. Laroche CM, Mier AK, Moxham J, Green M. Diaphragm strength in patients with recent hemidiaphragm paralysis. Thorax 1988; 43:170–174.

247. Hart N, Nickol AH, Cramer D, Ward SP, Lofaso F, Pride NB, Moxham J, Polkey MI. Effect of severe isolated unilateral and bilateral diaphragm weakness on exercise performance. Am J Respir Crit Care Med 2002; 165: 1265–1270.

248. McCool FD, Mead J. Dyspnea on immersion: mechanisms in patients with bilateral diaphragm paralysis. Am Rev Respir Dis 1989; 139:275–276.

249. Mier AK, Brophy C, Green M. Out of depth, out of breath. Br Med J 1986; 292:1495–1496.

250. Loh L, Goldman M, Newsom Davis J. Assessment of diaphragm function. Medicine 1977; 56:165–169.

251. Mier-Jedrzejowicz A, Brophy C, Moxham J, Green M. Assessment of diaphragm weakness. Am Rev Respir Dis 1988; 137:877–883.

252. Lisboa C, Pare PD, Pertuze J, Contreras G, Moreno R, Guillemi S, Cruz E. Inspiratory muscle function in unilateral diaphragmatic paralysis. Am Rev Respir Dis 1986; 134:488–492.

253. Martinez FJ, Strawderman RL, Flaherty KR, Cowan M, Orens JB, Wald J. Respiratory response during arm elevation in isolated diaphragm weakness. Am J Respir Crit Care Med 1999; 160:480–486.

254. Alexander C. Diaphragm movement and the diagnosis of diaphragm paralysis. Clin Radiol 1966; 17:79.

255. Houston JG, Fleet M, Cowan MD, McMillan NC. Comparison of ultrasound with fluoroscopy in the assessment of suspected hemidiaphragmatic movement abnormality. Clin Radiol 1995; 50:95–98.

256. Gerscovich EO, Cronan M, McGaham JP, Jain K, Jones CD, McDonald C. Ultrasonographic evaluation of diaphragmatic motion. J Ultrasound Med 2001; 20:597–604.

257. Gottesman E, McCool FD. Ultrasound evaluation of the paralyzed diaphragm. Am J Respir Crit Care Med 1997; 155:1570–1574.

258. Hillman DR, Finucane KE. Respiratory pressure partitioning during quiet inspiration in unilateral and bilateral diaphragmatic weakness. Am Rev Respir Dis 1988; 137:1401–1405.

259. Gibson GJ. Diaphragmatic paresis: pathophysiology, clinical features, and investigation. Thorax 1989; 44:960–970.

260. Chan CK, Loke J, Virgulto JA, Mohsenin V, Ferranti R, Lammertse T. Bilateral diaphragmatic paralysis: clinical spectrum, prognosis, and diagnostic approach. Arch Phys Med Rehabil 1988; 69:976–979.

261. Oo T, Watt JW, Soni BM, Sett PK. Delayed diaphragm recovery in 12 patients after high cervical spinal cord injury. A retrospective review of the diaphragm status of 107 patients ventilated after acute spinal cord injury. Spinal Cord 1999; 37:117–122.

262. Winterholler M, Erbguth FJ. Tick bite induced respiratory failure. Diaphragm palsy in Lyme disease. Intensive Care Med 2001; 27:1095.

263. Fujibayashi S, Shikata J, Yoshitomi H, Tanaka C, Nakamura K, Nakamura T. Bilateral phrenic nerve palsy as a complication of anterior decompression and fusion for cervical ossification of the posterior longitudinal ligament. Spine 2001; 26:E281–E286.

264. Commare MC, Kurstjens SP, Barois A. Diaphragmatic paralysis in children: a review of 11 cases. Pediatr Pulmonol 1994; 18:187–193.

265. Valls-Sole J, Solans M. Idiopathic bilateral diaphragmatic paralysis. Muscle Nerve 2002; 25:619–623.

266. Pamuk ON, Dogutan H, Pamuk GE, Cakir N. Unilateral phrenic nerve paralysis in a patient with Wegener's granulomatosis. Rheumatol Int 2003; 23:201–203.

267. Dureuil B, Viires N, Pariente R, Desmonts JM, Aubier M. Effects of phrenic nerve cooling on diaphragmatic function. J Appl Physiol 1987; 63:1763–1769.

268. Mills GH, Khan ZP, Moxham J, Desai J, Forsyth A, Ponte J. Effects of temperature on phrenic nerve and diaphragmatic function during cardiac surgery. Br J Anaesth 1997; 79:726–732.

269. Tripp HF, Sees DW, Lisagor PG, Cohen DJ. Is phrenic nerve dysfunction after cardiac surgery related to internal mammary harvesting? J Card Surg 2001; 16:228–231.

270. Canbaz S, Turgut N, Halici U, Balci K, Ege T, Duran E. Electrophysiological evaluation of phrenic nerve injury during cardiac surgery—a prospective, controlled, clinical study. BMC Surg 2004; 4:2.

271. Dimopoulou I, Daganou M, Dafni U, Karakatsani A, Khoury M, Geroulanos S, Jordanoglou J. Phrenic nerve dysfunction after cardiac operations: electrophysiologic evaluation of risk factors. Chest 1998; 113:8014.

272. De Vita JA, Robinson LR, Rehder J, Hattler B, Cohen C. Incidence and natural history of phrenic neuropathy occurring during open heart surgery. Chest 1993; 103:850–856.

273. Efthimiou J, Butler J, Woodham C, Westaky S, Benson MK. Phrenic nerve and diaphragm function following open heart surgery; a prospective study with and without topical hypothermia. Q J Med 1992; 85:845–853.

274. Diehl JL, Lofaso F, Deleuze P, Similowski T, Lemaire F, Brochard L. Clinically relevant diaphragmatic dysfunction after cardiac operations. J Thorac Cardiovasc Surg 1994; 107:487–498.

275. Chandler KW, Rozas CJ, Kory RC, Goldman AL. Bilateral diaphragmatic paralysis complicating local cardiac hypothermia during open heart surgery. Am J Med 1984; 77:243–249.

276. Ferdinande P, Bruyninckx F, Van Raemdonck D, Daenen W, Verleden G, Leuven Lung Transplant Group. Phrenic nerve dysfunction after heart–lung and lung transplantation. J Heart Lung Transplant 2004; 23:105–109.

277. Raffa H, Kayali MT, Al-Ibrahim K, Mimish L. Fatal bilateral phrenic nerve injury following hypothermic open heart surgery. Chest 1994; 105:1268–1269.

278. Wilcox PG, Pare D, Pardy RL. Recovery after unilateral phrenic injury associated with coronary artery revascularization. Chest 1990; 98:661–666.

279. Katz MG, Katz R, Schachner A, Cohen AJ. Phrenic nerve injury after coronary artery bypass grafting: will it go away? Ann Thorac Surg 1998; 65:32–35.

280. Mulvey DA, Aquilina RJ, Elliott MW, Moxham J, Green M. Diaphragmatic dysfunction in neuralgic amyotrophy: an electrophysiologic evaluation of 16 patients presenting with dyspnea. Am Rev Respir Dis 1993; 147:66–71.

281. Lahrmann H, Grisold W, Authier FJ, Zifko UA. Neuralgic amyotrophy with phrenic nerve involvement. Muscle Nerve 1999; 22:437–442.

282. Tsairis P, Dyck PJ, Mulder DW. Natural history of brachial plexus neuropathy. Report on 99 patients. Arch Neurol 1972; 27:109–117.

283. Pierre PA, Laterre CE, Van den Bergh PY. Neuralgic amyotrophy with involvement of cranial nerves IX, X, XI, and XII. Muscle Nerve 1990; 13:704–707.

284. Hughes PD, Polkey MI, Moxham J, Green M. Long-term recovery of diaphragm strength in neuralgic amyotrophy. Eur Respir J 1999; 13:379–384.

285. Hardy K, Herry I, Attali V, Cadranel J, Similowski T. Bilateral phrenic paralysis in a patient with systemic lupus erythematosis. Chest 2001; 119:1274–1277.

286. Wilcox PG, Stein HB, Clarke SD, Pare PD, Pardy RL. Phrenic nerve function in patients with diaphragmatic weakness and systemic lupus erythematosis. Chest 1988; 93:352–358.

287. Laroche CM, Mulvey DA, Hawkins PN, Walport MJ, Strickland B, Moxham J, Green M. Diaphragm strength in the shrinking lung syndrome of systemic lupus erythematosis. Q J Med 1989; 71:429–439.

288. Rubin LA, Urowitz MB. Shrinking lung syndrome in SLE: a clinical pathologic study. J Rheumatol 1983; 10:973–976.

289. Wright C, Williams J, Ogilvie C, Donnelly R. Results of diaphragmatic plication for unilateral diaphragmatic paralysis. J Thorac Cardiovasc Surg 1985; 90:195.

290. Graham D, Kaplan D, Evans C, Hind CR, Donnelly R. Diaphragmatic plication for unilateral diaphragmatic plication for unilateral diaphragmatic paralysis: a 10-year experience. Ann Thorac Surg 1990; 49:248.

291. Stolk J, Versteegh MI. Long-term effect of bilateral plication of the diaphragm. Chest 2000; 117:786–789.

292. Lai DT, Paterson HS. Mini-thoracotomy for diaphragmatic plication with thoracoscopic assistance. Ann Thorac Surg 1999; 68:2364–2365.

293. Huttl TP, Wichmann MW, Reichart B, Geiger TK, Schildberg FW, Meyer G. Laparoscopic diaphragmatic plication: long-term results of a novel surgical technique for postoperative phrenic nerve palsy. Surg Endosc 2004 (Epub ahead of print).

294. Simansky DA, Paley M, Refaely Y, Yellin A. Diaphragm plication following phrenic nerve injury: a comparison of paediatric and adult patients. Thorax 2002; 57:613–616.

295. Higgs SM, Hussain A, Jackson M, Donnelly RJ, Berrisford RG. Long term results of diaphragmatic plication for unilateral diaphragm paralysis. Eur J Cardiothorac Surg 2002; 21:294–297.

296. Hill N. Noninvasive ventilation. Am Rev Respir Dis 147:1050.

297. Hines MH. Video-assisted diaphragm plication in children. Ann Thorac Surg 2003; 76:234–236.

298. Brouillette RT, Marzocchi M. Diaphragm pacing: clinical and experimental results. Biol Neonate 1994; 65:265–271.

299. Elefteriades JA, Quin JA. Diaphragm pacing. Ann Thorac Surg 2002; 73:691.

300. Morgan JA, Morales DL, John R, Ginsberg M, Kherani A, Vigilance D. Endoscopic, robotically assisted implantation of phrenic pacemakers. J Thorac Cardiovasc Surg 2003; 126:582.

301. DiMarco AF, Onders RP, Kowalski KE, Miller M, Ferek S, Mortimer J. Phrenic nerve pacing in a tetraplegic patient via intramuscular diaphragm electrodes. Am J Respir Crit Care Med 2002; 166:1604.

302. Glenn WWL, Hogan JF, Loke JSO, Ciesielski T, Phelps M, Rowedder R. Ventilatory support by pacing of the conditioned diaphragm in quadriplegia. N Engl J Med 1984; 310:1150.

303. Elefteriades JA, Quin JA, Hogan JF, Holcomb W, Letson G, Chlasta W, Glenn, W. Long-term follow-up of pacing of the conditioned diaphragm in quadriplegia. Pacing Clin Electrophysiol 2002; 25:897.

304. Mehta S, Hill NS. Noninvasive ventilation. Am J Respir Care Med 2001; 163:540–577.

305. Rowland LP, Shneider NA. Amyotrophic lateral sclerosis. N Engl J Med 2001; 344:1688–1700.

306. Talbot K. Motor neurone disease. Postgrad Med J 2002; 78:513–519.

307. Patel SA, Maragakis NJ. Amyotrophic lateral sclerosis: pathogenesis, differential diagnoses, and potential interventions. J Spinal Cord Med 2002; 25:262–273.

308. Jackson CE, Bryan WW. Amyotrophic lateral sclerosis. Semin Neurol 1998; 18:27–39.

309. Kaplan LM, Hollander D. Respiratory dysfunction in amyotrophic lateral sclerosis. Clinics in Chest Medicine 1994; 15:675–681.

310. Braun SR. Respiratory system in amyotrophic lateral sclerosis. Neurol Clin 1987; 5:9–31.

311. Fromm GB, Wisdom PJ, Block AJ. Amyotrophic lateral sclerosis presenting with respiratory failure in motor neurone disease. Chest 1977; 71:612–614.

312. Hill R, Martin J, Hakin A. Acute respiratory failure in motor neurone disease. Arch Neurol 1983; 40:30–32.

313. Ross MA, Miller RG, Berchert L, Parry G, Barohn RJ, Armon C, Bryan WW, Petajan J, Stromatt S, Goodpasture J, McGuire D. Toward earlier diagnosis of amyotrophic lateral sclerosis: revised criteria. RhCNTF ALS Study Group. Neurology 1998; 50:768–772.

314. Bensimon G, Lacomblez L, Meininger V, ALS/Riluzole Study Group. A controlled trial of riluzole in amyotrophic lateral sclerosis. N Engl J Med 1994; 330:585–591.

315. Lacomblez L, Bensimon G, Leigh PN, Guillet P, Powe L, Durrleman S, Delumean J, Meininger V. A confirmatory dose-ranging study of riluzole in ALS. Neurology 1996; 47S:S242–S250.

316. Riviere M, Meininger V, Zeisser P, Munsat T. An analysis of extended survival in patients with amyotrophic lateral sclerosis treated with riluzole. Arch Neurol 1998; 55:526–528.

317. Lai EC, Felice KJ, Festoff BW, Gawel MJ, Gelinas DF, Kratz R, Murphy MF, Natter HM, Norris FH, Rudnicki SA. Effect of recombinant human insulin-like growth factor-I on progression of ALS. A placebo-controlled study. The North America ALS/IGF-I Study Group. Neurology 1997; 49:1621–1630.

318. Borasio GD, Robberecht W, Leigh PN, Emile J, Guiloff RJ, Jerusalem F, Silani V, Vos PE, Wokke JH, Dobbins T. A placebo-controlled trial of insulin-like growth factor-I in amyotrophic lateral sclerosis. European ALS/IGF-I Study Group. Neurology 1998; 51:583–586.

319. Dib M. Amyotrophic lateral sclerosis: progress and prospects for treatment. Drugs 2003; 63:289–310.

320. Lechtzin N, Rothstein J, Clawson L, Diette GB, Wiener CM. Amyotrophic lateral sclerosis: evaluation and treatment of respiratory impairment. Amyotroph Lateral Scler Other Motor Neuron Disord 2002; 3:5–13.

321. Hardiman O. Symptomatic treatment of respiratory and nutritional failure in amyotrophic lateral sclerosis. J Neurol 2000; 247:245–251.

322. Escarrabill J, Estopa R, Farrero E, Monasterio C, Manresa F. Long-term mechanical ventilation in amyotrophic lateral sclerosis. Respir Med 1998; 92:438–441.

323. Desport JC, Preux PM, Truong CT, Courat L, Vallat JM, Couratier P. Nutritional assessment and survival in ALS patients. Amyotroph Lateral Scler Other Motor Neuron Disord 2000; 1:91–96.

324. Howard RS, Orrell RW. Management of motor neurone disease. Postgrad Med J 2002; 78:736–741.

325. Raymond M. Paralysie essentielle de l'enfance, atrophile musculaire consecutive. C Rendus Heb Seances Mem Soc Biol 1875; 27:158–160.

326. Dalakas MC. Post-polio syndrome 12 years later: how it all started. Ann N Y Acad Sci 1995; 753:11–18.

327. Halstead LS, Rossi CD. New problems in old polio patients: results of a survey of 539 polio survivors. Orthopedics 1985; 8:845–850.

328. Dalakas MC. Pathogenetic mechanisms of post-polio syndrome: morphological, electrophysiological, virological, and immunological correlations. Ann N Y Acad Sci 1995; 753:167–185.

329. Jubelt B. Post-polio syndrome. Curr Treat Options Neurol 2004; 6:87–93.

330. Thorsteinsson G. Management of post-polio syndrome. Mayo Clin Proc 1997; 72:627–638.

331. Bach JR. Management of post-polio respiratory sequelae. Ann N Y Acad Sci 1995; 753:96–102.

332. Halstead LS, Rossi CD. Post-polio syndrome: clinical experience with 132 consecutive outpatients. Birth Defects 1987; 23:13–26.

333. Agre JC, Rodriguez AA, Sperling KB. Symptoms and clinical impressions of patients seen in a post-polio clinic. Arch Phys Med Rehabil 1989; 70:367–370.

334. Lonnberg F. Late onset polio sequelae in Denmark: presentation and results of a nation-wide survey of 3,607 polio survivors. Scand J Rehabil Med Suppl 1993; 28:7–15.

335. Abaza MM, Sataloff RT, Hawkshaw MJ, Mandel S. Laryngeal manifestations of post-poliomyelitis syndrome. J Voice 2001; 15:291–294.

336. Dean AC, Graham BA, Dalakas M, Sato S. Sleep apnea in patients with post-polio syndrome. Ann Neurol 1998; 43:661–664.

337. Agre JC. The role of exercise in the patient with post-polio syndrome. Ann N Y Acad Sci 1995; 753:321–334.

338. Halstead LS. Assessment and differential diagnosis for post-polio syndrome. Orthopedics 1991; 14:1209–1217.

339. Birk TJ. Poliomyelitis and the post-polio syndrome: exercise capacities and adaptation—current research, future directions, and widespread applicability. Med Sci Sports Exerc 1993; 25:466–472.

340. Young GR. Energy conservation, occupational therapy, and the treatment of post-polio sequelae. Orthopedics 1991; 14:1233–1239.

341. Howard RS, Wiles CM, Hirsch NP, Spencer GT. Respiratory involvement in primary muscle disorders: assessment and management. Q J Med 1993; 86:175–1889.

342. Hoffman EP, Brown RH Jr, Kunkel LM. Dystrophin: the protein product of the Duchenne muscular dystrophy locus. Cell 1987; 51:519.

343. Hoffman EP. Genotype/phenotype correlations in Duchenne/Becker dystrophy. In: Partridge TA, ed. Molecular and Cellular Biology of Muscular Dystrophy, London: Chapman and Hall, 1991.

344. Monckton G, Hoskin V, Warren S. Prevalence and incidence of muscular dystrophy in Alberta, Canada. Clin Genet 1982; 21:19.

345. Gardner-Medwin D. Clinical features and classification of the muscular dystrophies. Br Med Bull 1980; 36:109.

346. Bradley WG, Jones MZ, Mussini JM. Becker-type muscular dystrophy. Muscle Nerve 1978; 1:111.

347. Phillips MF, Quinlivan RC, Edwards RH, Calverley PM. Changes in spirometry over time as a prognostic marker in patients with Duchenne muscular dystrophy. Am J Respir Crit Care Med 2001; 164:2191–2194.

348. Raphael JC, Chevret S, Chastang C, Bouvet F. Randomised trial of preventive nasal ventilation in Duchenne muscular dystrophy. French Multicentre Cooperative Group on Home Mechanical Ventilation Assistance in Duchenne de Boulogne Muscular Dystrophy. Lancet 1994; 343:1600–1604.

349. Mendell JR, Moxley RT, Griggs RC, Brooke M, Fenichel G, Miller J, King W, Signore L, Pandya S, Florence J, Robinson J. Randomized, double-blind six-month trial of prednisone in Duchenne's muscular dystrophy. N Engl J Med 1989; 320:1592.

350. Griggs RC, Moxley RT, Mendell JR, Fenichel G, Brooke M, Pestronk A, Miller J, Cwik V, Pandya S, Robinson J. Duchenne dystrophy: randomized, controlled trial of prednisone (18 months) and azathioprine (12 months). Neurology 1993; 43:520.

351. Wanke T, Toifl K, Merkle M, Formanek D, Lahrmann H, Swick H. Inspiratory muscle training in patients with Duchenne muscular dystrophy. Chest 1994; 105:475–482.

352. Harper PS. Myotonic dystrophy, Vol. 21, 2nd ed. In: Major Problems in Neurology. London: WB Saunders, 1989.

353. Begin P, Mathieu J, Almirall J, Grassino A. Relationship between chronic hypercapnia and inspiratory-muscle weakness in myotonic dystrophy. Am J Respir Crit Care Med 1997; 156:133–139.

354. Zifko UA, Hahn AF, Remtulla H, George CF, Wihlidal W, Bolton CF. Central and peripheral respiratory electrophysiological studies in myotonic dystrophy. Brain 1996; 119:1911–1922.

355. Begin R, Bureau MA, Lupien L, Lemieux B. Control and modulation of respiration in Steinert's myotonic dystrophy. Am Rev Respir Dis 1980; 121:281–289.

356. Mathieu J, Allard P, Potvin L, Prevost C, Begin P. A 10-year study of mortality in a cohort of patients with myotonic dystrophy. Neurology 1999; 52:1658–1662.

357. Robertson PL, Roloff DW. Chronic respiratory failure in limb-girdle muscular dystrophy: successful long-term therapy with nasal bilevel positive airway pressure. Pediatr Neurol 1994; 10:328–331.

358. Ryan MM, Schnell C, Strickland CD, Shield LK, Morgan G, Iannaccone ST, Laing NG, Beggs AH, North KN. Nemaline myopathy: a clinical study of 143 cases. Ann Neurol 2001; 50:312–320.

359. Zeman AZ, Dick DJ, Anderson JR, Watkin SW, Smith IE, Shneerson JM. Multicore myopathy presenting in adulthood with respiratory failure. Muscle Nerve 1997; 20:367–369.

360. Hirano M, DiMauro S. Metabolic myopathies. Adv Neurol 2002; 88:217–234.

361. Vladutiu GD. Laboratory diagnosis of metabolic myopathies. Muscle Nerve 2002; 25:649–663.

362. Vorgerd M, Zange J. Carbohydrate oxidation disorders of skeletal muscle. Curr Opin Clin Nutr Metab Care 2002; 5:611–617.

363. Raben N, Plotz P, Byrne BJ. Acid alpha-glucosidase deficiency (glycogenosis type II, Pompe disease). Curr Mol Med 2002; 2:145–166.

364. Rosenow III EC, Engel AG. Acid maltase deficiency in adults presenting as respiratory failure. Am J Med 1978; 64:485–491.

365. Moufarrej NA, Bertorini TE. Respiratory insufficiency in adult-type acid maltase deficiency. South Med J 1993; 86:560–567.

366. Mellies U, Ragette R, Schwake C, Baethmann M, Voit T, Teschler H. Sleep-disordered breathing and respiratory failure in acid maltase deficiency. Neurology 2001; 57:1290–1295.

367. Ausems MG, Lochman P, van Diggelen OP, Ploos van Amstel HK, Reuser AJ, Wokke JH. A diagnostic protocol for adult-onset glycogen storage disease type II. Neurology 1999; 52:851–853.

368. Pichiecchio A, Uggetti C, Ravaglia S, Egitto MG, Rossi M, Sandrini G. Danesino C. Muscle MRI in adult-onset maltase deficiency. Neuromuscul Disord 2004; 14:51–55.

369. Reuser AJ, Van Den Hout H, Bijvoet AG, Kroos MA, Verbeet MP, Van Der Ploeg AT. Enzyme therapy for Pompe disease: from science to industrial enterprise. Eur J Pediatr 2002; 161(suppl):S106–S111.

370. Pfeiffer G, Winkler G, Neunzig P, Wolf W, Thayssen G, Kunze K. Long-term management of acute respiratory failure in metabolic myopathy. Intensive Care Med 1996; 22:1406–1409.

371. Stedwell RE, Allen KM, Binder LS. Hypokalemic paralyses: a review of the etiologies, pathophysiology, presentation, and therapy. Am I Emerg Med 1992; 10:143–148.

372. Renner DR, Ptacek LJ. Periodic paralyses and nondystrophic myotonias. Adv Neurol 2002; 88:235–252.

373. Lehmann-Horn F, Jurkat-Rott K, Rudel R. Periodic paralysis: understanding channelopathies. Curr Neurol Neurosci Rep 2002; 2:61–69.

374. Ahlawat SK, Sachdev A. Hypokalameic paralysis. Postgrad Med J 1999; 75:193–197.

375. Gutmann L. Periodic paralyses. Neurol Clin 2000; 18:195–202.

376. Griggs RC, Engel WK, Resnick JS. Acetazolamide treatment of hypokalemic periodic paralysis. Ann Int Med 1970; 73:39–48.

377. Dalakas MC. Polymyositis, dermatomyositis, and inclusion-body myositis. N Engl J Med 1991; 325:1487–1498.

378. Marie I, Hatron PY, Levesque H, Hachulla E, Hellot M, Michon-Pasture U, Cortois H, Devulder B. Influence of age on characteristics of polymyositis and dermatomyositis in adults. Medicine (Baltimore) 1999; 78:139.

379. Schiavi EA, Roncoroni AJ, Puy RJ. Isolated bilateral diaphragmatic paresis with interstitial lung disease. An unusual presentation of dermatomyositis. Am Rev Respir Dis 1984; 129:337–339.

380. Selva-O'Callaghan A, Sanchez-Sitjes L, Munoz-Gall X, Mijares-Boeckh-Behrens T, Solans-Laque R, Angel Bosch-Gil J, Morell-Brotad F, Vilardell-Tarres M. Respiratory failure due to muscle weakness in inflammatory myopathies: maintenance therapy with home mechanical ventilation. Rheumatology (Oxford) 2000; 39:914–916.

381. Tymms KE, Webb J. Dermatopolymyositis and other connective tissue diseases: a review of 105 cases. J Rheumatol 1985; 12:1140.

382. Fafalak RG, Peterson MGE, Kagen LJ. Strength in polymyositis and dermatomyositis: best outcome in patients treated early. J Rheumatol 1994; 21:643.

383. Drake LA, Dinehart SM, Farmer ER, Goltz R, Graham G, Hordinsky M, Lewis C, Pariser D, Skouge J, Webster S, et al. Guidelines of care for dermatomyositis. J Am Acad Dermatol 1996; 34:824.

384. Dalakas MC. Current treatment of the inflammatory myopathies. Curr Opin Rheumatol 1994; 6:595.

385. Bunch TW. Prednisone and azathioprine for polymyositis. Long-term follow-up. Arthritis Rheum 1981; 24:45.

386. Newman ED, Scott DW. The use of low-dose oral methotrexate in the treatment of polymyositis and dermatomyositis. J Clin Rheumatol 1995; 1:99.

387. Cherin P, Pelletier S, Teixeira A, Laforet P, Genereau T, Simon A, Maisonobe T, Eymard B, Herson S. Results and long-term follow-up of intravenous immunoglobulin infusions in chronic, refractory polymyositis: an open study with thirty-five adult patients. Arthritis Rheum 2002; 46:467.

388. Qushmaq KA, Chalmers A, Esdaile JM. Cyclosporin A in the treatment of refractory adult polymyositis/dermatomyositis: population based experience in 6 patients and literature review. [In Process Citation.] J.Rheumatol 2000; 27:2855.

389. Amato AA, Gronseth GS, Jackson CE, Wolfe G, Katz J, Bryan W, Barohn R. Inclusion body myositis: clinical and pathological boundaries. Ann Neurol 1996; 40:581.

390. Cohen R, Lipper S, Dantzker DR. Inclusion body myositis as a cause of respiratory failure. Chest 1993; 104:975–977.

391. Czerwinski SM, Zak R, Kurowski TT, Falduto MT, Hickson RC. Myosin heavy chain turnover and glucocorticoid deterrence by exercise in muscle. J Appl Physiol 1989; 67:2311–2315.

392. Lofberg E, Gutierrez A, Wernerman J, Anderstam B, Mitch WE, Price SR, Bergstrom J, Alverstrand A. Effects of high doses of glucocorticoids on free amino acids, ribosomes and protein turnover in human muscle. Eur J Clin Invest 2002; 32:345–353.

393. Auclair D, Garrel DR, Zerouala AC, Ferland LH. Activation of the ubiquitin pathway in rat skeletal muscle by catabolic doses of glucocorticoids. Am J Physiol Cell Physiol 1997; 272:C1007–C1016.

394. Dekhuijzen PNR, Gayan-Ramirez G, de Bock V, Dom R, Decramer M. Triamcinolone and prednisolone affect contractile properties and histopathology of rat diaphragm differently. J Clin Invest 1993; 92:1534–1542.

395. Eason JM, Dodd SL, Powers SK, Martin AD. Detrimental effects of short-term glucocorticoid use on the rat diaphragm. Phys Ther 2000; 80:160–167.

396. Van Balkomo RH, van der Heijden HF, van Moerkerk HT, Veerkamp JH, Fransen JA, Ginsel LA, Folgering HT, van Herwaarden CL, Dekhuijzen PN. Effects of different treatment regimens of methylprednisolone on rat diaphragm contractility, immunohistochemistry, and biochemistry. Eur Respir J 1996; 9:1217–1223.

397. Decramer M, deBock V, Dom R. Functional and histological picture of steroid-induced myopathy in chronic obstructive pulmonary disease. Am J Respir Crit Care Med 1996; 153:1958–1964.

398. Decramer M, Gosselink R, Troosters T, Verschueren M, Evers G. Muscle weakness is related to utilization of health care resources in COPD patients. Eur Respir J 1997; 10:417–423.

399. Decramer M, Lacquet LM, Fagard R, Rogiers P. Corticosteroids contribute to muscle weakness in chronic airflow obstruction. Am J Respir Crit Care Med 1994; 150:11–16.

400. Decramer M, Stas KJ. Corticosteroid-induced myopathy involving respiratory muscles in patients with chronic obstructive pulmonary disease or asthma. Am Rev Respir Dis 1992; 146:800–822.

401. Weiner P, Azgad Y, Weiner M. The effect of corticosteroids on inspiratory muscle performance in humans. Chest 1993; 104:1788–1791.

402. Picado C, Fiz JA, Montserrat JM, Grau JM, Fernandez-Sola J, Luengo MT, Casademont J, Agusti-Vidal A. Respiratory and skeletal muscle function in steroid-dependent bronchial asthma. Am Rev Respir Dis 1990; 141:14–20.

403. Wang Y, Zintel T, Vasquez A, Gallagher CG. Corticosteroid therapy and respiratory muscle function in humans. Am Rev Respir Dis 1991; 144:108–112.

404. Decramer M, Ludovic ML, Fagard R, Rogiers P. Corticosteroids contribute to muscle weakness in chronic airflow obstruction. Am J Respir Crit Care Med 1994; 150:11–16.

8

Acute Coronary Syndrome

KUANG-YUH CHYU and BOJAN CERCEK

Division of Cardiology, Cedars–Sinai Medical Center
Geffen School of Medicine at UCLA
Los Angeles, California, U.S.A.

I. Changing Face of Acute Coronary Syndrome

Acute coronary syndrome (ACS) encompasses two major categories—ST elevation myocardial infarction (STEMI) and non-ST elevation myocardial infarction/unstable angina (NSTEMI/UA). Its treatment, patient demographics, and characteristics have evolved greatly in the past decades. According to the National Registry of Myocardial Infarction (NRMI) database (1), from 1994 to 1999 the mean age of patients increased from 66.5 to 68.0 years, and the proportion of female patients increased from 37.7% to 39.3%. Patients became more obese, and the prevalence of traditional atherosclerosis risk factors, such as diabetes, hypertension, and hypercholesterolemia, also increased. In the same period of time, the prevalence of STEMI decreased from 36.4% to 27.1%, with a concomitant rise of NSTEMI from 45% to 63%. However, due to the implementation of published guidelines, the door-to-drug time for STEMI significantly reduced from 47 minutes in 1994 to 38 minutes in 1999, with a significant increase in the use of aspirin, beta-blockers, and angiotensin-converting enzyme inhibitors (ACEI) during the first 24 hours after presentation. Overall, these treatments led to a 48% reduction in hospital days, a 16% reduction of hospital mortality (from 11.2% in 1990 to 9.4% in 1999), and varying degrees of reduction of post-MI complications, such as ventricular tachycardia, reinfarction, and cardiac rupture.

II. Pathophysiology of ACS

Although rare entities such as spontaneous dissection of coronary artery, vasospasm, anomalous origin of coronary artery, or coronary ostial stenosis after radiation therapy can cause ACS, the major cause of ACS is in situ thrombus formation due to atherosclerotic plaque rupture. The mechanisms responsible for plaque rupture are not entirely known, but factors such as hemodynamic stress, thinning fibrous cap of the plaques, degradation of collagen matrix in the plaque and apoptosis of vascular smooth muscle cells, activation of immune responses, and release of inflammatory cytokines are believed to be involved (2). The exposure of thrombogenic components of the plaque, such as tissue factors in the lipid gruel, results in platelet activation, aggregation, and subsequent thrombus formation. The magnitude of thrombus formation, complete or subtotal lumen occlusion, the duration of occlusion, and formation of collateral flow account for the differences in clinical presentation (STEMI vs. NSTEMI/UA).

III. Diagnosis of ACS

Any patient presenting to the Emergency Department or physician's office with the complaint of chest pain, with or without associated symptoms such as dyspnea, nausea/vomiting or diaphoresis, should be evaluated promptly with 12-lead ECG recording. Treating physicians should pay particular attention to patients with old age (especially >75 yr of age) and diabetes mellitus (DM) because they may present with atypical symptoms, such as dyspnea and altered mental status. Treating physicians should also quickly rule out patients with other potential catastrophic disorders, such as aortic dissection, pulmonary embolism, pneumothorax, or pneumonia (3–7).

After focused history-taking, physical examination, and initial laboratory tests (CBC, Chem-I, ECG, CXR, and cardiac enzymes), a reasonable clinical impression whether the patient has ACS can be made. Patients who are identified to have STEMI are candidates for immediate reperfusion therapy by thrombolytic therapy or primary percutaneous coronary intervention (PCI) if no contraindication exists. Patients who are suspected to have NSTEMI or unstable angina should be further assessed for short-term risk of cardiac events (death or nonfatal myocardial infarction [MI]). Patients who have accelerating ischemic symptoms in the preceding 48 hours, prolonged ongoing (>20 min) resting chest pain, dynamic ST-segment changes with chest pain, clinical signs of congestive heart failure, hypotension, or positive cardiac enzymes should be considered high-risk and require more aggressive treatment (see subsequent paragraphs). In the high-risk group, the rate of nonfatal MI and death varies from approximately 10–20%, depending on the definition of MI employed in the study/registry (clinical event/ECG changes with positive troponin or positive troponin only).

IV. Management of ACS

The management of ACS consists of two main categories: routine measures and reperfusion-therapy related measures. The management of ACS patients can be summarized in an algorithm in Figure 1.

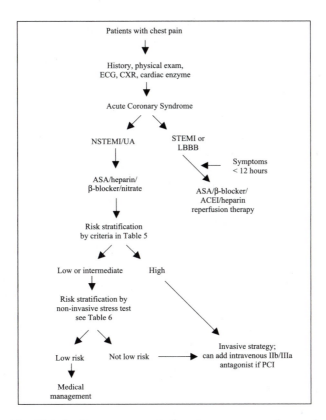

Figure 1 Algorithm for the management of acute coronary syndrome. *Source*: From Refs. 4, 74, and 110.

A. Routine Measures

Routine measures in the management of acute coronary syndrome include oxygen, analgesia, aspirin, beta-blockers, angiotensin converting enzyme inhibitors (ACEI), lipid lowering therapy, and, in selected patients, nitroglycerin and antiarrhythmics. Use of these agents is similar in STEMI and NSTEMI/UA patients.

Aspirin

The anti-thrombotic effect of aspirin is due to its irreversible inhibition of cyclo-oxygenase activity in platelets, causing reduced thromboxane A_2 production and reduced platelet activation and aggregation. Randomized clinical trials had shown convincingly that early initiation of aspirin reduced 35-day mortality compared to placebo after acute myocardial infarction (8). Although there is no consensus regarding the optimal dose of aspirin, it is a common practice to start aspirin in the range of 162–325 mg upon admission and continue such a dose daily (3). It was not proven in a properly-sized randomized trial that aspirin provides long-term mortality benefit. However, it is also a common practice to continue aspirin at a lower dose indefinitely in patients with ACS due to its low price and good safety profile. Another common practice is to give additional aspirin to ACS patients who have already been on aspirin, although again the data from randomized clinical trials are lacking.

Beta Blockers

Early prethrombolysis studies suggested a 22% relative risk reduction of all-cause mortality and a 27% relative risk reduction for reinfarction at seven days (9,10). In the TIMI IIB trial (11), for patients receiving thrombolytic therapy, early use of iv metoprolol (within two hours of rt-PA) was associated with decreased reinfarction rate (2.7% vs. 5.1%) and recurrent ischemia (18.8% vs. 24.1%) compared to delayed treatment (metoprolol started at day 6), but there was no benefit in improving left ventricular function or reducing mortality. Besides improvement in ischemic symptoms and decreased rate of reinfarction, early use of beta-blockers may increase long-term utilization. Long-term use of beta-blockers after acute myocardial infarction (AMI) has been shown in a meta-analysis to convey a 23% reduction in mortality (12). We recommend the use of beta-blockers in all patients with ACS to be started early (within 24 hours) and to continue indefinitely unless contraindicated. Common precautions and contraindications of the use of beta-blocker are listed in Table 1. In patients without contraindications, beta-blockers can be started with Atenolol 25 mg bid or Metoprolol 50–100 mg bid, followed by weekly titration with target dose of Atenolol 50 mg bid or Metoprolol 100 mg bid (13).

Beta-blockers can be used in patients with reactive airway disease without use of beta-agonists (14) and in patients with mild to moderate peripheral

Table 1 Contraindicaitons and Precautions to Beta-Blocker Therapy in Acute Coronary Syndrome

Contraindications
1. Heart rate <50–60 bpm
2. Systolic BP <90–100 mmHg
3. Severe CHF or cardiogenic shock requiring IV diuretics or inotropes
4. Severe reactive airway disease requiring bronchodilator
5. Second or third degree AV block

Precautions
1. CHF
2. COPD
3. DM
4. Peripheral vascular disease
5. First degree AV block

Source: From Refs. 3 and 13.

vascular disease (15). It should be started in a low dose and increased as tolerated with frequent monitoring (13).

Angiotensin Converting Enzyme Inhibitor/Angiotensin Receptor Blocker

Intravenous use of enalapril in the earlier trial (CONSENSUS II Trial) was associated with increased incidence of hypotensive episodes with increased mortality. In subsequent trials (GISSI-3, ISIS-4), careful titration of angiotensin converting enzyme inhibitors (ACEIs) to avoid hypotension was associated with modest reduction in all-cause mortality (16). The benefit was more impressive in patients with anterior MI and in patients with decreased left ventricular (LV) function (LVEF <40%). ACEIs are recommended in patients with signs of congestive heart failure (CHF) or decreased left ventricular ejection fraction (LVEF) below 40%, with careful attention to dosing to prevent hypotensive reaction. Another approach is to start the treatment with ACEI in all patients and discontinue it at discharge in patients with preserved LVEF.

Oral ACEI should be started with low dose and titrated to achieve a full dose within 24–48 hours if patient tolerates (3). For example, Captopril can be initiated at a dose of 6.25 mg, followed by 12.5 mg two hours later, 25 mg 10–12 hours later, and then 50 mg twice a day (3,17). To improve the patient's compliance, Captopril can be switched to a single daily dose of ACEI before discharge.

Valsartan, when used with or without captopril, is not superior to captopril alone in reducing all cause mortality in patients after acute myocardial infarction complicated with left ventricular systolic dysfunction. The combination of Valsartan and Captopril actually had more drug-related adverse effects (17a).

Calcium Channel Blockers

Calcium channel blockers (CCBs) have not been shown to improve outcome in patients with ACS (18). In contrast, in patients with LV dysfunction or CHF, a harmful effect was observed. Diltiazem is the only calcium channel blocker that has benefits on clinical outcome in selected patients with ACS (non-Q wave infarction, normal left ventricular function) (18).

Nitrates

No benefit on mortality with routine use of nitrates was observed in the GISSI-3 and ISIS-4 trials (17,19). Nitrates remain, however, the mainstay of therapy for management of ischemia, pulmonary congestion, or hypertension. They should be used with caution in patients with inferior and/or right ventricular wall myocardial infarction for risk of hypotension and bradycardia mediated through decreased preload or vagally-mediated Bezold-Jarisch reflex.

Lipid-Lowering Therapy

Lipid-lowering therapy using statins during hospital admissions for ACS may be associated with a decreased rate of recurrent myocardial infarction and less need for revascularization. Such benefit was thought to be due to plaque stabilization, reduction of inflammation, and improvement of endothelial function, independently of lipid levels. There is no consensus as to how low the lipid should be lowered; however, the emerging view supported by latest results of PROVE-IT trial suggest that there is probably no lower limit for high-risk patients (20,21).

B.   Reperfusion-Therapy Related Measures

Reperfusion strategies and use of antithrombotic/antiplatelet therapies differ in STEMI and NSTEMI/UA.

V.   ST-Elevation Myocardial Infarction

A.   Reperfusion Therapy

Currently the golden rule in treating patients with STEMI is to initiate reperfusion therapy as soon as possible after diagnosis (within 12 hours after onset of symptoms), provided there is no contraindication. The choice of reperfusion therapy between thrombolytic therapy and primary PCI largely depends on the availability of an on-site catheterization laboratory and an interventional team.

Thrombolytic Therapy

Thrombolytic agents can be largely categorized into nonfibrin-specific and fibrin-specific agents. The former includes streptokinase and anisoylated plasminogen streptokinase activator complex (Anistreplase, APSAC), whereas the latter includes tissue plasminogen activator (t-PA) and its derivatives (Reteplase, r-PA; Tenecteplase, TNK-tPA). In general, t-PA achieved higher patency rate (TIMI grade 2 and 3 flow, Table 2) in the infarct-related artery 90 minutes after administration when compared to nonfibrin-specific agents. However, this benefit does not translate to a significant better mortality outcome in the major

Table 2 Thrombolysis in Myocardial Infarction Grading System of Coronary Flow in the Infarct-Related Artery

Grade 0: Complete occlusion of the infarct-related artery
Grade 1: Some penetration of the contrast material beyond the point of obstruction but without perfusion of the distal coronary bed
Grade 2: Perfusion of the entire infarct vessel into the distal bed but with delayed flow compared with a normal artery
Grade 3: Full perfusion of the infarct vessel with normal flow

Source: From Refs. 111 and 112.

clinical trials. Hence, in the authors' opinion, the choice of thrombolytic agents primarily depends on ease of use, cost, and history of prior use of streptokinase. Streptokinase is immunogenic, and pre-existing antibodies may decrease the lytic effects or provoke allergic response when repeatedly administered.

The criteria for thrombolytic therapy are ST elevation greater than 0.1 mV in two or more contiguous leads or left bundle branch block (LBBB), new or old, within 12 hours of onset of symptoms (3). The contraindications for thrombolytic therapy are listed in Table 3. Clinically successful reperfusion can be determined by (22–24):

1. Resolution of ischemic related symptoms (chest pain, dyspnea).
2. Greater than 50% decline in ST-segment elevation within 45–60 minutes from the onset of the first noticeable decrease in ST-segment elevation.
3. Reperfusion arrhythmia, such as accelerated idioventricular rhythm or Bezold–Jarisch reflex.
4. Early rate of rise and time to peak of cardiac enzymes CK and CK isoenzymes or troponin.

A meta-analysis of nine trials with 58,600 patients has demonstrated that the earlier the treatment, the higher the reduction of 35-day mortality rate (25). If the therapy is started within one hour of symptom onset, there is an 3.5% absolute reduction of mortality, whereas there is virtually minimal mortality benefit if the therapy is started after 12 hours of symptom onset.

Table 3 Absolute and Relative Contraindication to Thrombolytic Therapy

Absolute contraindication
1. Active internal bleeding (melena)
2. CVA within the past two months (in many institutions within six months or at anytime)
3. Known CNS neoplasm
4. Recent severe trauma or major surgery within the past two weeks
5. Pregnancy

Relative contraindication
1. Severe hypertension (SBP > 180 mmHg or DBP > 110 mmHg) that does not respond to pharmacological treatment
2. Prolonged CPR (>5–10 min)
3. Diabetic retinopathy
4. Age >75 years

Source: From Ref. 3.

Thrombolytic therapy results in a "lytic state" characterized by hypo-fibrinogenemia, elevated level of fibrinogen degradation products, and depletion of factors V and VIII (26). This "lytic state" puts patients at risk for bleeding complication, which often occurs at vascular puncture sites (about 70%) but can also be spontaneous (27). Intracranial hemorrhage occurs less than 1% in the major clinical trials. It is the most feared complication; it usually occurs within 24 hours of administration of thrombolytic agents and is deadly in half of the inflicted patients (25,26,28,29). The independent predictors associated with intracranial hemorrhage are age >65 years, low body weight (<70 kg), hypertension on presentation, and use of alteplase (3,29,30). The laboratory tests to predict bleeding complication are lack of sensitivity and specificity, hence routine coagulation testing in patients receiving thrombolytic agents without complication is not recommended (26). The best way to reduce bleeding complication is by careful selection of patients for thrombolytic therapy, frequent monitoring by medical personnel, high index of suspicion of bleeding complication, and avoidance of unnecessary procedures. An algorithm for managing bleeding complication should be readily available in the intensive care unit (ICU) (Fig. 2).

Special Patient Groups

>75 *Years of Age.* Age is a powerful independent predictor for in-hospital or six-month postdischarge mortality in patients with ACS (31–33). Patients older than 75 years constitute less than 15% of patients enrolled in trials. The choice of reperfusion therapy in this group of patients is crucial since they tend to have more medical comorbidities and a higher incidence of bleeding complication with thrombolytic therapy. In the GUSTO IIb study, the incidence of bleeding (disabling stroke, hemodynamic compromise, or requiring transfusion) after thrombolysis was about 20% in patients older than 75 years, whereas it was only 9–10% in patients less than 65 years old (34). A large retrospective cohort study suggested thrombolysis could be detrimental in patients older than 75 (35). Several small randomized studies suggested that primary angioplasty had a better clinical outcome (combined end-point of death, nonfatal MI, or stroke) when compared to thrombolytic therapy in this group of patient (32,36).

Patients with Prior Coronary Bypass Graft Surgery. This group constitutes about 3–4% of AMI patients (37,38). Analysis from GUSTO-1 trial indicated that higher mortality in this group of patients compared to STEMI patients without history of coronary bypass graft surgery (CABG) (37). The poorer outcome with thrombolytic therapy may be due to higher thrombus burden or lack of side branch in the vein graft (39). Primary percutaneous intervention (PCI including angioplasty, stenting) may be preferable in this group, although data from randomized trials are lacking.

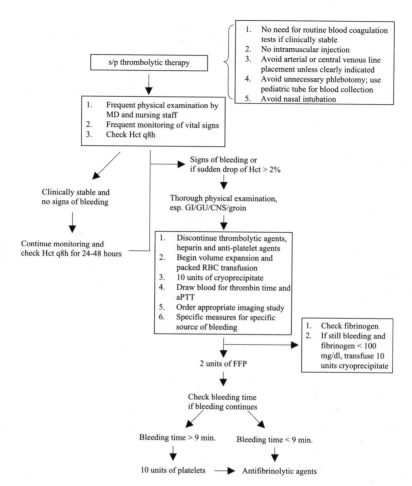

Figure 2 Algorithm for the management of bleeding complication after thrombolytic therapy. *Source*: Based on the authors' experience and adapted from Ref. 26.

Primary PCI

Primary PCI as an initial reperfusion therapy for STEMI depends on the availability of a catheterization laboratory and dedicated interventional teams around the clock. In the U.S., 46.6% of the hospitals contributing to the NRMI-2 database had the capability to perform PCI, but even in these hospitals no more than one-third of these reperfusion attempts were by primary PCI (40).

Primary PCI achieves higher patency rate of infarct-related artery and is associated with less recurrent myocardial ischemia/infarction and less bleeding complication compared to thrombolytic therapy (41,42). With coronary stenting, the incidence of recurrent ischemic events and repeat target vessel revascularization is even less (43–46).

Since most hospitals do not have the capacity to perform primary PCI, the question of how to best reperfuse STEMI patients who presented to a hospital without on-site cardiac catheterization facility often arises. Transfer of patients during AMI is feasible with a low mortality or complication rate (47–50). In these trials (PRAGUE, PRAGUE-2, DANAMI), the mean transport time was less than one hour and resulted in a reduction of the combined end-point of death/reinfarction/stroke at 30 days when compared to thrombolytic therapy (47–49). Wide implementation of transfer strategy with transport time less than one hour would be difficult to achieve in many instances in the U.S.

PCI After Thrombolysis

Successful thrombolytic therapy achieving TIMI 3 flow in the infarct-related artery only occurs in about 50–60% of patients, and 30-day mortality is highest among patients with persistence of complete occlusion (51). Invasive strategies such as "rescue PCI" have been developed to manage this subset of patients who failed thrombolysis. A recent meta-analysis including nine randomized clinical trials and four contemporary registries suggested that PCI after failed thrombolysis (TIMI 0 to 1 flow in the infarct-related artery) appears to reduce the rate of congestive heart failure and improve one-year survival (52).

The efficacy of rescue PCI in patients with sluggish TIMI 2 flow post-thrombolysis is unclear due to limited data from the randomized clinical trials (52).

In several studies, the use of routine balloon angioplasty after successful thrombolysis (TIMI 3 flow) offered no clinical benefit and potentially increased bleeding complication and early re-occlusion of infarct-related artery (53–55). The effect of more recent coronary intervention with stents and GP IIb/IIIa inhibitors has not been adequately studied.

B. Glycoprotein IIb/IIIa Inhibitor

Four randomized trials showed that patients treated with thrombolytic agents (t-PA, streptokinase or reteplase) and glycoprotein (GP) IIb/IIIa inhibitor (abciximab or eptifibatide) experienced higher TIMI 3 flow rate in the infarct-related artery compared to patients receiving thrombolytic agents alone (56–59). However, higher patency rate did not translate to a better 30-day mortality rate (60) but led to a higher bleeding complication (60,61).

The use of GP IIb/IIIa inhibitors with primary PCI for STEMI was tested in four randomized trials (62–65). These trials consistently showed that use of GP IIb/IIIa inhibitors reduced the composite end point of death, recurrent MI, and urgent target vessel revascularization, primarily by the reduction in the rate of urgent target revascularization (66).

C. Anti-Thrombotic Therapy

Due to lack of data from large randomized clinical trials, the role of unfractionated heparin (UFH) in the management of AMI has been controversial (67). Earlier meta-analysis suggested that use of UFH without aspirin reduced short-term mortality (average follow up of 10 days) by 25%. The benefit decreased to 6% when compared to aspirin alone, with a small nonsignificant excess of bleeding complication (68). In elderly STEMI patients who did not receive reperfusion therapy, use of UFH did not decrease the 30-day mortality rate (69). In another randomized trial of STEMI patients not treated with reperfusion therapy but receiving aspirin, UFH or enoxaparin with or without additional GP IIb/IIIa inhibitor treatment had similar 30-day combined end-point of death, reinfarction, and recurrent angina (70).

UFH is therefore recommended during percutaneous or surgical revascularization and in conjunction with thrombolytic agents. In patients receiving alteplase, UFH is started at initiation of alteplase infusion, then maintained for 48 hours with aPTT at 1.5–2.0 times control (50–70 sec). In patients treated with nonselective thrombolytic agents (streptokinase, anistreplase, urokinase) who are at high risk for systemic emboli (large or anterior MI, atrial fibrillation, previous embolus, or known LV thrombus), intravenous UFH heparin is started six hours after thrombolytic therapy. Patients not at high risk for thromboembolic events are treated with subcutaneous injection of UFH or low molecular weight heparin (LMWH). Guidelines also recommend deep vein thrombosis prophylaxis with sq UFH (7500 U bid) (3) or LMWH (enoxaparin 40 mg qd).

VI. NSTEMI/UA

Patients with NSTEMI/UA are a heterogeneous group with distinct clinical outcomes based on their risk profile (71,72). Its treatment is dictated by risk stratification, which aims to detect the presence of adverse characteristics, allowing utilization of different management strategies. Traditional characteristics used for risk stratification, including the history, physical examination, electrocardiogram, and serum markers of myocardial injury, are usually sufficient enough to establish the risk categories. Occasionally, determination of left ventricular function and extent of wall motion abnormalities with echocardiography may help this process.

From the history and physical examination, the risk is increased for a patient who has (1) prolonged rest pain over two hours and still continues at the time of the presentation, (2) patients over 65 years of age, (3) presence of the hemodynamic instability, pulmonary edema, hypotension, ventricular gallop, new or worsening mitral regurgitation, and ventricular arrhythmias. A recent analysis of data of 26,090 patients revealed that Killip classification (Table 4) based on physical examination at presentation of STEMI applies to this group of patients as well. Higher Killip class is associated with higher mortality rate at 30 days and six months (73).

Table 4 Killip Classification of In-Patients with ST
Elevation Myocardial Infarction

Class 1: No evidence of congestive heart failure on physical examination
Class 2: Physical findings consistent with mild to moderate CHF, such as jugular venous distention or lung rales less than half way up the posterior lung fields or an S_3
Class 3: Physical findings demonstrate overt pulmonary edema
Class 4: Patients in cardiogenic shock

Source: From Refs. 113 and 114.

The 12-lead electrocardiogram provides important prognostic information at patient's presentation (4,7,74). ECG should be obtained during a chest pain episode and compared to ECG obtained when symptoms have resolved and to a previous ECG if available. ECG features that are highly suggestive of NSTEMI/UA are (4,7,74):

1. Transient ST depression >1 mm in two contiguous leads associated with symptom (Fig. 3A).
2. Inverted T-wave (>1 mm) in leads with prominent R-wave.
3. Symmetrical and marked (≥ 2 mm) precordial T-wave inversion (Fig. 3B).

Nonspecific ST segment or T-wave changes (ST segment deviation <0.5 mm, T-wave inversion <2 mm) or established Q wave ≥ 0.04 sec are less specific for NSTEMI/UA. A completely normal ECG recorded during chest pain does not exclude the possibility of NSTEMI/UA, because approximately 5% of such patients will eventually develop myocardial infarction (75).

Cardiac troponin is a highly sensitive and specific cardiac enzyme that has been widely accepted as a marker for myocardial necrosis or damage. Although positive troponin can occur in the absence of new coronary occlusion in patients with pulmonary embolism, congestive heart failure, or sepsis, in the clinical context of patients with chest pains, with or without dynamic EKG changes, positive troponin increases the risk of subsequent myocardial infarction or coronary death (76). The interval from the beginning of symptoms to the blood sampling should be more than four hours. Before four hours, there can be up to 40% false negative results.

On the basis of the clinical examination, electrocardiographic findings, and biochemical markers, patients can be risk-stratified into low, intermediate or high short-term risk of death of nonfatal MI. The features of each risk categories are listed in Table 5. These criteria have been validated prospectively by several institutions (including ours) and have been found to be very useful. In our institution, more than 30% patients are of high risk, primarily due to old age; the largest group, with 50% of patients, is of intermediate risk, and approximately 15–20% are of low risk. High-risk patients should be admitted to a monitored

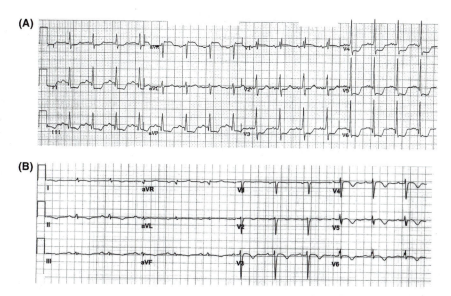

Figure 3 (**A**) 68-year-old male with history of heavy cigarette smoking, coronary artery disease and peripheral vascular disease (aortoiliac bypass and asymptomatic carotid stenosis) presented to ER with substernal tightness and dyspnea. Coronary angiogram showed subtotal distal left main stenosis and triple vessel disease. Troponin peaked at 3.3 ng/mL. Patient underwent successful coronary artery bypass graft surgery. (**B**) 70-year-old female with history of hypercholesterolemia and CABG now presented with recurrent chest pain. Coronary angiogram revealed patent LIMA graft to LAD, a closed RIMA graft to RCA and a nongrafted left circumflex artery (LCx). Angiogram also showed 90% left main stenosis at the bifurcation of LAD and LCx. Patient underwent successful high-risk PCI with placement of drug-eluting stent at distal left main and proximal circumflex artery.

bed/CICU and have a coronary angiography within 24–48 hours if stable with medical management (see below) or immediately when having recurrent episodes of ischemia, ECG changes, or increasing troponin levels.

A. Thrombolytic Therapy

There is no proven role for thrombolytic therapy as an initial reperfusion therapy for NSTEMI. In several randomized clinical trials in the early 1990s, thrombolytic therapy did not improve clinical outcomes (77–81).

B. Invasive vs. Conservative Strategies in Managing NSTEMI/UA

The questions addressed in various clinical trials were: (1) Is early invasive strategy a better management than conservative strategy and (2) if invasive strategy is better, what is the best timing for invasive management?

Table 5 Risk Categories for Patients with NSTEMI/UA

High risk
  1. Prolonged on-going chest pain over 20 minutes
  2. Age over 75
  3. Sustained VT
  4. Pulmonary congestion/edema
  5. Dynamic ST segment depression >1 mm with chest pain
  6. Hypotension
  7. Markedly elevation of cardiac enzymes

Intermediate risk
  1. No high risk features
  2. History of prior MI, PVD, CVA, CABG or prior asipirn use
  3. Rest angina relieved by rest or sublingual NTG
  4. Age over 70
  5. Pathological Q wave
  6. Normal or slightly elevated cardiac enzymes
  7. Dynamic T-wave inversion

Low risk
  1. No high or intermediate risk features
  2. New-onset angina in the past two weeks without greater than
     20 minutes rest pain
  3. Normal or unchanged ECG during chest pain
  4. Normal cardiac enzymes

Abbreviation: CABG, coronary bypass graft surgery.
Source: From Refs. 4 and 74.

Earlier randomized trials such as TIMI IIIb (82) or VANQWISH trials (83) suggested that early invasive strategy did not provide survival benefit. More contemporary studies—FRISC II (84), TACTICS-TIMI 18 (85), and RITA 3 (86)—consistently showed significant reduction of refractory angina (86) or myocardial infarction (84,85) at four- or six-month follow-up in patients receiving early invasive intervention. The FRISC II study showed additional mortality benefit at one-year follow-up (87). Subgroup analysis from TACTICS-TIMI 18 suggested that patients older than 65 years of age, with history of prior MI or diabetes, ST-segment changes on ECG, or positive cardiac enzymes, benefited more from early invasive strategy.

Similarly a 5-year follow up from RITA 3 study suggested routine invasive strategy reduced the risk of death or non-fatal myocardial infarction in high risk patients. (87a)

There is no consensus on the best timing of coronary angiography and PCI with invasive strategy (84,85). In a recent trial of high-risk patients (88), intensive medical treatment with antithrombotic and antiplatelet agents was associated with a higher rate of MI or death at 30 days follow-up compared to early intervention within six hours.

Routine use of early invasive strategy may be hampered by (1) the need for 24-hour availability of catheterization laboratory and personnel; (2) only patients with high risk features benefitting from such aggressive intervention; and (3) possible higher cost (89).

C. Unfractionated Heparin or Low Molecular Weight Heparin in NSTEMI/UA

An early study by Theroux et al. showed a reduction of death, MI, and recurrent ischemia with the use of UFH with or without aspirin compared to placebo (90). This therapy continues to be the cornerstone of the therapy for NSTEMI/UA. Recent studies have compared unfractionated heparin to LMWH. Although in the ESSENCE Trial (91) and TIMI 11B (92) there was a consistent positive effect on the combined endpoint of mortality, recurrent MI, and reduction in the urgent revascularization of the involved vessel, a recently presented larger trial, SYNERGY (93), failed to show any benefit of LMWH when compared to UFH. The study examining Fraxiparine and the Fragmin in ischemic syndromes also did not demonstrate an advantage of LMWH over UFH. When analyzed together, these studies suggest that there is a modest advantage of enoxaparine over UFH in high-risk patients.

Either UFH or LMWH can be discontinued within 24 hours in the absence of symptoms. Observation study has suggested that unstable angina symptoms may be reactivated after heparin is discontinued, but this "rebound phenomenon" can be prevented by concomitant use of aspirin (94). The long-term use of LMWH in outpatients has not proven to be beneficial. The use of LMWH in the treatment of ACS has been hampered by the concerns about its safety during coronary interventions, especially in conjunction with the GPIIb/IIIa inhibitors.

D. Platelet GP IIb/IIa Inhibitors

Platelet activation and aggregation via glycoprotein IIb/IIIa (GP IIb/IIIa) receptors play a pivotal role in the pathogenesis of ACS. Intravenous GP IIb/IIIa receptor inhibitors are abciximab, lamifiban, tirofiban, and eptifibatide, which were tested in four randomized clinical trials (abciximab in GUSTO-IV ACS, Tirofiban in PRISM [95] and PRISM-PLUS [96], Epitifibatide in PURSUIT [97], and Lamifiban in PARAGON [98]) to evaluate their efficacy in reducing clinical events (death, MI, or refractory angina) in patients with NSTEMI/UA. The GUSTO IV-ACS trial investigated the effect of intravenous abciximab on outcome in NSTEMI/UA patients without early coronary revascularization. At 30 days and one year, there was no survival benefit in patients receiving abciximab when compared to placebo. Subgroup analysis did not reveal any benefit in high-risk patients either (99,100). Earlier trials (PRISM, PRISM-PLUS with tirofiban, PURSUIT with eptifibatide, and PARAGON with lamifiban) have shown a small reduction of short-term event rates of combined end-points death, MI, or refractory angina. However, reduction in short-term mortality alone was not consistent. Subgroup analysis from these trials suggested that patients with high-risk features may benefit more from the use of IIb/IIIa inhibitors (95,97,100).

The efficacy of intravenous GPIIb/IIIa inhibitors in reducing clinical events in patients with NSTEMI/UA undergoing PCI was also tested in clinical trials—abciximab in EPILOG (101) and CAPTURE (102), Tirofiban in RESTORE (103). The EPILOG and CAPTURE trials with abciximab showed a reduction of 30-day composite end-point of death, MI, re-infarction, and urgent or repeat revascularization, whereas the RESTORE trial with tirofiban showed a reduction of combined event rates only in the first seven days after PCI. A recent meta-analysis of 19 trials with more than 20,000 patients showed a 31% relative reduction in 30-day mortality (absolute reduction from 1.37% in placebo group to 0.9% in treatment group) (104).

In contrast to the clinical benefit of intravenous GP IIb/IIIa antagonists, oral GP IIb/IIIa antagonists such as xemilofiban, orbofiban, and sibrafiban showed no clinical benefit but increased risk of bleeding (105).

Taking all these together, overall data suggest that use of intravenous GP IIb/IIIa inhibitors is beneficial in high-risk patients with NSTEMI/UA undergoing PCI.

E. Ticlopidine and Clopidogrel

Ticlopidine and clopidogrel belong to the thienopyridines class and are adenosine diphosphate (ADP) antagonists that can cause irreversible blockade of ADP-induced platelet-fibrinogen binding. Currently, clopidogrel is preferred to ticlopidine because of its faster inhibition of platelets and more favorable safety profile (less fatal neutropenia or thrombotic thrombocytopenic purpura) (4,106).

In the CURE trial, treatment with clopidogrel was associated with a 2.1% absolute reduction in the composite end-point of cardiovascular death, MI, and stroke compared to placebo for a mean duration of nine months. At 30 days, there was a 0.9% reduction in death or MI, an effect that was similar to the effects of GP IIb/IIIa inhibitors. There was a 1% increase in major bleeding. The use of clopidogrel is associated with a risk of excessive bleeding if the patient is referred for immediate surgical revascularization. In our institution, clopidogrel is withheld until diagnostic angiography is performed.

Current ACC/AHA guidelines recommend aspirin as the first line antiplatelet therapy, and clopidogrel is used in patients who are unable to take aspirin due to hypersensitity or major GI contraindication (recent significant bleeding from peptic ulcer or gastritis). Based on the CURE trial, use of clopidogrel with aspirin is also recommended in patients for whom an early noninterventional approach is planned (5). Many physicians prescribe clopidogrel to the majority of patients admitted for ACS, in part due to the obligatory use of clopidogrel in patients who received stents.

F. Predischarge Stress Testing

Patients treated medically and stable for >24–48 hours can be risk stratified prior to discharge with a noninvasive stress test. Those with high risk results (Table 6) should be referred to coronary angiography to delineate coronary anatomy and for possible PCI or surgical revascularization prior to discharge.

VII. Positive Cardiac Enzyme in Noncardiac Critically Ill Patients

Not uncommonly, noncardiac critically ill patients in the ICU have an elevated level of cardiac troponin (107,108), usually not higher than 10-fold of the detection limit. The mechanism(s) underlying this increase is likely related to release of the cytoplasmic portion of troponin with hypotension. This troponin "leak" is often not associated with significant flow-limiting coronary artery disease but is nevertheless associated with higher mortality rate, lower left ventricular ejection fraction, and sepsis, and it is associated with the more frequent need for mechanical ventilation or longer ICU stay (109).

The management of this subset of patients is complicated because these patients often have multiple medical comorbidities with complex and critical acute illness. The management decision should be made on an individual basis. In the authors' opinion, early reperfusion therapy with PCI as the preferred reperfusion strategy may be beneficial in patients with clinical evidence of myocardial ischemia (ST elevation or depression on ECG) or hemodynamic instability from ACS, provided there is no contraindication to procedures and aggressive anticoagulation and antiplatelet regimen mandated by PCI. Otherwise, cardiac risk stratification should await stabilization of the patient's noncardiac medical conditions. Risk stratification can be done either before discharge or on an early outpatient basis. In the interim, antiplatelet and antithrombotic therapy can be initiated if there is no contraindication.

Table 6 High Risk Features on Risk Stratification by Noninvasive Stress Test

1. Resting LV dysfunction with LVEF <35%
2. Signs of ischemia at low level of exercise (angina during exercise, exercise capacity <6 METS, stress-induced LV dysfunction)
3. Stress-induced large perfusion defect or multiple perfusion defects of moderate size
4. Hypotension during exercise
5. Ventricular tachycardia during exercise
6. Increased pulmonary radiotracer uptake after exercise
7. Transient LV dilatation immediately after exercise

Source: From Refs. 4 and 74.

VIII. Summary

With the advancement of treatment strategies, the mortality of ACS has been decreasing. However, there are still many patients suffering from ACS due to the high prevalence of atherosclerosis. Each ACS patient should be counseled for aggressive risk factors modification, including lipid lowering, smoking cessation, DM and hypertension control, exercise, and diet.

References

1. Rogers WJ, Canto JG, Lambrew CT, Tiefenbrunn AJ, Kinkaid B, Shoultz DA, Frederick PD, Every N. Temporal trends in the treatment of over 1.5 million patients with myocardial infarction in the US from 1990 through 1999: the National Registry of Myocardial Infarction 1, 2 and 3. J Am Coll Cardiol 2000; 36:2056–2063.
2. Falk E, Shah PK, Fuster V. Coronary plaque disruption. Circulation 1995; 92: 657–671.
3. Ryan TJ, Anderson JL, Antman EM, Braniff BA, Brooks NH, Califf RM, Hillis LD, Hiratzka LF, Rapaport E, Riegel BJ, Russell RO, Smith EEJ, Weaver WD. ACC/AHA guidelines for the management of patients with acute myocardial infarction. A report of the American College of Cardiology/American Heart Association Task Force on Practice Guidelines (Committee on Management of Acute Myocardial Infarction). J Am Coll Cardiol 1996; 28:1328–1428.
4. Braunwald E, Antman EM, Beasley JW, Califf RM, Cheitlin MD, Hochman JS, Jones RH, Kereiakes D, Kupersmith J, Levin TN, Pepine CJ, Schaeffer JW, Smith EE, Steward DE, Theroux P, Alpert JS, Eagle KA, Faxon DP, Fuster V, Gardner TJ, Gregoratos G, Russell RO, Smith SCJ. ACC/AHA guidelines for the management of patients with unstable angina and non-ST-segment elevation myocardial infarction. A report of the American College of Cardiology/American Heart Association Task Force on Practice Guidelines (Committee on the Management of Patients With Unstable Angina). J Am Coll Cardiol 2000; 36:970–1062.
5. Braunwald E, Antman EM, Beasley JW, Califf RM, Cheitlin MD, Hochman JS, Jones RH, Kereiakes D, Kupersmith J, Levin TN, Pepine CJ, Schaeffer JW, Smith EE, Steward DE, Theroux P, Gibbons RJ, Alpert JS, Faxon DP, Fuster V, Gregoratos G, Hiratzka LF, Jacobs AK, Smith SCJ. ACC/AHA 2002 guideline update for the management of patients with unstable angina and non-ST-segment elevation myocardial infarction—summary article: a report of the American College of Cardiology/American Heart Association task force on practice guidelines (Committee on the Management of Patients With Unstable Angina). J Am Coll Cardiol 2002; 40:1366–1374.
6. Ryan TJ, Antman EM, Brooks NH, Califf RM, Hillis LD, Hiratzka LF, Rapaport E, Riegel B, Russell RO, Smith EE, Weaver WD, Gibbons RJ, Alpert JS, Eagle KA, Gardner TJ, Garson AJ, Gregoratos G, Smith SCJ. 1999 update: ACC/AHA guidelines for the management of patients with acute myocardial infarction. A report of the American College of Cardiology/American Heart Association Task Force on Practice Guidelines (Committee on Management of Acute Myocardial Infarction). J Am Coll Cardiol 1999; 34:890–911.

7. Bertrand ME, Simoons ML, Fox KA, Wallentin LC, Hamm CW, McFadden E, de FP, Specchia G, Ruzyllo W. Management of acute coronary syndromes: acute coronary syndromes without persistent ST segment elevation; recommendations of the Task Force of the European Society of Cardiology. Eur Heart J 2000; 21: 1406–1432.

8. ISIS-2.ISIS-2 (Second International Study of Infarct Survival) Collaborative Group. Randomized trial of intravenous streptokinase, oral aspirin, both, or neither among 17,187 cases of suspected acute myocardial infarction. J Am Coll Cardiol 1988; 12:3A–13A.

9. The MIAMI Trial Research Group. Metoprolol in acute myocardial infarction (MIAMI). A randomised placebo-controlled international trial. Eur Heart J 1985; 6:199–226.

10. First International Study of Infarct Survival Collaborative Group. Randomised trial of intravenous atenolol among 16,027 cases of suspected acute myocardial infarction: ISIS-1. Lancet 1986; 2:57–66.

11. Roberts R, Rogers WJ, Mueller HS, Lambrew CT, Diver DJ, Smith HC, Willerson JT, Knatterud GL, Forman S, Passamani E. Immediate versus deferred beta-blockade following thrombolytic therapy in patients with acute myocardial infarction. Results of the Thrombolysis in Myocardial Infarction (TIMI) II-B Study. Circulation 1991; 83:422–437.

12. Freemantle N, Cleland J, Young P, Mason J, Harrison J. Beta-blockade after myocardial infarction: systematic review and meta regression analysis. Brit Med J 1999; 318:1730–1737.

13. Gheorghiade M, Goldstein S. Beta-blockers in the post-myocardial infarction patient. Circulation 2002; 106:394–398.

14. Chen J, Radford MJ, Wang Y, Marciniak TA, Krumholz HM. Effectiveness of beta-blocker therapy after acute myocardial infarction in elderly patients with chronic obstructive pulmonary disease or asthma. J Am Coll Cardiol 2001; 37:1950–1956.

15. Radack K, Deck C. Beta-adrenergic blocker therapy does not worsen intermittent claudication in subjects with peripheral arterial disease. A meta-analysis of randomized controlled trials. Arch Intern Med 1991; 151:1769–1776.

16. Opie LH. The new trials: AIRE, ISIS-4, and GISSI-3. Is the dossier on ACE inhibitors and myocardial infarction now complete? Cardiovasc Drugs Ther 1994; 8:469–472.

17. ISIS-4 (Fourth International Study of Infarct Survival) Collaborative Group. ISIS-4: a randomised factorial trial assessing early oral captopril, oral mononitrate, and intravenous magnesium sulphate in 58,050 patients with suspected acute myocardial infarction. Lancet 1995; 345:669–685.

17a. Marc A. Pfeffer, John J.V. McMurray, Eric J. Velazquez, Jean-Lucien Rouleau, Lars Køber, Aldo P. Maggioni, Scott D. Solomon, Karl Swedberg, Frans Van de Werf, Harvey White, Jeffrey D. Leimberger, Marc Henis, Susan Edwards, Steven Zelenkofske, D.O., Mary Ann Sellers, M.S.N., Robert M. Califf. Valsartan in acute myocardial infarction trial investigators. Valsartan, captopril, or both in myocardial infarction complicated by heart failure, left ventricular dysfunction, or both. N Engl J Med. 2003; 13:1893–1906.

18. Gibson RS. Current status of calcium channel-blocking drugs after Q wave and non-Q wave myocardial infarction. Circulation 1989; 80:IV107–IV119.

19. Gruppo Italiano per lo Studio della Sopravvivenza nell'infarto Miocardico. GISSI-3: effects of lisinopril and transdermal glyceryl trinitrate singly and together on 6-week mortality and ventricular function after acute myocardial infarction. Lancet 1994; 343:1115–1122.

20. Pepine CJ. Optimizing lipid management in patients with acute coronary syndromes. Am J Cardiol 2003; 91:30B–35B.

21. Spin JM, Vagelos RH. Early use of statins in acute coronary syndromes. Curr Cardiol Rep 2002; 4:289–297.

22. Shah PK, Cercek B, Lew AS, Ganz W. Angiographic validation of bedside markers of reperfusion. J Am Coll Cardiol 1993; 21:55–61.

23. de Lemos J, Morrow DA, Gibson CM, Murphy SA, Rifai N, Tanasijevic M, Giugliano RP, Schuhwerk KC, McCabe CH, Cannon CP, Antman EM, Braunwald E. Early noninvasive detection of failed epicardial reperfusion after fibrinolytic therapy. Am J Cardiol 2001; 88:353–358.

24. de Lemos J, Braunwald E. ST segment resolution as a tool for assessing the efficacy of reperfusion therapy. J Am Coll Cardiol 2001; 38:1283–1294.

25. Fibrinolytic Therapy Trialists' (FTT) Collaborative Group. Indications for fibrinolytic therapy in suspected acute myocardial infarction: collaborative overview of early mortality and major morbidity results from all randomised trials of more than 1000 patients. Lancet 1994; 343:311–322.

26. Sane DC, Califf RM, Topol EJ, Stump DC, Mark DB, Greenberg CS. Bleeding during thrombolytic therapy for acute myocardial infarction: mechanisms and management. Ann Intern Med 1989; 111:1010–1022.

27. Rao AK, Pratt C, Berke A, Jaffe A, Ockene I, Schreiber TL, Bell WR, Knatterud G, Robertson TL, Terrin ML. Thrombolysis in Myocardial Infarction (TIMI) Trial—phase I: hemorrhagic manifestations and changes in plasma fibrinogen and the fibrinolytic system in patients treated with recombinant tissue plasminogen activator and streptokinase. J Am Coll Cardiol 1988; 11:1–11.

28. Levine MN, Goldhaber SZ, Gore JM, Hirsh J, Califf RM. Hemorrhagic complications of thrombolytic therapy in the treatment of myocardial infarction and venous thromboembolism. Chest 1995; 108:291S–301S.

29. De Jaegere P, Arnold AA, Balk AH, Simoons ML. Intracranial hemorrhage in association with thrombolytic therapy: incidence and clinical predictive factors. J Am Coll Cardiol 1992; 19:289–294.

30. Simoons ML, Maggioni AP, Knatterud G, Leimberger JD, de JP, van DR, Boersma E, Franzosi MG, Califf R, Schroder R. Individual risk assessment for intracranial haemorrhage during thrombolytic therapy. Lancet 1993; 342:1523–1528.

31. Maggioni AP, Maseri A, Fresco C, Franzosi MG, Mauri F, Santoro E, Tognoni G. Age-related increase in mortality among patients with first myocardial infarctions treated with thrombolysis. The Investigators of the Gruppo Italiano per lo Studio della Sopravvivenza nell'Infarto Miocardico (GISSI-2). N Engl J Med 1993; 329:1442–1448.

32. Holmes DRJ, White HD, Pieper KS, Ellis SG, Califf RM, Topol EJ. Effect of age on outcome with primary angioplasty versus thrombolysis. J Am Coll Cardiol 1999; 33:412–419.

33. Granger CB, Goldberg RJ, Dabbous O, Pieper KS, Eagle KA, Cannon CP, Van DW, Avezum A, Goodman SG, Flather MD, Fox KA. Predictors of hospital

mortality in the global registry of acute coronary events. Arch Intern Med 2003; 163:2345–2353.

34. White HD, Barbash GI, Califf RM, Simes RJ, Granger CB, Weaver WD, Kleiman NS, Aylward PE, Gore JM, Vahanian A, Lee KL, Ross AM, Topol EJ. Age and outcome with contemporary thrombolytic therapy. Results from the GUSTO-I trial. Global Utilization of Streptokinase and TPA for Occluded coronary arteries trial. Circulation 1996; 94:1826–1833.

35. Thiemann DR, Coresh J, Schulman SP, Gerstenblith G, Oetgen WJ, Powe NR. Lack of benefit for intravenous thrombolysis in patients with myocardial infarction who are older than 75 years. Circulation 2000; 101:2239–2246.

36. de BM, Ottervanger JP, Van't Hof AW, Hoorntje JC, Suryapranata H, Zijlstra F. Reperfusion therapy in elderly patients with acute myocardial infarction: a randomized comparison of primary angioplasty and thrombolytic therapy. J Am Coll Cardiol 2002; 39:1723–1728.

37. Labinaz M, Sketch MHJ, Ellis SG, Abramowitz BM, Stebbins AL, Pieper KS, Holmes DRJ, Califf RM, Topol EJ. Outcome of acute ST-segment elevation myocardial infarction in patients with prior coronary artery bypass surgery receiving thrombolytic therapy. Am Heart J 2001; 141:469–477.

38. Zahger D, Behar S, Harpaz D, Leor J, Weiss AT, Gottlieb S. Characteristics, management and outcome of patients with prior coronary bypass surgery presenting with acute myocardial infarction. Cardiology 2003; 99:105–110.

39. Zahger D, Cercek B, Cannon CP, Jordan M, Shah PK. Thrombolytic therapy for acute myocardial infarction in patients with prior coronary bypass surgery: results from the Thrombolysis in Myocardial Infarction (TIMI) 4 trial. J Thromb Thrombolysis 1995; 2:45–50.

40. Rogers WJ, Canto JG, Barron HV, Boscarino JA, Shoultz DA, Every NR. Treatment and outcome of myocardial infarction in hospitals with and without invasive capability. Investigators in the National Registry of Myocardial Infarction. J Am Coll Cardiol 2000; 35:371–379.

41. Weaver WD, Simes RJ, Betriu A, Grines CL, Zijlstra F, Garcia E, Grinfeld L, Gibbons RJ, Ribeiro EE, DeWood MA, Ribichini F. Comparison of primary coronary angioplasty and intravenous thrombolytic therapy for acute myocardial infarction: a quantitative review. J Am Med Assoc 1997; 278:2093–2098.

42. Zijlstra F, Hoorntje JC, de BM, Reiffers S, Miedema K, Ottervanger JP, van, Suryapranata H. Long-term benefit of primary angioplasty as compared with thrombolytic therapy for acute myocardial infarction. N Engl J Med. 1999; 341:1413–1419.

43. Le MM, Labinaz M, Davies RF, Marquis JF, Laramee LA, O'Brien ER, Williams WL, Beanlands RS, Nichol G, Higginson LA. Stenting versus thrombolysis in acute myocardial infarction trial (STAT). J Am Coll Cardiol 2001; 37:985–991.

44. Goldenberg I, Matetzky S, Halkin A, Roth A, Di SE, Freimark D, Elian D, Agranat O, Har ZY, Guetta V, Hod H. Primary angioplasty with routine stenting compared with thrombolytic therapy in elderly patients with acute myocardial infarction. Am Heart J 2003; 145:862–867.

45. Schomig A, Kastrati A, Dirschinger J, Mehilli J, Schricke U, Pache J, Martinoff S, Neumann FJ, Schwaiger M. Coronary stenting plus platelet glycoprotein IIb/IIIa

blockade compared with tissue plasminogen activator in acute myocardial infarction. Stent versus Thrombolysis for Occluded Coronary Arteries in Patients with Acute Myocardial Infarction Study Investigators. N Engl J Med 2000; 343:385–391.

46. Kastrati A, Mehilli J, Dirschinger J, Schricke U, Neverve J, Pache J, Martinoff S, Neumann FJ, Nekolla S, Blasini R, Seyfarth M, Schwaiger M, Schomig A. Myocardial salvage after coronary stenting plus abciximab versus fibrinolysis plus abciximab in patients with acute myocardial infarction: a randomised trial. Lancet 2002; 359:920–925.

47. Zijlstra F, Van't Hof AW, Liem AL, Hoorntje JC, Suryapranata H, de BM. Transferring patients for primary angioplasty: a retrospective analysis of 104 selected high risk patients with acute myocardial infarction. Heart 1997; 78:333–336.

48. Vermeer F, Oude OA, vd BE, Brunninkhuis LG, Werter CJ, Boehmer AG, Lousberg AH, Dassen WR, Bar FW. Prospective randomised comparison between thrombolysis, rescue PTCA, and primary PTCA in patients with extensive myocardial infarction admitted to a hospital without PTCA facilities: a safety and feasibility study. Heart 1999; 82:426–431.

49. Widimsky P, Groch L, Zelizko M, Aschermann M, Bednar F, Suryapranata H. Multicentre randomized trial comparing transport to primary angioplasty vs immediate thrombolysis vs combined strategy for patients with acute myocardial infarction presenting to a community hospital without a catheterization laboratory. The PRAGUE study. Eur Heart J 2000; 21:823–831.

50. Andersen HR, Nielsen TT, Rasmussen K, Thuesen L, Kelbaek H, Thayssen P, Abildgaard U, Pedersen F, Madsen JK, Grande P, Villadsen AB, Krusell LR, Haghfelt T, Lomholt P, Husted SE, Vigholt E, Kjaergard HK, Mortensen LS. A comparison of coronary angioplasty with fibrinolytic therapy in acute myocardial infarction. N Engl J Med 2003; 349:733–742.

51. The GUSTO Angiographic Investigators. The effects of tissue plasminogen activator, streptokinase, or both on coronary-artery patency, ventricular function, and survival after acute myocardial infarction. N Engl J Med 1993; 329:1615–1622.

52. Ellis SG, Da SE, Spaulding CM, Nobuyoshi M, Weiner B, Talley JD. Review of immediate angioplasty after fibrinolytic therapy for acute myocardial infarction: insights from the RESCUE I, RESCUE II, and other contemporary clinical experiences. Am Heart J 2000; 139:1046–1053.

53. Topol EJ, Califf RM, George BS, Kereiakes DJ, Abbottsmith CW, Candela RJ, Lee KL, Pitt B, Stack RS, O'Neill WW. A randomized trial of immediate versus delayed elective angioplasty after intravenous tissue plasminogen activator in acute myocardial infarction. N Engl J Med 1987; 317:581–588.

54. The TIMI Research Group. Immediate vs delayed catheterization and angioplasty following thrombolytic therapy for acute myocardial infarction. TIMI II A results. JAMA 1988; 260:2849–2858.

55. Simoons ML, Arnold AE, Betriu A, De BD, Col J, Dougherty FC, von ER, Lambertz H, Lubsen J, Meier B. Thrombolysis with tissue plasminogen activator in acute myocardial infarction: no additional benefit from immediate percutaneous coronary angioplasty. Lancet 1988; 1:197–203.

56. Antman EM, Gibson CM, de Lemos J, Giugliano RP, McCabe CH, Coussement P, Menown I, Nienaber CA, Rehders TC, Frey MJ, Van dW, Andresen D, Scherer J, Anderson K, Van DW, Braunwald E. Combination reperfusion therapy with abciximab and reduced dose reteplase: results from TIMI 14. The Thrombolysis in Myocardial Infarction (TIMI) 14 Investigators. Eur Heart J 2000; 21:1944–1953.

57. Ohman EM, Kleiman NS, Gacioch G, Worley SJ, Navetta FI, Talley JD, Anderson HV, Ellis SG, Cohen MD, Spriggs D, Miller M, Kereiakes D, Yakubov S, Kitt MM, Sigmon KN, Califf RM, Krucoff MW, Topol EJ. Combined accelerated tissue-plasminogen activator and platelet glycoprotein IIb/IIIa integrin receptor blockade with Integrilin in acute myocardial infarction. Results of a randomized, placebo-controlled, dose-ranging trial. IMPACT-AMI Investigators. Circulation 1997; 95:846–854.

58. Brener SJ, Zeymer U, Adgey AA, Vrobel TR, Ellis SG, Neuhaus KL, Juran N, Ivanc TB, Ohman EM, Strony J, Kitt M, Topol EJ. Eptifibatide and low-dose tissue plasminogen activator in acute myocardial infarction: the integrilin and low-dose thrombolysis in acute myocardial infarction (INTRO AMI) trial. J Am Coll Cardiol 2002; 39:377–386.

59. Strategies for Patency Enhancement in the Emergency Department (SPEED) Group. Trial of abciximab with and without low-dose reteplase for acute myocardial infarction. Circulation 2000; 101:2788–2794.

60. Topol EJ. Reperfusion therapy for acute myocardial infarction with fibrinolytic therapy or combination reduced fibrinolytic therapy and platelet glycoprotein IIb/IIIa inhibition: the GUSTO V randomised trial. Lancet 2001; 357:1905–1914.

61. Efficacy and safety of tenecteplase in combination with enoxaparin, abciximab, or unfractionated heparin: the ASSENT-3 randomised trial in acute myocardial infarction. Lancet 2001; 358:605–613.

62. Brener SJ, Barr LA, Burchenal JE, Katz S, George BS, Jones AA, Cohen ED, Gainey PC, White HJ, Cheek HB, Moses JW, Moliterno DJ, Effron MB, Topol EJ. Randomized, placebo-controlled trial of platelet glycoprotein IIb/IIIa blockade with primary angioplasty for acute myocardial infarction. ReoPro and Primary PTCA Organization and Randomized Trial (RAPPORT) Investigators. Circulation 1998; 98:734–741.

63. Neumann FJ, Kastrati A, Schmitt C, Blasini R, Hadamitzky M, Mehilli J, Gawaz M, Schleef M, Seyfarth M, Dirschinger J, Schomig A. Effect of glycoprotein IIb/IIIa receptor blockade with abciximab on clinical and angiographic restenosis rate after the placement of coronary stents following acute myocardial infarction. J Am Coll Cardiol 2000; 35:915–921.

64. Montalescot G, Barragan P, Wittenberg O, Ecollan P, Elhadad S, Villain P, Boulenc JM, Morice MC, Maillard L, Pansieri M, Choussat R, Pinton P. Platelet glycoprotein IIb/IIIa inhibition with coronary stenting for acute myocardial infarction. N Engl J Med 2001; 344:1895–1903.

65. Stone GW, Grines CL, Cox DA, Garcia E, Tcheng JE, Griffin JJ, Guagliumi G, Stuckey T, Turco M, Carroll JD, Rutherford BD, Lansky AJ. Comparison of angioplasty with stenting, with or without abciximab, in acute myocardial infarction. N Engl J Med 2002; 346:957–966.

66. Eisenberg MJ, Jamal S. Glycoprotein IIb/IIIa inhibition in the setting of acute ST-segment elevation myocardial infarction. J Am Coll Cardiol 2003; 42:1–6.

67. Rich MW. Heparin for acute myocardial infarction: the controversy continues. J Am Coll Cardiol 1998; 31:964–966.

68. Collins R, MacMahon S, Flather M, Baigent C, Remvig L, Mortensen S, Appleby P, Godwin J, Yusuf S, Peto R. Clinical effects of anticoagulant therapy in suspected acute myocardial infarction: systematic overview of randomised trials. Brit Med J 1996; 313:652–659.

69. Krumholz HM, Hennen J, Ridker PM, Murillo JE, Wang Y, Vaccarino V, Ellerbeck EF, Radford MJ. Use and effectiveness of intravenous heparin therapy for treatment of acute myocardial infarction in the elderly. J Am Coll Cardiol 1998; 31:973–979.

70. Cohen M, Gensini GF, Maritz F, Gurfinkel EP, Huber K, Timerman A, Krzeminska-Pakula M, Danchin N, White HD, Santopinto J, Bigonzi F, Hecquet C, Vittori L. The safety and efficacy of subcutaneous enoxaparin versus intravenous unfractionated heparin and tirofiban versus placebo in the treatment of acute ST-segment elevation myocardial infarction patients ineligible for reperfusion (TETAMI): a randomized trial. J Am Coll Cardiol 2003; 42:1348–1356.

71. Prasad A, Mathew V, Holmes DRJ, Gersh BJ. Current management of non-ST-segment-elevation acute coronary syndrome: reconciling the results of randomized controlled trials. Eur Heart J 2003; 24:1544–1553.

72. Braunwald E. Application of current guidelines to the management of unstable angina and non-ST-elevation myocardial infarction. Circulation 2003; 108: III28–III37.

73. Khot UN, Jia G, Moliterno DJ, Lincoff AM, Khot MB, Harrington RA, Topol EJ. Prognostic importance of physical examination for heart failure in non-ST-elevation acute coronary syndromes: the enduring value of Killip classification. J Am Med Assoc 2003; 290:2174–2181.

74. Mody VH, Faxon DP. Management of unstable angina: integrating the new approaches. Rev Cardiovasc Med 2000; 1:104–119.

75. Rouan GW, Lee TH, Cook EF, Brand DA, Weisberg MC, Goldman L. Clinical characteristics and outcome of acute myocardial infarction in patients with initially normal or nonspecific electrocardiograms (a report from the Multicenter Chest Pain Study). Am J Cardiol 1989; 64:1087–1092.

76. Antman EM, Tanasijevic MJ, Thompson B, Schactman M, McCabe CH, Cannon CP, Fischer GA, Fung AY, Thompson C, Wybenga D, Braunwald E. Cardiac-specific troponin I levels to predict the risk of mortality in patients with acute coronary syndromes. N Engl J Med 1996; 335:1342–1349.

77. Williams DO, Topol EJ, Califf RM, Roberts R, Mancini GB, Joelson JM, Ellis SG, Kleiman NS. Intravenous recombinant tissue-type plasminogen activator in patients with unstable angina pectoris. Results of a placebo-controlled, randomized trial. Circulation 1990; 82:376–383.

78. Schreiber TL, Rizik D, White C, Sharma GV, Cowley M, Macina G, Reddy PS, Kantounis L, Timmis GC, Margulis A. Randomized trial of thrombolysis versus heparin in unstable angina. Circulation 1992; 86:1407–1414.

79. Bar FW, Verheugt FW, Col J, Materne P, Monassier JP, Geslin PG, Metzger J, Raynaud P, Foucault J, de ZC. Thrombolysis in patients with unstable angina improves the angiographic but not the clinical outcome. Results of UNASEM, a

multicenter, randomized, placebo-controlled, clinical trial with anistreplase. Circulation 1992; 86:131–137.

80. Freeman MR, Langer A, Wilson RF, Morgan CD, Armstrong PW. Thrombolysis in unstable angina. Randomized double-blind trial of t-PA and placebo. Circulation 1992; 85:150–157.

81. Effects of tissue plasminogen activator and a comparison of early invasive and conservative strategies in unstable angina and non-Q-wave myocardial infarction. Results of the TIMI IIIB Trial. Thrombolysis in Myocardial Ischemia. Circulation 1994; 89:1545–1556.

82. Anderson HV, Cannon CP, Stone PH, Williams DO, McCabe CH, Knatterud GL, Thompson B, Willerson JT, Braunwald E. One-year results of the Thrombolysis in Myocardial Infarction (TIMI) IIIB clinical trial. A randomized comparison of tissue-type plasminogen activator versus placebo and early invasive versus early conservative strategies in unstable angina and non-Q wave myocardial infarction. J Am Coll Cardiol 1995; 26:1643–1650.

83. Boden WE, O'Rourke RA, Crawford MH, Blaustein AS, Deedwania PC, Zoble RG, Wexler LF, Kleiger RE, Pepine CJ, Ferry DR, Chow BK, Lavori PW. Outcomes in patients with acute non-Q-wave myocardial infarction randomly assigned to an invasive as compared with a conservative management strategy. Veterans Affairs Non-Q-Wave Infarction Strategies in Hospital (VANQWISH) Trial Investigators. N Engl J Med 1998; 338:1785–1792.

84. FRISC: FRagmin and Fast Revascularisation during InStability in Coronary artery disease Investigators. Invasive compared with non-invasive treatment in unstable coronary-artery disease: FRISC II prospective randomised multicentre study. Lancet 1999; 354:708–715.

85. Cannon CP, Weintraub WS, Demopoulos LA, Vicari R, Frey MJ, Lakkis N, Neumann FJ, Robertson DH, DeLucca PT, DiBattiste PM, Gibson CM, Braunwald E. Comparison of early invasive and conservative strategies in patients with unstable coronary syndromes treated with the glycoprotein IIb/IIIa inhibitor tirofiban. N Engl J Med 2001; 344:1879–1887.

86. Fox KA, Poole-Wilson PA, Henderson RA, Clayton TC, Chamberlain DA, Shaw TR, Wheatley DJ, Pocock SJ. Interventional versus conservative treatment for patients with unstable angina or non-ST-elevation myocardial infarction: the British Heart Foundation RITA 3 randomised trial. Randomized Intervention Trial of unstable Angina. Lancet 2002; 360:743–751.

87. Wallentin L, Lagerqvist B, Husted S, Kontny F, Stahle E, Swahn E. Outcome at 1 year after an invasive compared with a non-invasive strategy in unstable coronary-artery disease: the FRISC II invasive randomised trial. FRISC II Investigators. Fast Revascularisation during Instability in Coronary artery disease. Lancet 2000; 356:9–16.

87a. Fox KA, Poole-Wilson P, Clayton TC, Henderson RA, Shaw TR, Wheatley DJ, Knight R, Pocock, SJ. 5-year outcome of an interventional strategy in non-ST-elevation acute coronary syndrome: the British Heart Foundation RITA 3 randomised trial. Lancet. 2005; 10:914–920.

88. Neumann FJ, Kastrati A, Pogatsa-Murray G, Mehilli J, Bollwein H, Bestehorn HP, Schmitt C, Seyfarth M, Dirschinger J, Schomig A. Evaluation of prolonged antithrombotic pretreatment ("cooling-off" strategy) before intervention in

patients with unstable coronary syndromes: a randomized controlled trial. J Am Med Assoc 2003; 290:1593–1599.

89. Mahoney EM, Jurkovitz CT, Chu H, Becker ER, Culler S, Kosinski AS, Robertson DH, Alexander C, Nag S, Cook JR, Demopoulos LA, DiBattiste PM, Cannon CP, Weintraub WS. Cost and cost-effectiveness of an early invasive vs conservative strategy for the treatment of unstable angina and non-ST-segment elevation myocardial infarction. J Am Med Assoc 2002; 288:1851–1858.

90. Theroux P, Ouimet H, McCans J, Latour JG, Joly P, Levy G, Pelletier E, Juneau M, Stasiak J, deGuise P. Aspirin, heparin, or both to treat acute unstable angina. N Engl J Med 1988; 319:1105–1111.

91. Cohen M, Demers C, Gurfinkel EP, Turpie AG, Fromell GJ, Goodman S, Langer A, Califf RM, Fox KA, Premmereur J, Bigonzi F. A comparison of low-molecular-weight heparin with unfractionated heparin for unstable coronary artery disease. Efficacy and Safety of Subcutaneous Enoxaparin in Non-Q-Wave Coronary Events Study Group. N Engl J Med 1997; 337:447–452.

92. Antman EM, McCabe CH, Gurfinkel EP, Turpie AG, Bernink PJ, Salein D, Bayes dL, Fox K, Lablanche JM, Radley D, Premmereur J, Braunwald E. Enoxaparin prevents death and cardiac ischemic events in unstable angina/non-Q-wave myocardial infarction. Results of the thrombolysis in myocardial infarction (TIMI) 11B trial. Circulation 1999; 100:1593–1601.

93. Presented at late breaking clinical trials at the ACC meeting, New Orleans Califf RM. The Superior Yield of the New Strategy of Enoxaparin, Revascularization and Glycoprotein IIb/IIIa Inhibitors (SYNERGY) Trial: primary results, LA, 2004 (Abstract).

94. Theroux P, Waters D, Lam J, Juneau M, McCans J. Reactivation of unstable angina after the discontinuation of heparin. N Engl J Med 1992; 327:141–145.

95. Platelet Receptor Inhibition in Ischemic Syndrome Management (PRISM) Study Investigators. A comparison of aspirin plus tirofiban with aspirin plus heparin for unstable angina. N Engl J Med 1998; 338:1498–1505.

96. Platelet Receptor Inhibition in Ischemic Syndrome Management in Patients Limited by Unstable Signs and Symptoms (PRISM-PLUS) Study Investigators. Inhibition of the platelet glycoprotein IIb/IIIa receptor with tirofiban in unstable angina and non-Q-wave myocardial infarction. N Engl J Med 1998; 338:1488–1497.

97. The PURSUIT Trial Investigators. Inhibition of platelet glycoprotein IIb/IIIa with eptifibatide in patients with acute coronary syndromes. Platelet glycoprotein IIb/IIIa in unstable angina: receptor suppression using integrilin therapy. N Engl J Med 1998; 339:436–443.

98. The PARAGON Investigators. International, randomized, controlled trial of lamifiban (a platelet glycoprotein IIb/IIIa inhibitor), heparin, or both in unstable angina. Platelet IIb/IIIa antagonism for the reduction of acute coronary syndrome events in a global organization network. Circulation 1998; 97:2386–2395.

99. Klootwijk P, Langer A, Meij S, Green C, Veldkamp RF, Ross AM, Armstrong PW, Simoons ML. Non-invasive prediction of reperfusion and coronary artery patency by continuous ST segment monitoring in the GUSTO-I trial. Eur Heart J. 1996; 17:689–698.

100. Ottervanger JP, Armstrong P, Barnathan ES, Boersma E, Cooper JS, Ohman EM, James S, Topol E, Wallentin L, Simoons ML. Long-term results after the glycoprotein IIb/IIIa inhibitor abciximab in unstable angina: one-year survival in the

GUSTO IV-ACS (Global Use of Strategies To Open Occluded Coronary Arteries IV–Acute Coronary Syndrome) Trial. Circulation 2003; 107:437–442.

101. The EPILOG Investigators. Platelet glycoprotein IIb/IIIa receptor blockade and low-dose heparin during percutaneous coronary revascularization. N Engl J Med 1997; 336:1689–1696.

102. Randomised placebo-controlled trial of abciximab before and during coronary intervention in refractory unstable angina: the CAPTURE investigators. Lancet 1997; 349:1429–1435.

103. The RESTORE Investigators. Effects of platelet glycoprotein IIb/IIIa blockade with tirofiban on adverse cardiac events in patients with unstable angina or acute myocardial infarction undergoing coronary angioplasty. Randomized Efficacy Study of Tirofiban for Outcomes and REstenosis. Circulation 1997; 96:1445–1453.

104. Karvouni E, Katritsis DG, Ioannidis JP. Intravenous glycoprotein IIb/IIIa receptor antagonists reduce mortality after percutaneous coronary interventions. J Am Coll Cardiol 2003; 41:26–32.

105. Chew DP, Bhatt DL, Sapp S, Topol EJ. Increased mortality with oral platelet glycoprotein IIb/IIIa antagonists: a meta-analysis of phase III multicenter randomized trials. Circulation 2001; 103:201–206.

106. Behan MW, Storey RF. Antiplatelet therapy in cardiovascular disease. Postgrad Med J 2004; 80:155–164.

107. Guest TM, Ramanathan AV, Tuteur PG, Schechtman KB, Ladenson JH, Jaffe AS. Myocardial injury in critically ill patients. A frequently unrecognized complication. J Am Med Assoc 1995; 273:1945–1949.

108. Arlati S, Brenna S, Prencipe L, Marocchi A, Casella GP, Lanzani M, Gandini C. Myocardial necrosis in ICU patients with acute non-cardiac disease: a prospective study. Intensive Care Med 2000; 26:31–37.

109. Ammann P, Maggiorini M, Bertel O, Haenseler E, Joller-Jemelka HI, Oechslin E, Minder EI, Rickli H, Fehr T. Troponin as a risk factor for mortality in critically ill patients without acute coronary syndromes. J Am Coll Cardiol 2003; 41: 2004–2009.

110. Shah PK, Chyu KY. Unstable angina, In: Crawford MH, ed. Current diagnosis and Treatment in Cardiology. Lange Medical Books/McGraw-Hill, 2003:44–56.

111. TIMI Study Group. The Thrombolysis in Myocardial Infarction (TIMI) trial. Phase I findings. N Engl J Med 1985; 312:932–936.

112. Chesebro JH, Knatterud G, Roberts R, Borer J, Cohen LS, Dalen J, Dodge HT, Francis CK, Hillis D, Ludbrook P. Thrombolysis in Myocardial Infarction (TIMI) Trial, Phase I. a comparison between intravenous tissue plasminogen activator and intravenous streptokinase. Clinical findings through hospital discharge. Circulation 1987; 76:142–154.

113. Killip T, Kimball JT. Treatment of myocardial infarction in a coronary care unit. A two year experience with 250 patients. Am J Cardiol 1967; 20:457–464.

114. DeGeare VS, Boura JA, Grines LL, O'Neill WW, Grines CL. Predictive value of the Killip classification in patients undergoing primary percutaneous coronary intervention for acute myocardial infarction. Am J Cardiol 2001; 87:1035–1038.

9

Management of Congestive Heart Failure with a Focus on the Role of B-Type Natriuretic Peptide

VIKAS BHALLA and ALAN MAISEL

Division of Cardiology, La Jolla VA Medical Center and University of California
San Diego School of Medicine
La Jolla, California, U.S.A.

I. Introduction

Congestive heart failure (CHF), owing to the drastic increase in cardiovascular risk factors such as obesity and diabetes and improved survival rate after acute myocardial infarction (and subsequent development of CHF), with the prevalence of 4.9 million and an incidence of 550,000 cases per year, is a major and increasing cause of death and disability in the U.S. Heart failure (HF) accounts for 999,000 hospital discharges annually (a 165% increase since 1979), and its in-hospital mortality and readmission rates are extremely high (1–4). While sudden cardiac death (SCD) is a major cause of death in patients with CHF, many individuals also die from progressive pump failure and shock (defined as cardiac death with preceding symptomatic or hemodynamic deterioration) (5,6).

II. Etiology and Pathogenesis

CHF is a complex clinical syndrome characterized by dysfunction of the left, right, or both ventricles, which results in the impairment of the heart's ability to circulate blood at a rate sufficient to maintain the metabolic needs of peripheral tissues and various organs. The causes for the loss of a critical amount of functioning myocardium could be acute myocardial infarction (MI), prolonged cardiovascular stress (hypertension, valvular disease), toxins (e.g., alcohol abuse), or infection; in some cases, there is no apparent cause (idiopathic cardiomyopathy).

This syndrome is accompanied by exercise intolerance, shortness of breath (orthopnea, paroxysmal nocturnal dyspnea, dyspnea at rest and during exertion), fluid retention due to compensatory hemodynamic and neurohumoral mechanisms resulting in jugular vein distention, peripheral pitting edema, sinus tachycardia, basal rales or coarse bubbling rales throughout both lung fields, cardiomegaly, S_3 gallop sound, liver enlargement, and shortened survival. The occurrence of HF often indicates that all reserve capacity and compensatory mechanisms of the myocardium and peripheral circulation have been exhausted.

Several complex interactions between myocardial hemodynamic and neurohumoral compensatory events follow the initial cardiac damage, together giving rise to a clinical syndrome characterized by elevated intracardiac pressures, cardiac hypertrophy, reduced cardiac output, and diminished functional reserve. These mechanisms include activation of the renin-angiotensin-aldosterone system (RAAS), natriuretic peptide system, sympathetic nervous system (SNS), endothelins, and other neurohormonal factors. Thus, cardiorenal, hemodynamic, and neurohormonal factors all play a role in the pathogenesis of HF. Activation of these compensatory mechanisms leads to progressive worsening of left ventricular function, in part by increasing remodeling and overall work of the heart.

III. Diagnosis

The American College of Cardiology/American Heart Association (ACC/AHA) practice guidelines formulating committee decided to take a new approach to the classification of HF that emphasized both the evolution and progression of the disease (7). Table 1 depicts stages of HF with examples and recommended treatment strategies. Stage A identifies the patient who is at high risk for developing HF but has no structural disorder of the heart; Stage B refers to a patient with a structural disorder of the heart but who has never developed symptoms of HF; Stage C denotes the patient with past or current symptoms of HF associated with underlying structural heart disease; and Stage D designates the patient with end-stage disease who requires specialized treatment strategies such as mechanical circulatory support, continuous inotropic infusions, cardiac transplantation, or hospice care. The New York Heart Association (NYHA) classification of course applies to Stages C and D in this classification. Also, the common signs and symptoms that aid in the diagnosis of CHF (Stages C and D) are orthopnea, paroxysmal nocturnal dyspnea, dyspnea at rest and during exertion, jugular vein distention, peripheral pitting edema, sinus tachycardia, basal rales or coarse bubbling rales throughout both lung fields, cardiomegaly, S_3 gallop sound, and liver enlargement.

The common diagnostic studies that are performed are electrocardiography, exercise stress testing, chest radiograph, echocardiography, radionuclide ventriculography, and cardiac catheterization. Of these, the echocardiographic examination is considered the gold standard test in establishing the diagnosis, type of HF (systolic and diastolic), and type of cardiomyopathy (dilated,

Table 1 Stages of HF and Their Management

Stage	Description	Examples	Treatment of heart failure
A	Patients at high risk for HF because of the presence of conditions strongly associated with the development of HF; no identified structural or functional abnormalities of the pericardium, myocardium, or cardiac valves; no current or previous history of signs or symptoms of HF	Systemic hypertension; coronary artery disease; diabetes mellitus; history of cardiotoxic drug therapy or alcohol abuse; personal history of rheumatic fever; family history of cardiomyopathy	Treat hypertension Encourage smoking cessation Treat lipid disorders Encourage regular exercise Discourage alcohol intake, illicit drug use Prescribe ACE inhibitors if appropriate
B	Patients with structural heart disease that is strongly associated with the development of HF but who have no current or previous history of signs or symptoms of HF	Left ventricular hypertrophy or fibrosis; left ventricular dilatation or hypocontractility; asymptomatic valvular heart disease; previous myocardial infarction	All measures used for Stage A ACE inhibitors if appropriate β-Blockers if appropriate
C	Patients who currently have or who in the past have had symptoms of HF associated with underlying structural heart disease	Dyspnea or fatigue due to left ventricular systolic dysfunction; asymptomatic patients who are undergoing treatment for prior symptoms of HF	All measures used for Stage A Drugs for routine use: ACE inhibitors β-Blockers Digitalis Dietary salt restriction
D	Patients with advanced structural heart disease and marked symptoms of HF at rest despite maximal medical therapy; need for specialized interventions	Patients who are frequently hospitalized for HF and cannot be safely discharged from the hospital; patients in the hospital awaiting heart transplantation; patients at home receiving continuous intravenous support for symptom relief or being supported with a mechanical circulatory assist device; patients in a hospice setting for the management of HF	All measures used for Stages A, B, and C Mechanical assist devices Heart transplantation Continuous (not intermittent) I.V. inotropic infusions for palliation Hospice care

Abbreviation: HF, heart failure.
Source: From http://www.acc.org/clinical/guidelines/failure/hf_index.htm.

restrictive, hypertrophic) and in evaluating the possible primary or secondary causes (valvular disease, LV aneurysm, intracardiac shunts) of HF.

Recently, the Food and Drug Administration (FDA) approved a new biomarker (B-type natriuretic peptide) for the diagnosis of CHF.

A. Types of HF

It is important to identify the type of HF (systolic and diastolic), as the prognosis and the management may differ considerable between the two (7). Table 2 shows the differences in the characteristics of systolic and diastolic HF. Although controlled studies have been performed with digitalis, angiotensin converting enzyme (ACE) inhibitors, angiotensin receptor antagonists, β-Blockers, and calcium channel blockers in patients with HF who had a normal left ventricular ejection fraction, these trials have been small or have produced inconclusive results in contrast to the treatment of HF due to systolic dysfunction. Nevertheless, many patients with diastolic HF are treated with these drugs because of the presence of comorbid conditions (i.e., atrial fibrillation, hypertension, diabetes, and coronary artery disease). Hence the management of patients with diastolic dysfunction is based on the control of physiological factors (blood pressure,

Table 2 Characteristics of Diastolic HF Versus Systolic HF

Characteristic	Diastolic HF	Systolic HF
Clinical features:		
Symptoms (e.g., dyspnea)	Yes	Yes
Congestive state (e.g., edema)	Yes	Yes
Neurohormonal activation (e.g., brain natriuretic peptide)	Yes	Yes
Left ventricular structure and function:		
Ejection fraction	Normal	Decreased
Left ventricular mass	Increased	Increased
Relative wall thickness	Increased	Decreased
End diastolic volume	Normal	Increased
End diastolic pressure	Increased	Increased
Left atrial size	Increased	Increased
Exercise:		
Exercise capacity	Decreased	Decreased
Cardiac output augmentation	Decreased	Decreased
End diastolic pressure	Increased	Increased

Abbreviation: HF, heart failure.
Source: From Aurigemma GP, Gaasch WH. Clinical practice. Diastolic heart failure. N Engl J Med 2004; 351:1097–1105.

heart rate, blood volume, and MI) that are known to exert important effects on ventricular relaxation (7) (Table 3). In addition, recommendations regarding the use of anticoagulation and antiarrhythmic agents apply to both systolic and diastolic HF (7).

Table 3 Management Principles for Patients with Diastolic HF

Goal	Treatment	Daily dose of medication
Reduce the congestive state	ACE inhibitors Diuretics Salt restriction Angiotensin II–receptor blockers	<2 g of sodium/day Enalapril, 2.5–40 mg Losartan, 25–100 mg Furosemide, 10–120 mg Lisinopril, 10–40 mg Hydrochlorothiazide, 12.5–25 mg Candesartan, 4–32 mg
Maintain atrial contraction and prevent tachycardia	Cardioversion of atrial fibrillation Sequential atrioventricular pacing β-Blockers Calcium-channel blockers Radiofrequency ablation modification of atrioventricular node and pacing	Atenolol, 12.5–100 mg Metoprolol, 25–100 mg Verapamil, 120–360 mg Diltiazem, 120–540 mg
Treat and prevent myocardial ischemia	Nitrates β-Blockers Calcium-channel blockers Coronary-artery bypass surgery, percutaneous coronary intervention	Isosorbide dinitrate, 30–180 mg Isosorbide mononitrate, 30–90 mg Atenolol, 12.5–100 mg Diltiazem, 120–540 mg Verapamil, 120–360 mg Metoprolol, 25–200 mg
Control hypertension	Antihypertensive agents	Chlorthalidone, 12.5–25 mg Hydrochlorothiazide, 12.5–50 mg Atenolol, 12.5–100 mg Metoprolol, 12.5–200 mg Amlodipine, 2.5–10 mg Felodipine, 2.5–20 mg Enalapril, 2.5–40 mg Lisinopril, 10–40 mg Candesartan, 4–32 mg Losartan, 50–100 mg

Abbreviation: HF, heart failure.
Source: From Aurigemma GP, Gaasch WH. Clinical practice. Diastolic heart failure. N Engl J Med 2004; 351:1097–1105.

IV. Quantifying the Severity of HF: Natriuretic Peptide, Its History, Structure, and Physiology

Accurately classifying (or "grading") the severity of CHF is a valuable goal in determining prognosis. Recent studies have caused a great deal of excitement over the use of natriuretic peptides for this purpose.

The history surrounding the development of natriuretic peptides as diagnostic markers for CHF is summarized in Table 4. Although the principal peptide is named BNP (for "brain" natriuretic peptide), its primary site of synthesis has since been localized to the ventricular myocardium.

Three major natriuretic peptides have now been identified and all—atrial natriuretic peptide (ANP), BNP, and C natriuretic peptide (CNP)—share a 17-amino-acid ring structure (Fig. 1). ANP and BNP originate in myocardial cells, while CNP is of endothelial origin (15). Natriuretic peptides are secreted by the heart in response to wall stress, such as from CHF, and result in increased myocardial relaxation (lusitropy) as well as opposition to the vasoconstrictive, sodium retaining, and antidiuretic effects of the neurohormonal imbalance initiated by activation of RAAS, SNS, endothelins, and other neurohormonal factors. Specific stimuli vary for the secretion of each natriuretic peptide. BNP is synthesized, stored and released primarily by the ventricular myocardium in response to volume expansion and pressure overload (16–19), while ANP is released by atrial as well as ventricular tissue in response to volume overload. At the cellular level, volume stretch leads to pulsatile bursts in pre–pro-BNP synthesis, which is then cleaved progressively to pro-BNP and, finally, to BNP and inactive N-terminal pro-BNP. Since BNP is more stable than ANP and other neurohormones, and because it originates in the ventricles, it is more sensitive to left ventricular dysfunction than ANP and other neurohormones (20). BNP has been hypothesized to play an important regulatory role in response to acute changes in ventricular volume (21).

Table 4   Developmental History of BNP as a Marker for CHF and Wall Strain

1956	Henry and Pearce first observed BNP as a response to balloon stretch of the canine left atrium (8)
1981	De Bold et al. injected homogenized atrial tissue into rats and noted a potent natriuretic response (9)
1984	Kangawa et al. identified the structure of atrial natriuretic peptide (ANP) (10)
1988	Sudoh et al. isolated a compound from pig brain that caused natriuretic and diuretic responses similar to ANP (11)
1990	Sudoh et al. isolated a structurally distinct member of the natriuretic peptide family, C-type natriuretic peptide (CNP), from pig brain (12)
1991	Minamino et al. reported that CNP is expressed to a much greater extent in central nervous system and vascular tissues than in the heart (13)
1991	The primary site of BNP synthesis was localized to the ventricular myocardium (14)

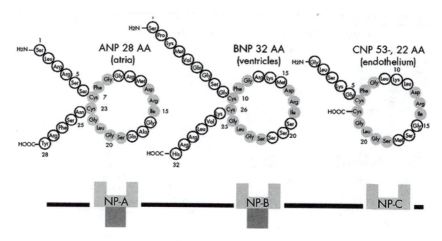

Figure 1 Structure of the three major natriuretic peptides. *Abbreviations*: ANP, atrial natriuretic peptide; BNP, brain natriuretic peptide; CNP, C natriuretic peptide.

V. Role of Natriuretic Peptides in CHF

The correlation of serum BNP concentrations with elevated end-diastolic pressure (18,19) closely parallels dyspnea in heart failure, suggesting that this peptide is uniquely suited for use as a neurohormonal index of progressive heart failure (22). BNP concentrations also parallel NYHA clinical status (23,24) more than does ANP. Thus, BNP has emerged as a strong diagnostic and prognostic indicator of left ventricular dysfunction and heart failure.

VI. Role of BNP in the Emergency-Care Setting

Several studies have established the role of BNP in the clinical diagnosis of CHF. In 1586 patients presenting to the emergency room with acute dyspnea, admission BNP exceeding 100 pg/mL had a sensitivity of 90% and a specificity of 76% for CHF as opposed to other causes of dyspnea, while BNP exceeding 50 pg/mL had a negative predictive value for CHF of 96% (23) (Fig. 2). In another study of 321 patients presenting to the emergency room with dyspnea of unknown etiology, BNP accurately separated CHF (mean BNP 759 ± 798 pg/mL) from pulmonary disease (61 ± 10 pg/mL) with a high specificity, sensitivity, and accuracy of 91%. Moreover, comparing patients with heart failure whose dyspnea was due to chronic obstructive pulmonary disease (COPD) (mean BNP 47 ± 23 pg/mL), to COPD patients whose dyspnea was due to heart failure (731 ± 764 pg/mL), a BNP value of 94 pg/mL yielded a sensitivity and specificity of 86% and 98%, respectively, and differentiated HF from lung disease with an accuracy of 91% (25).

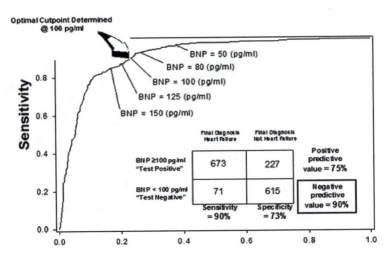

Figure 2 Sensitivity versus specificity for heart failure by BNP levels. *Abbreviation*: BNP, brain natriuretic peptide. *Source*: From Breathing Not Properly Multinational Study.

BNP has been shown in several studies to be an accurate and independent index of HF. Moreover, in the studies mentioned above, BNP predicted CHF in multivariate analyses of history, symptoms, signs, and radiological and laboratory studies.

Combining these results, Maisel and colleagues have proposed an algorithm for using BNP in the diagnosis and management of CHF that is in use at the La Jolla VA Medical Center. In patients presenting with acute dyspnea, a serum BNP value less than 100 pg/mL essentially excludes CHF as the cause of dyspnea, whereas values greater than 400 pg/mL provide a 95% likelihood for CHF. Values between 100–400 pg/mL warrant further investigation (26).

In a recent study, Mueller et al. (27) extended the value ascertained from the Breathing Not Properly Multinational Study in terms of cost-effectiveness of using BNP levels throughout the diagnostic and hospitalization phases of HF. In the study, the investigators studied patients presenting to the emergency department with acute dyspnea who were randomly assigned to undergo either a single measurement of B-type natriuretic peptide or no such measurement. Participating clinicians were advised that a level of B-type natriuretic peptide below 100 pg/mL made the diagnosis of congestive heart failure unlikely, whereas a level above 500 pg/mL made it highly likely. For intermediate levels, use of clinical judgment and adjunctive testing were encouraged. In this single-blind trial of 452 patients, rapid measurement of B-type natriuretic peptide in the emergency department was associated with decreases in the rate of hospital admission by 10 percentage points, the median length of stay by three days, and the mean total cost of treatment by about $1800, with no adverse effects on mortality or the rate of subsequent hospitalization. This carefully performed trial suggests that the use of an inexpensive blood test for B-type natriuretic peptide in the emergency evaluation of acute dyspnea can significantly improve both the efficiency and the quality of care. These results are consistent with the Breathing Not Properly study and showed that the use of an improved diagnostic test in the emergency department can reduce the use of hospital resources and associated costs by eliminating the need for other, more expensive tests, or by establishing an alternative diagnosis that does not require hospitalization. This finding is similar to our REDHOT trial (28), which showed that the use of BNP would have decreased unnecessary hospitalization by ~10%, which would result in saving of $400 million per year in the U.S. alone if extrapolated according to diagnosis-related groups (DRGs).

VII. BNP and CHF Screening

Not only is BNP useful in diagnosis and prognostication, a threshold BNP level ≥ 20 pg/mL has been shown by Atishta et al. (29) to be useful in screening and in forming a pretest probability in patients undergoing echocardiograpy. They found a high sensitivity and negative predictive value especially in patients with systolic and combined systolic and diastolic HF. Heidenreich et al. (30) also found that screening with BNP using a threshold BNP level of 24 pg/mL followed by echocardiography in those with an abnormal test was economically attractive for 60-year-old men and possibly for women in groups with at least a 1% prevalence of moderate or greater LV systolic dysfunction (EF < 40%). Screening all patients with echocardiography was expensive, but the sequential BNP-echocardiography screening strategy was economically attractive.

VIII. BNP and CHF Prognosis

Studies are increasingly showing that serum BNP levels are highly predictive of subsequent cardiac events. In a study of 325 patients presenting with dyspnea to the emergency department, patients with BNP levels greater than 480 pg/mL had a 51% cumulative probability of death (cardiac and noncardiac), hospital admissions (cardiac), or repeat emergency-department visits over the next six months. In contrast, only 2.5% of patients with BNP levels <230 pg/mL suffered one of these events (31).

Recently, Wang et al. (32), the investigators from the Framingham Offspring Study, examined the long-term prognostic importance of the levels of atrial natriuretic peptide and B-type natriuretic peptide in asymptomatic middle-aged persons. After adjusting for traditional risk factors, Wang and colleagues found that the level of B-type natriuretic peptide was independently predictive of the risk of death, heart failure, atrial fibrillation, and stroke over a mean follow-up period of about five years. Levels of B-type natriuretic peptide above the 80th percentile in this cohort (i.e., >20 pg/mL) were associated with an increase by more than 60% in the long-term risk of death. Furthermore, there was a significant prognostic gradient with respect to the risk of heart failure, atrial fibrillation, and stroke among the three levels of B-type natriuretic peptide (low, intermediate, and high) examined. This remarkable finding suggests that, in the asymptomatic community based cohort, there are important prognostic data even in the range of B-type natriuretic peptide levels below 100 pg/mL, the level used to rule out HF in 90% of acutely dyspneic patients. Echocardiographic measurements of left ventricular mass, left atrial diameter, and left ventricular systolic function did statistically explain the association between the level of B-type natriuretic peptide and the risk of death. These associations persisted even after adjustment for standard risk factors and echocardiographic measurements, suggesting that slight elevations of B-type natriuretic peptide may reflect very early stages of pathologic processes that precede the development of apparent cardiac manifestations (such as measurable left ventricular hypertrophy).

In this community cohort, only 2.2% of the participating men and 1.5% of the women had levels above 80 pg/mL, which would be expected as these are asymptomatic patients without any signs of overt heart failure.

IX. BNP and the Prediction of Sudden Cardiac Death

Recent studies raise the exciting possibility that BNP may indicate risk for ventricular arrhythmias and SCD, likely by reflecting volume overload and ventricular wall stretch. This association was most impressively demonstrated by Berger et al. (33) who found that BNP levels independently predicted SCD in 452 ambulatory patients with mild to moderate heart failure (NYHA classes I and II) and left ventricular ejection fraction less than 35%. In that study, BNP above 130 pg/mL separated patients with high from those with low rates of SCD. Furthermore, only 1% (1 of 110) of patients with a BNP level <130 pg/mL died suddenly, compared with 19% (43 of 227) of patients with BNP levels >130 pg/mL.

X. Management of HF

Apart from the behavioral modifications as in preventive strategies, changes in activity and diet (sodium restriction); and correction of precipitating factors (valvular dysfunction, intracardiac shunts, and other high-output states; bradyarrhythmias or tachyarrhythmias; infectious or ischemic events. Reversible causes of diastolic dysfunction) the mainstays of pharmacologic treatment include diuretics (thiazides, loop diuretics, potassium-sparing agents), inotropic drugs (direct and indirect; digitalis glycosides; sympathomimetics—dopamine and dobutamine; phosphodiesterase inhibitors—amrinone, milrinone, and enoximone), vasoactive drugs (venous vasodilators—nitrates and β-blockers; arterial vasodilators—hydralazine and minoxidil), and calcium channel blockers. A number of studies (CONSENSUS, SOLVD, AIRE) have proven the efficacy of ACE inhibitors in heart failure patients, and they are now the first-line therapy for all patients with LV dysfunction and heart failure (NYHA I-IV). In these patients, inhibition of the angiotensin-converting enzyme has been shown to produce a moderate increase in cardiac output (increased stroke work and cardiac index) and a significant decrease in right and left ventricular filling pressures, pulmonary and systemic vascular resistances, and mean arterial pressure, all without increasing the heart rate. Lately the angiotensin II receptor blockers (ARB) provide direct blockade of angiotensin II type-1 (AT1) receptor activation. In addition, this blockade does not result in accumulation of bradykinin, which is considered to be responsible for adverse reactions associated with the use of ACEI, such as persistent cough, angioedema, and significant hypotension. Table 5 provides additional information on the commonly used drugs, their utility in heart failure and their doses (7,34). Even with these therapies, the management of heart failure remains far from perfect, as there remains ambiguity in objectively assessing and titrating these therapies for optimal outcome.

XI. BNP-Guided Therapy and Prognosis in Acutely Ill Patients

Another important study (35) demonstrated that BNP levels in shock patients admitted to the intensive care unit (ICU) might provide powerful information in mortality prediction. In this study, the median BNP levels were higher in those who died than those who survived (943 pg/mL vs. 378 pg/mL, $p < 0.001$). Also using multivariate analysis, they showed that BNP level in the highest log-quartile was the strongest predictor of mortality (odds ratio = 4.50). They showed no correlation between a single BNP value and pulmonary capillary wedge pressure (PCWP) in interpatient analysis. This lack of correlation could be explained by variation of individual patients, age, gender, ethnicity, baseline and dry BNP level, and to some extent by renal function, and it is clear that a BNP <350 pg/mL had a very high negative predictive value (95%) for the diagnosis of cardiogenic shock. This study supports the study published in 2001 by Kazanegra et al. (36) involving 20 patients with decompensated NYHA class III–IV CHF undergoing tailored therapy, which showed significant correlation between percent change in wedge pressure from baseline per hour and the percent change of BNP from baseline per hour (Fig. 3). In this study they also showed that the patients who died had higher final BNP levels (1078 ± 123 pg/mL vs. 701 ± 107 pg/mL). They concluded that although using BNP levels will not obviate the need for invasive hemodynamic monitoring, it may be a useful adjunct in tailoring therapy to these patients and may improve the in-hospital management of patients admitted with decompensated CHF. Even though

Table 5 Medications Used to Treat Patients with HF

Medication	Starting dose (oral unless indicated)	Maximum dose	Comments
Diuretics			
Furosemide	20–40 mg q d or bid	Up to 600 mg/day in divided doses; high doses limited by toxicity	IV or oral depending on severity of pulmonary edema, IV usually produces more effective diuresis. Continuous infusion (10–20 mg/hr; max 40 mg/hr)
Bumetanide	0.5–1.0 mg q d or bid	Up to 10 mg/day	IV infusion: 1 mg/hr up to 2 mg/hr
Toresmide	50 mg q d or bid	Up to 200 mg/day	IV infusion: 10 mg/hr up to 20 mg/hr
Metolazone	1.25 mg 30 min prior to loop diuretic	Up to 5 mg bid	Add when furosemide not effective
Spironolactone	25 mg q d or qod	25 mg bid, rarely higher	Add to difficult chronic cases and use only with a loop diuretic; caution to avoid hyperkalemia
Hydrochlorothiazide	25–100 mg prior to loop diuretic	Same	Use if less potent effect than metolazone desired
Digitalis			
Digoxin	0.125–0.25 mg q d or qod	Limited by toxicity; especially in patients with renal insufficiency	Improves contractility, slows ventricular rate in atrial fibrillation. May be harmful in acute myocardial infarction, hypertrophic cardiomyopathy or aortic stenosis. Load with 1 mg IV or oral (0.5 mg, then 0.25 mg q 6 hr), early benefit noted in rapid atrial fibrillation.

ACE inhibitors			Class effect: Decreases afterload, improves symptoms and exercise capacity; survival benefit; lower doses if on a diuretic; caution in renal failure
Captopril	6.25 mg bid	50–100 mg qid	
Enalapril maleate	2.5 mg bid	10–20 mg bid	
Enalaprilat	0.625–1.25 mg IV q 6 hr	5 mg IV q 6 hr	IV ACE inhibitor; 1.25 mg equivalent to 5 mg oral
Fosinopril sodium	5–10 mg q d	40–80 mg q d	
Lisinopril	2.5–5 mg q d	20–40 mg q d	
Quinapril hydrochloride	10 mg bid	20 mg bid	
Ramipril	1.25–2.5 mg q d	10 mg q d	
β-Blockers			Bisoprolol and carvedilol decreases all cause mortality and sudden death, independent of the severity or cause of heart failure
Bisoprolol	1.25 mg q d	10 mg q d	
Carvedilol	3.125 mg bid	25–50 mg bid	
Labetalol			Higher doses used in hypertension
Metoprolol tartrate	6.25 mg bid	75 mg bid	
Metoprolol CR/XL	12.5–25 mg q d	200 mg q d	
Metoprolol	5 mg IV	15 mg IV q 3–6 hr	15 mg over 15 min in acute coronary syndrome; NOT generally recommended acute heart failure
Vasodilators			
Nitroglycerin tablets	0.4 mg sublingual		Repeat every 5 min
Nitroglycerin ointment	1″ topically q 6 hr	3″ topically q 6 hr	Rapid removal if adverse effects

(Continued)

Table 5 Medications Used to Treat Patients with HF *(Continued)*

Medication	Starting dose (oral unless indicated)	Maximum dose	Comments
Nitroglycerin infusion	5 µgm/min IV, increase by 5 µgm/min q 3–5 min, up to 20 µgm/min; then increase 10–20 µgm/min	200 µgm/min	IV nitroglycerin may provide short term benefit with decrease in preload, afterload, and systemic vascular resistatance; effects limited by headache and hypotension; caution with tachyphylaxis
Isosorbide dinitrate	10 mg tid oral	80 mg tid	Tachyphylaxis
Hydralazine	25 mg tid or 10 mg IV	150 mg qid	Use with nitrates; caution with reflex tachycardia
Inotropes			
Dobutamine	2.5 µgm/kg/min	Up to 20 µgm/kg/min	Caution with tachyarrhythmias and ischemia Infusions may improve symptoms but does not impact survival; limit to short term use (2–3 days)
Amrinone	0.75 mg/kg IV load over 3 minutes, then 5 µgm/kg/min IV	Up to 15 µgm/kg/min	Limited by tachyarrhythmias, ischemia, thrombocytopenia, and hypotension; can be use in conjunction with dobutamine
Milrinone	50 µgm/kg IV load over 10 min, then 0.375 µgm/kg/min	0.75 µgm/kg/min	Limited by tachyarrhymias, ischemia, and hypotension; can be use in conjuction with dobutamine

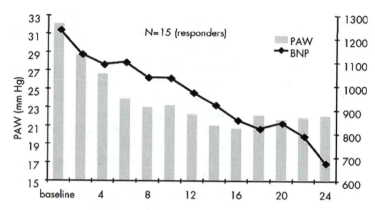

Figure 3 The correlation of treatment-induced change in pulmonary artery wedge pressure (PAW) with change in BNP from baseline. *Abbreviations*: PAW, pulmonary artery wedge pressure; BNP, brain natriuretic peptide. *Source*: From Ref. 34.

Tung et al. (35) could not differentiate cardiogenic from noncardiogenic shock using BNP, because BNP levels have been a useful surrogate of wedge pressure and are useful in differentiating heart failure from lung disease, it may be useful not only in excluding cardiogenic shock but in differentiating cardiogenic from noncardiogenic pulmonary edema. In a study by Berman et al. (37), BNP levels were obtained in 35 patients with acute respiratory distress syndrome (ARDS) and from 42 patients hospitalized for severe dyspnea with the diagnosis of CHF. The median BNP level in patients with CHF of 773 pg/mL was significantly higher than patients with ARDS (123 pg/mL ($p < 0.001$) (Fig. 4). The area under the receiver-operated characteristic curve using BNP to differentiate CHF from ARDS was 0.90 (0.83–0.98; $p < 0.001$). At a cut point of 360 pg/mL, there was 90% sensitivity, 86% specificity, 89% positive predictive value, and a 94% negative predictive value (accuracy = 88%) for ARDS versus CHF. Thus, BNP may be accurate enough to differentiate noncardiogenic from cardiogenic

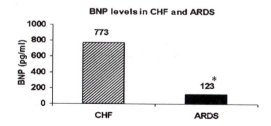

Figure 4 Comparison of the BNP levels in CHF and ARDS patients. *$p < 0.001$. *Abbreviations*: BNP, brain natriuretic peptide; CHF, congestive heart failure; ARDS, acute respiratory distress syndrome. *Source*: From Berman, Maisel et al. AHA 106:19, II-647, S3191, 2002.

pulmonary edema such that invasive hemodynamic catheter placement may not always be necessary. Hence BNP levels >360 pg/mL suggest CHF as the diagnosis of pulmonary edema.

The merit of these studies demonstrates that low BNP levels in a single inexpensive point of care assay can exclude cardiogenic shock (a high PCWP or low Cardiac Index) in the ICU setting and may be useful to avoid pulmonary artery catheterization, along with the risks associated with its placement and the necessity of an ICU bed. Also, elevated BNP levels may offer superior prognostic information to the critical care practitioner to help identify patients at highest risk for mortality. Cheng et al. (38) followed the course of 72 patients admitted with decompensated CHF with daily BNP levels and their relationship to 30-day read-mission rates or death. Patients who were most likely to have a cardiac event had higher BNP levels both at the times of admission and discharge. Figure 5 shows the relationship between a rise or fall in the BNP level with treatment and sub-sequent endpoints. Only 16% of patients with a fall in BNP levels during hospi-talization had a subsequent cardiac event, while 52% of those with rising BNP levels during treatment had either readmission or cardiac death. Patients whose discharge BNP levels fell below 430 pg/mL had a reasonable likelihood of not being readmitted within the following 30 days. This data was supported by a recent study by Bettencourt et al. (39), who found that failure of BNP levels to fall over the hospitalization predicted death/rehospitalization and that discharge levels <250 pg/mL predicted event-free survival.

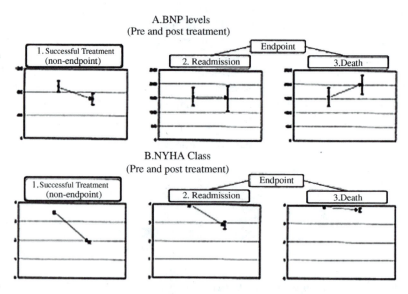

Figure 5   The relationship between a rise or fall in the BNP level with treatment and subsequent endpoints. *Abbreviation*: BNP, brain natriuretic peptide.

Measurement of serum BNP levels thus shows promise in monitoring patients with CHF, in tailoring management and titrating their therapy, and in predicting adverse cardiac events and readmissions.

XII. BNP Level-Guided Therapy and Prognosis in Ambulatory Patients

Since BNP levels have been shown to predict prognosis in ambulatory patients, it is possible that a BNP-guided treatment strategy may reduce mortality in such patients. Indeed, in the Acute Infarction Ramipril Efficacy (AIRE) trial, 45% of patients who died suddenly had severe or worsening CHF prior to their death (40). Although the monitoring of serum BNP in the outpatient setting has yet to be proven effective in tailoring CHF treatment, several ongoing studies are testing this hypothesis. In a small study, Troughton et al. showed that patients who had therapy tailored by BNP levels had less hospitalizations and lower mortality than those treated without knowledge of BNP levels (41). Less directly, the fact that effective CHF treatments correlate with falling BNP levels also bodes well for future attempts to tailor therapy in this way (42,43). Lee et al. found that BNP levels in outpatients rose in those showing signs of decompensation, yet BNP levels fell in those showing improvement in NYHA class (44). BNP levels may also have value in indicating a number of outpatient states that are indirectly linked with SCD, including volume overload from renal failure or decompensated valvular heart disease, and silent myocardial ischaemia in diabetics (44).

XIII. BNP as a Drug: Treating Decompensated HF with Nesiritide

While there are many possibilities, including dietary indiscretion, medical non-compliance, ischemia, and arrhythmias, it is almost always the disturbed balance between vasoconstrictors and vasodilators (natriuretic peptides) that leads to decompensation in the stable CHF patient. Exogenous BNP may be helpful in these patients. The question as to why should we give a patient exogenous BNP when endogenous levels are also high has not been fully explained. It is probably analogous to giving insulin for insulin resistance. The high levels of endogenous BNP may be released as a "distress hormone," and there may or may not be an altered potency of this hormone due to structural or chemical abnormality. These levels are no longer effective in maintaining the balance of vasoconstriction and vasodilation. Hence it makes intuitive and practical sense that giving back BNP in the form of exogenous nesiritide might restore neurohormonal homeostasis. Nesiritide not only has the ideal properties of a good vasodilator, but it has an ability to interrupt the vicious cycle of decompensation (Fig. 6).

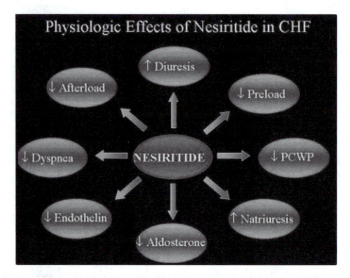

Figure 6   Physiologic effects of nesiritide (Natrecor®).

XIV.   Efficacy of Nesiritide

Colucci et al. (46) reported the efficacy of nesiritide in two trials, the Efficacy Trial and the Comparative Trial. Nesiritide administration produced a dose-related decrease in PCWP, systemic vascular resistance (SVR), mean right arterial pressure, dyspnea, and fatigue, plus a significant increase in cardiac index. Global status improved significantly more in nesiritide patient groups. The most common side effect, which has been noted in most follow-up studies, was dose-related hypotension. The Comparative Trial was longer term and evaluated nesiritide against a variety of other cardiovascular agents considered standard therapy (47). These agents included dobutamine, milrinone, nitroglycerin, dopamine, and amrinone. Global clinical status, fatigue, and dyspnea improved in all groups, with no significant differences between patients receiving nesiritide and patients receiving standard therapy. The most common side effects were bradycardia and dose-related hypotension.

In 1998, Burger et al. (48) conducted the Prospective Randomized Evaluation of Cardiac Ectopy with Dobutamine or Nesiritide Therapy (PRECEDENT) study. They demonstrated significantly fewer arrhythmias and no increase in heart rate (hence myocardial oxygen demand, the risk of ischemia, and mortality) in patients treated with nesiritide compared with patients treated with a low dose of dobutamine. Furthermore, the 21-day readmission rate and six-month mortality rate were higher for the dobutamine group. They concluded that nesiritide might be a safer drug than dobutamine for short-term management of decompensated CHF, especially in patients with tachycardia, a history of atrial or ventricular arrhythmias, or evidence of ventricular irritability.

Scios Inc. sponsored the Vasodilation in the Management of Acute Congestive Heart Failure (VMAC) trial (49) in 1999 to address safety criteria necessary for FDA approval of nesiritide. The investigators found that nesiritide had a more rapid onset and greater reduction in PCWP than IV nitroglycerin. The improvement in global clinical status and dyspnea was similar in both treatment groups. They concluded that when added to standard care, nesiritide improved hemodynamic function more effectively than IV nitroglycerin or placebo. Shortly after the VMAC trial, nesiritide was approved by the FDA for the treatment of acutely decompensated HF.

XV. Nesiritide: The Drug of Choice for the Treatment of Decompensated CHF?

Few guidelines exist for adequately treating patients admitted with decompensated CHF. As clinicians, we need to determine the cause of the decompensation, effectively treat the patient until not only stability has occurred but the patient is also euvolemic, and take steps to insure that early readmission does not occur. Here is a perspective on why nesiritide may be the most rational drug for treating decompensated HF.

> *Neurohormonal improvement.* Unlike most drugs, nesiritide mitigates many of the vasoconstrictor and water-retaining effects that help drive the vicious cycle of heart failure. (50,51)
>
> *Comparison to diuretics.* While diuretics are often the initial treatment, and sometimes the only treatment used for the decompensated CHF, by themselves they may actually do more harm than good (52). Additionally, diuretics often further impair renal blood flow, lowering glomerular filtration rate (GFR). Nesiritide, by its direct "priming" action on the kidney, appears to mitigate the need for high doses of diuretics as well as to mitigate the effects of vasoconstrictive neurohormones (53,54).
>
> *Comparison to vasodilators.* Vasodilators, while the mainstay of CHF treatment in the hospital, have their share of problems (55). These include hypotension, tachyphylaxis, and production of toxic metabolites. Also, some drugs like nitroprusside need to be handled with special care, and patients need to be in a monitored bed with an arterial line. One major advantage to using nesiritide is its ease of use—no need for an ICU bed, no arterial line, and only a 4% incidence of clinically significant hypotension.
>
> *Comparison with inotropes.* Parenteral inotropes have never been shown to be effective except in very-short-term symptom improvement. Furthermore, inotropes cause significant mortality, which has lessened their use considerably (56–58). The fact that Nesiritide increases cardiac output without increasing the heart rate or causing arrhythmias when given to decompensated patients makes it much more attractive for use than inotropic agents (59).

XVI. Indications of Nesiritide

The ideal patient profile for nesiritide therapy is as follows:

1. Patients with high BNP levels that do not decrease with one day of hospital treatment. Along with renal dysfunction and lack of diuresis, this appears to place the patient at high risk for negative outcomes.
2. Elevated filling pressures either measured through direct measurement or clinical estimation—these patients almost always have elevated BNP levels.
3. Patient not in cardiogenic shock.
4. Systolic blood pressure not consistently <90 mmHg. Some physicians (Uri Elkayam, personal communication, September 2003) have found nesiritide to be effective in patients with systolic blood pressures hovering a few millimeters below 90 mmHg. In such cases, holding off on diuretics, and even bypassing the bolus initially, may be tried. If the blood pressure is secondary to a primary decrease in stroke volume, author has found that 2.5–5 ug/kg/min dobutamine just before nesiritide infusion might be helpful.
5. Nesiritide has the advantage over other cardiac drugs that it can be used in patients with renal disease, acute coronary syndromes, diastolic dysfunction, and serious arrhythmias, and also in those taking concurrent β-blocker therapy.

Table 6 shows a sample order of nesiritide. Figure 7 shows an algorithm that can be followed for initiating nesiritide therapy and guidelines for managing patients thereafter.

XVII. How Often Should One Obtain a BNP Level in the Hospital?

This is an often-asked question with no one right answer. One author (ASM) obtains a BNP level after 24 hours of treatment. Failure of BNP levels to fall in a 24-hour period may delineate a high-risk patient who should receive more vigorous treatment. If a very sick patient is being treated in the ICU without a pulmonary arterty catheter placement and guidance, perhaps more frequent assessment of BNP levels (every four to six hours) is warranted. During nesiritide infusion, BNP levels (measure would be sum of endogenous plus exogenous) or NTpro BNP can help monitoring therapy.

XVIII. BNP Levels and Nesiritide in the Outpatient Management of CHF

Elevations of BNP have been shown to be a powerful marker for prognosis and risk stratification in the setting of HF (60). In addition, changes in plasma BNP

Table 6 Sample Orders for Nesiritide (Natrecor®)

Sample Natrecor dosing orders

Start Natrecor infusion:
    Administer bolus of 2 mcg/kg over 60 sec then
    infuse at 0.01 mcg/kg/min
Example: For 80 kg patient: Bolus 27 mL then start
    infusion at 8 mL/hr

Increase Natrecor infusion:
    Rebolus at 1 mcg/kg over 60 sec then increase
    infusion to 0.015 mcg/kg/min
Example: For above patient: Bolus at 13 mL then start
    infusion at 12 mL/hr

Increase Natrecor infusion
    Rebolus at 1 mcg/kg over 60 sec then increase
    infusion to 0.020 mcg/kg/min
Example: For above patient: Bolus at 13 mL then start
    infusion at 16 mL/hr

Hold Natrecor infusion till SBP >90 mmHg:
    Then restart Natrecor infusion at 30% lower dose
Example: For above patient: Decrease infusion to
    11 mL/hr (0.014 mcg/kg/min)

levels were significantly related to changes in limitations of physical activities and were a powerful predictor of the functional status deterioration.

Figure 8 suggests a possible algorithm for using BNP levels along with nesiritide infusion in the emergency department. The Algorithm for Nesiritide Success in the Emergency Room (ANSWER) has not yet been tested.

XIX. Outpatient Management Using BNP Levels: Implications for Partnership Between the Level and the Drug

Perhaps the best way to keep a person out of the hospital is not to let the discharge BNP level go up. This will be tested in the multicenter Rapid Assessment of Bedside BNP In Treatment of HF (RABBIT) trial. But perhaps more importantly, is there an outpatient level of BNP we should aim for? It is evident that patients with poor ejection fraction but with BNP levels that are under 200 pg/mL have a very good prognosis (33). Using BNP levels to identify a patient population with a higher risk of sudden death can help to tailor their treatment and extend survival.

It also appears that ACE inhibitors, angiotensin receptor blocker agents, spironolactone, and perhaps β-blockers drive BNP levels down, though it is unclear whether this is a true marker of clinical improvement. The current

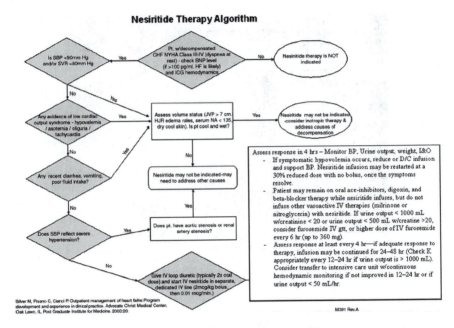

Figure 7   Nesiritide treatment algorithm.

practice of this author (ASM) is to aim for BNP levels under 200–300 pg/mL with standard therapy of ACE inhibitors and β-Blockers and diuretics. Patients with BNP levels between 200 and 500 pg/mL are often NYHA class II/III and may require more diuretics, especially spironolactone. These theories will be tested in RABBIT as well as the BNP-assisted Treatment to Lessen Serial Cardiac Readmissions and Death (BATTLE-SCARRED) trial. Patients who, despite standard medical treatment, have advanced symptoms along with high BNP levels (>400–600 pg/mL) might be candidates for outpatient infusions of inotropes or nesiritide, biventricular pacing (if QRS >120–130 milliseconds) or cardiac transplantation, an assist device, or perhaps even gene therapy.

As is the practice at San Diego VA healthcare system, when a patient comes to the urgent care center with symptoms that could represent a decompensated state, a BNP level is drawn. If no different from baseline values, then decompensation is unlikely. As BNP is not a stand-alone test, it should be used in conjunction with other features of the exam. In our experience, clinical features of decompensation along with an increase of 50% or more from baseline are often associated with decompensation.

XX.   Toward Earlier Attention to Rising BNP Levels: Implications for Outpatient Nesiritide Infusions

The Follow Up Serial Infusions of Natrecor (FUSION) trial (61) was a multi-center, randomized, open-label study of 210 CHF patients at high risk for

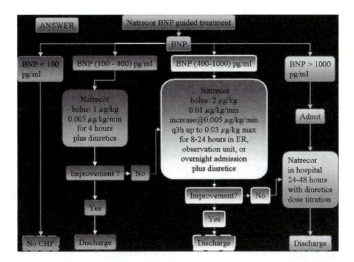

Figure 8 Treatment of heart failure with nesiritide guided by BNP levels. *Abbreviations*: BNP, brain natriuretic peptide; CHF, congestive heart failure.

hospitalization. The study demonstrated that weekly infusions of nesiritide in the outpatient setting were well tolerated and associated with few deaths and hospitalizations as well as improvement in NYHA class and overall clinical status. If the benefits seen in the FUSION trial on clinical outcomes such as mortality and hospitalizations are replicated in a larger trial, nesiritide has the potential to become an effective outpatient treatment for hundreds of thousands of patients with advanced chronic heart failure. The likely trigger for outpatient infusions would include symptoms of decompensation along with a rising BNP level.

XXI. Summary

BNP is the first biomarker to prove its value in (1) screening for LVD, (2) in assessing prognosis while monitoring patients, (3) in tailoring management and titrating therapy, (4) providing objectivity in assessing discharge and admission criteria, (5) predicting and decreasing adverse cardiac events and readmissions in heart failure inpatients, and (6) characterization and prognostication of ICU patients in shock.

To conclude, this rapid, inexpensive, point-of-care test, which is simple to administer in a variety of clinical settings, can enable care providers to facilitate and optimize the care of heart failure patients. As with everything, there are limitations to BNP testing, as it is not a stand-alone test, but when used judiciously, it could be a powerful tool in the hands of clinicians. Emerging clinical data will help further refine biomarker-guided therapeutic and monitoring strategies involving BNP.

References

1. American Heart Association. Heart Disease and Stroke Statistics—2003 Update. Dallas, Texas: American Heart Association, 2002.
2. Cohn JN, Levine TB, Olivari MT, Garberg V, Lura D, Francis GS, Simon AB, Rector T. Plasma norepinephrine as a guide to prognosis in patients with chronic congestive heart failure. N Engl J Med 1984; 311:819–823.
3. Vinson JM, Rich MW, Sperry JC, Shah AS, McNamara T. Early readmission of elderly patients with heart failure. J Am Geriatr Soc 1990; 38:1290–1295.
4. Krumholz HM, Wang Y, Parent EM, Mockalis J, Petrillo M, Radford MJ. Readmission after hospitalization for congestive heart failure among Medicare beneficiaries. Arch Intern Med 1997; 157:99–104.
5. The CONSENSUS Trial Study Group. Effects of enalapril on mortality in severe congestive heart failure. Results of the Cooperative North Scandinavian Enalapril Survival Study (CONSENSUS). N Engl J Med 1987; 316:1429.
6. The SOLVD Investigators. Effect of enalapril on survival in patients with reduced left ventricular ejection fractions and congestive heart failure. N Engl J Med 1991; 325:293.
7. Hunt SA, Baker DW, Chin MH, Cinquegrani MP, Feldman AM, Francis GS, Ganiats TG, Goldstein S, Gregoratos G, Jessup ML, Noble RJ, Packer M, Silver MA, Stevenson LW. ACC/AHA guidelines for the evaluation and management of chronic heart failure in the adult: a report of the American College of Cardiology/American Heart Association Task Force on Practice Guidelines (Committee to Revise the 1995 Guidelines for the Evaluation and Management of Heart Failure). 2001. American College of Cardiology website available at: http://www.acc.org/clinical/guidelines/failure/hf_index.htm.
8. Henry JP, Pearce JW. The possible role of cardiac stretch receptors in the induction of changes in urine flow. J Physiol 1956; 131:572–594.
9. De Bold AJ, Borenstein HB, Veress AT, Sonnenberg H. A rapid and potent natriuretic response to intravenous injection of atrial myocardial extract in rats. Life Sci 1981; 28:89–94.
10. Kangawa K, Fukuda A, Minamino N, Matsuo H. Purification and complete amino acid sequence of beta-rat atrial natriuretic polypeptide (beta-rANP) of 5000 daltons. Biochem Biophys Res Commun 1984; 119:933–940.
11. Sudoh T, Kangawa K, Minamino N, Matsuo H. A new natriuretic peptide in porcine brain. Nature 1988; 332:78–81.
12. Sudoh T, Minamino N, Kangawa K, Matsuo H. C-type natriuretic peptide (CNP): a new member of natriuretic peptide family identified in porcine brain. Biochem Biophys Res Commun 1990; 168:863–870.
13. Minamino N, Makino Y, Tateyama H, Kangawa K, Matsuo H. Characterization of immunoreactive human C-type natriuretic peptide in brain and heart. Biochem Biophys Res Commun 1991; 179:535–542.
14. Hosoda K, Nakao K, Mukoyama M, Saito Y, Jougasaki M, Shirakami G, Suga S, Ogawa Y, Yasue H, Imura H. Expression of brain natriuretic peptide gene in human heart: production in the ventricle. Hypertension 1991; 17:1152–1155.
15. Stingo AJ, Clavell AL, Heublein DM, Wei CM, Pittelkow MR, Burnett JC Jr. Presence of C-type natriuretic peptide in cultured human endothelial cells and plasma. Am J Physiol 1992; 263:H1318–H1321.

16. Klinge R, Hystad M, Kjekshus J, Karlberg BE, Djoseland O, Aakvaag A, Hall C. An experimental study of cardiac natriuretic peptides as markers of development of heart failure. Scand J Clin Lab Invest 1998; 58:683–691.

17. Luchner A, Stevens TL, Borgeson DD, Redfield M, Wei CM, Porter JG, Burnett JC. Differential atrial and ventricular expression of myocardial BNP during evolution of heart failure. Am J Physiol 1998; 274:H1684–H1689.

18. Maeda K, Tsutamoto T, Wada A, Hisanaga T, Kinoshita M. Plasma brain natriuretic peptide as a biochemical marker of high left ventricular end-diastolic pressure in patients with symptomatic left ventricular dysfunction. Am Heart J 1998; 135:825–832.

19. Muders F, Kromer EP, Griese DP, Pfeifer M, Hense HW, Riegger GA, Elsner D. Evaluation of plasma natriuretic peptides as markers for left ventricular dysfunction. Am Heart J 1997; 134:442–449.

20. Yasue H, Yoshimura M, Sumida H, Kikuta K, Kugiyama K, Jougasaki M, Ogawa H, Okumura K, Mukoyama M, Nakao K. Localization and mechanism of secretion of B-type natriuretic peptide in comparison with those of A-type natriuretic peptide in normal subjects and patients with heart failure. Circulation 1994; 90:195–203.

21. Nakagawa O, Ogawa Y, Itoh H, Suga S, Komatsu Y, Kishimoto I, Nishino K, Yoshimasa T, Nakao K. Rapid transcriptional activation and early mRNA turnover of BNP in cardiocyte hypertrophy. Evidence for BNP as an "emergency" cardiac hormone against ventricular overload. J Clin Invest 1995; 96:1280–1287.

22. Grantham JA, Borgeson DD, Burnett JC. BNP: pathophysiological and potential therapeutic roles in acute congestive heart failure. Am J Physiol 1997; 92:R1077–R1083.

23. Dao Q, Krishnaswamy P, Kazanegra R, Harrison A, Amirnovin R, Lenert L, Clopton P, Alberto J, Hlavin P, Maisel AS. Utility of B-type natriuretic peptide (BNP) in the diagnosis of heart failure in an urgent care setting. J Am Coll Cardiol 2001; 37:379–385.

24. Maisel AS, Krishnaswamy P, Nowak RM, McCord J, Hollander JE, Duc P, Omland T, Storrow AB, Abraham WT, Wu AH, Clopton P, Steg PG, Westheim A, Knudsen CW, Perez A, Kazanegra R, Herrmann HC, McCullough PA. Rapid measurement of B-type natriuretic peptide in the emergency diagnosis of heart failure. N Engl J Med 2002; 347:161–167.

25. Morrison LK, Harrison A, Krishnaswamy P, Kazanegra R, Clopton P, Maisel A. Utility of rapid B-type natriuretic peptide in differentiating congestive heart failure from lung disease. J Am Coll Cardiol 2002; 39(2):202–209.

26. Maisel A. B-type natriuretic peptide measurements in diagnosing congestive heart failure in the dyspneic emergency department patient. Rev Cardiovasc Med 2002; 3(suppl 4):S10–S17.

27. Mueller C, Scholer A, Laule-Kilian K, Martina B, Schindler C, Buser P, Pfisterer M, Perruchoud AP. Use of B-type natriuretic peptide in the evaluation and management of acute dyspnea. N Engl J Med 2004; 350(7):647–654.

28. Maisel A, Hollander JE, Guss D, McCullough P, Nowak R, Green G, Saltzberg M, Ellison SR, Bhalla MA, Bhalla V, Clopton P, Jesse R. Rapid Emergency Department Heart Failure Outpatient Trial investigators. Primary results of the Rapid Emergency Department Heart Failure Outpatient Trial (REDHOT). A multicenter study of B-type natriuretic peptide levels, emergency department decision making, and outcomes in patients presenting with shortness of breath. J Am Coll Cardiol 2004; 44(6):1328–1333.

29. Atisha D, Bhalla MA, Morrison LK, Felicio L, Clopton P, Gardetto N, Kazenegra R, Chiu A, Maisel AS. A prospective study in search of an optimal BNP level to screen patients for cardiac dysfunction. Am Heart J 2004; 148(3):518–523.

30. Heidenreich PA, Gubens MA, Fonarow GC, Konstam MA, Stevenson LW, Shekelle PG. Cost-effectiveness of screening with B-type natriuretic peptide to identify patients with reduced left ventricular ejection fraction. J Am Coll Cardiol 2004; 43(6):1019–1026.

31. Harrison A, Morrison LK, Krishnaswamy P, Kazanegra R, Clopton P, Dao Q, Hlavin P, Maisel AS. B-type natriuretic peptide predicts future cardiac events in patients presenting to the emergency department with dyspnea. Ann Emerg Med 2002; 39:131–138.

32. Wang TJ, Larson MG, Levy D, Benjamin EJ, Leip EP, Omland T, Wolf PA, Vasan RS. Plasma natriuretic peptide levels and the risk of cardiovascular events and death. N Engl J Med 2004; 350:655–663.

33. Berger R, Huelsman M, Strecker K, Bojic A, Moser P, Stanek B, Pacher R. B-type natriuretic peptide predicts sudden death in patients with chronic heart failure. Circulation 2002; 105:2392–2397.

34. Nohria A, Lewis E, Stevenson LW. Medical management of advanced heart failure. JAMA 2002; 287(5):628–640.

35. Tung RH, Garcia C, Morss AM, Pino RM, Fifer MA, Thompson BT, Lewandrowski K, Lee-Lewandrowski E, Januzzi JL. Utility of B-type natriuretic peptide for the evaluation of intensive care unit shock. Crit Care Med 2004; 32(8):1643–1647.

36. Kazanegra R, Cheng V, Garcia A, Krishnaswamy P, Gardetto N, Clopton P, Maisel A. A rapid assay for B-type natriuretic peptide correlates with falling wedge pressures in patients treated for decompensated heart failure: a pilot study. J Card Fail 2001; 7(1):21–29.

37. Berman B, Spragg R, Maisel A. B-type natriuretic peptide (BNP) levels in differentiating congestive heart failure from acute respiratory distress syndrome (ARDS). Abstracts from the 75th Annual Scientific Meeting of the American Heart Association. Circulation 2002; 106:S3191.

38. Cheng V, Kazanagra R, Garcia A, Lenert L, Krishnaswamy P, Gardetto N, Clopton P, Maisel A. A rapid bedside test for B-type natriuretic peptide predicts treatment outcomes in patients admitted with decompensated heart failure. J Am Coll Cardiol 2001; 37:386–391.

39. Bettencourt P, Ferreira S, Azevedo A, Ferreira A. Preliminary data on the potential usefulness of B-type natriuretic peptide levels in predicting outcomes after hospital discharge in patients with heart failure. Am J Med 2002; 113(3):215–219.

40. Cleland JG, Erhardt L, Murray G, Hall AS, Ball SG. on behalf of the AIRE Study Investigators. Effect of ramipril on morbidity and mode of death among survivors of acute myocardial infarction with clinical evidence of heart failure. A report from the AIRE Study Investigators. Eur Heart J 1997; 18:41.

41. Troughton RW, Frampton CM, Yandle TG, Espiner EA, Nicholls MG, Richards AM. Treatment of heart failure guided by plasma amino terminal brain natriuretic peptide (N-BNP) concentrations. Lancet 2000; 355:1126–1130.

42. Tsutamoto T, Wada A, Maeda K, Mabuchi N, Hayashi M, Tsutsui T, Ohnishi M, Sawaki M, Fujii M, Matsumoto T, Matsui T, Kinoshita M. Effect of spironolactone

on plasma brain natriuretic peptide and left ventricular remodeling in patients with congestive heart failure. J Am Coll Cardiol 2001; 37(5):1228–1233.

43. Anand IS, Fisher LD, Chiang Y-T, Latini R, Masson S, Maggioni AP, Glazer RD, Tognoni G, Cohn JN, for the Val-HeFT Investigators. Changes in brain natriuretic peptide and norepinephrine over time and mortality and morbidity in the Valsartan Heart Failure Trial (Val-HeFT). Circulation 2003; 107:1278–1283.

44. Lee SC, Stevens TL, Sandberg SM, Heublein DM, Nelson SM, Jougasaki M, Redfield MM, Burnett JC Jr. The potential of brain natriuretic peptide as a biomarker for New York Heart Association class during the outpatient treatment of heart failure. J Card Fail 2002; 8(3):149–154.

45. Bhalla V, Willis S, Maisel AS. B-type natriuretic peptide: the level and the drug—partners in the diagnosis of congestive heart failure. Congest Heart Fai 2004; 10:3–27.

46. Colucci WS, Elkayam U, Horton DP, Abraham WT, Bourge RC, Johnson AD, Wagoner LE, Givertz MM, Liang CS, Neibaur M, Haught WH, LeJemtel TH. Intravenous nesiritide, a natriuretic peptide, in the treatment of decompensated congestive heart failure. N Engl J Med 2000; 343:246–253.

47. Silver MA, Horton DP, Ghali JK, Elkayam U. Effect of nesiritide versus dobutamine on short-term outcomes in the treatment of patients with acutely decompensated heart failure. J Am Coll Cardiol 2002; 39(5):798–803.

48. Burger A, Horton D, Le Jemtel T. Effects of nesiritide (B-type natriuretic peptide) and dobutamine on ventricular arrhythmias in the treatment of patients with acutely decompensated congestive heart failure: the PRECEDENT study. Am Heart J 2002; 144(6):1102–1108.

49. Publication Committee for the VMAC Investigators (Vasodilators in the Management of Acute CHF). Intravenous nesiritide vs nitroglycerin for treatment of decompensated congestive heart failure: a randomized controlled trial. JAMA 2002; 287:1531–1540.

50. Colucci WS, Elkayam U, Horton DP, Abraham WT, Bourge RC, Johnson AD, Wagoner LE, Givertz MM, Liang CS, Neibaur M, Haught WH, LeJemtel TH. Intravenous nesiritide, a natriuretic peptide, in the treatment of decompensated congestive heart failure. Nesiritide Study Group. N Engl J Med 2000; 343(4):246–253.

51. Abraham WT, Lowes BD, Ferguson DA, Odom J, Kim JK, Robertson AD, Bristow MR, Schrier RW. Systemic hemodynamic, neurohormonal, and renal effects of a steady-state infusion of human brain natriuretic peptide in patients with hemodynamically decompensated heart failure. J Card Fail 1998; 4(1):37–44.

52. Mehta RL, Pascual MT, Soroko S, Chertow GM; PICARD Study Group. Diuretics, mortality, and nonrecovery of renal function in acute renal failure. JAMA 2002; 288(20):2547–2553.

53. Jensen KT, Carstens J, Pedersen EB. Effect of BNP on renal hemodynamics, tubular function and vasoactive hormones in humans. Am J Physiol 1998; 274(1 Pt 2): F63–F72.

54. Jensen KT, Eiskjaer H, Carstens J, Pedersen EB. Renal effects of brain natriuretic peptide in patients with congestive heart failure. Clin Sci (Lond) 1999; 96(1):5–15.

55. Remme WJ. Vasodilator therapy without converting-enzyme inhibition in congestive heart failure—usefulness and limitations. Cardiovasc Drugs Ther 1989; 3(3):375–396 (Review).

56. Ewy GA. Inotropic infusions for chronic congestive heart failure: medical miracles or misguided medicinals? J Am Coll Cardiol 1999; 33(2):572–575 (Review).

57. Felker GM, O'Connor CM. Inotropic therapy for heart failure: an evidence-based approach. Am Heart J 2001; 142(3):393–401 (Review).

58. Felker GM, Benza RL, Chandler AB, Leimberger JD, Cuffe MS, Califf RM, Gheorghiade M, O'Connor CM; OPTIME-CHF Investigators. Heart failure etiology and response to milrinone in decompensated heart failure: results from the OPTIME-CHF study. J Am Coll Cardiol 2003; 41(6):997–1003.

59. Burger AJ, Horton DP, LeJemtel T, Ghali JK, Torre G, Dennish G, Koren M, Dinerman J, Silver M, Cheng ML, Elkayam U; Prospective Randomized Evaluation of Cardiac Ectopy with Dobutamine or Natrecor Therapy. Effect of nesiritide (B-type natriuretic peptide) and dobutamine on ventricular arrhythmias in the treatment of patients with acutely decompensated congestive heart failure: the PRECEDENT study. Am Heart J 2002; 144(6):1102–1108.

60. Koglin J, Pehlivanli S, Schwaiblmair M, Vogeser M, Cremer P, vonScheidt W. Role of brain natriuretic peptide in risk stratification of patients with congestive heart failure. J Am Coll Cardiol 2001; 38:1934–1941.

61. Yancy CW, Saltzberg MT, Berkowitz RL, Bertolet B, Vijayaraghavan K, Burnham K, Oren RM, Walker K, Horton DP, Silver MA. Safety and feasibility of using serial infusions of nesiritide for heart failure in an outpatient setting (from the FUSION I trial). Am J Cardiol 2004; 94(5):595–601.

10

Sepsis

DAVID L. BALFE

Division of Pulmonary and Critical Care Medicine
Cedars–Sinai Medical Center
Los Angeles, California, U.S.A.

I. Introduction

Sepsis, septic shock, and their sequelae are unquestionably a major contributor to morbidity and mortality in hospitalized patients worldwide. Severe sepsis often punctuates the terminal phase of illness due to a multitude of underlying disease conditions in patients both young and old. Severe sepsis/septic shock is recognized as one of the leading causes of death in developed countries (1), and the frequency of severe sepsis is clearly increasing in North America, Europe, and many other countries throughout the world (1,2). The problem of sepsis has been recognized for over a century by astute clinicians who recognized that many patients were dying from severe infection as a result of a deleterious host response to the infection, rather than from direct invasion of the microbial pathogen into the tissues of the patient. As a result of innovations and advances in medicine and surgical technique, sepsis has become "a disease of medical progress." The ever-increasing incidence of sepsis is related in large part to improved survival rates from other reversible causes of lethality, such as blood loss, volume depletion, trauma, many cancers, and a variety of other disease processes that were rapidly fatal even a few human generations ago. These advances in medicine and surgery provide a large number of severely injured, hospitalized patients who remain susceptible to morbidity and mortality from severe sepsis/septic shock (3,4).

Significant resources have been invested in developing and evaluating potential treatments. After numerous unsuccessful trials of anti-inflammatory agents in patients with sepsis, investigators doubted that mortality could be decreased. Advances in unraveling the pathophysiology and genetic basis for the host response to sepsis have changed the prevailing understanding of the syndrome, and several therapies have demonstrated surprising efficacy (5).

II. Overview of the Extent of the Problem

Sepsis represents a substantial health care burden as the leading cause of death in critically ill patients in the U.S. Care of patients with sepsis costs as much as $50,000 per patient (6), resulting in an economic burden of nearly $17 billion annually in the U.S. alone (1,7). Sepsis is often lethal, killing 20–50% of severely affected patients (8). Furthermore, sepsis substantially reduces the quality of life of those who survive (9,10). It has been projected that sepsis will continue to increase at a rate of 1.5% per year on the basis of growth and aging of the U.S. population (7). Care of patients with sepsis costs as much as $50,000 per patient (6), resulting in an economic burden of nearly $17 billion annually in the U.S. alone (7). Sepsis is often lethal, killing 20–50% of severely affected patients (8). It is the second leading cause of death among patients in non-coronary intensive care units (ICUs) (11) and the tenth leading cause of death overall in the U.S. (12). Furthermore, sepsis substantially reduces the quality of life of those who survive (1,9,10).

III. Definition

The systemic response to infection has been termed sepsis (13–15). A prevailing theory has been that sepsis represents an uncontrolled inflammatory response (15–17). A similar, or even identical, response can arise in the absence of infection; this has been termed the systemic inflammatory response syndrome (SIRS), and is manifested by two or more of the following manifestations (which represent a change from the physiological baseline): Body temperature $>38°C$ or $<36°C$, heart rate greater than 90 beats per minute, respiratory rate greater than 20 breaths per minute, $PaCO_2$ of less than 32 mmHg, white blood cell count $>12,000/mm^3$ or $<4000/mm^3$, or $>10\%$ band forms (15). Severe sepsis is defined as sepsis associated with organ dysfunction, sepsis-induced hypotension, or hypoperfusion abnormalty (lactic acidosis, oliguria, altered mental status).

Septic shock is a subset of severe sepsis and is defined as sepsis-induced hypotension, persisting despite adequate fluid resuscitation, along with the presence of hypoperfusion abnormalities or organ dysfunction (15) (Fig. 1).

The presence of hypotension is defined as one of the following: a reduction of systolic pressure to less than 90 mmHg, a 50% reduction in hypertensive patients, or a systemic manifestation of peripheral hypoperfusion, such as lactic acidosis, oliguria, or acute alteration of mental status. Septic shock is

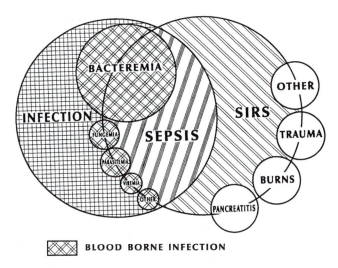

BLOOD BORNE INFECTION

Figure 1   The relationship between infection, systemic inflammatory response syndrome, and sepsis. *Source*: From Ref. 15.

defined as a patient with hypotension not responsive to at least 500-mL intravenous fluid challenge plus manifestations of peripheral hypoperfusion. Patients without hypotension but requiring more than 5 μgm/kg/min of dopamine or any other vasopressor agent are also considered to be in shock (15). A progressively higher mortality rate was observed in patients with increasing severity of sepsis. If no SIRS criteria are noted, the 28 day mortality is 3%, two SIRS criteria 7%, three SIRS criteria 10%, and four SIRS criteria 17%. The mortality for patients with sepsis is 16%, severe sepsis 20%, and septic shock 46%, a significant increase (18).

IV.   Definitions of End-Organ Dysfunction

Every organ is affected in sepsis as can be appreciated by the following definitions. Acute lung injury can progress to acute respiratory distress syndrome (ARDS), which is defined as the presence of respiratory insufficiency (PaO_2/FIO_2 ratio <200) and bilateral infiltrates consistent with pulmonary edema on chest radiology, in the absence of heart failure (if measured, a pulmonary capillary wedge pressure <18 mmHg) or primary pulmonary disease. Acute renal failure is defined as an acute increase in the serum creatinine concentration greater than 2.0 mg/dL (180 μmol/L), a doubling in the admission creatinine level in a patient with chronic renal failure, or the requirement for acute dialysis or ultrafiltration. Oliguria is defined as a urinary output less than 0.5 mL/kg per hour for at least one hour or less than 30 mL for two hours. Lactic acidosis is diagnosed if the plasma lactate level is greater than 2.0 mmol/L. Disseminated intravascular coagulation was defined as a decrease in the platelet count of 25% or more from the baseline with any increase in prothrombin time. Mental status changes have been scored using the Glasgow Coma Scale (GCS), with altered mental status specifically defined as a GCS score of 11 or less (18).

Effective therapy of organ failure is essential because it is the cumulative burden of organ failure that is associated with increasing mortality, the average risk of death increasing by 15–20% with each additional failing organ (8). It has been noted that in patients with multiple organ failure, intensive care support did not result in improved long term survival, but merely delayed death (19). Patients 65 years and older with three or more organ failures lasting more than two days have mortality rates exceeding 90% (19).

In 2001, the Society of Critical Care Medicine, the European Society of Intensive Care Medicine, the American College of Chest Physicians, the American Thoracic Society, and the Surgical Infection Society held a conference (the SCCM/ESICM/ACCP/ATS/SIS International Sepsis Definitions Conference) with the aim of revisiting the definitions for sepsis and related conditions. The overall goals of the conference were three-fold and began with a view of the strengths and weaknesses of the current definitions of sepsis and related conditions. The second goal focused on the identification of ways to improve the current definitions. The final goal sought to identify methodologies for increasing the accuracy, reliability, and/or clinical utility of the diagnosis of sepsis (20).

V. Staging System for Sepsis

Despite the above mentioned definitions for sepsis, severe sepsis, and septic shock (outlined in Table 1), the SCCM/ESICM/ACCP/ATS/SIS International Sepsis Definitions Conference felt these terms did not allow for precise characterization and staging of patients with this condition. The conference developed a classification scheme for sepsis—called PIRO—that aims to stratify patients on the basis of their Predisposing conditions, the nature and extent of the insult (in the case of sepsis, Infection), the nature and magnitude of the host Response, and the degree of concomitant Organ dysfunction (Table 2). It was emphasized at the conference that the PIRO concept is rudimentary; extensive testing and further refinement will be needed before it can be considered ready for routine application in clinical practice. The potential utility of the proposed PIRO model lies in being able to discriminate morbidity arising from infection and morbidity arising from the response to infection. Interventions that modulate the response may impact adversely on the ability to contain an infection; conversely, interventions that target the infection are unlikely to be beneficial if the morbidity impact is being driven by the host response. Premorbid conditions establish a baseline risk, independent of the infectious process, while acquired organ dysfunction is an outcome to be prevented (20).

Table 1 Diagnostic Criteria for Sepsis (2001 SCCM/ESICM/ACCP/ATS/SIS International Sepsis Definitions Conference)

Infection, documented or suspected, and some of the following general variables:
Fever (core temperature >38.3°C)
Hypothermia (core temperature <36°C)
Heart rate >90 per min or >2 SD above the normal value for age
Tachypnea
Altered mental status
Significant edema or positive fluid balance (>20 mL/kg over 24 hr)
Hyperglycemia (plasma glucose >120 mg/dL or 7.7 mmol/L) in the absence of diabetes
Inflammatory variables
Leukocytosis (WBC count >12,000 per microliter)
Leukopenia (WBC count <4000 per microliter)
Normal WBC count with >10% immature forms
Plasma C-reactive protein >2 SD above the normal value
Plasma procalcitonin >2 SD above the normal value

Hemodynamic variables:
Arterial hypotension$b$ (SBP < 90 mmHg, MAP < 70, or an SBP decrease >40 mmHg in adults or <2 SD below normal for age)
Mixed venous O_2 < 70%
Cardiac index <3.5 L/min/m^2

Organ dysfunction variables:
Arterial hypoxemia (P_aO_2/F_1O_2 ratio <300)
Acute oliguria (urine output <0.5 mL/kg/hr)
Creatinine increase >0.5 mg/dL
Coagulation abnormalities (INR > 1.5 or aPTT > 60 sec)
Ileus (absent bowel sounds)
Thrombocytopenia (platelet count <100,000 per microliter)
Hyperbilirubinemia (plasma total bilirubin >4 mg/dL or 70 mmol/L)

Tissue perfusion variables:
Hyperlactatemia (>1 mmol/L)
Decreased capillary refill or mottling

Abbreviations: ACCP, American College of Chest Physicians; ATS, American Thoracic Society; aPTT, activated partial thromboplastin time; ESICM, European Society of Intensive Care Medicine; INR, international normalized ratio; MAP, mean arterial blood pressure; SBP, systolic blood pressure; SCCM, Society of Critical Care Medicine; SIS, Surgical Infection Society; SvO$_2$, mixed venous oxygen saturation; WBC, white blood cell.
Source: From Ref. 20.

Table 2 PIRO Classification System (2001 SCCM/ESICM/ACCP/ATS/SIS International Sepsis Definitions Conference)

Domain	Current model	Future consideration	Rationale
Predisposition	Premorbid illness with reduced probability of short term survival. Cultural or religious beliefs, age, sex.	Genetic polymorphisms in components of inflammatory response; enhanced understanding of specific interactions between pathogens and host diseases.	Premorbid factors impact on the potential attributable morbidity and mortality of an acute insult; deleterious consequences of insult heavily dependent on genetic predisposition.
Infection	Culture and sensitivity of infecting pathogens; detection of disease amenable to source control.	Assay of microbial products (LPS, galactomannan, bacterial DNA); gene transcript profiles.	Specific therapies directed against inciting insult require demonstration and characterization of that insult.
Response	SIRS, other signs of sepsis, shock, CRP.	Nonspecific markers of activated inflammation (e.g., PCT or IL-6) or impaired host responsiveness (e.g., HLA-DR); specific detection of target of therapy (e.g., protein C, TNF, PAF).	Both mortality risk and potential to respond to therapy vary with nonspecific measures of disease severity; specific mediator-targeted therapy is predicated on presence and activity of mediator.
Organ dysfunction	Organ dysfunction as number of failing organs or composite score (e.g., MODS, SOFA, LODS, PEMOD, PELOD).	Dynamic measures of cellular response to insult: apoptosis, cytopathic hypoxia, cell stress.	Response to preemptive therapy (e.g., targeting microorganism or early mediator) not possible if damage already present; therapies targeting the injurious cellular process require that it be present.

Abbreviations: CRP, C-reactive protein; HLA-DR, human leukocyte antigen-DR; IL, interleukin; LODS, logistic organ dysfunction system; LPS, lipopolysaccharide; MODS, multiple organ dysfunction syndrome; PAF, platelet-activating factor; PCT, procalcitonin; PELOD, pediatric logistic organ dysfunction; PEMOD, pediatric multiple organ dysfunction; SIRS, systemic inflammatory response syndrome; SOFA, sepsis-related organ failure assessment; TLR, Toll-like receptor; TNF, tumor necrosis factor.
Source: From Ref. 20

The PIRO concept: *Predisposition.* Premorbid factors have a substantial impact on outcome in sepsis, modifying both the disease process and the approach taken to therapy. This point is emphasized by recent data showing that genetic factors play a greater role in determining the risk of premature mortality due to sepsis than they do in influencing the risk of premature death from other common conditions, such as cancer or cardiovascular diseases (21). Beyond genetic variability, however, the management of patients with sepsis, and hence the outcome of the disease, is clearly influenced by factors such as the premorbid health status of the patient, the reversibility of concomitant diseases, and a host of religious and cultural forces that shape the approach toward therapy. It was noted by the conference that these multiple predisposing factors could influence both the incidence and the outcome in similar or conflicting ways. They could also pose separate or different risks for each of the different stages of infection, response, and organ dysfunction. For example, immunosuppression may increase a person's risk of infection, decrease the magnitude of that person's inflammatory response, and have no direct influence on organ dysfunction. Similarly, a genetic polymorphism such as the TNF2 allele may result in a more aggressive inflammatory response to an invading organism. This might decrease a person's risk of infection but increase that person's risk of an overly exuberant, and potentially harmful, inflammatory response should that patient become infected (20).

Infection. The site, type, and extent of the infection have a significant impact on prognosis. By studying mortality rates among patients randomized to receive placebo in recent randomized clinical trials of new agents for the adjuvant treatment of sepsis, it is apparent that pneumonia and intra-abdominal infections are associated with a higher risk of mortality than are urinary tract infections. Patients with secondary nosocomial bacteremia experience a higher mortality than those with catheter-related or primary bacteremia (22). Similarly, there is evidence that the endogenous host response to gram-positive organisms differs from that evoked by gram-negative organisms (20,23).

Response. In general, current targeted therapies for sepsis are aimed at the host response, rather than the infecting organism. The host response has proven to be difficult to characterize. Putative biologic markers of response severity include circulating levels of procalcitonin (24,25), IL-6 (26,27), and many others. When a new mediator is identified, epidemiologic studies will be required to determine whether measurements of the compound can be useful for staging patients. Furthermore, the optimal set of biologic markers for staging sepsis may depend on the nature of the therapeutic decision to be made. For example, an indicator of dysregulation of the coagulation system might be more valuable for making a decision about whether to institute therapy with drotrecogin alfa (activated) (28), whereas a marker of adrenal dysfunction might be more useful for determining whether to institute therapy with hydrocortisone (20,29).

Organ dysfunction. By analogy with the TNM system, the presence of organ dysfunction in sepsis is similar to the presence of metastatic disease in cancer. Certainly, the severity of organ dysfunction is an important determinant of prognosis in sepsis (30,31). Whether the severity of organ dysfunction can aid in therapeutic stratification is less clear (20). Nevertheless, there is evidence that activated protein C may provide more benefit to patients with greater, as compared with lesser, disease burden (32). The modern organ failure scores can be used to quantitatively describe the degree of organ dysfunction developing over the course of critical illness (20,33). Using this concept, a systematic literature review covering 30 years demonstrated that both the nature of the organism and the site of infection have a significant impact on survival from sepsis and that there is a significant interaction between them (34).

VI.   Epidemiology

Sepsis develops in over 750,000 people annually, and more than 210,000 of them die (5,7,35). Sepsis is now among the 10 leading causes of death in the U.S. (1,36), having previously been ranked as the 13th leading cause of death in 1993 (37). It is the second leading cause of death among patients in noncoronary intensive care units (ICUs). A previous prospective observational study noted that 68% of ICU admissions met the criteria for the systemic inflammatory response syndrome. Of those patients, 26% were noted to develop sepsis, and 4% of these developed septic shock (18,38). A similar study described a population at eight academic medical centers with an occurrence rate of sepsis of 2.8 patients per 1000 patient days (39). A wide range of occurrence rates of sepsis has been noted in various studies, with rates of severe sepsis ranging from 2.1% (15) to 6.3% (40). In a recent study of 22 French hospitals over an eight-year period, the overall frequency of septic shock per admission was 8.2/100 admissions. It increased from seven to 9.7 admissions (from 1993 to 2000) (37). In a large study of all hospital discharge data from seven large states, 192,980 cases of severe sepsis were identified, 2.9% of all admissions. The mean age of the cases was 63.8 years, and 49.6% were male. Fifty-five percent of patients had underlying comorbidity and 21.4% were surgical. The incidence of severe sepsis was high in infants: 5.3/1000 (age <1 year), decreased in older children: 0.2/1000 (age 5–14 years), and increased throughout adulthood, increasing sharply in the elderly: 26.2/1000 (age ≥85 years). The overall hospital mortality rate was 28.6% (representing 215,000 deaths nationally). Mortality rates were higher for patients with preexisting conditions or receiving ICU care, and they correlated with increasing numbers of organ failure and with increasing age (from 10% in children to 38.4% in patients ≥85 years). Mortality rates were higher in men than women (29.3% vs. 27.9%) (38).

In an analysis of the occurrence of sepsis using a nationally representative sample of all nonfederal acute care hospitals in the U.S., it was noted that the population-adjusted incidence of sepsis had increased significantly over the past two decades. During the 22-year study period, there were 10,319,418 reported cases of sepsis (accounting for 1.3% of all hospitalizations). The number of patients with sepsis per year increased from 164,072 in 1979 to 659,935 in 2000 (an increase of 13.7% per year). After normalization to the population distribution in the 2000 U.S. Census, the incidence of sepsis increased over the 22-year period from 82.7 cases per 100,000 population to 240.4 cases per 100,000 population, for an annualized increase of 8.7% (1). During the study period, there were a total of approximately 750 million hospitalizations in the U.S. The average age of patients with sepsis increased consistently over time, from 57.4 years in the first part of the study to 60.8 years in the last part of the study. Sepsis developed later in life in female patients than in male patients; the mean age among women was 62.1 years, as compared with 56.9 years among men. There was a similar pattern to the increases in incidence among men and among women, although the incidence among women increased more rapidly during the study period (an annualized increase of 8.7% vs. 8.0%) (Fig. 2) (1). Although men accounted for 48.1% of cases of sepsis on average per year, adjustment for sex in the population of the U.S. reveals that in every year, men were more likely to have sepsis than women (mean annual relative risk, 1.28). Whites had the lowest rates of sepsis during the study period, with both blacks and other nonwhite groups having a similarly elevated risk as compared with whites (mean annual relative risk, 1.89 and 1.90, respectively). Black men had the highest rate of sepsis during the study period (330.9 cases per 100,000), the youngest age at onset (mean age, 47.4 years), and the highest mortality (23.3%) (1).

It has been noted that fungal pathogens (25) and gram-positive organisms have become more significant (41,42). Other risk factors for mortality in sepsis

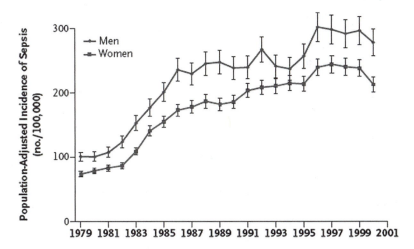

Figure 2 Population-adjusted incidence of sepsis, according to sex, 1979–2000. Points represent the annual incidence rate, and I bars the standard error. *Source*: From Ref. 1.

include adequacy of antibiotics, source and type of infection, presence of shock, need for vasopressors, multiple organ failure, and neutropenia (43). Blood-borne infection associated with candida and enterococcus species is associated with the highest attributable mortality (30–40%), while bacteremia associated with coagulase negative staphylococci is associated with the lowest attributable mortality (15–20%) (39,44). In addition, the proportion of septic shock due to staphylococcus resistant to methicillin and pseudomonas has increased dramatically with time, reaching a proportion between one fifth and a quarter in a large French study (37). The site of infection can also influence the outcome of sepsis, increased mortality being noted with intra-abdominal or lower respiratory tract infections (45). Early mortality from sepsis (<3 days) was associated with arterial pH < 7.33, increasing number of failing organs, shock, multiple sources of sepsis, and higher Simplified Acute Physiology II (SAPS II) scores.

Of note is that the mortality from septicemia decreased from 31% to 25.5% from 1979 to 1989 (39,46). In a recent study of 22 French hospitals over an eight-year period, septic shock mortality (crude and adjusted) decreased from 63% to 58% (from 1993 to 2000) (37). This has been attributed to changes in the susceptible population developing sepsis and, possibly, to improvements in supportive care and antimicrobial and other therapy. Of note is that initial use of inappropriate antibiotics is associated with a worse outcome, and in addition, failure to provide adequate surgical drainage of infected areas is associated with increased mortality (39,47). Between 1979 and 1987, gram-negative bacteria were the predominant organisms causing sepsis, whereas gram-positive bacteria were reported most commonly in each subsequent year. Among the organisms reported to have caused sepsis in 2000, gram-positive bacteria accounted for 52.1% of cases, with gram-negative bacteria accounting for 37.6%, polymicrobial infections for 4.7%, anaerobes for 1.0%, and fungi for 4.6%. Specific organisms causing sepsis were recorded in 51% of all discharge records over the 22-year period, with the rate increasing during the first subperiod and remaining static thereafter. The greatest relative changes were observed in the incidence of gram-positive infections, which increased by an average of 26.3% per year. The number of cases of sepsis caused by fungal organisms increased by 207%, from 5231 cases in 1979 to 16,042 cases in 2000 (1).

VII. Pathogenesis of Sepsis

The idea that sepsis was caused by an overwhelming reaction of the patient to invading microorganisms was probably at least partially based on the observation that, on many occasions, no clinical evidence for infection (e.g., positive bacterial blood cultures) was found in patients with septic symptoms (48). In 1972, Lewis Thomas (49) noted that "it is our response that makes the disease" and that the patient was, therefore, more endangered by this response than by the invading micro-organisms. The response of the patient's immune system is determined by many factors, including the virulence of the organism, the size of the innoculum, and the patient's coexisting conditions, nutritional status, age, and polymorphisms in cytokine genes or other immune-effector molecules or their receptors (5).

A. Innate Immunity

The innate immune system is the initial line of defense against infection and is activated when a pathogen crosses the host's natural defense barriers (50,51). It consists of:

1. soluble elements (the alternative and mannan-binding lectin pathways of the complement system, acute phase proteins, and cytokines);
2. cellular elements (macrophages, monocytes, neutrophils, and dendritic cells in addition to natural killer cells) (50).

Innate immune responses must be tightly regulated because unbalanced inflammatory and immune reactions can result in either uncontrolled growth of invading organisms or overwhelming inflammatory responses with tissue injury, vascular collapse, and multi-organ failure (50). Detection of invading micro-organisms is mediated by pattern recognition receptors expressed on the surface of innate immune cells. Pattern recognition receptors recognize structures common to many microbial pathogens. These structures are called pathogen-associated molecular patterns and include endotoxins (lipopolysaccharide), peptidoglycan, lipoteichoic acid, lipopeptides, flagellin, mannan, and viral RNA (50). The structures are essential for survival of the micro-organisms and therefore do not undergo major mutations (50). When a pathogen-associated molecular pattern binds to a pattern recognition receptor, it activates several intracellular signaling pathways, resulting in the activation of transcription factors (NF-kappaB, AP-1, Fos, Jun) (50). The transcription factors control the expression of immune response genes and the release of numerous effector molecules, such as cytokines. Cytokines have an essential role in orchestrating the innate and acquired immune responses to an invading pathogen (50,52). Gram-negative bacilli (mainly *Enterobacteriaceae* and *Pseudomonas aeruginosa*) and gram-positive cocci (mainly staphylococci and streptococci) are the most common microbes isolated from patients with severe sepsis and septic shock (53). Fungi, mostly Candida, account for only about 5% of all cases of severe sepsis.

B. Gram-Negative Sepsis

Most cases of gram-negative sepsis are caused by *Enterobacteriaceae* (*E. coli* and *Klebsiella*) species. *Pseudomonas aeruginosa* is the third commonest cause. Gram-negative infections usually occur in the lung, abdomen, bloodstream, or urinary tract. Lipopolysaccharide is a key component of the outer membrane of gram-negative bacteria and has an important role in the pathogenesis of gram-negative sepsis (54). Lipopolysaccharide binding protein in host cells binds to lipopolysaccharide in the bacteria and transfers it to CD14 (55). CD14, a protein anchored in the outer leaflet of the plasma membrane, also exists as a soluble plasma protein that attaches lipopolysaccharide to CD14-negative cells (e.g., endothelial cells). CD14 is located in the extracellular space and therefore cannot induce cellular activation without a transmembrane signal transducing coreceptor (55).

Toll receptors were first discovered in the fruit fly, where they were found to have a role in the defense against fungi and gram-positive bacteria (56). Toll-like receptors (TLR) were subsequently identified in other species. Human TLR, like their homologues in insects and other mammalian species, are type I transmembrane proteins with an extracellular leucine-rich repeat domain and an intracellular domain homologous to the interleukin 1 receptor. Previous genetic studies in mice have shown that mutations in the TLR4 gene were linked to resistance to lipopolysaccharide, providing evidence that TLR4 was an essential component of the lipopolysaccharide receptor complex (57). MD-2, a secreted protein associated with the extracellular domain of TLR4, has also recently been shown to have an important role in responsiveness to lipopolysaccharide (58).

C. Gram-Positive Sepsis

Staphylococci (mainly Staph aureus and coagulase-negative staphylococci) and streptococci (Strep pyogenes, viridans streptococci, Strep pneumoniae) are the commonest causes of gram-positive sepsis. They are usually responsible for infections of skin and soft tissues, infections associated with intravascular devices, primary bloodstream infections, or respiratory infections. Gram-positive organisms can cause sepsis by at least two mechanisms:

1.   by producing exotoxins that act as superantigens;
2.   by components of their cell walls stimulating immune cells (59).

Superantigens are molecules that bind to MHC class II molecules of antigen-presenting cells and to Vß chains of T cell receptors. In doing so, they activate large numbers of T cells to produce massive amounts of pro-inflammatory cytokines. Staphylococcal enterotoxins, toxic shock syndrome toxin-1, and streptococcal pyrogenic exotoxins are examples of bacterial superantigens. Gram-positive bacteria without exotoxins can also induce shock, probably by stimulating innate immune responses through similar mechanisms to those in gram-negative sepsis. Indeed, Toll-like receptor 2 (TLR2) has been shown to mediate cellular responses to heat-killed gram-positive bacteria and their cell wall structures (peptidoglycan, lipoproteins, lipoteichoic acid, and phenol soluble modulin) (60).

The clinical manifestations of sepsis produced by different gram-positive and gram-negative bacteria vary. For example, the clinical pictures of streptococcal toxic shock syndrome and meningococcaemia are very different. In addition, *E. coli* urosepsis follows a more benign course than nosocomial pneumonia due to *P. aeruginosa*. Gram-positive and gram-negative sepsis result in different expression and release of pro-inflammatory mediators, such as the cytokine tumor necrosis factor-α (61). These observations suggest that there are specific host immune responses to each pathogen mediated by various sets of pathogen-associated molecular patterns and pattern recognition receptors.

D. Toll Like Receptors

Of the 10 human TLRs identified so far, seven interact with microbial motifs (51). For example, TLR2 binds components of the cell wall of gram-positive bacteria as well as ligands derived from other pathogens, TLR5 is the receptor for bacterial flagellin (62), and TLR9 is required for cellular activation by unmethylated CpG motifs of bacterial DNA (63). Cooperation between TLRs is necessary to respond to certain pathogens, such as gram-positive bacteria in addition to yeast (zymosan) (64). Several signal-transducing pathways are activated after microbial ligands bind to TLRs (65). The fact that different microbial products bind to different TLRs, the existence of receptor-specific signaling pathways, and the idea of differential expression of TLRs by tissues and organs strongly suggest that the innate immune system is tailored in a pathogen- and tissue-specific manner (50). Expression of immune genes and host responses to infections will vary depending on the structural and biochemical composition of the invading pathogen (50). If confirmed, these hypotheses point to the need to develop pathogen-specific approaches to treatment (50). Other soluble and membrane-associated proteins have recently been shown to be involved in recognizing bacteria or microbial products. These include peptidoglycan recognition proteins and triggering receptor expressed on myeloid cells (TREM-1) (50).

E. Coagulation Abnormalities and Other Inflammatory Mediators

Coagulation abnormalities, especially disseminated intravascular coagulation, are common in patients with sepsis and microvascular thrombosis (50). The ensuing tissue damage may have an important role in the pathophysiology of organ dysfunction. Treatment with activated protein C, a protein that has antithrombotic, profibrinolytic, and anti-inflammatory effects, reduces mortality from severe sepsis at the price of a slight increase in bleeding events (50,66). Glucocorticoids exert broad metabolic and immunomodulating effects and have been used to treat several inflammatory diseases. Although high doses of steroids have no clinical benefit (50,67), a previous multicenter trial found that a seven-day course of low doses of hydrocortisone and fludrocortisone reduced mortality in patients with septic shock and relative adrenal insufficiency (29,50).

A marker that is able to distinguish the inflammatory response to infection from other types of inflammation would be of great clinical use. Unfortunately, the availability of a highly specific and sensitive marker of infection is still unsatisfied (68,69). The proinflammatory cytokines tumor necrosis factor (TNF) and interleukin (IL)-1, the most proximal mediators of this cascade, are evoked by bacterial cell wall components such as endotoxin, lipo teichoic acid, and peptido-glycan (70–77). These cytokines activate multiple downstream inflammatory pathways, triggering the release of both pro- and anti-inflammatory mediators, activating coagulation, and inhibiting fibrinolysis (78–81). IL-6, released in response to TNF and IL-1 (82), is consistently detected in the blood of patients with sepsis, and elevated levels are associated with adverse outcome (83). Elevated plasma concentrations of a variety of cytokines and chemokines, such as TNF-α (84), interleukin (IL)-1 (85), IL-6 (86), IL-8 (87), and the monocyte chemotactic proteins-1 and -2 (88), have been described in septic patients and often correlate with the severity of the disease (68). In addition, the complement system is activated in patients suffering from sepsis and SIRS (68). Increased plasma concentrations of either protein complement 3a (C3a) or the terminal complement complex have been found, which are attributable to either a direct or indirect interaction of microorganisms with the complement system and the subsequent activation of either the alternative or classic pathway (68,89). In addition, it may be in part the result of C-reactive protein (CRP)-mediated complement activation (68,90). CRP is an acute phase protein released in both infective and noninfective inflammatory processes, such as trauma or neoplasm (68,91). The proinflammatory cytokines TNF-α, IL-1, and, most important, IL-6 trigger synthesis and release of CRP from hepatocytes (68). A recent study revealed that determination of plasma procalcitonin, IL-6, and C3a is more reliable to differentiate between sepsis and SIRS than the variables CRP and elastase (68).

VIII.   Failure of Clinical Trials in Sepsis

The failure of clinical trials investigating anti-inflammatory strategies for the treatment of sepsis has been referred to as a "graveyard" for pharmaceutical companies, since almost none of these strategies have resulted in significantly improved survival of patients (48). Although cytokines are considered to be culprits, they also have beneficial effects in sepsis. Studies in an animal model of peritonitis demonstrated that blocking TNF-α worsens survival (5,92,93). In clinical trials, a TNF antagonist increased mortality (94). The role of TNF-α in combating infection has recently been underscored by the finding that sepsis and other infectious complications developed in patients with rheumatoid arthritis who were treated with TNF antagonists (95). The debate about the merits of inhibiting cytokines in patients with sepsis has been rekindled by a recent trial that indicated that a subgroup of patients with sepsis who had therapy directed against TNF-α had improved survival (96). Also, a meta-analysis of clinical trials of anti-inflammatory agents in patients with sepsis showed that although high doses of anti-inflammatory agents were generally harmful in such patients, a subgroup of patients (approximately 10%) benefited (Fig. 3) (97).

Retrospectively, a crucial problem in most of the clinical trials investigating anti-inflammatory agents appears to be the nonhomogeneity of the patient

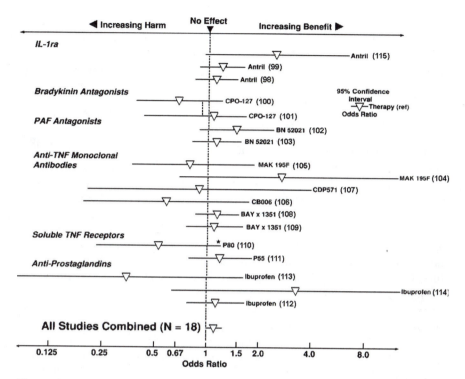

Figure 3 Odds ratios and 95% confidence intervals for survival in 18 clinical trials of nonglucocorticoid anti-inflammatory agents in patients with sepsis and septic shock. The odds of surviving equals the probability of surviving divided by the probability of dying. In this figure, the odds ratios were determined by calculating the odds of surviving in the treatment group and dividing this by the odds of surviving in the control group. (*This odds ratio includes low, medium, and high doses of P-80-soluble tumor necrosis factor receptor.) *Abbreviations*: IL-1ra, interleukin-1 receptor antagonist; PAF, platelet-activating factor; TNF, tumor necrosis factor. Figures in parentheses reflects the reference number of the study. *Source*: From Ref. 97.

population enrolled, which partially stems from an inability to more effectively classify the immune status of the septic patient (5).

IX. Management of Severe Sepsis and Septic Shock

In 2003, critical care and infectious disease experts representing 11 international organizations developed management guidelines for severe sepsis and septic shock (116). The results of the conference, which were based on evidence-based recommendations, will form the basis for the discussion of the management of severe sepsis and septic shock (116). Shock occurs when the circulatory system fails to maintain adequate cellular perfusion, resulting in cellular and ultimately organ dysfunction (117). The resuscitation of a patient in severe sepsis or sepsis-induced tissue hypoperfusion (hypotension or elevated serum lactate) should begin as soon as the condition is recognized, not delayed until the patient is admitted to an ICU.

A. Initial Resuscitation

During the first six hours of resuscitation, the goals of initial resuscitation of sepsis-induced hypotension should include all of the following: Central venous pressure: 8–12 mmHg, mean arterial pressure ≥65 mmHg, urine output ≥0.5 mL/kg/hr, mixed venous oxygen saturations ≥70%. Early goal-directed therapy has been shown to improve survival in patients with severe sepsis and septic shock (116).

In a landmark paper, Rivers and colleagues (118) conducted a randomized controlled study in an emergency room setting. Patients were assigned to receive either six hours of early goal-directed therapy or standard therapy. Early hemodynamic assessment on the basis of physical findings, vital signs, central venous pressure (119), and urinary output (120) have previously been noted to inadequately detect persistent global tissue hypoxia (118). The objective of early goal-directed therapy is to provide a more definitive resuscitation strategy involving goal-oriented manipulation of cardiac preload, afterload, and contractility to achieve a balance between systemic oxygen delivery and oxygen demand (118,119). Patients in the intervention arm of the study were treated in a nine-bed unit in the emergency room (for at least six hours), staffed by an emergency room physician, two residents, and three nurses. Patients underwent peripheral arterial catheterization in addition to central venous catheterization with a catheter capable of measuring central venous oxygen saturation continuously. Early goal-directed therapy was as follows (Fig. 4): A 500 mL bolus of crystalloid was administered every 30 minutes to achieve a central venous pressure of 8–12 mmHg. If the mean arterial pressure was less than 65 mmHg, vasopressors were given to maintain a mean arterial pressure of at least 65 mmHg. If the mean arterial pressure was greater than 90 mmHg, vasodilators were given until it was 90 mmHg or below. If the central venous oxygen saturation was less than 70%, a red blood cell transfusion was administered to maintain a hematocrit of at least 30%. If after the central venous pressure, mean arterial pressure and hematocrit were optimized as described, the central venous oxygen saturation was less than 70%, dobutamine administration was administered at a starting dose of 2.5 μgm/kg of body weight per minute, the dose being increased by 2.5 μgms/kg per minute every 30 minutes until the central venous oxygen saturation was greater than or equal to 70% (or until a maximal dobutamine dose of 20 μgm/Kg of body weight per minute was given). Note the dobutamine was decreased in dose or discontinued if the mean arterial pressure was less than 65 mmHg or if the heart rate was greater than 120 per minute. In patients in

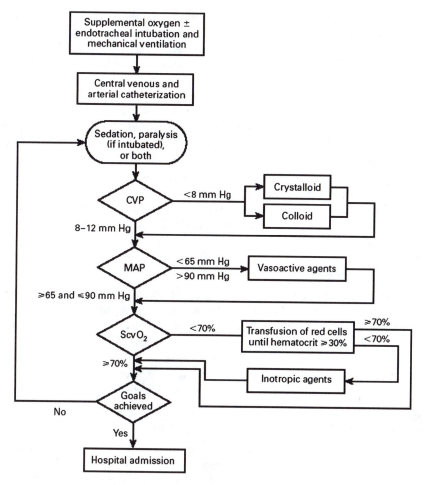

Figure 4 Protocol for early goal-directed therapy. CVP denotes central venous pressure, MAP mean arterial pressure, and $ScvO_2$ central venous oxygen saturation. *Source*: From Ref. 118.

whom hemodynamic optimization could not be achieved, mechanical ventilation with sedation was initiated. The in-hospital mortality of patients in the intervention arm was 30.5%, as compared to 46.5% in the control arm ($p = 0.009$). Of note is that the patients in the early goal-directed therapy arm of the study received significantly more intravenous fluid than the control arm in the first six hours; however, during the first 72 hours of hospitalization, there was no significant, difference in intravenous fluid administration (118).

Although the specific approach that is used may vary, there are critical elements that should be incorporated in any resuscitative effort. A 2004 update to practice parameters for hemodynamic support of sepsis in adult patients noted that therapy should be guided by parameters that reflect the adequacy of tissue and organ perfusion. Although patients with shock and mild hypovolemia may be treated successfully with rapid fluid administration, right heart catheterization may be useful to provide a diagnostic hemodynamic assessment. Fluid infusion should be the initial step in hemodynamic support, being titrated to clinical end points (central venous pressure 8–12 mmHg, pulmonary artery occlusion pressure 12–15 mmHg). More important than the specific method of monitoring is that the method should be used in a dynamic fashion (117). Dopamine and norepinephrine are both effective for increasing arterial blood pressure. It is imperative to ensure that patients are adequately fluid-resuscitated. Dopamine raises cardiac output more than norepinephrine, but its use may be limited by tachycardia. Norepinephrine may be a more effective vasopressor in some patients. Administration of low doses of dopamine to maintain renal function is not recommended (117,121).

B. Diagnosis

Appropriate cultures should always be obtained before antimicrobial therapy is initiated. To optimize the identification of causative organisms, at least two blood cultures should be obtained, with at least one drawn percutaneously and one drawn through each vascular access device (unless the device was inserted within 48 hours). Cultures of other sites such as urine, cerebrospinal fluid, wounds, respiratory secretions, or other body fluids should be obtained before antibiotic therapy is initiated as the clinical situation dictates (116).

C. Antibiotic Therapy

Intravenous antibiotic therapy should be started within the first hour of recognition of severe sepsis, after appropriate cultures have been obtained. Initial empirical anti-infective therapy should include one or more drugs that are likely to be effective against the patient's suspected pathogens. In addition, such therapy should penetrate into the presumed site of origin of the sepsis syndrome. The initial choice of antibiotics should be broad enough, covering all likely pathogens, since there is no margin for error in critically ill patients (116). It is important to note that significant delay in administering appropriate antibiotics is associated with increased hospital mortality (122). Inadequate empirical antimicrobial therapy for patients with sepsis has been shown to increase mortality (123). In a recent large randomized controlled sepsis trial (anti-TNF–MONARCS trial), 91% of enrolled patients received adequate antibiotic support, and the overall mortality rate was 34%, with rates of 33% and 43% for patients receiving adequate and inadequate antibiotic treatment, respectively. A 10% decrease in the overall crude mortality rate was associated with adequate early empiric antibiotic treatment. With the exception of a small group of patients infected with *P. aeruginosa*, no subgroup had a prognosis so poor that adequate empiric antibiotic treatment was not beneficial. In fact, reductions in mortality rates were apparent even among patients with septic shock and positive blood culture results (124). Although restricting the use of antibiotics, particularly broad spectrum antibiotics, is important for limiting super-infection and for decreasing the development of antibiotic resistant pathogens, patients with severe sepsis or septic shock warrant broad spectrum anti-infective agents until the causative organism and its antimicrobial sensitivities are defined. The anti-infective regimen should always be reassessed after 48–72 hours on the basis of microbiological and clinical data (116).

D. Source Control

Every patient presenting with severe sepsis should be evaluated for the presence of a focus of infection amenable to source control measures, specifically the drainage of an abscess or local focus of infection, the debridement of infected necrotic tissue, the removal of a potentially infected device, or the definitive control of a source of ongoing microbial contamination (116,125). The selection of optimal source control methods must weigh the potential risks and benefits of the proposed intervention, which may cause further complications such as bleeding, fistulas, or inadvertent injury to other structures (116,126). Case series and expert opinion support the principle that rapid correction of a source of microbial contamination is essential to maximize survival of the severely septic patient (116,127).

E. Fluid Therapy

Fluid infusion should be the initial step in hemodynamic support, being titrated to clinical end points (central venous pressure 8–12 mmHg, pulmonary artery occlusion pressure 12–15 mmHg). More important than the specific method of monitoring is that the method should be used in a dynamic fashion. Isotonic crystalloids or iso-oncotic colloids are equally effective when titrated to the same hemodynamic end points (117). In a large muticenter, double blind, randomized trial comparing the use of 4% albumin to normal saline for intravascular volume resuscitation in a heterogeneous ICU population, equivalent rates of death from any cause during the 28-day study period were noted (128). Requirements for mechanical ventilation and renal-replacement therapy, time spent in the ICU and in the hospital during the 28-day study period, and the time until death (among the patients who died) were also equivalent. The proportion of patients in the two groups in whom new single-organ or multiple-organ failure developed were similar. However, it should be noted that in subgroup analysis, there was a nonsignificant trend suggesting benefit with colloid therapy in those patients with sepsis. Albumin and saline were not found to be equipotent intravascular volume expanders; patients who were resuscitated with albumin received less fluid than those who were resuscitated with saline. During the first four days of the study, the ratio of albumin administered to saline administered was approximately 1:1.4

(128). There was no significant difference in mean arterial pressure between the groups, and the differences in central venous pressure and heart rate were small. Patients who were assigned to the albumin group received a significantly greater volume of packed red cells during the first two days of the study. The reasons for this difference may have been greater hemodilution with albumin than with saline or increased blood loss with albumin due to transient alterations in coagulation (128). As the volume of distribution is much larger for crystalloids than for colloids, resuscitation with crystalloids requires more fluid to achieve the same end points and results in more edema. Fluid challenge inpatients with suspected hypovolemia may be given at a rate of 500–1000 mL of crystalloids or 300–500 mL of colloids over 30 minutes and repeated based on response and tolerance, avoiding intravascular volume overload. Fluid challenge must be clearly separated from an increase in maintenance fluid administration. Fluid challenge is a term used to describe the initial volume expansion period in which the response of the patient to fluid administration is carefully evaluated (116).

F. Blood Product Administration

Once tissue hypoperfusion has resolved in the absence of extenuating circumstances, such as significant coronary artery disease, acute hemorrhage, or lactic acidosis (see recommendations for initial resuscitation), red blood cell transfusion should occur only when hemoglobin decreases to ≤7.0 g/dL to target a hemoglobin of 7.0–9.0 g/dL (116). Erythropoietin is not recommended as a specific treatment of anemia associated with severe sepsis but may be used when septic patients have other accepted reasons for administration of erythropoietin, such as renal failure induced compromise of red blood cell production (116). Using the early goal-directed approach in the initial resuscitation of patients, if the central venous oxygen saturation was less than 70%, a red blood cell transfusion was administered to maintain the hematocrit of at least 30% (118).

G. Vasopressor and Ionotropic Therapy

Dopamine and norepinephrine are both effective for increasing arterial blood pressure. Vasopressor agents should be given through a central line as soon as available. It is imperative to ensure that patients are adequately fluid resuscitated. When a fluid challenge fails to restore adequate blood pressure and tissue perfusion, therapy with vasopressor agents should be started (116). Dopamine raises cardiac output more that norepinephrine, but its use may be limited by tachycardia. Norepinephrine may be a more effective vasopressor in some patients. Administration of low doses of dopamine to maintain renal function is not recommended (117).

   A large randomized trial and a meta-analysis comparing low dose dopamine to placebo in critically ill patients found no difference in either primary outcomes (peak serum creatinine, need for renal replacement therapy, urine output, time to recovery of normal renal function) or secondary outcomes (survival to either ICU or hospital discharge, ICU stay, hospital stay, arrhythmias) (116,121,129).

Vasopressin use can be considered in patients with refractory shock despite adequate fluid resuscitation and high dose conventional vasopressors. It is not recommended as a replacement for norepinephrine or dopamine as a first line agent (116). Plasma vasopressin levels are in most cases increased at the initial phase of septic shock, contributing to the maintenance of arterial pressure; however, a relative vasopressin deficiency is likely to occur after 36 hours from the onset of septic shock, probably resulting from decreased secretion rather than an increased clearance from the plasma (130). In adults it should be administered at infusion rates of 0.01–0.04 units per minute. It should be used with caution in patients with cardiac dysfunction (cardiac index less than 2–2.5 L/min/m^2), as it has been shown to reduce stroke volume. Doses of vasopressin >0.04 units/min have been associated with decreases in cardiac output and cardiac arrest (116,131–133). In patients with low cardiac output despite adequate fluid resuscitation, dobutamine is the first choice ionotrope to increase cardiac output. If used in the presence of low blood pressure, it should be combined with other vasopressor therapy (116).

H. Mechanical Ventilation of Sepsis-Induced Acute Lung Injury/ARDS

High tidal volumes that are coupled with high plateau pressures should be avoided in acute lung injury (ALI) and in the ARDS. Clinicians should use as a starting point a reduction in tidal volumes over one to two hours to a "low" tidal volume (6 mL/kg of predicted body weight) as a goal in conjunction with the goal of maintaining the end inspiratory plateau pressures ≤30 cmH$_2$O. Hypercapnia (allowing $P_a CO_2$ to increase above normal, so-called permissive hypercapnia) can be tolerated in patients with ALI/ARDS if required to minimize plateau pressures and tidal volumes. A minimum amount of positive end expiratory pressure should be set to prevent lung collapse at end-expiration. Setting positive end-expiratory pressure based on severity of oxygenation deficit and guided by the $F_I O_2$ required to maintain adequate oxygenation is one acceptable approach. Some experts titrate positive end-expiratory pressure according to bedside measurements of thoracopulmonary compliance (to obtain the highest compliance, reflecting lung recruitment) (116,134). The management of patients with ARDS is reviewed in detail in a separate chapter.

The semirecumbent position has been demonstrated to decrease the incidence of ventilator-required pneumonia (135). Patients are laid flat for procedures, hemodynamic measurements, and during episodes of hypotension. Consistent return to semirecumbent position should be viewed as a quality indicator in patients receiving mechanical ventilation. A weaning protocol should be in place, and mechanically ventilated patients should undergo a spontaneous breathing trial to evaluate the ability to discontinue mechanical ventilation when they satisfy the following criteria: (1) arousable; (2) hemodynamically stable (without vasopressor agents); (3) no new potentially serious conditions; (4) low ventilatory and end-expiratory pressure requirements; and (5) requiring levels of FIO_2 that could be safely delivered with a face mask or nasal cannula. If the spontaneous breathing trial is successful, consideration should be given for extubation (116).

I. Renal Replacement Therapy

Acute renal failure occurs in approximately 19% of patients with moderate sepsis, 23% with severe sepsis, and 51% with septic shock when blood cultures are positive (18,136,137). The combination of acute renal failure and sepsis is associated with a 70% mortality, as compared with a 45% mortality among patients with acute renal failure alone (136). The cytokine-mediated induction of nitric oxide synthesis that occurs in sepsis decreases systemic vascular resistance (138). This arterial vasodilatation predisposes patients with sepsis to acute renal failure, the need for mechanical ventilation, and ultimately, increased mortality (136). Patients with sepsis and acute renal failure are hypercatabolic. Studies suggesting that increased doses of dialysis improve survival in patients who are hypercatabolic and have acute renal failure are persuasive (136). In a study comparing aggressive hemodialysis with peritoneal dialysis, survival was markedly improved in patients receiving aggressive hemodialysis who had heat-stroke, rhabdomyolysis, and acute renal failure (139). Hemofiltration has been shown to produce better survival rates than peritoneal dialysis in patients with acute renal failure associated with malaria and other infections (140). A recent study showed that daily hemodialysis as compared with alternate-day hemodialysis was associated with significantly less systemic inflammatory response syndrome or sepsis (22% vs. 46%), significantly lower mortality (28% vs. 46%) and a significantly shorter duration of acute renal failure (mean nine vs. 16 days) (141). Continuous renal-replacement therapy has increasingly been used to treat acute renal failure. A randomized study using continuous venovenous hemofiltration suggested that the ultrafiltration rate of 35 or 45 mL/kg per hour as compared with 20 mL/kg per hour improves survival in acute renal failure ($p < 0.001$) (142). In addition, for patients with sepsis-related acute renal failure, better survival was observed with an ultrafiltration rate of 45 mL/kg per hour than with a rate of 35 mg/kg per hour (136,142). Meta-analysis of hemodialysis as compared with continuous renal-replacement therapy in acute renal failure, however, has not yet shown an advantage for either mode of renal-replacement therapy (143). The benefit of the removal of cytokines by continuous renal-replacement therapy also remains to be proven as a method for improving survival in patients with sepsis and acute renal failure (136).

J. Steroids

An increase in tissue corticosteroid levels during acute illness is an important protective response. Many diseases and their treatments interfere with the normal corticosteroid response to illness and thus induce tissue corticosteroid insufficiency (144). Cortisol is the predominant corticosteroid secreted from the adrenal cortex in humans. In a healthy, unstressed subject, cortisol is secreted according to a diurnal pattern under the influence of corticotropin released from the pituitary gland (144). Corticotropin secretion, in turn, is under the influence of hypothalamic corticotropin-releasing hormone, and both hormones are subject to negative feedback control by cortisol itself (144). Circulating cortisol is bound to corticosteroid-binding globulin, with less than 10% in the free (bioavailable) form (144). With severe infection, trauma, burns, illness, or surgery, there is an increase in cortisol production by as much as a factor of six that is roughly proportional to the severity of the illness (144–147). Diurnal variation in cortisol secretion is also lost under conditions of severe illness. These effects are due to increased production of corticotropin-releasing hormone and corticotropin and a reduction in negative feedback from cortisol (144,148). Stimulation of the hypothalamic–pituitary–adrenal axis in the context of severe illness is caused by elevated levels of circulating cytokines, among other factors (144,149). Adrenal responsiveness to exogenous corticotropin is normally maintained during acute illness (144,150,151).

During severe illness, many factors can impair the normal corticosteroid response. These factors include pre-existing conditions affecting the hypothalamic–pituitary–adrenal axis (152), but corticosteroid insufficiency can also occur during the course of acute illness. Responses involving corticotropin-releasing hormone and corticotropin can be impaired by head injury, central nervous system depressants, or pituitary infarction (153). Adrenal cortisol synthesis can be impaired by multiple mechanisms (150,152). Medications such as etomidate and the ketoconazole inhibit the activity of enzymes involved in cortisol synthesis (144,154).

Adrenal hemorrhage can occur in sick patients, especially those with septicemia and underlying coagulopathy, and adrenal insufficiency can occur when there is extensive destruction of adrenal tissue caused by tumors or infection (144). The high levels of inflammatory cytokines in patients with sepsis can also directly inhibit adrenal cortisol synthesis (155). Exogenous corticosteroid administration suppresses the production of corticotropin-releasing hormone and corticotropin and can induce adrenal atrophy that may persist for months after the cessation of corticosteroid treatment (144,156). This effect depends on the dose and duration of treatment and varies greatly from person to person but should be anticipated in any patient who has been receiving more than 30 mg of hydrocortisone per day (or 7.5 mg of prednisolone or 0.75 mg of dexamethasone per day) for more than three weeks (144). Similar suppression of the hypothalamic–pituitary–adrenal axis has been reported with medroxyprogesterone and megestrol acetate treatment (144,157,158). The hepatic metabolism of cortisol may be enhanced by drugs such as rifampin or phenytoin (144).

Several factors complicate investigation of the hypothalamic–pituitary–adrenal axis in patients with critical illness. Expected cortisol levels vary with the type and severity of disease, making it difficult to define normal ranges. Since the highest levels of cortisol are found in patients with the severest illness, both high and low cortisol levels have been shown to be associated with a poor prognosis (144,159,160).

Assessment of corticosteroid sufficiency can be made on the basis of randomly measured cortisol levels or the corticotropin stimulation test. Despite the correlation between cortisol levels and the severity of illness, it is difficult to estimate usefully what an appropriate response should be in a critically ill patient. More useful would be the identification of a minimal threshold level below which adrenal insufficiency is likely and a maximal threshold level above which insufficiency is unlikely (144). Many threshold levels have been proposed for the definition of an insufficient cortisol level (measured at any time of day) during acute illness (151,161). Proposed minimal levels have ranged from 10 μgm/dL (276 nmol/L) (162) to 34 μgm/dL (938 nmol/L), but several studies suggest that a threshold of 15 μgm/dL (414 nmol/L) best identifies persons with clinical features of corticosteroid insufficiency or who would benefit from corticosteroid replacement (144,163–166).

The corticotropin stimulation test has also been evaluated in patients with critical illness [with the intramuscular or intravenous administration of 250 μgm of cosyntropin (a synthetic peptide consisting of the first 24 amino acids of corticotropin), with plasma cortisol levels measured 0, 30, and sometimes 60 minutes after administration]. The use of the test in this setting remains controversial, but the incremental response after the administration of corticotropin (in contrast to the response found in patients who are not critically ill) may have prognostic implications, with a small increase [less than 9 μgm/dL (250 nmol/L)] from the base-line cortisol level to the highest cortisol level (measured at 30 or 60 minutes) associated with an increased risk of death (29,160). It is felt that adrenal insufficiency appears to be unlikely when a random cortisol measurement is greater than 34 μgm/dL (136). Conversely, adrenal insufficiency is likely if the serum cortisol level is below 15 μgm/dL during acute severe illness (Fig. 5) (144). For persons with cortisol levels between these two values, a poor response on a corticotropin test would indicate the possibility of adrenal insufficiency and a need for supplemental corticosteroids. At least among patients in septic shock, these criteria appear to identify many patients who will benefit from supplemental corticosteroid treatment (29). Such cutoffs are somewhat arbitrary however, since levels of circulating cortisol only partly mediate corticosteroid action at the tissue level. Ideally, a corticotropin test should be performed at the outset, rather than wait for the results of random measurements of cortisol. The corticotropin test, however, has clear limitations when hypoadrenalism occurs secondary to recent hypothalamic or pituitary insults, and caution is necessary. A low-dose (1-μgm) corticotropin stimulation test has been proposed, with the suggestion that it may be more sensitive than the 250-μgm test (167,168). It is important to be aware

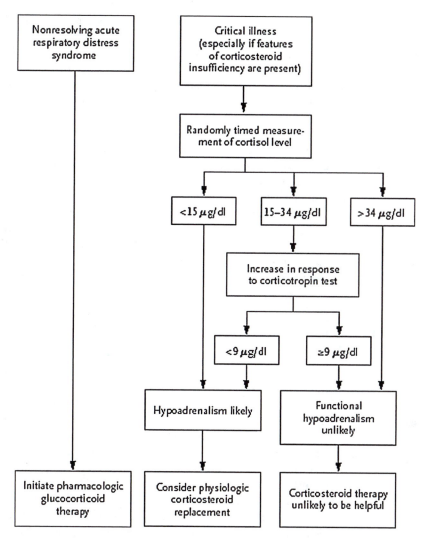

Figure 5 Investigation of adrenal corticosteroid function in critically ill patients on the basis of cortisol levels and response to the corticotropin stimulation test. The scheme has been evaluated for patients with septic shock. It must be borne in mind, however, that no cutoff value will be entirely reliable. *Source:* From Ref. 144.

that even in patients who have normal test results, adrenal insufficiency may develop later in the illness. It is unclear how often one should perform such tests, but the development of new clinical features suggesting corticosteroid insufficiency or a deterioration in clinical condition should prompt further testing (136).

The prevalence of adrenal insufficiency in septic shock is about 50% (169). Initial studies with corticosteroid administration in patients with sepsis and septic shock used short courses of high dose steroids and did not show any significant benefit (170,171). A recent systematic review and meta-analysis including all trials of steroids regardless of the dose or duration noted that more recent studies (after 1992) favored steroids as being associated with a lower risk of death. More recent studies used lower doses of corticosteroids with the aim of treating adrenal insufficiency. The preferred dosing was 200–300 mg daily in divided doses tapered over approximately a week, which parallels the cortisol concentrations achieved at maximum exercise in healthy people (169,172–174).

One multicenter, randomized, controlled trial with patients in severe septic shock showed a significant shock reversal and reduction in mortality rate in patients with relative adrenal insufficiency (post adrenocorticotropic hormone cortisol increase of $\leq 9\,\mu\mathrm{gm/dL}$) (29). Some experts suggest using a $250\,\mu\mathrm{gm}$ adrenocorticotropic hormone test (cortisol response $>9\,\mu\mathrm{gm/dL}$ after 30–60 minutes) to discontinue steroids in those patients with such significant response. However, clinicians would not wait for the results of such testing prior to starting the steroids (116).

K. Recombinant Human Activated Protein C

Coagulopathy and inflammation are both parts of the innate host response to infection. The combined anticoagulant, profibrinolytic, anti-inflammatory, and antiapoptotic activities of the protein C pathway have for a long time been recognized as an attractive combination for treating severe sepsis. In severe sepsis, in which control of these systems is altered, the extent of their dysfunction correlates with disease severity and mortality (5,175,176). The protein C (PC) pathway serves as a major system for controlling thrombosis, limiting the inflammatory response, and potentially decreasing endothelial cell apoptosis in response to inflammatory cytokines (177). The key feature of this pathway is its ability to respond to the presence of thrombin. As the thrombin concentration rises, much of the thrombin binds to thrombomodulin, an endothelial-surface glycoprotein (178), leading to both rapid thrombin inactivation and a change in the substrate preference of thrombin from procoagulants such as fibrinogen and factor V to anticoagulants such as PC, especially in the capillaries. Conversely, once thrombin generation reverts to homeostatic levels, the PC activation complex slows the rate of generation of activated PC (APC) down to physiologic levels. PC activation is enhanced when PC is bound to another endothelial surface protein, the endothelial cell PC receptor (Fig. 6) (175,179). Additional details of the mechanism of action is included in the legend.

A rapid and prolonged depletion of PC occurs in human sepsis, presumably due to increased consumption, degradation, or decreased hepatic synthesis, and contributes to sepsis-induced coagulopathy and correlates with a poor prognosis (5,175,176). Endogenous PC activation is blunted in severe meningococcal

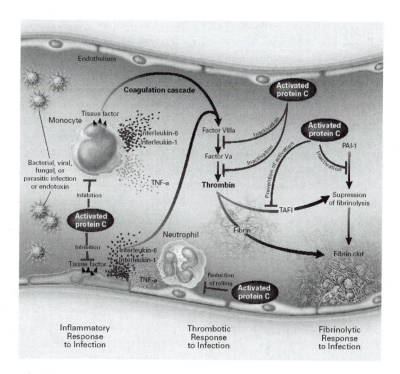

Figure 6   Proposed actions of activated protein C in modulating the systemic inflammatory, procoagulant, and fibrinolytic host responses to infection. Infectious agents and inflammatory cytokines such as TNF-α and interleukin-1 activate coagulation by stimulating the release of tissue factor. The presentation of tissue factor leads to the formation of thrombin and a fibrin clot. Inflammatory cytokines and thrombin impair the endogenous fibrinolytic potential by stimulating the release of PAI-1. PAI-1 is a potent inhibitor of tissue plasminogen activator, an endogenous fibrinolytic. In addition, thrombin can stimulate multiple inflammatory pathways and further suppress the endogenous fibrinolytic system by activating TAFI. The conversion of protein C, by thrombin bound to thrombomodulin, to the serine protease activated protein C is impaired by the inflammatory response. Endothelial injury results in decreased thrombomodulin levels. The end result of the host response to infection may be diffuse endovascular injury, microvascular thrombosis, organ ischemia, multiorgan dysfunction, and death. Activated protein C exerts an antithrombotic effect by inactivating factors Va and VIIIa, limiting the generation of thrombin. This reduces the inflammatory, procoagulant, and antifibrinolytic response induced by thrombin. Activated protein C exerts an anti-inflammatory effect by inhibiting the production of inflammatory cytokines (TNFα, interleukin-1, and interleukin-6) and limiting the rolling of monocytes and neutrophils on injured endothelium by binding selectins. Activated protein C indirectly increases the fibrinolytic response by inhibiting PAI-1. *Abbreviations*: TNFα, tumor necrosis factor α; PAI 1, plasminogen activator inhibitor 1; TAFI, thrombin-activatable fibrinolysis inhibitor. *Source*: From Ref. 179.

infection (175,180). APC is recommended for use in patients at high risk of death [Acute Physiology and Chronic Health Evaluation (APACHE) II ≥ 25, sepsis induced multiple organ failure, septic shock, or sepsis-induced ARDS] (116). It should only be used in patients with no absolute contraindications that outweigh the potential benefit of APC. It is administered as an infusion at a rate of 24 μgm/kg/hr for 96 hours. APC has been shown to significantly reduce the 28-day mortality rate in a randomized, double blind, placebo-controlled, multicenter study (PROWESS). The mortality rate in the treatment group was 24.7%, with a placebo group mortality of 30.8% (a 19.4% reduction in the relative risk of death). The incidence of severe bleeding was 3.5% in the APC treated patients (179). Significantly more APC patients than controls survived to hospital discharge, and more of these survivors are discharged home (181). Exclusion criteria in the study included age <18, weight >135 kg, platelet count $<30,000$ per μL, conditions associated with an increased risk of bleeding, known hypercoagulable state, moribund state, not expected to survive 28 days because of underlying condition, HIV with CD4 <50 per μL, chronic renal failure on dialysis, organ transplantation (except kidney and heart), and significant liver disease (179).

The ENHANCE U.S. study was an open-label, nonrandomized trial that allowed investigators to collect additional data about drotrecogin alfa (activated) APC in U.S. patients with severe sepsis within a controlled clinical trial setting. Recognizing the limitations associated with comparing results across trials, treatment with APC in the ENHANCE U.S. trial resulted in a 28-day mortality rate that was similar to that of the APC group in the PROWESS U.S. trial. Consistent with a previous analysis of data from the global PROWESS trial, the treatment effects of APC were similarly observed among almost all subgroups in the ENHANCE U.S. trial (i.e., patients were segregated according to the number of organ failures, the use of a mechanical ventilator or vasopressor, and thrombocytopenia status), regardless of disease severity (182). The incidence of serious bleeding in the study was 4% in the APC group (182).

To minimize the risk of bleeding, the infusion of APC should be discontinued two hours before the patient undergoes invasive procedures, and should be resumed 12 hours following major procedures and after ensuring adequate hemostasis (179). Following uncomplicated invasive procedures, infusion may be resumed immediately. Because bleeding risk is increased during procedures that involve the instrumentation of large blood vessels or highly vascular organs, physicians should show special caution before, during, and after such procedures. Meningitis associated with coagulopathy or severe thrombocytopenia (i.e., platelet count, $\leq 30,000$ cells/μL) may also potentially increase the risk of bleeding associated with APC (182). Post hoc subgroup analysis of the PROWESS study data revealed that no significant survival benefit was noted in the use of APC in patients with an initial APACHE II score of <25 (181). A recent multicenter study, the ADDRESS study, involving subjects with sepsis and an APACHE II score of <25 was stopped because of a lack of benefit with APC in these less severely ill patients (181).

L. Intensive Insulin Therapy for Hyperglycemia

Hyperglycemia associated with insulin resistance (183–186) is common in critically ill patients, even those who have not previously had diabetes. It has been reported that pronounced hyperglycemia may lead to complications in such patients (183,187–191). In diabetic patients with acute myocardial infarction, therapy to maintain blood glucose at a level below 215 mg/dL (11.9 mmol/L) improves the long-term outcome (183,192–194). In nondiabetic patients with protracted critical illnesses, high serum levels of insulin-like growth factor-binding protein 1, which reflect an impaired response of hepatocytes to insulin, increase the risk of death (183,195,196).

A large single-center trial of predominantly post-operative surgical patients demonstrated that intensive insulin therapy that maintained the blood glucose level at 80 to 110 mg/dL (4.4–6.1 mmol/L) resulted in lower morbidity and mortality among critically ill patients (regardless of whether they had a history of diabetes) than did conventional therapy that maintained the blood glucose level at 180–200 mg/dL (10.0–11.1 mmol/L) (5,183). Almost all the patients in the intensive insulin therapy group required exogenous insulin. In the conventional treatment group, only 39% of patients required exogenous insulin. The study was terminated early because of the significant difference in mortality.

Intensive insulin therapy reduced the frequency of episodes of sepsis by 46%. Patients with bacteremia who were treated with intensive insulin therapy had lower mortality than those who received conventional therapy (12.5% vs. 29.5%). Insulin therapy reduced the rate of death from multiple-organ failure among patients with sepsis, regardless of whether they had a history of diabetes. There was a significantly higher occurrence of hypoglycemia [<40 mg/dL (2.2 mmol/L)] in the intensive insulin therapy group (5.1%), compared to less than 1% in the conventionally treated group (183).

The protective mechanism of insulin in sepsis is unknown. The phagocytic function of neutrophils is impaired in patients with hyperglycemia, and correcting hyperglycemia may improve bacterial phagocytosis. Another potential mechanism involves the antiapoptotic effect of insulin (197). Insulin prevents apoptotic cell death from numerous stimuli by activating the phosphatidylinositol 3-kinase-Akt pathway (198). Regardless of mechanism, it seems reasonable to control blood glucose more tightly in critically ill patients. Clinicians must avert hypoglycemic brain injury in attempting to maintain the blood glucose level at 80–110 mg per deciliter. Frequent monitoring of blood glucose is imperative, and studies are needed to determine whether less tight control of blood glucose [e.g., a blood glucose level of 120–160 mg/dL (6.7–8.9 mmol/L)], provides similar benefits (5). It is important to note that the landmark study on the role of an aggressive approach to glycemic control was conducted in predominantly surgical patients. Further study of this approach is essential to confirm its benefits; until then, widespread adoption of this approach would be premature (199).

X. Future Treatment Strategies

The success of APC provides new hope that other new therapeutic strategies for the treatment of sepsis may be introduced into the clinic in the near future. The main target groups for anti-inflammatory treatment, according to the lessons learned, will likely be patients with severe sepsis or septic shock. Some new developments in the area of sepsis research appear to be particularly promising (48).

A. Apoptosis Inhibition

Programmed cell death (apoptosis) is differentiated from cell necrosis by typical features such as DNA fragmentation, condensation of chromatin, membrane blebbing, and cell shrinkage. Several proinflammatory mediators (such as TNFα) produced during experimental sepsis are known inducers of apoptosis involving various cell types (48). During sepsis, lymphocytes have been shown to undergo rapid apoptosis, whereas other cells, like neutrophils, demonstrate delayed apoptosis (48,200,201). Hotchkiss and colleagues (201–203) recently demonstrated that the prevention of lymphocyte cell death during sepsis could improve outcome (48). Caspase inhibitors were found to be an effective tool to protect animals from death during pneumonia-induced sepsis (48,204). These findings led to the hypothesis that immunodepression resulting from the loss of lymphocytes could represent a central pathogenic event in sepsis. Further studies have suggested that inhibition of intestinal epithelial apoptosis (by selective Bcl-2 overexpression) significantly improved outcomes in two different models of sepsis in mice (48,204,205). The underlying mechanisms of these studies are not yet understood. Treatment of septic patients with apoptosis inhibitors has to overcome several problems, including the selectivity of such inhibitors and potential uncontrolled cell growth. However, the concept of regulated apoptosis warrants further investigation (48).

B. Microbial Drugs and Pattern Recognition Molecules

Designing new drugs to neutralize microbial products or block their interaction with specific receptors on immune cells is an attractive concept. Potential targets include lipopolysaccharide binding protein, CD14, TLR4, and MD-2 for gram-negative sepsis, and CD14, TLR2, and TLR6 for gram-positive sepsis. Monoclonal antibodies against CD14 are being evaluated in phase II studies. Several intracellular signaling molecules, such as MyD88 and the mitogen-activated protein kinase, are other possible therapeutic targets. However, inactivating molecules that are pivotal to innate immunity can be harmful, as shown by the increased sensitivity to bacterial sepsis in mice with mutations of the TLR4 gene (50,206). Careful selection of patients with severe infections associated with a high probability of death will therefore be essential.

C. Macrophage Migration Inhibitory Factor

Macrophage migration inhibitory factor is a cytokine that has recently been shown to be important in innate immunity and sepsis (207). It is constitutively expressed in large amounts by immune, endocrine, and epithelial cells and is rapidly released after exposure to microbial products and pro-inflammatory cytokines. Macrophage migration inhibitory factor regulates innate immune responses to endotoxin and gram-negative bacteria by modulating the expression of TLR4, enabling macrophages and other cells at the front line of defenses to respond quickly (208). High levels of macrophage migration inhibitory factor have been detected in patients with inflammatory and infectious diseases, including severe sepsis and septic shock (209). Immunoneutralization of macrophage migration inhibitory factor or deletion of the Mif gene protects mice against lethal endotoxaemia, gram-positive toxic shock syndromes, and experimental bacterial peritonitis. Conversely, mice injected with macrophage migration inhibitory factor together with live bacteria or microbial toxins have increased death rates (50,203,210,211). This factor thus has the potential to endanger life when expressed in excess during sepsis. Development of drugs to block the production of macrophage migration inhibitory factor or inhibit its function may help treat severe sepsis and other inflammatory diseases (50).

D. High Mobility Group Protein 1

High mobility group protein 1, a protein previously known as DNA-binding protein regulating gene transcription and stabilizing nucleosome formation, has recently been described as a "late" mediator of inflammation and sepsis (50,212). Patients with septic or haemorrhagic shock have raised serum concentrations of high mobility group protein 1, and concentrations are associated with patient's outcome. Use of polyclonal antibodies to block high mobility group protein 1 in mice protects them against lipopolysaccharide induced acute lung injury and lethal endotoxaemia (50,213).

E. Genetic Studies of Susceptibility to Sepsis

Several gene polymorphisms have been associated with increased susceptibility to sepsis. Testing for polymorphisms of important genes may help to identify people who are at increased risk of sepsis when exposed to virulent bacteria and who may benefit from targeted immunomodulatory therapies (50).

XI. Conclusion

A major shift has occurred in the way investigators view the problem of sepsis. Sepsis may not be attributable solely to an immune system abnormality but may indicate an immune system that is severely compromised and unable to eradicate pathogens. Mechanisms of organ failure and death in patients with sepsis remain unknown, and autopsy studies do not reveal widespread necrosis. Current clinical advances in the treatment of sepsis include therapy with activated protein C, tight control of blood glucose, and early goal-directed therapy to treat sepsis-induced hypotension with correction of the cellular oxygen deficit. Other important components of therapy include using ventilatory techniques that minimize high plateau pressure (allowing modest hypercapnea if necessary, setting a minimum amount of positive end expiratory pressure to prevent lung collapse at end expiration), adequate nutrition (preferably via the enteral route), adequate sedation using a sedation goal with a daily interruption, and prophylaxis against deep venous thrombosis and stress gastritis/ulcers in addition to renal replacement therapy if indicated.

The next phase of the Surviving Sepsis Campaign, in conjunction with the Institute of Healthcare Improvement collaborative system, is the targeted implementation of a core set of recommendations in hospital environments where change in behavior and clinical impact can be measured. The first step in this next phase is to deploy a "change bundle" based on a core set of the previous recommendations (116). The change bundles are divided into the six-hour sepsis bundle and the 24-hour sepsis bundle. The six-hour sepsis bundle focuses on early identification of organ dysfunction (hypotension, elevated lactate), adequate initial resuscitation with early correction of the organ dysfunction, obtaining early blood cultures, and administering antibiotics within three hours of presentation (IHI.org). The 24-hour sepsis bundle focuses on adequate glucose control (<150 mg/dL or <8.3 mmol/L), administration of APC per hospital guidelines, and use of steroids in septic shock as described previously in the chapter, and use of a lung protective ventilatory strategy (including elevating the head of the bed to prevent nosocomial pneumonia).

Advance care planning, including the communication of likely outcomes and realistic goals of therapy, should be discussed with patients and their families. Decisions for less aggressive support or withdrawal of care may be in the patient's best interest (116). Future therapy may be directed at enhancing or inhibiting the patient's immune response, depending on genetic polymorphisms, the duration of disease, and the characteristics of the particular pathogen (5).

References

1. Martin GS, Mannino DM, Eaton S, Moss M. The epidemiology of sepsis in the United States from 1979–2000. N Engl J Med 2003; 348:1546–1554.
2. Abraham E, Matthay MA, Dinarello CA, Vincent JL, Cohen J, Opal SM, Glauser M, Parsons P, Fisher C, Repine JE. Consensus Conference Definitions for sepsis, acute lung injury, and ARDS—time for reevaluation. Crit Care Med 2000; 28:232–236.
3. Opal SM, Cross AS. Clinical trials for sepsis: past failures and future hopes. Infect Dis Clinics North Am 1999; 13:285–298.

4. Opal SM. Severe sepsis and septic shock: defining the clinical problem. Scand J Infect Dis 2003; 35:529–534.
5. Hotchkiss RS, Karl IE. The pathophysiology and treatment of sepsis. N Engl J Med 2003; 348:138–150.
6. Chalfin DB, Holbein ME, Fein AM, Carlon GC. Cost-effectiveness of monoclonal antibodies to gram-negative endotoxin in the treatment of gram-negative sepsis in ICU patients. J Am Med Assoc 1993; 269:249–254.
7. Angus DC, Linde-Zwirble WT, Lidicker J, Clermont G, Carcillo J, Pinsky MR. Epidemiology of severe sepsis in the United States: analysis of incidence, outcome, and associated costs of care. Crit Care Med 2001; 29:1303–1310.
8. Wheeler AP, Bernard GR. Treating patients with severe sepsis. N Engl J Med 1999; 340:207–214.
9. Perl TM, Dvorak L, Hwang T, Wenzel RP. Long-term survival and function after suspected gram-negative sepsis. J Am Med Assoc 1995; 274:338–345.
10. Heyland DK, Hopman W, Coo H, Tranmer J, McColl MA. Long-term health-related quality of life in survivors of sepsis: Short Form-36: a valid and reliable measure of health-related quality of life. Crit Care Med 2000; 28: 3599–3605.
11. Parrillo JE, Parker MM, Natanson C, et al. Septic shock in humans: advances in the understanding of pathogenesis, cardiovascular dysfunction, and therapy. Ann Intern Med 1990; 113:227–242.
12. Hoyert DL, Arias E, Smith BL, Murphy SL, Kochanek KD. Deaths: final data for 1999. National vital statistics reports. Vol. 49. No. 8. Hyattsville, MD: National Center for Health Statistics, 2001. (DHHS publication no. (PHS) 2001-1120 PRS 01-0573.) cohort study. Intensive Care Med 2002; 28:108-121. [Erratum, Intensive Care Med 2002; 28:525–526.]
13. Balk RA, Bone RC. The septic syndrome: definition and clinical implications. Crit Care Clin 1989; 5:1–8.
14. Ayres SM. SCCM's New Horizons Conference on Sepsis and Septic Shock. Crit Care Med 1985; 13:864–866.
15. Bone RC, Balk RA, Cerra FB, Dellinger RP, Fein AM, Knaus WA, Schein RMH, Sibbald WJ. Definitions for sepsis and organ failure and guidelines for the use of innovative therapies in sepsis: The ACCP/SCCM Consensus Conference Committee. Chest 1992; 101:1644–1655.
16. Warren HS. Strategies for the treatment of sepsis. N Engl J Med 1997; 336: 952–953.
17. Stone R. Search for sepsis drugs goes on despite past failures. Science 1994; 264:365–367.
18. Rangel-Frausto MS, Pittet D, Costigan M, et al. The natural history of the systemic inflammatory response syndrome (SIRS). A prospective study. J Am Med Assoc 1995; 273: 117–123.
19. Knaus WA, Draper EA, Wagner DP, Zimmerman JE. Prognosis in acute organ-system failure. Ann Surg 1985; 202:685–693.
20. Levy MM, Fink MP, Marshall JC, Abraham E, Angus, D, Cook D, Cohen J, Opal SM, Vincent JL, Ramsay G. For the International Sepsis Definitions Conference. 2001 SCCM/ESICM/ACCP/ATS/SIS International Sepsis Definitions Conference. Crit Care Med 2003; 31:1250–1256.
21. Gospodarowicz M, Benedet L, Hutter RV, et al. History and international developments in cancer staging. Cancer Prev Cont 1998; 2:262–268.

22. Renaud B, Brun-Buisson C, ICU-Bacteremia Study Group. Outcomes of primary and catheter-related bacteremia. A cohort and casecontrol study in critically ill patients. Am J Respir Crit Care Med 2001; 163:1584–1590.

23. Opal SM, Cohen J. Clinical gram-positive sepsis: does it fundamentally differ from gram-negative bacterial sepsis? Crit Care Med 1999; 27:1608–1616.

24. Harbarth S, Holeckova K, Froidevaux C, et al. Diagnostic value of procalcitonin, interleukin-6, and interleukin-8 in critically ill patients admitted with suspected sepsis. Am J Respir Crit Care Med 2001; 3:396–402.

25. Hausfater P, Garric S, Ayed SB, et al. Usefulness of procalcitonin as a marker of systemic infection in emergency department patients: a prospective study. Clin Infect Dis 2002; 34:895–901.

26. Damas P, Ledoux D, Nys M, et al. Cytokine serum level during severe sepsis in human IL-6 as a marker of severity. Ann Surg 1992; 215:356–362.

27. Panacek EA, Kaul M. IL-6 as a marker of excessive TNF-alpha activity in sepsis. Sepsis 1999; 3:65–73.

28. Bernard GR, Vincent J-L, Laterre PF, et al. Efficacy and safety of recombinant human activated protein C for severe sepsis. N Engl J Med 2001; 344:699–709.

29. Annane D, Sébille V, Charpentier C, et al. Effect of treatment with low doses of hydrocortisone and fludrocortisone on mortality in patients with septic shock. J Am Med Assoc 2002; 288:862–871.

30. Marshall JC, Cook DJ, Christou NV, et al. Multiple organ dysfunction score: a reliable descriptor of a complex clinical outcome. Crit Care Med 1995; 23:1638–1652.

31. Vincent J-L, Moreno R, Takala J, et al. The SOFA (Sepsis-related Organ Failure Assessment) score to describe organ dysfunction/failure. Intensive Care Med 1996; 22:707–710.

32. Eli Lilly and Company. Briefing document for XIGRIS for the treatment of severe sepsis. http:www.fda.gov/ohrms/dockets/ac/01/briefing/3797b1_01_Sponsor.htm, August 6, 2001.

33. Cook R, Cook DJ, Tilley J, et al. Multiple organ dysfunction: baseline and serial component scores. Crit Care Med 2001; 29:2046–2050.

34. Cohen J, Cristofaro P, Carlet J, Opal S. New method of classifjing infections in critically ill patients. Crit Care Med 2004; 32:1510–1526.

35. Murphy SL. Deaths: final data for 1998. National vital statistics report. Vol. 48. No. 11. Hyattsville, MD: National Center for Health Statistics, 2000. (DHHS publication no. (PHS) 2000-1120 0-0487.)

36. Hoyert DL, Arias E, Smith BL, Murphy SL, Kochanek KD. Deaths: final data for 1999. National vital statistics reports. Vol. 49. No. 8. Hyattsville, MD: National Center for Health Statistics, 2001. (DHHS publication no. (PHS) 2001-1120 PRS 01-0573.)

37. Annane D, Aegerter P, Jars-Guincestre MC, Guidet B. Current epidemiology of septic shock. Am J Respir Crit Care Med 2003; 168:165–172.

38. Angus DC, Linde-Zwirble WT, Lidicker J, Clermont G, Carcillo J, Pinsky MR. Epidemiology of severe sepsis in the United States: analysis of incidence, outcome, and associated costs of care. Crit Care Med 2001; 29:1303–1310.

39. Angus DC, Wax RS. Epidemiology of sepsis: an update. Crit Care Med 2001; 29:S109–S116.

40. Brun-Buisson C, Doyon F, Carlet J, et al. Incidence, risk factors, and outcome of severe sepsis and septic shock in adults: A multicenter prospective study in intensive care units. J Am Med Assoc 1995; 274:968–974.

41. Kieft H, Hoepelman AI, Zhou W, Rozenberg-Arska M, Struyvenberg A, Verhoef J. The sepsis syndrome in a Dutch university hospital: clinical observations. Arch Intern Med 1993; 153:2241–2247.

42. Bone RC. Toward an epidemiology and natural history of SIRS (systemic inflammatory response syndrome). J Am Med Assoc 1992; 268:3452–3455.

43. Barriere SL, Lowry SF. An overview of mortality risk prediction in sepsis. Crit Care Med 1995; 23:376–393.

44. Rangel-Frausto MS. The epidemiology of bacterial sepsis. Infect Dis Clin North Am 1999; 13:299–312.

45. Rello J, Ricart M, Mirelis B, et al. Nosocomial bacteremia in a medical-surgical intensive care unit: epidemiologic characteristics and factors influencing mortality in 111 episodes. Intensive Care Med 1994; 20:94–98.

46. Center for Disease Control. Increase in national hospital discharge survey rates for septicemia: United States, 1979–1987. MMWR Morb Mortal Wkly Rep 1990; 39:31–34.

47. Angus DC. Discourse on method: Measuring the value of new therapies in intensive care. In: Vincent J-L, ed. 1998 Yearbook of Intensive Care and Emergency Medicine. Berlin: Springer-Verlag, 1998:265.

48. Riedemann NC, Guo R-F, Ward PA. The enigma of sepsis. J Clin Invest 2003; 112:460–467.

49. Thomas L. Germs. N Eng J Med 1972; 287:553–555.

50. Bochud P-Y, Calandra T. Pathogenesis of sepsis: new concepts and implications for future treatment. BMJ 2003; 326:262–266.

51. Janeway CA Jr, Medzhitov R. Innate immune recognition. Annu Rev Immunol 2002; 20:197–216.

52. Calandra T, Bochud PY, Heumann D. Cytokines in septic shock. In: Remington JS, Swartz MN, eds. Current Clinical Topics in Infectious Diseases. Oxford: Blackwell Publishing, 2002:1–23.

53. Bochud PY, Glauser MP, Calandra T. Antibiotics in sepsis. Intensive Care Med 2001; 27(suppl 1):S33–S48.

54. Alexander C, Rietschel ET. Bacterial lipopolysaccharides and innate immunity. J Endotoxin Res 2001; 7:167–202.

55. Ulevitch RJ, Tobias PS. Recognition of gram-negative bacteria and endotoxin by the innate immune system. Curr Opin Immunol 1999; 11:19–22.

56. Hoffmann JA, Reichhart JM. Drosophila innate immunity: an evolutionary perspective. Nat Immunol 2002; 3:121–126.

57. Poltorak A, He X, Smirnova I, Liu MY, Huffel CV, Du X, et al. Defective LPS signalling in C3H/HeJ and C57BL/10ScCr mice: mutations in Tlr4 gene. Science 1998; 282:2085–2088.

58. Nagai Y, Akashi S, Nagafuku M, Ogata M, Iwakura Y, Akira S, et al. Essential role of MD-2 in LPS responsiveness and TLR4 distribution. Nat Immunol 2002; 3: 667–672.

59. Calandra T. Pathogenesis of septic shock: implications for prevention and treatment. J Chemother 2001; 13:173–180.

60. Takeuchi O, Hoshino K, Kawai T, Sanjo H, Takada H, Ogawa T, et al. Differential roles of TLR2 and TLR4 in recognition of gram-negative and gram-positive bacterial cell wall components. Immunity 1999; 11:443–451.

61. Cohen J, Abraham E. Microbiologic findings and correlations with serum tumor necrosis factor-alpha in patients with severe sepsis and septic shock. J Infect Dis 1999; 180:116–121.

62. Hayashi F, Smith KD, Ozinsky A, Hawn TR, Yi EC, Goodlett DR, et al. The innate immune response to bacterial flagellin is mediated by Toll-like receptor 5. Nature 2001; 410:1099–1103.

63. Hemmi H, Takeuchi O, Kawai T, Kaisho T, Sato S, Sanjo H, et al. A Toll-like receptor recognizes bacterial DNA. Nature 2000; 408:740–745.

64. Ozinsky A, Underhill DM, Fontenot JD, Hajjar AM, Smith KD, Wilson CB, et al. The repertoire for pattern recognition of pathogens by the innate immune system is defined by cooperation between toll-like receptors. Proc Natl Acad Sci USA 2000; 97:13766–13771.

65. Kaisho T, Akira S. Toll-like receptors as adjuvant receptors. Biochim Biophys Acta 2002; 1589:1–13.

66. Calandra T, Bochud PY, Heumann D. Cytokines in septic shock. In: Remington JS, Swartz MN, eds. Current Clinical Topics in Infectious Diseases. Oxford: Blackwell Publishing, 2002:1–23.

67. Vincent JL, Sun Q, Dubois MJ. Clinical trials of immunomodulatory therapies in severe sepsis and septic shock. Clin Infect Dis 2002; 34:1084–1093.

68. Selberg O, Hecker H, Martin M, Klos A, Bautsch W, Köhl J. Discrimination of sepsis and systemic inflammatory response syndrome by determination of circulating plasma concentrations of procalcitonin, protein complement 3a, and interleukin-6. Crit Care Med 2000; 28:2793–2798.

69. Luzzani A, Polati E, Dorizzi R, Rungatscher A, Pavan R, Merlini A. Comparison of procalcitonin and C-reactive protein as markers of sepsis. Crit Care Med 2003; 31:1737–1741.

70. Panacek EA, Marshall JC, Albertson TE, Johnson DH, Johnson S, MacArthur RD, Miller M, Barchuk WT, Fischkoff S, Kaul M, Teoh L, Van Meter L, Daum L, Lemeshow S, Hicklin G, Doig C. Efficacy and safety of the monoclonal anti-tumor necrosis factor antibody F(ab')2 fragment afelimomab in patients with severe sepsis and elevated interleukin-6 levels. Crit Care Med 2004; 32:2173–2182.

71. Cannon JG, Tompkins RG, Gelfand JA, et al. Circulating interleukin-1 and tumor necrosis factor in septic shock and experimental endotoxin fever. J Infect Dis 1990; 161:79–84.

72. Michie H, Manogue K, Springs D. Detection of circulating tumor necrosis factor after endotoxin administration. N Engl J Med 1988; 318:1481–1486.

73. Natanson C, Eichenholz PW, Danner RL, et al. Endotoxin and tumor necrosis factor challenges in dogs simulate the cardiovascular profile of human septic shock. J Exp Med 1989; 169:823–832.

74. Tracey KJ, Beutler B, Lowry SF, et al. Shock and tissue injury induced by human recombinant cachectin. Science 1986; 234:470–474.

75. Dinarello CA, Wolff, Sheldon M. Mechanisms of disease: the role of interleukin-1 in disease. N Engl J Med 1993; 328:106–113.

76. Fast DJ, Schlievert PM, Nelson RD. Toxic shock syndrome-associated staphylococcal and streptococcal pyogenic toxins are potent inducers of tumor necrosis factor production. Infect Immun 1989; 57:291–294.

77. Kusunoki T, Haliman E, Juan TS, et al. Molecules from Staphylococcal aureus that bind CD 14 and stimulate innate immune responses. J Exp Med 1995; 182:1673–1682.

78. Hack C, Aarden L, Thijis L. Role of cytokines in sepsis. Adv Immunol 1997; 66:101–195.

79. Vervloet MG, Thijs LG, Hack CE. Derangements of coagulation and fibrinolysis in critically ill patients with sepsis and septic shock. Semin Thromb Hemost 1998; 24:33–44.

80. Suffredini AF, Harpel PC, Parrillo JE. Promotion and subsequent inhibition of plasminogen activation after administration of intravenous endotoxin to normal subjects. N Engl J Med 1989; 320:1165–1172.

81. De Boer JP, Creasey AA, Chang A, et al. Activation patterns of coagulation and fibrinolysis in baboons following infusion with lethal or sublethal dose of Escherichia coli. Circ Shock 1993; 39:59–67.

82. Thijs LG, Hack CE. Time course of cytokine levels in sepsis. Intensive Care Med 1995; 21:S258–S263.

83. Casey L, Balk R, Bone R. Plasma cytokine and endotoxin levels correlate with survival in patients with the sepsis syndrome. Ann Intern Med 1993; 119:771–778.

84. Waage A, Brandtzaeg P, Halstensen A, et al. The complex pattern of cytokines in serum from patients with meningococcal septic shock. Association between interleukin 6, interleukin 1, and fatal outcome. J Exp Med 1989; 169:333–338.

85. Waage A, Halstensen A, Espevik T. Association between tumour necrosis factor in serumvand fatal outcome in patients with meningococcal disease. Lancet 1987; i:355–357.

86. Hack CE, de Groot ER, Felt-Bersma RJ, et al. Increased plasma concentrations of interleukin-6 in sepsis. Blood 1989; 74:1704–1710.

87. Hack CE, Hart M, van Schijndel RJ, et al. Interleukin-8 in sepsis: relation to shock and inflammatory mediators. Infect Immun 1992; 60:2835–2842.

88. Bossink AW, Paemen L, Jansen PM, et al. Plasma concentrations of the chemokines monocyte chemotactic proteins-1 and -2 are elevated in human sepsis. Blood 1995; 86:3841–3847.

89. Ember JA, Jagels MA, Hugli TE. Characterization of complement anaphylatoxins and their biological responses. In: Volanakis JE, Frank MM, eds. The Human Complement System in Health and Disease. New York: Marcel Dekker, 1998: 241–284.

90. Wolbink GJ, Bossink AW, Groeneveld AB, et al. Complement activation in patients with sepsis is in part mediated by C reactive protein. J Infect Dis 1998; 177:81–87.

91. Steel DM, Whitehead AS. The major acute phase reactants: C-reactive protein, serum amyloid P component and serum amyloid A protein. Immunol Today 1994; 15:81–88.

92. Eskandari MK, Bolgos G, Miller C, Nguyen DT, DeForge LE, Remick DG. Anti-tumor necrosis factor antibody therapy fails to prevent lethality after cecal ligation and puncture or endotoxemia. J Immunol 1992; 148:2724–2730.

93. Echtenacher B, Weigl K, Lehn N, Mannel DN. Tumor necrosis factor-dependent adhesions as a major protective mechanism early in septic peritonitis in mice. Infect Immun 2001; 69:3550–3555.

94. Fisher CJ Jr, Agosti JM, Opal SM, et al. Treatment of septic shock with the tumor necrosis factor receptor: Fc fusion protein. N Engl J Med 1996; 334:1697–1702.

95. Keane J, Gershon S, Wise RP, et al. Tuberculosis associated with infliximab, a tumor necrosis factor a-neutralizing agent. N Engl J Med 2001; 345:1098–1104.

96. Reinhart K, Karzai W. Anti-tumor necrosis factor therapy in sepsis: update on clinical trials and lessons learned. Crit Care Med 2001; 29(suppl):S121–S125.

97. Zeni F, Freeman BF, Natanson C. Antiinflammatory therapies to treat sepsis and septic shock: a reassessment. Crit Care Med 1997; 25:1095–1100.

98. Opal SM, Fisher CJ Jr, Dhainaut J-FA, et al. Confirmatory interleukin-1 receptor antagonist trial in severe sepsis: a phase III, randomized, double-blind, placebo-controlled, multicenter trial. Crit Care Med 1997; 25:1115–1124.

99. Fisher CJ, Dhainaut JFA, Opal SM. Recombinant human interleukin-1 receptor antagonist in the treatment of patients with sepsis syndrome. J Am Med Assoc 1994; 271: 1836–1843.

100. Rodell TC, Foster C. Sepsis data show negative trend in second phase II sepsis trial. July 18, 1995. Press Release: Cortech Inc., 7000 North Broadway, Denver, CO 80221.

101. Fein AM, Bernard GR, Criner GJ, et al. Treatment of severe systemic inflammatory response syndrome and sepsis with a novel bradykinin antagonist, Deltibant (CP-0127). J Am Med Assoc 1997; 277:482–487.

102. Dhainaut JFA, Tenaillon A, LeTuizo Y. Platelet-activating factor receptor antagonist BN 52021 in the treatment of severe sepsis: a randomized, double-blind, placebo-controlled, multicenter clinical trial. Crit Care Med 1994; 22:1720–1728.

103. Dhainaut JFA, Tenaillon A, Hemmer M. Confirming phase III clinical trial to study the efficacy of a PAF antagonist, BN 52021, in reducing mortality of patients with severe Gram-negative sepsis. Abstr Am J Respir Crit Care Med 1995; 151:A447.

104. Kay CA. Can better measures of cytokine responses be obtained to guide cytokine inhibition? Knoll AG, Ludwigshafen, Germany. Presentation and handout. Cambridge Health Institutes' Designing Better Drugs & Clinical Trials for Sepsis/SIRS: Reducing Mortality to Patients and Suppliers. Washington, DC, February 20–21, 1996 (unpublished).

105. Reinhart K, Wiegand-Lohnert C, Grimminger F. Assessment of the safety and efficacy of the monoclonal anti-tumor necrosis factor antibody fragment, MAK 195, in patients with sepsis and septic shock: a multicenter, randomized, placebo-controlled, dose-ranging study. Crit Care Med 1996; 24:733–742.

106. Fisher CJ, Opal SM, Dhainaut JF. Influence of anti-tumor necrosis factor monoclonal antibody on cytokine levels in patients with sepsis. Crit Care Med 1993; 21:318–327.

107. Dhainaut JFA, Vincent JL, Richard C. CDP571, a humanized antibody to human tumor necrosis factor-alpha: safety, pharmacokinetics, immune response, and influence of the antibody on cytokine concentrations in patients with septic shock. Crit Care Med 1995; 23:1461–1469.

108. Abraham E, Wunderink R, Silverman H. Efficacy and safety of monoclonal antibody to human tumor necrosis factor-alpha in patients with sepsis syndrome. J Am Med Assoc 1995; 273:934–941.

109. Cohen J, Carlet J. INTERSEPT: an international, multicenter, placebo-controlled trial of monoclonal antibody to human tumor necrosis factor-alpha in patients with sepsis. International Sepsis Trial Study Group. Crit Care Med 1996; 24:1431–1440.

110. Fisher CJ, Agosti JM, Opal SM. Treatment of septic shock with the tumor necrosis factor receptor: Fc fusion protein. N Engl J Med 1996; 334:1697–1702.

111. Abraham E, Glauser M, Gelmont D, et al. Ro 45-2081 (TNFR55-1gG1) in the treatment of patients with severe sepsis and septic shock: preliminary results. [Abstract] International Autumnal Thematic Meeting on Sepsis, Deauville, France, November 5–7, 1995.

112. Bernard GB, Wheeler AP, Russell JA, et al. The effects of ibuprofen on the physiology and survival of patients with sepsis. N Engl J Med 1997; 336:912–918.

113. Haupt MT, Jastremski MS, Clemmer TP, et al. Effect of ibuprofen in patients with severe sepsis: a randomized, double-blind, multicenter study. Crit Care Med 1991; 19:1339–1347.

114. Bernard GR, Reines HD, Halushka PV, et al. Prostacyclin and thromboxane A sub 2 formation is increased in human sepsis syndrome. Am Rev Respir Dis 1991; 144:1095–1101.

115. Fisher CJ, Slotman GJ, Opal SM. Initial evaluation of human recombinant interleukin-1 receptor antagonist in the treatment of sepsis syndrome: a randomized, open-label, placebo-controlled multicenter trial. Crit Care Med 1994; 22:12–21.

116. Dellinger RP, Carlet JM, Masur H, Gerlach H, Calandra T, Cohen J, Gea-Banacloche J, Keh D, Marshall JC, Parker MM, Ramsay G, Zimmerman JL, Vincent JL, Levy MM; for the Surviving Sepsis Campaign Management Guidelines Committee. Surviving Sepsis Campaign guidelines for management of severe sepsis and septic shock. Crit Care Med 2004; 32, 858–872.

117. Hollenberg SM, Ahrens TS, Annane D, Astiz ME, Chalfin DB, Dasta JF, Heard SO, Martin C, Napolitano LM, Susla GM, Totaro R, Vincent JL, Zanotti-Cavazzoni S. Practice parameters for hemodynamic support of sepsis in adult patients: 2004 update. Crit Care Med 2004; 32:1928–1948.

118. Rivers E, Nguyen B, Havstad S, Ressler J, Muzzin A, Knoblich B, Peterson E, Tomlanovich M, For the Early Goal-Directed Therapy Collaborative Group. Early goal-directed therapy in the treatment of severe sepsis and septic shock. N Engl J Med 2001; 345:1368–1377.

119. Rady MY, Rivers EP, Nowak RM. Resuscitation of the critically ill in the ED: responses of blood pressure, heart rate, shock index, central venous oxygen saturation, and lactate. Am J Emerg Med 1996; 14:218–225.

120. Cortez A, Zito J, Lucas CE, Gerrick SJ. Mechanism of inappropriate polyuria in septic patients. Arch Surg 1977; 112:471–476.

121. Bellomo R, Chapman M, Finfer S, et al. Low-dose dopamine in patients with early renal dysfunction: a placebo-controlled randomised trial. Australian and New Zealand Intensive Care Society (ANZICS) Clinical Trials Group. Lancet 2000; 356:2139–2143.

122. Ward IM, Fraser VJ, Kollef MH. Clinical importance of delays in the initiation of appropriate antibiotic treatment for ventilator-associated pneumonia. Chest 2002; 122:262–268.

123. Garnacho-Montero J, Garcia-Garmendia JL, Barrero-Almodovar A, Jiminez-Jiminez FJ, Perez-Paredes C, Ortiz-Leyba C. Impact of adequate empirical antibiotic therapy on the outcome of patients admitted to the intensive care unit with sepsis. Crit Care Med 2003; 31:2742–2751.

124. MacArthur RD, Miller M, Albertson T, Panacek E, Johnson D, Teoh L, Barchuk W. Adequacy of early empiric antibiotic treatment and survival in severe sepsis: experience from the MONARCS trial. CID 2004; 38:284–288.

125. Jimenez MF, Marshall JC. Source control in the management of sepsis. Intensive Care Med 2001; 27:S49–S62.

126. Bufalari A, Giustozzi G, Moggi L. Postoperative intraabdominal abscesses: percutaneous versus surgical treatment. Acta Chir Belg 1996; 96:197–200.

127. Moss RL, Musemeche CA, Kosloske AM. Necrotizing fasciitis in children: prompt recognition and aggressive therapy improve survival. J Pediatr Surg 1996; 31: 1142–1146.

128. The SAFE Study Investigators [The Saline versus Albumin Fluid Evaluation (SAFE) Study]. A comparison of albumin and saline for fluid resuscitation in the Intensive Care Unit. N Engl J Med 2004; 350:2247–2256.

129. Kellum J, Decker J. Use of dopamine in acute renal failure: a meta-analysis. Crit Care Med 2001; 29:1526–1531.

130. Sharshar T, Blanchard A, Paillard M, Raphael JC, Gajdos P, Annane D. Circulating vasopressin levels in septic shock. Crit Care Med 2003; 31:1752–1757.

131. Holmes CL, Patel BM, Russell JA, et al. Physiology of vasopressin relevant to management of septic shock. Chest 2001; 120:989–1002.

132. Malay MB, Ashton RC, Landry DW, et al. Low-dose vasopressin in the treatment of vasodilatory septic shock. J Trauma 1999; 47:699–705.

133. Holmes CL, Walley KR, Chittock DR, et al. The effects of vasopressin on hemodynamics and renal function in severe septic shock: a case series. Intensive Care Med 2001; 27:1416–1421

134. The Acute Respiratory Distress Syndrome Network. Ventilation with lower tidal volumes as compared with traditional tidal volumes for acute lung injury and the acute respiratory distress syndrome. N Engl J Med 2000; 342:1301–1308.

135. Drakulovic M, Torres A, Bauer T, et al. Supine body position as a risk factor for nosocomial pneumonia in mechanically ventilated patients: a randomised trial. Lancet 1999; 354:1851–1858.

136. Schrier RW, Wang W. Mechanisms of disease: acute renal failure and sepsis. N Engl J Med 2004; 351:159–169.

137. Riedemann NC, Guo RF, Ward PA. The enigma of sepsis. J Clin Invest 2003; 112:460–467.

138. Landry DW, Oliver JA. The pathogenesis of vasodilatory shock. N Engl J Med 2001; 345:588–595.

139. Schrier RW, Henderson HS, Tisher CC, Tannen RL. Nephropathy associated with heat stress and exercise. Ann Intern Med 1967; 67:356–376.

140. Phu NH, Hien TT, Mai NTH, et al. Hemofiltration and peritoneal dialysis in infection-associated acute renal failure in Vietnam. N Engl J Med 2002; 347: 895–902.

141. Schiffl H, Lang SM, Fischer R. Daily hemodialysis and the outcome of acute renal failure. N Engl J Med 2002; 346:305–310.

142. Ronco C, Bellomo R, Homel P, et al. Effects of different doses in continuous veno-venous haemofiltration on outcomes of acute renal failure: a prospective randomised trial. Lancet 2000; 356:26–30.

143. Tonelli M, Manns B, Feller-Kopman D. Acute renal failure in the intensive care unit: a systematic review of the impact of dialytic modality on mortality and renal recovery. Am J Kidney Dis 2002; 40:875–885.

144. Cooper MS, Stewart, PM. Corticosteroid insufficiency in acutely ill patients. N Engl J Med 2003; 348:727–734.

145. Esteban NV, Loughlin T, Yergey AL, et al. Daily cortisol production rate in man determined by stable isotope dilution/mass spectrometry. J Clin Endocrinol Metab 1991; 72:39–45.

146. Barton RN, Stoner HB, Watson SM. Relationships among plasma cortisol, adrenocorticotrophin, and severity of injury in recently injured patients. J Trauma 1987; 27:384–392.

147. Chernow B, Alexander HR, Smallridge RC, et al. Hormonal responses to graded surgical stress. Arch Intern Med 1987; 147:1273–1278.

148. Perrot D, Bonneton A, Dechaud H, Motin J, Pugeat M. Hypercortisolism in septic shock is not suppressible by dexamethasone infusion. Crit Care Med 1993; 21: 396–401.

149. Chrousos GP. The hypothalamic–pituitary–adrenal axis and immune-mediated inflammation. N Engl J Med 1995; 332:1351–1362.

150. Lamberts SWJ, Bruining HA, de Jong FH. Corticosteroid therapy in severe illness. N Engl J Med 1997; 337:1285–1292.

151. Burchard K. A review of the adrenal cortex and severe inflammation: quest of the "eucorticoid" state. J Trauma 2001; 51:800–814.

152. Ten S, New M, Maclaren N. Clinical review 130: Addison's disease 2001. J Clin Endocrinol Metab 2001; 86:2909–2922.

153. Case records of the Massachusetts General Hospital (Case 15-2001). N Engl J Med 2001; 344:1536–1542.

154. Wagner RL, White PF, Kan PB, Rosenthal MH, Feldman D. Inhibition of adrenal steroidogenesis by the anesthetic etomidate. N Engl J Med 1984; 310:1415–1421.

155. Catalano RD, Parameswaran V, Ramachandran J, Trunkey DD. Mechanisms of adrenocortical depression during Escherichia coli shock. Arch Surg 1984; 119:145–150.

156. Salem M, Tainsh RE Jr, Bromberg J, Loriaux DL, Chernow B. Perioperative glucocorticoid coverage: a reassessment 42 years after emergence of a problem. Ann Surg 1994; 219:416–425.

157. Malik KJ, Wakelin K, Dean S, Cove DH, Wood PJ. Cushing's syndrome and hypothalamic-pituitary adrenal axis suppression induced by medroxyprogesterone acetate. Ann Clin Biochem 1996; 33:187–189.

158. Subramanian S, Goker H, Kanji A, Sweeney H. Clinical adrenal insufficiency in patients receiving megestrol therapy. Arch Intern Med 1997; 157:1008–1011.

159. Sibbald WJ, Short A, Cohen MP, Wilson RF. Variations in adrenocortical responsiveness during severe bacterial infections: unrecognized adrenocortical insufficiency in severe bacterial infections. Ann Surg 1977; 186:29–33.

160. Annane D, Sebille V, Troche G, Raphael JC, Gajdos P, Bellissant E. A 3-level prognostic classification in septic shock based on cortisol levels and cortisol response to corticotropin. J Am Med Assoc 2000; 283:1038–1045.

161. Beishuizen A, Thijs LG. Relative adrenal failure in intensive care: an identifiable problem requiring treatment? Best Pract Res Clin Endocrinol Metab 2001; 15:513–531.

162. Knowlton AL. Adrenal insufficiency in the intensive care setting. J Intensive Care Med 1989; 4:35–41.

163. Jacobs HS, Nabarro JD. Plasma 11-hydroxycorticosteroid and growth hormone levels in acute medical illnesses. Br Med J 1969; 2:595–598.

164. Barquist E, Kirton O. Adrenal insufficiency in the surgical intensive care unit patient. J Trauma 1997; 42:27–31.

165. Kidess AI, Caplan RH, Reynertson RH, Wickus GG, Goodnough DE. Transient corticotropin deficiency in critical illness. Mayo Clin Proc 1993; 68:435–441.

166. Bouachour G, Tirot P, Varache N, Govello JP, Harry P, Alquier P. Hemodynamic changes in acute adrenal insufficiency. Intensive Care Med 1994; 20:138–141.

167. Oelkers W. Dose-response aspects in the clinical assessment of the hypothalamo-pituitary-adrenal axis, and the low dose adrenocorticotropin test. Eur J Endocrinol 1996; 135:27–33.

168. Zaloga GP, Marik P. Hypothalamic-pituitary-adrenal insufficiency. Crit Care Clin 2001; 17:25–41.

169. Annane D, Bellissant E, Bollaert PE, Briegel J, Keh D, Kupfer Y. Corticosteroids for severe sepsis and septic shock: a systematic review and meta-analysis. BMJ, doi:10.1136/bmj.38181.482222.55 (published 2 August 2004).

170. Lefering R, Neugebauer EAM. Steroid controversy in sepsis and septic shock: a metaanalysis. Crit Care Med 1995; 23:1294–1303.

171. Cronin L, Cook DJ, Carlet J, Heyland DK, King D, Lansang MA, et al. Corticosteroid treatment for sepsis: a critical appraisal and meta-analysis of the literature. Crit Care Med 1995; 23:1430–1439.

172. Bollaert PE, Charpentier C, Levy B, Debouverie M, Audibert G, Larcan A. Reversal of late septic shock with supraphysiologic doses of hydrocortisone. Crit Care Med 1998; 26:645–650.

173. Briegel J, Forst H, Haller M, Schelling G, Kilger E, Kuprat G, et al. Stress doses of hydrocortisone reverse hyperdynamic septic shock: a prospective, randomized, doubleblind, single-center study. Crit Care Med 1999; 27:723–732.

174. Keh D, Boehnke T, Weber-Cartens S, Schulz C, Ahlers O, Bercker S, et al. Immunologic and hemodynamic effects of "low-dose" hydrocortisone in septic shock: a double-blind, randomized, placebo-controlled, crossover study. Am J Resp Crit Care Med 2003; 167:512–520.

175. Dhainaut JF, Yan B, Claessens Y. Protein C/activated protein C pathway: overview of clinical trial results in severe sepsis. Crit Care Med 2004; 32:S194–S201.

176. Aird WC. The role of the endothelium in severe sepsis and multiple organ dysfunction syndrome. Blood 2003; 101:3765–3777.

177. Esmon CT. The protein C pathway. Chest 2003; 124(3 suppl):26S–32S.

178. Esmon CT. Thrombomodulin as a model of molecular mechanisms that modulate protease specificity and function at the vessel surface. FASEB J 1995; 9:946–955.

179. Bernard GR, Vincent JL, Laterre PF, Larosa SP, Dhainaut J-F, Lopez-Rodriguez A, Steingrub JS, Garber GE, Helterbrand JD, Ely W, Fisher CJ; for the Recombinant

Human Activated Protein C Worldwide Evaluation in Severe Sepsis (PROWESS) Study Group. N Engl J Med 2001; 344:699–709.

180. Faust SN, Levin M, Harrison OB, et al. Dysfunction of endothelial protein C activation in severe meningococcal sepsis. N Engl J Med 2001; 345:408–416.

181. Angus DC, Laterre P-F, Helterbrand J, Ely W, Ball DE, Garg Rekha, Weissfeld LA, Bernard GR; for the PROWESS Investigators. The effect of drotrecogin alfa (activated) on long-term survival after severe sepsis. Crit Care Med 2004; 32:2199–2218.

182. Bernard GR, Margolis DB, Shanies HM, Ely EW, Wheeler AP, Levy H, Wong K, Wright TJ; for the ENHANCE US Investigators. Extended Evaluation of Recombinant Human Activated Protein C United States Trial (ENHANCE US). A single-arm, phase 3B, multicenter study of drotrecogin alfa (activated) in severe sepsis. Chest 2004; 125:2206–2216.

183. Van den Berghe G, Wouters P, Weekers F, et al. Intensive insulin therapy in critically ill patients. N Engl J Med 2001; 345:1359–1367.

184. Wolfe RR, Allsop JR, Burke JF. Glucose metabolism in man: responses to intravenous glucose infusion. Metabolism 1979; 28:210–220.

185. Wolfe RR, Herndon DN, Jahoor F, Miyoshi H, Wolfe M. Effect of severe burn injury on substrate cycling by glucose and fatty acids. N Engl J Med 1987; 317:403–408.

186. Shangraw RE, Jahoor F, Miyoshi H, et al. Differentiation between septic and post-burn insulin resistance. Metabolism 1989; 38:983–989.

187. Mizock BA. Alterations in carbohydrate metabolism during stress: a review of the literature. Am J Med 1995; 98:75–84.

188. McCowen KC, Malhotra A, Bistrian BR. Stress-induced hyperglycemia. Crit Care Clin 2001; 17:107–124.

189. Fietsam R Jr, Bassett J, Glover JL. Complications of coronary artery surgery in diabetic patients. Am Surg 1991; 57:551–557.

190. O'Neill PA, Davies I, Fullerton KJ, Bennett D. Stress hormone and blood glucose response following acute stroke in the elderly. Stroke 1991; 22:842–847.

191. Scott JF, Robinson GM, French JM, O'Connell JE, Alberti KG, Gray CS. Glucose potassium insulin infusions in the treatment of acute stroke patients with mild to moderate hyperglycemia: the Glucose Insulin in Stroke Trial (GIST). Stroke 1999; 30:793–799.

192. Malmberg K, Norhammar A, Wedel H, Ryden L. Glycometabolic state at admission: important risk marker of mortality in conventionally treated patients with diabetes mellitus and acute myocardial infarction: long-term results from the Diabetes and Insulin-Glucose Infusion in Acute Myocardial Infarction (DIGAMI) study. Circulation 1999; 99:2626–2632.

193. Malmberg K. Prospective randomised study of intensive insulin treatment on long term survival after acute myocardial infarction in patients with diabetes mellitus. BMJ 1997; 314:1512–1515.

194. Malmberg K, Ryden L, Efendic S, et al. A randomized trial of insulin-glucose infusion followed by subcutaneous insulin treatment in diabetic patients with acute myocardial infarction (DIGAMI study): effects of mortality at 1 year. J Am Coll Cardiol 1995; 26:57–65.

195. Van den Berghe G, Wouters P, Weekers F, et al. Reactivation of pituitary hormone release and metabolic improvement by infusion of growth hormone-releasing peptide and thyrotropin-releasing hormone in patients with protracted critical illness. J Clin Endocrinol Metab 1999; 84:1311–1323.

196. Van den Berghe G, Baxter RC, Weekers F, Wouters P, Bowers CY, Veldhuis JD. A paradoxical gender dissociation within the growth hormone/insulin-like growth factor I axis during protracted critical illness. J Clin Endocrinol Metab 2000; 85:183–192.

197. Gao F, Gao E, Yue TL, et al. Nitric oxide mediates the antiapoptotic effect of insulin in myocardial ischemia-reperfusion: the roles of PI3-kinase, Akt, and endothelial nitric oxide synthase phosphorylation. Circulation 2002; 105: 1497–1502.

198. Siegel JP. Assessing the use of activated protein C in the treatment of severe sepsis. N Engl J Med 2002; 347:1030–1034.

199. Evans W. Hemodynamic and metabolic therapy in critically ill patients. N Engl J Med 2001; 345:1417–1418.

200. Oberholzer C, Oberholzer A, Clare-Salzler M, Moldawer LL. Apoptosis in sepsis: a new target for therapeutic exploration. FASEB J 2001; 15:879–892.

201. Hotchkiss RS, et al. Overexpression of Bcl-2 in transgenic mice decreases apoptosis and improves survival in sepsis. J Immunol 1999; 162:4148–4156.

202. Hotchkiss RS, et al. Prevention of lymphocyte cell death in sepsis improves survival in mice. Proc Natl Acad Sci USA 1999; 96:14541–14546.

203. Hotchkiss RS, et al. Caspase inhibitors improve survival in sepsis: a critical role of the lymphocyte. Nat Immunol 2000; 1:496–501.

204. Coopersmith CM, et al. Inhibition of intestinal epithelial apoptosis and survival in a murine model of pneumonia-induced sepsis. J Am Med Assoc 2002; 287:1716–1721.

205. Coopersmith, CM, et al. Overexpression of Bcl-2 in the intestinal epithelium improves survival in septic mice. Crit Care Med 2002; 30:195–201.

206. Cross AS, Sadoff JC, Kelly N, Bernton E, Gemski P. Pretreatment with recombinant murine tumor necrosis factor alpha/cachectin and murine interleukin 1 alpha protects mice from lethal bacterial infection. J Exp Med 1989; 169: 2021–2027.

207. Froidevaux C, Roger T, Martin C, Glauser MP, Calandra T. Macrophage migration inhibitory factor and innate immune responses to bacterial infections. Crit Care Med 2001; 29:S13–S15.

208. Roger T, David J, Glauser MP, Calandra T. MIF regulates innate immune responses through modulation of Toll-like receptor 4. Nature 2001; 414:920–924.

209. Calandra T, Echtenacher B, Roy DL, Pugin J, Metz CN, Hultner L, et al. Protection from septic shock by neutralization of macrophage migration inhibitory factor. Nat Med 2000; 6:164–170.

210. Bernhagen J, Calandra T, Mitchell RA, Martin SB, Tracey KJ, Voelter W, et al. MIF is a pituitary-derived cytokine that potentiates lethal endotox-aemia. Nature 1993; 365:756–759.

211. Bozza M, Satoskar AR, Lin G, Lu B, Humbles AA, Gerard C, et al. Targeted disruption of migration inhibitory factor gene reveals its critical role in sepsis. J Exp Med 1999; 189:341–346.

212. Wang H, Yang H, Czura CJ, Sama AE, Tracey KJ. HMGB1 as a late mediator of lethal systemic inflammation. Am J Respir Crit Care Med 2001; 164:1768–1773.
213. Wang H, Bloom O, Zhang M, Vishnubhakat JM, Ombrellino M, Che J, et al. HMG-1 as a late mediator of endotoxin lethality in mice. Science 1999; 285:248–251.

11

Management of Acute Gastrointestinal Hemorrhage

GORDON V. OHNING

Department of Medicine, VA Greater Los Angeles Healthcare System-West
   Los Angeles, California; CURE Digestive Diseases Research Center
   Center for Neurovisceral Sciences and Women's Health
Geffen School of Medicine at UCLA
Los Angeles, California, U.S.A.

I. Introduction

Gastrointestinal hemorrhage remains a common and serious clinical problem, accounting for more than 300,000 hospitalizations per year in the U.S.A. (1), and is a frequent indication for admission to the intensive care unit (ICU). Upper gastrointestinal (UGI) bleeding, defined as a bleeding source proximal to the ligament of Treitz, is more common than lower gastrointestinal (LGI) bleeding, with an estimated annual hospitalization rate in the U.S. of 100–150 per 100,000 adults (2,3) versus 20 per 100,000 adults (4), respectively. Although diagnostic and treatment modalities have markedly improved over the past several decades, the mortality for acute UGI bleeding has remained relatively constant at 5–10% (1,2). This static mortality rate is likely due to the successful improvement in overall life expectancy, resulting in an increased average age, and comorbid medical conditions for patients presenting with acute UGI bleeding (1,3). Mortality for LGI bleeding is currently less than 5%, having benefiting from improved diagnostic/therapeutic techniques and intensive care management (4). It should be emphasized that the majority of patients presenting with acute GI blood loss will resolve the initial bleed spontaneously. Therefore, the primary benefit and clinical success are derived from noninterventional therapies delivered within the ICU setting. The cornerstones of effective management for patients presenting with acute, significant GI blood loss continues to be rapid assessment combined with early and effective resuscitation and recognition of potential complicating factors that can impact the hospital course. Successful outcome is a product of team effort, with admission to an ICU for all patients presenting with significant bleeding and timely consultation of gastroenterologists, radiologists, and surgeons.

II. Assessment

The initial assessment should be directed towards determining the urgency and location of the blood loss. Urgency is correlated with the degree of volume depletion, signs of ongoing blood loss, and the presence of comorbid conditions that are adversely affected by the circulatory compromise associated with significant blood loss. The degree of volume depletion will dictate the presentation and can vary from modest alterations in vital signs to frank shock. Assessment of the location of GI bleeding typically focuses on differentiating UGI and LGI sources, but it is prudent to consider non-GI sources of blood loss in appropriate circumstances. Approximately 80% of patients presenting with acute GI blood loss will resolve the initial bleeding event spontaneously (5,6). Intervention is therefore directed towards diagnosis of the underlying cause and reducing the risk of late rebleeding. Conversely, patients who present with persistent or early recurrent bleeding represent a high mortality group, and early identification of such patients will permit timely therapeutic intervention to achieve hemostasis (7,8). Although discussed separately, the history, physical examination, and resuscitation efforts should be done concurrently in actual practice.

A. Medical History and Physical Examination

The history and physical examination should be concise and not delay the initial resuscitation efforts. The most urgent attention should be placed on determining the patient's hemodynamic stability. The presence of agitation, pallor, tachycardia, and hypotension warrants immediate and aggressive resuscitation to restore the intravascular volume. Important clues from the medical history concerning the source of bleeding and potential comorbidity should be identified. Any prior history of GI bleeding should be determined, as recurrent bleeding from the same etiology occurs in over 50% of patients (9). This is particularly true for rare hereditary conditions associated with GI bleeding, such as hereditary hemorrhagic telangiectasia (Osler–Weber–Rendu syndrome) (10). Any prior history of abdominal surgery (particularly repair of abdominal aortic aneurysm), recent gastrointestinal illness (such as pancreatitis), or any endoscopic procedures, particularly if performed in the immediate one to two weeks prior to presentation, should be documented. Any known history of liver, renal, or cardiopulmonary disease should be elicited, although these conditions may be present even if the medical history is unremarkable. A focused review of symptoms correlated with GI disease should also be performed, including the quality and localization of abdominal pain, antecedent vomiting or retching, heartburn, dysphagia, abdominal pain, weight loss, and any change in stools, particularly the presence of melena or hematochezia. Medication history should specifically question the use of aspirin, nonsteroidal anti-inflammatory drugs (NSAIDs) or anticoagulants as such medications are of immediate significance in management decisions.

As with the medical history, physical examination should initially be directed at determining the degree of hemodynamic compromise. Orthostatic hypotension is defined as a decrease in systolic blood pressure of >20 mmHg or diastolic blood pressure of >10 mmHg associated with an increase in the pulse of >20 beats per minute (bpm) that occurs by moving the patient from a supine to standing position and is associated with a 15–20% loss of blood volume (11). Typically, a patient with this degree of volume loss also presents with a resting tachycardia (>100 bpm); however, supine hypotension (shock) is usually associated with more substantial blood loss (12). These physical exam findings are not always reliable as a patient's age, medication use, and comorbid medical conditions can dramatically alter their accuracy. The examiner should interpret orthostatic findings with particular caution in the elderly or patients with significant diabetes, cardiovascular disease, or autonomic dysfunction (13). Conversely, younger and healthier patients have an enhanced ability to compensate, and findings of volume depletion may underestimate the actual degree of blood loss (14). Examination should assess the patient for stigmata of chronic liver disease, including spider angiomata, jaundice, nodular liver edge, splenomegaly, or ascites, as such findings would raise the possibility of variceal bleeding. Hyperactive bowel sounds are frequently heard due to the cathartic affect of intralumenal blood. A rectal examination should always be performed to determine if hematochezia, melena, or heme-positive stools are present. Hematochezia usually signifies a LGI source; however, 11% of patients with hematochezia will have an UGI source associated with massive bleeding (15). Conversely, melenic stools are typically associated with UGI bleeding, but they can occur from distal small bowel or proximal colon sources if the bleeding is not brisk and large bowel motility has not been accelerated.

Although chronic GI blood loss typically presents with iron-deficiency anemia and heme-positive stools, severe chronic anemia can also present with pallor, dizziness, angina, and dyspnea. This can be a diagnostic challenge, particularly in elderly patients, as the presence of postural vital signs may be present due to comorbidity unrelated to the GI blood loss (13). Obviously, it would be prudent to treat such patients as though in an acute GI bleed until the clinical situation is clarified.

B. Laboratory Tests

Measurement of the initial hematocrit (HCT) should be performed; however, the value must be interpreted with caution. In acute bleeding, the initial HCT does not adequately reflect the degree of blood loss, as bleeding occurs without adequate time to permit fluid redistribution from the extravascular compartment. Serial measurement of subsequent HCTs to monitor the response to transfusion therapy also requires cautious interpretation as volume expansion frequently occurs during resuscitation and results in transient dilutional effects. Redistribution of fluid between the intra- and extravascular compartments requires up to 72 hours before the HCT accurately reflects the vascular blood volume (9). The initial HCT and mean corpuscular volume (MCV), if abnormal, may suggest an underlying cause for the patient's presentation (such as cancer in an elderly patient with an underlying iron-deficiency anemia). For underlying chronic anemia, the MCV and serum iron studies are superior to the HCT for estimating the degree of chronic blood loss.

Additional laboratory testing should include measurement of coagulation parameters [platelets, prothrombin time (PT), and partial thromboplastin time (PTT)], renal function [blood urea nitrogen (BUN) and creatinine], and hepatic function parameters, including the serum albumin level. In the absence of renal disease, an elevation in the BUN and/or BUN: creatinine ratio suggests an UGI source of bleeding as blood tracking through the small bowel provides a good protein source (16). This can be of particular importance in patients with cirrhosis as a harbinger of hepatic encephalopathy. A type and crossmatch for transfusion should also be obtained upon admission in all cases of significant bleeding.

An EKG and serial serum creatinine kinase or troponin levels should be obtained to evaluate for myocardial ischemia, especially in patients presenting with massive blood loss. This is particularly important in elderly patients, as the incidence of concomitant myocardial infarction upon presentation is high even in the absence of a prior history of coronary artery disease (17). The implications of myocardial disease and GI bleeding are discussed further in a subsequent section.

C. Nasogastric Tube Aspiration

A nasogastric tube (NGT) should be placed to assess for an UGI source of bleeding in all patients presenting with severe gastrointestinal hemorrhage. Even if a history of recent hematemesis (coffee grounds or blood) unequivocally indicates an UGI source, it is important to access the patient for continuing blood loss. A sole exception might be the patient with active hematemesis during examination. NGT placement should be performed using room temperature tap water for lavage. If the available water is safe to consume, it is adequate for NGT lavage, and the use of sterile saline merely adds expense without benefit (18). The use of iced solutions for NGT lavage should also be avoided (19). Although historically advocated as a method of inducing arterial spasm within ulcers, the intragastric infusion of cold solutions is both uncomfortable for the patient and adversely affects platelet function and the coagulation cascade (20). NGT aspiration should be performed gently because vigorous manipulation causes mucosal injury from suction artifact and complicates the interpretation of findings during subsequent diagnostic endoscopy. Suspected varices (or even know varices) are not a contraindication to a diagnostic NGT. The utility of determining the presence of active UGI bleeding outweighs any theoretical concern regarding induction of variceal bleeding due to NGT use. The NGT should be removed once the diagnostic aspiration is complete as prolonged NGT placement can cause erosions at the LES with an increased risk of causing bleeding (particularly if esophageal varices are present) and produce additional artifacts to annoy the endoscopist.

A positive NGT aspirate will vary from coffee grounds to frank blood, both of which indicate an UGI source of bleeding. A clear color does not necessarily since exclude an UGI source since bleeding in the duodenum may not reflux into the gastric lumen (21). Although the presence of bile staining in the NGT aspirate provides a degree of reassurance that an UGI source has been excluded, UGI bleeding is typically intermittent and a "negative" NGT aspirate may simply be a matter of timing (22). The color of the NGT aspirate has prognostic value (21) and, when considered in conjunction with the stool color, has a strong correlation with the risk of rebleeding and overall mortality. A clear NGT aspirate correlates with a mortality of 6–10%, while red blood in the NGT aspirate associated with hematochezia carries a 30% mortality. NGT aspirates should be evaluated solely by visual inspection. Hemmocult testing adds no value (23) and will result in confusion, if such "data" is improperly reported. Finally, the NGT is a diagnostic device and should not be used to clear blood and clots the stomach for endoscopy, as it is routinely ineffective for this purpose.

III. Initial Therapy

Resuscitation is the single most effective intervention in the successful treatment of gastrointestinal hemorrhage, and its importance cannot be overstated. Patients should be admitted to an ICU to provide adequate support and monitoring during resuscitation and the initial diagnostic and therapeutic efforts. Adequate intravenous (iv) catheter access should be obtained using a minimum of two large bore catheters, typically 14 or 16 gauge. If peripheral access is problematic or brisk bleeding requires rapid infusion of fluids and blood products, central venous access should be obtained. One common error is to equate "many" small-bore iv catheters with a single large-bore iv catheter. A review of the Poiseuille's equation regarding the resistance to fluid flow in tubes (24) indicates that one 16-gauge iv catheter is equivalent to four 18-gauge, nine 20-gauge, or 30 22-gauge iv catheters. Although this might be an oversimplification of the physical principal, it does emphasize the practical point concerning the bore diameter of iv catheters used in resuscitation efforts: bigger is better. Once iv catheter access is established, fluid resuscitation should commence immediately using normal saline (or Ringers lactate, if preferred) to normalize the vascular volume and restore end-organ perfusion. The use of vasopressors should be avoided, as these medications will only worsen end-organ perfusion and their use should only be considered if the response to aggressive fluid resuscitation is inadequate (9). Continued monitoring of the patient's vital signs must be performed and adjustments to fluid resuscitation therapy should be individualized to the patient's needs and response to treatment. An inadequate response may be a sign of continued bleeding, and reassessment should be performed, including repeated NGT aspiration of the stomach. General measures that are of value include providing supplemental oxygen to maximize the oxygen-carrying capacity of the remaining blood. Supplemental oxygen should be used cautiously in patients with underlying chronic pulmonary disease to prevent carbon dioxide retention and precipitate respiratory failure (25). Urine output should be measured and stool output should be monitored for continued melena or hematochezia. Patients should be kept NPO in anticipation of early endoscopy. In patients with a history of congestive heart failure, end-stage renal disease, or cirrhosis, fluid resuscitation requires careful monitoring to prevent overzealous volume expansion and the precipitation of pulmonary edema. Placement of a Swan–Ganz catheter may improve monitoring in selected patients at high risk of complications.

A. Blood Products

Replacement of erythrocytes, platelets, and coagulation factors should be individualized to the patient's needs. Transfusion with packed-red blood cells (PRBCs) is the preferred method for replacing blood loss and should be initiated rapidly to improve oxygen transport and reduce the risk of end-organ damage. The use of whole blood is rarely indicated and should be reserved for patients with uncontrolled massive bleeding requiring immediate surgery. The degree of erythrocyte replacement should be tailored to the clinical setting; however, most patients with substantial bleeding should achieve a target HCT of approximately 30% to both minimize the systemic effects of anemia and provide a reserve for potential rebleeding. The major considerations for transfusion requirements include age >60, the presence of cardiopulmonary comorbidity, and evidence of continuing blood loss (26). This can be modified for younger patients without significant comorbid conditions, particularly the absence of cardiovascular disease, and targeting a HCT of 20–25% may be more appropriate if high-risk lesions are not subsequently identified on endoscopy (27). An inadequate response to transfusion may be a manifestation of ongoing blood loss, and the patient should be reassessed for recurrent bleeding. Each unit of PRBC should elevate the HCT by 3–4% (28), although ongoing volume replacement with fluids may temper this general approximation. Overzealous transfusion to higher hematocrits should be avoided. This is especially important in patients with varices as overexpansion of the vascular volume increases the risk of bleeding (29).

Platelets and fresh-frozen plasma (FFP) may be required to maintain an adequate state of coagulation and promote hemostasis. Both are frequently compromised in patients with underlying liver disease; however, massive blood loss may consume these factors and require replacement in patients without a baseline coagulopathy. It is important to achieve and maintain the PT below 15 seconds (INR < 1.5) to both promote hemostasis and allow for therapeutic intervention during endoscopy (30). A typical "rule of thumb" is to expect one unit of FFP for every four units of PRBCs (31); however, monitoring the patient's PT/PTT should provide a more exact guide. Platelet number and function can be compromised patients with a variety of disorders, including disseminated intravascular coagulation (DIC) and chronic renal failure, in addition to the sequestering observed in patients with underlying cirrhosis and portal hypertension. Typically, the platelet count should be maintained above 50,000. Pre-admission medications can adversely affect coagulation properties and include both platelet active drugs, such as aspirin, NSAIDs, and ticlopidine, as well as anticoagulants, such as warfarin and heparin. These medications should be discontinued and their effects reversed in patients with life-threatening GI bleeding.

Other considerations may arise when extreme transfusion requirements are encountered. The use of citrate in PRBC preparation may lead to chelation of circulating calcium, and the free calcium should be measured in cases requiring massive amounts of PRBC transfusions with replacement of calcium as needed (32,33). Large volumes of transfusion products infused at or below room temperature may lower the patient's body temperature, and the use of warming for subsequent infusions may be required to prevent hypothermia (34).

Successful resuscitation efforts should target a heart rate of <100 bpm, systolic blood pressure >100 mmHg, adequate replacement of erythrocytes, and correction of any coagulopathy in anticipation of further diagnostic and therapeutic interventions.

IV. Post-Resuscitation Management

Post-resuscitation efforts should be directed at diagnosing and treating the underlying cause of bleeding in an effort to provide hemostasis for ongoing bleeding or to reduce the risk of recurrent bleeding. Early consultation from a gastroenterologist should be obtained, as the need for endoscopy is virtually universal in patients presenting with GI bleeding. Surgical consultation should be obtained in most patients with significant GI bleeding, particularly if patients present with evidence of volume depletion or shock. Specific etiologies requiring surgical consultation include a history of recent GI surgery or prior repair of an abdominal aortic aneurysm, suspected ischemic bowel or perforation, and high-risk lesions identified on subsequent endoscopy.

A. Pharmacologic Therapy

Since the majority of UGI lesions causing bleeding are acid-peptic disorders, empiric acid suppression should be instituted, as side effects are minimal (Table 1). Although divergent conclusions have been reported concerning the

Table 1   Medical Therapies for UGI Bleeding

Therapy	Action	Uses[a]	Typical dosing[b,c]
H-2 blockers			
Cimetidine	Acid suppression (histamine-2 receptor antagonist)	Second line agents for acute bleeding, ulcer healing, and prophylaxis	37.5 mg/hr (iv); 400–800 mg q12 (po)
Ranitidine			6.25 mg/hr (iv); 150 mg q12 (po)
Famotidine			20 mg q12 (iv) 20–40 mg q12 (po)
Nizatidine			150–300 mg q12 (po)
PPIs			
Omeprazole	Acid suppression (direct inhibition of parietal cell proton pump)	First line agents for acute bleeding, ulcer healing, and prophylaxis	80 mg bolus, 8 mg/hr (iv); 20 mg q6 or 40 mg q12 (po)
Pantoprazole			80 mg bolus 8 mg/hr (iv); 40 mg q12 (po)
Rabeprazole			20–40 mg q12 (po)
Lansoprazole			30–60 mg q12 (po)
Esomeprazole			20–40 mg q12 (po)
Sucralfate	Barrier (growth factor adhesion?)	Third line agent for ulcer healing and prophylaxis	1 g q4 (po)
Antacids	Acid neutralization	Breakthrough symptom control; fourth line agent for prophylaxis	30–60 cc q2 (po) or "as need" for symptom control
Vasopressin[d]	Reduce splanchnic blood flow	Second line agent for variceal bleeding	0.2–0.4 U bolus, then 0.4–1.0 U/hr (iv)
Octreotide	Reduce splanchnic blood flow	First line agent for variceal bleeding	50 ug bolus, then 50 ug/hr (iv)

[a]General characterization of use; other factors may alter importance in any particular patient.
[b]FDA approved and unapproved doses reported in various studies; consult pharmacist regarding current recommendations for dosing and application.
[c]For the acute GI bleed setting, recommend continuous infusion iv agents and target intragastric pH >4.5 (see text).
[d]Should be used in conjunction with iv nitroglycerin (10–50 ug/min).
Abbreviation: PPIs, proton pump inhibitors.

effectiveness of H-2 receptor antagonists in acute GI bleeding (35,36), both H-2 receptor antagonists and proton pump inhibitors (PPIs) have been shown to decrease the risk of recurrent bleeding when therapy targets an intragastric pH above 4.5 (37). Intravenous preparations should be used as they are more effective in maintaining continuous acid suppression, and oral administration will likely be poorly absorbed in the setting of an acute UGI bleed (38). Antacids and sucralfate are not effective in preventing early rebleeding, and their use in the acute setting may complicate endoscopic interpretation of mucosal lesions. Sucralfate may be useful in prophylaxis for stress ulcers and in the treatment of radiation colitis.

Suspected variceal hemorrhage can be empirically treated with octreotide, which has supplanted vasopressin due to its similar efficacy and markedly improved safety profile (39). Additionally, limited data suggest that octreotide therapy may be beneficial for nonvariceal etiologies of UGI bleeding (40). If variceal hemorrhage is suspected on the basis of the history or physical examination, initial dosing with 50 ug followed by continuous infusion at 50 ug/hr can be started in the emergency room and continued for up to five to seven days as an adjunctive treatment to subsequent endoscopic therapy (41,42). Discontinuation of octreotide after hemostasis has been achieved does not require tapering; however, octreotide treatment is only a temporizing measure and definitive endoscopic, radiographic, or surgical therapy should be aggressively pursued to reduce the risk of rebleeding. The combination of octreotide with endoscopic therapy has been shown to be more effective than either therapy alone and can achieve hemostasis in up to 90% of patients (42,43).

B. Endoscopy

Endoscopy is the primary diagnostic modality, and radiographic barium studies play absolutely no role in the diagnosis of acute upper or lower GI bleeding. Early endoscopy contributes to both the diagnostic and therapeutic capabilities and has been shown to reduce overall mortality (44) by confirming the site of bleeding, providing endoscopic risk stratification, and allowing the use of therapeutic modalities to control bleeding. Patients are initially stratified according to the pre-endoscopic assessment of potential etiologies and comorbidity (Table 2). In high-risk patients with significant bleeding, endoscopy should be performed after the patient has been adequately stabilized. Low-risk patients with significant, but self-limited, bleeding should undergo endoscopy within the first 12–24 hours. Endoscopy allows for further risk stratification by both identifying the cause of bleeding and assessing the risk of recurrent hemorrhage. For upper GI lesions, endoscopic stigmata for hemorrhage have been primarily directed towards peptic ulcer disease. Endoscopic stigmata that confer a higher risk include the presence of active arterial bleeding, a visible vessel, or adherent clot and benefit from immediate therapeutic endoscopic treatment (Table 3). Conversely, ulcers with a clean base or only a flat spot have less than a 5%

Table 2   Poor Prognostic Indicators for UGI Bleeding

Age >60
Comorbid medical conditions (especially cardiopulmonary)
Onset of bleeding during hospitalization
Hemodynamic instability
Red NG aspirate
High transfusion requirements (>5 units PRBCs)
Continued or recurrent bleeding
Emergency surgery

risk of rebleeding within the first 72 hours and do not benefit from therapeutic intervention. Although the use of early endoscopy in the emergency department has been shown to reduce costs by avoiding hospitalization of patients with low risk nonvariceal lesions (45), the decision regarding the appropriate location and timing of endoscopy should also account for the availability of trained endoscopy staff, appropriate therapeutic equipment, and the availability of surgical backup (30). Conversely, high risk patients or those with ulcer stigmata on endoscopy should be admitted to an ICU for monitoring, and patients with severe hemodynamic compromise may require endoscopy in the operating room (30). ICU monitoring should continue until the patient has demonstrated adequate hemostasis.

Endoscopy is directed towards the suspected site of bleeding; however, both upper and lower endoscopy may be required if the location of bleeding is unclear. Use of therapeutic modalities during endoscopy requires correction of any coagulopathy prior to initiating endoscopy (PT < 15 sec, platelets >50,000) (30). Endotracheal intubation to provide airway protection should be performed prior to upper endoscopy in patients with active bleeding, altered

Table 3   Prognostic Significance of Endoscopic Stigmata of Ulcer Hemorrhage

Endoscopic findings	Prevalence[a]	Rebleed rate[b] (untreated)	Rebleed rate[b] (treated)
Active arterial bleed	12	90	15–30
Visible vessel	22	50	15–30
Adherent clot	10	12–33	5
Oozing without stigmata	14	10–27	n/a
Flat spot	10	7	n/a
Clean base	32	3	n/a

Note: n/a, not available.
[a]Percentage with recurrent bleeding.
[b]Percentage of total at presentation.
Source: Ref. 30.

mental status, or at risk of aspiration. Alternatively, a large overtube can be used at the time of endoscopy (30). Upper panendoscopy should be performed after clearing blood or clots from the gastric lumen. Gastric lavage should be performed with a large-bore oro-gastric (Ewald) tube using gravity infusion and flushing or very gentle manual lavage to reduce mucosal injury and artifacts. Metoclopramide (10 mg, iv) can be given to promote gastric emptying if endoscopy is not performed immediately after successful resuscitation. The routine use of "second look" endoscopy has not been shown to be beneficial or cost-effective in the management of UGI bleeding; however, recurrent bleeding may warrant a repeated endoscopic examination.

Colonoscopy can be successfully preformed after a rapid purge (4 L of polyethylene glycol preparation given orally or via NG tube over two hours), and metoclopramide (10 mg) should be given to reduce the risk of nausea and decrease intestinal transit (15). The cecum can be reached in over 95% of patients, and the diagnostic accuracy is over 80% (15). Patients must be adequately resuscitated prior to endoscopy to permit sedation and controlled endoscopic examination and treatment. Patients with massive bleeding that is unresponsive to aggressive resuscitation will require emergency surgical consultation, and intraoperative endoscopy can be attempted to localize the source of bleeding.

V. Upper GI Bleeding

The common causes of UGI bleeding include peptic ulcer disease, varices, Mallory–Weiss (MW) tear, and erosive gastropathies, with a variety of less frequent, but important, etiologies (Table 4). The most critical prognostic indicator is the etiology of the bleed, with variceal bleeding being associated with a higher mortality compared to other causes (46). Other important prognostic indicators include the severity of the bleed, age >60, the number and severity of comorbid conditions (particularly cardiopulmonary disease), the onset of bleeding during hospitalization, the presence of giant ulcers (>2 cm diameter), and the need for emergency surgery (Table 2) (47). This discussion will briefly review the initial management, and the reader is directed to other in-depth reviews for more details concerning the diagnosis and treatment of specific disease entities. Variceal bleeding will be considered separately due to the unique differences in presentation, initial treatment, and prognosis compared to UGI bleeding from nonvariceal causes.

VI. Nonvariceal Bleeding

Peptic ulcer disease remains the most common cause (55%) of significant UGI bleeding (30). Despite the development of effective therapies for treating peptic ulcer disease, including development of effective eradication therapies for *Helicobacter pylori*, the hospitalization rate for bleeding ulcers has remained virtually

Table 4   Etiologies of Gastrointestinal Bleeding

Upper GI bleeding	
etiology	Incidence (range)[a]
Peptic ulcers (DU and GU)	50 (45–55)%
Varices (esophageal and gastric)	12 (10–14)%
Angiomata	4 (1–6)%
Mallory–Weiss tear	7 (5–8)%
Cancer	3 (3–4)%
Erosions	18 (4–27)%
Dieulafoy's	1
Hemobilia	<1
Aorto-enteric fistula	<1
Other/unknown causes	11 (10–12)%
Lower GI bleeding	
etiology	Incidence (range)[a]
Diverticulosis	32 (15–55)%
Angiodysplasia	15 (3–40)%
Cancer/polyp	15 (8–36)%
Colitis/ulcer	15 (6–22)%
Anorectal	5 (3–9)%
Other/unknown causes	18 (5–29)%

[a]Variable incidences due to differences in populations studied.
Source: Refs. 4, 66, 107–115.

unchanged (2). Bleeding can occur without significant antecedent peptic symptoms, and this may therefore represent the first presentation of *H. pylori*-associated disease (48). The use of aspirin and NSAIDs, which can cause ulcers in the absence of *H. pylori* infection, have increased substantially in the past few decades due to their easy availability coupled with an aging population requiring increased utilization (49). Although it is important to screen for *H. pylori* in patients presenting with UGI bleeding secondary to peptic ulcers because eradication therapy reduces the risk of recurrent disease, the presence of *H. pylori* does not significantly alter the initial treatment for acute UGI bleeding.

Gastritis is frequently listed as an endoscopic diagnosis, although this term is correctly applied only when the presence of mucosal inflammation has been confirmed by microscopic examination of biopsy specimens (a task beyond the capabilities of current endoscopes). Gastropathy more correctly describes the endoscopic finding of superficial erosive disease that is associated with NSAIDs, portal hypertension, or stress-induced mucosal lesions (47). UGI bleeding from gastropathies typically occurs as a result of diffuse mucosal involvement and endoscopic therapies are ineffective, unless a single or limited number of bleeding lesions can be identified (50). The initial management should be directed at supportive measures and rigorous correction of any existing coagulopathy.

Esophagitis with erosions or ulceration can infrequently present with significant bleeding, particularly in patients with extensive mucosal involvement or an underlying coagulopathy (51). Institution of acid suppression with high-dose proton-pump inhibitors and correction of any coagulopathy typically results in rapid resolution of symptoms. Therapeutic endoscopy has been used with caution for unresponsive lesions due to the increased risk of perforation (52).

MW tears occur in the distal esophagus at the level of the gastro-esophageal junction and typically present with brisk bleeding due to rupture of the underlying venous and/or arterial vessels. Although MW tears presumably occur due to vomiting or retching, a precedent history is frequently absent (53). Endoscopic treatment is very effective in controlling active hemorrhage, but is not typically employed for nonbleeding lesions. Most bleeding from MW tears is self-limited, with healing of the mucosal tear usually occurring within 48 hours. Patients with portal hypertension are at increased risk of massive bleeding, and rebleeding is frequently seen within the first 24 hours (54). Patients refractory to endoscopic treatment and correction of any underlying coagulopathy may require angiographic embolization to achieve adequate hemostasis.

Angiodysplasia is more commonly associated with LGI bleeding but can occur in the stomach and duodenum, particularly in elderly patients or in the presence of chronic renal insufficiency (55). Hereditary hemorrhagic telangiectasia (Osler–Weber–Rendu syndrome) frequently presents in younger patients without other risk factors for UGI bleeding. Endoscopic treatment is effective, but rebleeding rates are high due to the natural history of the diseases (56). A rare, but important, disorder due to vascular abnormalities is gastric antral vascular ectasia (GAVE). GAVE, or "watermelon stomach," can present with acute bleeding; however, chronic anemia is the more common presentation (57). Although idiopathic GAVE usually occurs in elderly (age >70) female patients, it can be associated with cirrhosis and should be differentiated from the more common portal hypertensive gastropathy as the response to treatment is markedly different. GAVE responds to endoscopic coagulation therapies (58), but is not improved by portal decompression with transjugular intrahepatic portosystemic shunt (TIPS) (59). Conversely, portal hypertensive gastropathy is responds to portal decompression, and endoscopic therapies are typically ineffective.

Aorto-enteric fistula is a rare, but lethal cause of UGI bleeding (60). Secondary fistulas due to Dacron graft repair of abdominal aortic aneurysm are far more common than primary fistulas due to atherosclerotic disease or infection (tuberculosis, syphilis). Secondary aorto-enteric fistulas can rarely occur due to trauma, penetrating peptic ulcers, or malignancy (61). Bleeding typically presents with a significant, but self-limited, "sentinel" bleed commonly originating in the third or fourth portion of the duodenum, followed by a massive exsanguinating bleed within hours to days of the initial presentation. In suspected cases of bleeding from aorto-enteric fistulas, upper endoscopy using an long endoscope and/or side-viewing duodenoscope should be performed to exclude other etiologies and possibly confirm the diagnosis. Early surgery is the only effective treatment (60) and should be aggressively pursued in the presence of severe, active bleeding in patients with documented or suspected aorto-enteric fistula.

Dieulafoy's lesion is a large, cavernous submucosal artery that typically occurs in the upper stomach along the lesser curvature near the gastroesophageal junction, although other locations (including the LGI tract) have been reported. Bleeding occurs by pressure necrosis into the gastric lumen without overlying mucosal disease and can be very difficult to diagnose with endoscopy, unless active bleeding occurs during the procedure or an adherent thrombus is present due to a recent bleeding activity (62). Although bleeding is usually self-limited, it almost invariably recurs and can present with massive blood loss. If repeated endoscopy fails to identify the lesion, endoscopic ultrasound (EUS) or radiographic techniques (angiography, CT scan) may be required to confirm the diagnosis. Endoscopic therapy can be effective at achieving hemostasis (63), but recurrent bleeding rates are high (up to 40%), and definitive surgical treatment by wedge resection may be required earlier in patients refractory to endoscopic treatment (64).

Hemobilia, or bleeding from a hepatobiliary tract source, can rarely present with acute UGI bleeding (65). Any recent history of endoscopic retrograde cholangio-pancreatography (ERCP), liver biopsy, or TIPS should increase suspicion, although gallstones, infection, and cancers are also potential causes. Diagnosis requires use of a side-viewing duodenoscope or ERCP, although arteriography is typically required to localize the lesion and provide embolization.

Malignant cancers can present with massive UGI bleeding when the tumor invades an artery. Early surgical treatment is usually required for uncontrolled or continued bleeding, although endoscopic hemostasis or angiographic embolization can be attempted as a temporizing measure. As bleeding is typically a late manifestation of GI malignancies, the prognosis is usually dismal (66), and decisions regarding the appropriate use of invasive procedures should be clarified. Conversely, benign tumors, such as leiomyomas, occasionally cause acute UGI bleeding due to central necrosis and can usually be surgically excised with an excellent prognosis (67).

Non-GI source should be considered if the history is appropriate and other UGI sources are not found on diagnostic endoscopy. Blood originating from oropharyngeal lesions, nasal sinuses, or lung lesions can present in a similar manner to UGI lesions after ingestion. Early recognition of these entities is important in mobilizing the appropriate teams and management to control bleeding.

A. Endoscopic Treatment

The ability to provide endoscopic therapy to achieve hemostasis of gastrointestinal lesions has had a substantial impact on the treatment of gastrointestinal lesions over the past few decades. Endoscopic therapies have become the primary treatment modality for most mucosal lesions and have diminished the need for emergency surgery to control hemostasis. The current modalities used to treat nonvariceal lesions can be generally characterized as thermal, injection, or mechanical techniques. In certain situations, a combination of modalities can provide better hemostasis. Specific techniques that are currently in common practice include use of bipolar or heater probes, injection of epinephrine, alcohol, ethanolamine, and glue, and use of band ligation or hemoclips. The type of endoscopic treatment method will vary, depending on the availability of the necessary equipment and local expertise. For a more detailed summary of the current state-of-the-art for endoscopic therapeutic modalities and their proper application, the reader is referred to a recent review of this topic (30).

VII. Variceal Bleeding

Variceal bleeding occurs in patients with underlying cirrhosis with portal hypertension when portal vein pressures is >12 mmHg (68) and has significantly higher morbidity and mortality than nonvariceal UGI bleeding (69). In sharp contrast to nonvariceal hemorrhage, varieal bleeding spontaneously resolves in only about 50% of patients (70). Early endoscopy should be performed in patients with suspected variceal bleeding to confirm the diagnosis and provide endoscopic therapy to achieve hemostasis. Over 50% of cirrhotic patients will have bleeding from a nonvariceal cause, and this is associated with substantially different treatment requirements and short-term mortality (44). Resuscitation efforts should avoid volume overexpansion as this increases the risk of variceal bleeding. Gastric varices, although less common than esophageal varices, respond poorly to most therapies and are associated with higher rates of rebleeding. The mortality associated with variceal bleeding is $\sim$40%, with one-year survival of approximately one-third of patients, and is usually associated with the degree of underlying end-organ failure.

A. Endoscopic Treatment

Treatment with octreotide should be initiated in patients with suspected variceal bleeding as a temporizing measure until endoscopy can be performed. Endoscopic techniques have significantly evolved over the past decade and now provide primary therapy for variceal hemorrhage. Esophageal variceal ligation (EVL), or "banding," is the current treatment of choice for esophageal varices and has been employed, albeit with less success, for gastric varices (71). The EVL device attaches to the end of the endoscope and applies small o-ring bands to occlude the superficial variceal vessels. Sclerotherapy can also be used, but has higher side effects (72), and is usually employed when banding is either not available or less efficacious (as with smaller varices). Endoscopic treatment is effective in controlling esophageal variceal bleeding in 80–90% of patients, although it does not affect long-term mortality (71).

B. Balloon Tamponade

If pharmacologic and endoscopic treatments are ineffective, balloon tamponade can be employed as a temporizing measure. It should be emphasized that use of balloon tamponade carries a substantial risk and should not be employed for the mere suspicion of variceal bleeding (73). Any failed attempt at therapeutic endoscopy should confirm the etiology and location of bleeding, as use of the esophageal balloon would depend on whether the source was identified as esophageal or gastric varices. Two types of balloon devices are available: the Sengstaken–Blakemore 4-lumen dual balloon (esophageal and gastric) device (Fig. 1) and

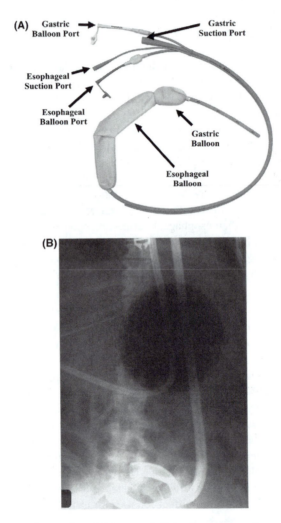

Figure 1 (**A**) The Sengstaken–Blakemore balloon has both esophageal and gastric balloons with separate ports for insufflation. Suction ports are also available for control of gastric and esophageal secretions. See text for indications and description of use. (**B**) Abdominal radiograph of patient with a Sengstaken–Blakemore tube in place. Note that only the inflated gastric balloon is visible. *Source*: Courtesy of Dr Margaret Lee, Olive View Medical Center, Sylmar, California, U.S.A.

the Linton 3-lumen single balloon (gastric) device (74). The complication rate is high, and use is limited by the potential for pressure necrosis and ulceration of the underlying mucosa (73). Balloon tamponade is not a definitive treatment for varices and merely provides transient pressure occlusion to control acute bleeding. More definite therapy should be pursued once initial hemostasis has been achieved, as the rate of rebleeding after balloon tamponade is high. Placement should be done after adequate airway protection has been established with endotracheal intubation (75). The balloon is well lubricated and passed perorally into the stomach (beyond 45 cm), while taking care to avoid passage into the pylorus or duodenum. The gastric balloon is then insufflated slowly with air (250–300 cc) and should be immediately deflated if pain occurs. A plain radiograph is obtained to confirm location in the stomach, and the balloon is gently pulled proximally until it engages the cardia/lower esophageal sphimeter (LES). Traction is applied (3 lb), and the balloon is typically retained in its position by use of a football helmet, attaching the tube to the face guard. Radiographs should be obtained at least daily or if any question arises concerning displacement of the balloon. The balloon should be immediately deflated if any chest pain or respiratory compromise occurs, and it is recommended that a pair of scissors be kept at the bedside for this purpose. Use of the esophageal balloon on the Sengstaken–Blakemore tube significantly increases the risk of esophageal rupture and should only be used if positioning of the gastric balloon does not provide adequate hemostasis for esophageal varices. Insufflation of the esophageal balloon to 25–45 mmHg should be performed using a pressure-monitoring device and should be limited to the absolute minimum balloon pressure required to obtain hemostasis. The esophageal balloon should be deflated at 24 hours and the gastric balloon should be deflated at 48 hours (76). The deflated balloon can be left in position for an additional 24 hours in case rebleeding occurs.

C. TIPS and Surgery

The use of portal decompression should be considered when medical treatment fails to control variceal hemorrhage. TIPS is an angiographic technique in which a shunt is created between the hepatic and portal veins using a fenestrated metal stent (77). The technique is over 90% successful and can be performed under moderate sedation (78). In patients with tense ascites, large volume paracentesis should be performed to reduce the upward dislocation of the liver and facilitate stent deployment (79). Successful stent placement is associated with a significant reduction in the size of esophageal varices within seven days, even if the portal venous pressure remains elevated (80). TIPS is much less effective for gastric varices, which often do not resolve and have a 20–50% risk of recurrent bleeding. Stent dysfunction due to displacement, stenosis, or kinking of the stent occurs in up to 10% of patients and is usually noted in the first few weeks. Long-term recurrence of varices approaches 80% and is frequently associated with bleeding (81). Surgical decompression of the portal system can be performed in patients who fail medical, endoscopic, and radiographic therapy. For patients with Childs B or C cirrhosis, orthotopic liver transplantation (OLT) should be considered in cases of refractory recurrent variceal bleeding (82).

VIII. Lower GI Bleeding

Acute LGI hemorrhage originates from a source distal to the ligament of Treitz, and significant bleeding usually presents with hematochezia and hemodynamic instability. Most of the clinically significant LGI bleeding arises from the colon (Table 4); however, the jejunum and ileum should be considered if lesions adequate to explain the degree of blood loss are not identified with standard upper and lower endoscopy, as additional diagnostic modalities will be required. Diverticulosis and angiodysplasia account for the majority of significant LGI bleeding in the U.S. population. Angiodysplasia is more common in elderly patients (age >65) (15), while inflammatory bowel disease (IBD) and infectious colitis are more common in younger patients. LGI bleeding is usually less severe compared to most UGI sources, but LGI bleeding typically occurs in elderly patients who are less tolerant of blood loss. The risk of LGI bleeding increases over 200-fold between the second and eighth decades (4).

Diverticuli typically occur at the site of vascular penetration of the colon wall and likely cause bleeding by erosion of the artery at the dome of the diverticulum. Bleeding is painless and self-limited in the majority of patients. The risk of continued bleeding or rebleeding is proportional to the degree of blood loss. In patients requiring transfusion with less than four units of blood, 99% will spontaneously resolve without recurrence, compared to only 75% of patients with more substantial transfusion requirements (83). Bleeding rarely occurs in the presence of diverticular inflammation (diverticulitis), and the presence of pain, fever, or leukocytosis should suggest an alternative diagnosis. Colonoscopy should be performed in an attempt to localize the source of bleeding, although the success rate in precisely identifying the offending diverticulum is disappointingly low. In the unusual case in which an actively bleeding diverticulum is located, thermal coagulation therapy can be successfully employed; however, the main contribution of colonoscopy is to exclude alternative diagnoses and evaluate the extent of the diverticular disease.

Angiodysplasia (vascular ectasia) commonly occur in the elderly or in chronic renal failure patients and typically present as occult bleeding or iron-deficiency anemia. When acute, significant bleeding occurs, it typically presents as painless bleeding and is therefore clinically indistinguishable from diverticular blood loss. Since angiodysplasia are more common in the right colon (6), a more modest rate of blood loss may present as melena rather than hemaotochezia. Therapeutic endoscopy is highly successful in controlling bleeding by employing a variety of techniques, including electrocautery, heater probe, and injection treatment (6,84). The risk of perforation is higher for right-sided lesions due to the thin colon wall and propensity for transmural iatrogenic injury. The recurrence rate for bleeding can be high, as endoscopic treatment does not modify the underlying factors that generate vascular ectasia.

Both Crohn's colitis and ulcerative colitis (UC) can present with bloody diarrhea or frank hematochezia, although additional symptoms are typically present to aid in the diagnosis. The associated bleeding is typically self-limited, responds to supportive management, and rarely requires direct intervention. Massive bleeding occurs in <6% of patients and cannot be treated endoscopically due to the diffuse mucosal inflammation (85). If bleeding does not respond to medical therapy, emergency colectomy may be required (86).

Infectious colitis associated with significant LGI bleeding can occur with invasive organisms, such as Salmonella, Shigella, and Campylobacter species. Citomegalovirus (CMV) colitis is more commonly associated with immunosuppression, as in patients who are post-organ transplantation or have HIV-infection. Clostridium difficile colitis is commonly encountered in patients receiving antibiotic therapy. The bleeding from infectious colitis is typically self-limited and requires only supportive care with treatment directed at the underlying etiology.

Ischemic colitis, although typically self-limited, can present with significant LGI blood loss and should be considered in patients with shock or a risk of systemic embolic events. The onset of bleeding is typically associated with cramp-like abdominal pain, defecation urgency, and tenderness to palpation on exam. Typical radiographic findings ("thumbprinting") on plain film or CT scan are suggestive of the diagnosis in the proper clinical setting. Flexible sigmoidoscopy or limited colonoscopy can be performed to confirm the diagnosis; however, luminal distention should be limited in order to reduce the risk of further contribution to the bowel wall ischemia. If the underlying perfusion deficit is corrected (reduced cardiac output due to sepsis or myocardial insufficiency), the bleeding is typically self-limited and requires only supportive therapy. In most cases, the degree of mucosal is modest and symptoms typically resolve within 48 hours.

Malignant lesions typically present with occult bleeding or iron deficiency anemia; however, significant LGI bleeding can occur when anti-platelet or anticoagulation has been instituted. Colon polyps rarely cause significant acute bleeding, but hemorrhage can occur as a complication of polypectomy. Early bleeding is associated with inadequate cautery of the stalk. Thermal injury, typically associated with removal of larger polyps, can result in ulceration and delayed bleeding up to three weeks post-polypectomy (87). The risk of bleeding is increased in patients who require reinstitution of anticoagulation or NSAID treatment prior to two weeks post-polypectomy.

Perianal disease, particularly hemorrhoids, commonly present with hematochezia, although the degree of blood loss is typically not severe. An unusual exception is the patient with chronic liver disease and portal hypertension who may present with massive bleeding secondary to rectal varices. Perianal lesions are a more common source of bleeding in younger patients (age <50), although hemorrhoids are frequently encountered in all age groups. Anoscopy is the diagnostic modality of choice because endoscopes only visualize the anal canal during the "slow pull-out" maneuver and do not allow for adequate visualization of the anal mucosa. Hemorrhoids should not be accepted as a source of significant blood loss until alternative lesions have been thoroughly excluded, particularly in patients over the age of 50.

Small bowel lesions are an uncommon source of significant LGI bleeding, but should be considered when standard upper and lower endoscopy fails to identify a causal lesion. Most small intestinal lesions present with iron-deficiency anemia or occult blood loss; however, significant acute bleeding can occur in the presence of severe mucosal ulceration or with underlying coagulopathy. Angiodysplasia can occur in the small bowel beyond the duodenum, particularly in association with hereditary hemorrhagic telangiectasia (Osler–Weber–Rendu). A Meckel's diverticulum containing gastric mucosa can cause significant bleeding due to ulceration of the adjacent ileal mucosa. Patients typically present during childhood; however, the diagnosis can be considered in patients under the age of 30 when alternative etiologies have been excluded.

A. LGI Bleeding Diagnostic and Therapeutic Modalities

Diagnostic colonoscopy should be performed in patients with significant LGI bleeding after resuscitation and rapid colon purge in an effort to localize the source of bleeding. In patients presenting with hemodynamic instability, it is extremely important to exclude an UGI source of bleeding. Radionuclide imaging using technetium sulfur colloid or tagged erythrocytes can be used when colonoscopy fails to localize a source of bleeding, but requires bleeding rates of 0.1–0.5 cc/min and commonly fails to precisely localize the lesion (88). Angiography is highly specific but requires bleeding rates above 1 cc/min and can be limited by the amount of contrast that can be given, particularly in patients with reduced renal function (89). If upper endoscopy and colonoscopy fail to identify a source of bleeding, push enteroscopy can be used to examine a longer segment of the proximal small bowel. Although capsule endoscopy has been used successfully for the diagnosis of small bowel lesions responsible for occult or obscure GI bleeding, the presence of active bleeding or residual luminal blood would substantially impair the ability to examine the mucosa. Any role as a diagnostic modality in the acute or subacute setting for GI bleeding has yet to be established. A radiolabeled technicium scan (Meckel's scan) can be considered in patients under the age of 30-years old, particularly if no other source can be identified for significant (typically painless) LGI bleeding.

Therapy for LGI bleeding should be first directed at correction of any underlying coagulopathy. Endoscopic treatment can be used for angiodysplasia and hemorrhoids with good success. Diverticular bleeding is usually self-limited and requires only supportive care. Recurrent bleeding should be managed surgically, although angiographic infusion of vasopressin or embolization can be considered in patients with poor surgical risk (90).

IX. Special Considerations

A. Secondary Acute Bleeding After Hospitalization

Gastrointestinal hemorrhage that starts during hospitalization carries a much worse prognosis than patients who are admitted for GI bleeding. Mortality can be as high as 30–40% and is due to both the pathogenesis of the bleeding disorders and the increased number and severity of any comorbid conditions (91). Although the initial management is similar to that described for other GI bleeding, the presentation of the bleed is substantially different. Symptoms commonly associated with other causes of GI bleeding are absent. Pain, when present, is more likely to be associated with ischemic bowel rather than peptic diseases. Onset of bleeding may be more subtle and only noted by the finding of coffee grounds or blood in the NG aspirate or onset of melena. The pathophysiology for this type of bleeding is usually related to poor perfusion of mucosa and reduction in mucosal defense/repair mechanisms. Gastric acid secretion is usually normal or reduced, except in patients with severe head trauma in which circulating hypergastrinemia occurs (92). For the UGI tract, upper panendoscopy remains the primary diagnostic modality, and lesions typically present as a diffuse gastropathy or esophageal erosions rather than discrete ulcers. This complicates the endoscopic treatment, as most therapies are successful in achieving hemostasis when applied to one or a few discrete lesions, and treatment of diffuse disease is typically disappointing. Prevention is the key to management, and patients with mechanical ventilation, coagulopathy, multiorgan failure, or major trauma are at significantly increased risk of stress bleeding and should receive prophylaxis (93). Acid reduction therapy with a target of maintaining intraluminal pH above 4.0 has been shown to effectively reduce the risk for UGI bleeding (93). Once bleeding has started, it is important to correct the underlying disorders leading to the poor tissue perfusion, as this will allow healing. LGI bleeding is less common and usually occurs secondary to nonocclusive ischemic bowel due to poor vascular perfusion or from the effect of anticoagulation on pre-existing lesions. The major diagnostic modality is angiography; however, CT scanning may demonstrate typical changes in the bowel mucosa. Endoscopy can identify areas of bowel in which injury has already occurred, but it provides no therapeutic option for this etiology. Bleeding is usually self-limited and responds to correction of the underlying coagulopathy or vascular perfusion disorder. Recurrent or uncontrolled bleeding may require surgery; however, angiographic infusion of vasopressin or embolization can be employed in patients with poor surgical risk.

B. Mechanical Ventilation

The use of mechanical ventilation (MV) provides life-preserving support to critically ill patients, but it is associated with a variety of systemic complications. Stress ulceration is commonly seen in patients requiring MV and is likely due to the associated changes in splanchnic circulation compounding the adverse mucosal effects arising from the underlying serious medical comorbid conditions (94). Mucosal injury occurs within hours of the onset of critical illness and initially affects the gastric fundus, although the development of late antral ulcers is associated with a higher risk of significant hemorrhage (95,96). As noted in the previous section, prophylaxis with acid suppression is the key to minimizing the risk of clinically significant bleeding from MV-associated stress ulcers, and MV is one of the recognized subsets of ICU patients in which such treatment is warranted (97). Earlier concerns regarding an increased incidence of pneumonia in MV patients on acid suppression therapy (98) were not confirmed in a subsequent randomized trial comparing ranitidine and sucralfate, and acid-suppression therapy was associated with a superior reduction in the risk of stress-associated hemorrhage (97).

Another concern in patients requiring prolonged periods of MV is the need for enteral access to provide nutrition and medications. Placement of a thin flexible feeding tube rather than use of a nasogsatric tube is preferred, for shorter periods appear to minimize the risk of injury due to acid-reflux and pressure-related injury to the lower esophageal mucosa. Prolonged use of an NG tube can lead to significant hemorrhage due to esophageal ulceration, particularly in patients with associated coagulopathy. Patients requiring MV are likely at greater risk due to their recumbent position, as this will exacerbate acid reflux across the lower esophageal sphincter that has been rendered incompetent by the indwelling NG tube. If prolonged periods (greater than four weeks) of enteral feeding are required, a feeding gastrostomy tube can be placed endoscopically or radiographically (99). The use of a balloon-tipped feeding tube can infrequently cause pressure necrosis of the opposing gastric mucosa, typically at or near the lesser curvature. If significant gastric hemorrhaging occurs, replacement of the feeding tube with one utilizing a flat internal button should reduce the risk of further mucosal injury and promote hemostasis.

C. Pregnancy

Pregnancy can complicate the management of GI bleeding, as two patients are involved: the mother and the fetus. The initial management, including resuscitation, is similar to other GI bleeding presentations, except that aggressive oxygen supplementation and fetal monitoring should be performed, as the fetus is particularly susceptible to maternal hypoxemia (100). Consultation by an obstetrician and neonatologist should be obtained early to assist in managing both patients. Most of the acid reduction medications are safe in pregnancy, with the exception being prostaglandin analogs, such as misoprostol (Cytotec), as teratotoxicity and the ability to induce contractions with premature delivery are serious side effects. Upper endoscopy can be safely performed, but should be reserved for the diagnosis of significant UGI bleeding (101). Pregnancy confers an increased risk from esophageal lesions, particularly MW tears, due to commonly associated nausea and vomiting. Therapeutic treatment of high-risk peptic disorders is not associated with worsened outcome (mother or fetus), but use of epinephrine should avoid direct injection into arterial vessels (100). Variceal bleeding in pregnancy should be treated endoscopically with EVL as other medical treatments, including octreotide, are less effective due to the physiological expansion of the vascular volume, particularly in the third trimester (102). Use of radiographs should be avoided due to the effects on the fetus, and this complicates the use of balloon tamponade in such patients. Less experience has been reported for colonoscopy, as significant LGI bleeding, other than obvious hemorrhoidal bleeding, is not a frequent indication during pregnancy. If colonoscopy is performed, the placement in the supine position should be avoided due to uterine compression of the vena cava with reduction in fetal blood flow (100).

D.　Elderly Patients

Elderly patients commonly present with a paucity of symptoms or with atypical presentations; GI bleeding, severe anemia, or bowel perforation may be the presenting feature. The presence of antecedent abdominal pain or dyspepsia with peptic disease is far less frequent compared to younger patients (103). The likelihood of significant comorbidity, even if absent in the medical history, increases the mortality in elderly patients (104). Particular attention should be paid to the risk of myocardial ischemia as the decrease in oxygenation due to blood loss, coupled with the increased oxygen demand due to increased cardiac output, commonly results in silent ischemic events.

E.　Myocardial Infarction

Cardiac ischemia is present in upwards of 14% of patients presenting with severe GI bleeding and frequently presents without anginal symptoms (105). Treatment of acute myocardial infarction (AMI) in this setting can be difficult, as use of thrombolytic agents or anticoagulation is contraindicated in the presence of acute GI bleeding. Risk factors include age >65, prior coronary artery disease (CAD), two or more CAD risk factors, an admission systolic blood pressure (SBP) <90 mmHg, and admission HCT <20% (106). AMI associated with GI bleeding confers a three-fold increased mortality over AMI alone and a five-fold increase in GI bleeding alone (105). Upper panendoscopy can be performed in the absence of hemodynamic instability, but should be reserved for patients with substantial bleeding who would clearly benefit from endoscopic intervention as the risk of serious cardiovascular events is increased (106).

X.　Summary

Gastrointestinal hemorrhage continues to be a significant cause of morbidity and mortality in clinical medicine. Significant advances in the diagnostic and therapeutic armamentarium have been tempered by a substantial increase in the age and severity of comorbid conditions of patients presenting with acute GI bleeding. Successful outcome requires rapid assessment, aggressive resuscitation, and early post-resuscitation diagnosis and treatment to achieve hemostasis and reduce the risk of recurrent bleeding.

References

1. Friedman LS, Martin P. The problem of gastrointestinal bleeding. Gastroenterol Clin North Am 1993; 22(4):717–721.
2. Longstreth GF. Epidemiology of hospitalization for acute upper gastrointestinal hemorrhage: a population-based study. Am J Gastroenterol 1995; 90(2):206–210.
3. Barkun A, Bardou M, Marshall JK. Consensus recommendations for managing patients with nonvariceal upper gastrointestinal bleeding. Ann Intern Med 2003; 139(10):843–857.
4. Longstreth GF. Epidemiology and outcome of patients hospitalized with acute lower gastrointestinal hemorrhage: a population-based study. Am J Gastroenterol 1997; 92(3):419–424.
5. Fleischer D. Etiology and prevalence of severe persistent upper gastrointestinal bleeding. Gastroenterology 1983; 84(3):538–543.
6. Gupta N, Longo WE, Vernava AM, III. Angiodysplasia of the lower gastrointestinal tract: an entity readily diagnosed by colonoscopy and primarily managed nonoperatively. Dis Colon Rectum 1995; 38(9):979–982.
7. Provenzale D, Sandler RS, Wood DR, Levinson SL, Frakes JT, Sartor RB, Jackson AL, Kinard HB, Wagner EH, Powell DW. Development of a scoring system to predict mortality from upper gastrointestinal bleeding. Am J Med Sci 1987; 294(1):26–32.
8. Vreeburg EM, Terwee CB, Snel P, Rauws EAJ, Bartelsman JFWM, Meulen JHP, Tytgat GNJ. Validation of the Rockall risk scoring system in upper gastrointestinal bleeding. Gut 1999; 44(3):331–335.
9. Kupfer Y, Cappell MS, Tessler S. Acute gastrointestinal bleeding in the intensive care unit. The intensivist's perspective. Gastroenterol Clin North Am 2000; 29(2):275–307, v.
10. Korzenik JR. Hereditary hemorrhagic telangiectasia and other intestinal vascular anomalies. Gastroenterologist 1996; 4(3):203–210.
11. The Consensus Committee of the American Autonomic Society and the American Academy of Neurology. Consensus statement on the definition of orthostatic hypotension, pure autonomic failure, and multiple system atrophy. Neurology 1996; 46(5):1470.
12. Baron BJ, Scalea TM. Acute blood loss. Emerg Med Clin North Am 1996; 14(1):35–55.
13. Goldstein DS, Robertson D, Esler M, Straus SE, Eisenhofer G. Dysautonomias: clinical disorders of the autonomic nervous system. Ann Intern Med 2002; 137(9):753–763.
14. Abou-Khalil B, Scalea TM, Trooskin SZ, Henry SM, Hitchcock R. Hemodynamic responses to shock in young trauma patients: need for invasive monitoring. Crit Care Med 1994; 22(4):633–639.

15. Jensen D, Machicado G. Diagnosis and treatment of severe hematochezia. The role of urgent colonoscopy after purge. Gastroenterology 1988; 95(6):1569–1574.

16. Stellato T, Rhodes RS, McDougal WS. Azotemia in upper gastrointestinal hemorrhage. A review. Am J Gastroenterol 1980; 73(6):486–489.

17. Cappell MS. A study of the syndrome of simultaneous acute upper gastrointestinal bleeding and myocardial infarction in 36 patients. Am J Gastroenterol 1995; 90(9):1444–1449.

18. Rudolph JP. Automated gastric lavage and a comparison of 0.9% normal saline solution and tap water irrigant. Ann Emerg Med 1985; 14(12):1156–1159.

19. Andrus CH, Ponsky JL. The effects of irrigant temperature in upper gastrointestinal hemorrhage: a requiem for iced saline lavage. Am J Gastroenterol 1987; 82(10):1062–1064.

20. Waterman NG, Walker JL. The effect of gastric cooling on hemostasis. Surg Gynecol Obstet 1973; 137(1):80–82.

21. Silverstein FE, Gilbert DA, Tedesco FJ, Buenger NK, Persing J. The national ASGE survey on upper gastrointestinal bleeding. II. Clinical prognostic factors. Gastrointest Endosc 1981; 27(2):80–93.

22. Gilbert DA, Silverstein FE, Tedesco FJ, Buenger NK, Persing J. The national ASGE survey on upper gastrointestinal bleeding. III. Endoscopy in upper gastrointestinal bleeding. Gastrointest Endosc 1981; 27(2):94–102.

23. Layne EA, Mellow MH, Lipman TO. Insensitivity of guaiac slide tests for detection of blood in gastric juice. Ann Intern Med 1981; 94(6):774–776.

24. Badeer HS. Hemodynamics for medical students. Advan Physiol Edu 2001; 25(1):44–52.

25. Cappell MS, Nadler SC. Increased mortality of acute upper gastrointestinal bleeding in patients with chronic obstructive pulmonary disease. A case controlled, multiyear study of 53 consecutive patients. Dig Dis Sci 1995; 40(2): 256–262.

26. Hebert PC, Wells G, Blajchman MA, Marshall J, Martin C, Pagliarello G, Tweeddale M, Schweitzer I, Yetisir E. A multicenter, randomized, controlled clinical trial of transfusion requirements in critical care. Transfusion Requirements in Critical Care Investigators, Canadian Critical Care Trials Group. N Engl J Med 1999; 340(6):409–417.

27. Johnston JH. Endoscopic risk factors for bleeding peptic ulcer. Gastrointest Endosc 1990; 36(5 suppl):S16–S20.

28. Wiesen AR, Hospenthal DR, Byrd JC, Glass KL, Howard RS, Diehl LF. Equilibration of hemoglobin concentration after transfusion in medical inpatients not actively bleeding. Ann Intern Med 1994; 121(4):278–230.

29. Kravetz D, Sikuler E, Groszmann RJ. Splanchnic and systemic hemodynamics in portal hypertensive rats during hemorrhage and blood volume restitution. Gastroenterology 1986; 90(5Pt 1):1232–1240.

30. Savides TJ, Jensen DM. Therapeutic endoscopy for nonvariceal gastrointestinal bleeding. Gastroenterol Clin North Am 2000; 29(2):465–487, vii.

31. Lieberman D. Gastrointestinal bleeding: initial management. Gastroenterol Clin North Am 1993; 22:723–736.

32. Dzik WH, Kirkley SA. Citrate toxicity during massive blood transfusion. Transfus Med Rev 1988; 2:76–94.

33. Abbott TR. Changes in serum calcium fractions and citrate concentrations during massive blood transfusions and cardiopulmonary bypass. Br J Anaesth 1983; 55:753–760.

34. Boyan CP. Cold or warmed blood for massive transfusions. Ann Surg 1964; 160:282–286.

35. Collins R, Langman M. Treatment with histamine H2 antagonists in acute upper gastrointestinal hemorrhage. Implications of randomized trials. N Engl J Med 1985; 313(11):660–666.

36. Walt RP, Cottrell J, Mann SG, Freemantle NP, Langman MJ. Continuous intravenous famotidine for haemorrhage from peptic ulcer. Lancet 1992; 340(8827):1058–1062.

37. Pisegna JR. Treating patients with acute gastrointestinal bleeding or rebleeding. Pharmacotherapy 2003; 23(10 Pt 2):81S–86S.

38. Morgan D. Intravenous proton pump inhibitors in the critical care setting. Crit Care Med 2002; 30(suppl 6):S369–S372.

39. Imperiale TF, Teran JC, McCullough AJ. A meta-analysis of somatostatin versus vasopressin in the management of acute esophageal variceal hemorrhage. Gastroenterology 1995; 109(4):1289–1294.

40. Imperiale TF, Birgisson S. Somatostatin or octreotide compared with H2 antagonists and placebo in the management of acute nonvariceal upper gastrointestinal hemorrhage: a meta-analysis. Ann Intern Med 1997; 127(12):1062–1071.

41. Jenkins SA, Shields R, Davies M, Elias E, Turnbull AJ, Bassendine MF, James OF, Iredale JP, Vyas SK, Arthur MJ, Kingsnorth AN, Sutton R. A multicentre randomised trial comparing octreotide and injection sclerotherapy in the management and outcome of acute variceal haemorrhage. Gut 1997; 41(4):526–533.

42. Besson I, Ingrand P, Person B, Boutroux D, Heresbach D, Bernard P, Hochain P, Larricq J, Gourlaouen A, Ribard D. Sclerotherapy with or without octreotide for acute variceal bleeding. N Engl J Med 1995; 333(9):555–560.

43. de Franchis R, Primignani M. Endoscopic treatments for portal hypertension. Semin Liver Dis 1999; 19(4):439–455.

44. Lee JG, Turnipseed S, Romano PS, Vigil H, Azari R, Melnikoff N, Hsu R, Kirk D, Sokolove P, Leung JW. Management of upper gastrointestinal bleeding in the patient with chronic liver disease. Med Clin North Am 1996; 80(5):1035–1068.

45. Lee JG, Turnipseed S, Romano PS, Vigil H, Azari R, Melnikoff N, et al. Endoscopy-based triage significantly reduces hospitalization rates and costs of treating upper GI bleeding: a randomized controlled trial. Gastrointest Endosc 1999; 50(6):755–761.

46. Smith JL, Graham DY. Variceal hemorrhage: a critical evaluation of survival analysis. Gastroenterology 1982; 82(5 Pt 1):968–973.

47. Elta GH. Approach to the patient with gross gastrointestinal bleeding. In: Yamada T, Alpers DH, Laine L, Owyang C, Powell DW, eds. Textbook of Gastroenterology. Philadelphia, PA: Lippincott, Williams & Wilkins, 1999:714–743.

48. Jorde R, Burhol PG, Johnson JA. Peptic ulcer bleeding in patients with and without dyspepsia. Scand J Gastroenterol 1988; 23(2):213–216.

49. Armstrong CP, Blower AL. Non-steroidal anti-inflammatory drugs and life threatening complications of peptic ulceration. Gut 1987; 28(5):527–532.

50. Beejay U, Wolfe MM. Acute gastrointestinal bleeding in the intensive care unit. The gastroenterologist's perspective. Gastroenterol Clin North Am 2000; 29(2):309–336.

51. Wilcox CM, Clark WS. Causes and outcome of upper and lower gastrointestinal bleeding: the Grady Hospital experience. South Med J 1999; 92(1):44–50.

52. van den BJ, van Hillegersberg R, Siersema PD, de Bruin RW, Tilanus HW. Endoscopic ablation therapy for Barrett's esophagus with high-grade dysplasia: a review. Am J Gastroenterol 1999; 94(5):1153–1160.

53. Graham DY, Schwartz JT. The spectrum of the Mallory-Weiss tear. Medicine (Baltimore) 1978; 57(4):307–318.

54. Schuman BM, Threadgill ST. The influence of liver disease and portal hypertension on bleeding in Mallory-Weiss syndrome. J Clin Gastroenterol 1994; 18(1):10–12.

55. Gunnlaugsson O. Angiodysplasia of the stomach and duodenum. Gastrointest Endosc 1985; 31(4):251–254.

56. Askin MP, Lewis BS. Push enteroscopic cauterization: long-term follow-up of 83 patients with bleeding small intestinal angiodysplasia. Gastrointest Endosc 1996; 43(6):580–583.

57. Borsch G. Diffuse gastric antral vascular ectasia: the "watermelon stomach" revisited. Am J Gastroenterol 1987; 82(12):1333–1334.

58. Ng I, Lai KC, Ng M. Clinical and histological features of gastric antral vascular ectasia: successful treatment with endoscopic laser therapy. J Gastroenterol Hepatol 1996; 11(3):270–274.

59. Kamath PS, Lacerda M, Ahlquist DA, McKusick MA, Andrews JC, Nagorney DA. Gastric mucosal responses to intrahepatic portosystemic shunting in patients with cirrhosis. Gastroenterology 2000; 118(5):905–911.

60. Antinori CH., Andrew CT, Santaspirt JS, Villanueva DT, Kuchler JA, deLeon ML, Cody WC, DiPaola DJ, Manuele VJ. The many faces of aortoenteric fistulas. Am Surg 1996; 62(5):344–349.

61. Walsh AK, Gwynn BR. Atypical aorto-enteric fistula. Eur J Vasc Endovasc Surg 1995; 9(3):353–354.

62. Kaufman Z, Liverant S, Shiptz B, Dinbar A. Massive gastrointestinal bleeding caused by Dieulafoy's lesion. Am Surg 1995; 61(5):453–455.

63. Matsui S, Kamisako T, Kudo M, Inoue R. Endoscopic band ligation for control of nonvariceal upper GI hemorrhage: comparison with bipolar electrocoagulation. Gastrointest Endosc 2002; 55(2):214–218.

64. Grisendi A, Lonardo A, Della Casa G, Frazzoni M, Pulvirenti M, Ferrari AM, Varoli M, Mezzanotte G, Melini L. Combined endoscopic and surgical management of Dieulafoy vascular malformation. J Am Coll Surg 1994; 179(2):182–186.

65. Bloechle C, Izbicki JR, Rashed MY, el Sefi T, Hosch SB, Knoefel WT, Rogiers X, Broelsch CE. Hemobilia: presentation, diagnosis, and management. Am J Gastroenterol 1994; 89(9):1537–1540.

66. Savides TJ, Jensen DM, Cohen J, Randall GM, Kovacs TO, Pelayo E, Cheng S, Jensen ME, Hsieh HY. Severe upper gastrointestinal tumor bleeding: endoscopic findings, treatment, and outcome. Endoscopy 1996; 28(2):244–248.

67. Wilson JM, Melvin DB, Gray G, Thorbjarnarson B. Benign small bowel tumor. Ann Surg 1975; 181(2):247–250.

68. Lebrec D, De Fleury P, Rueff B, Nahum H, Benhamou JP. Portal hypertension, size of esophageal varices, and risk of gastrointestinal bleeding in alcoholic cirrhosis. Gastroenterology 1980; 79(6):1139–1144.

69. Infante-Rivard C, Esnaola S, Villeneuve JP. Role of endoscopic variceal sclerotherapy in the long-term management of variceal bleeding: a meta-analysis. Gastroenterology 1989; 96(4):1087–1092.

70. Graham DY, Smith JL. The course of patients after variceal hemorrhage. Gastroenterology 1981; 80(4):800–809.

71. Laine L, el Newihi HM, Migikovsky B, Sloane R, Garcia F. Endoscopic ligation compared with sclerotherapy for the treatment of bleeding esophageal varices. Ann Intern Med 1993; 119(1):1–7.

72. Vlavianos P, Westaby D. Management of acute variceal haemorrhage. Eur J Gastroenterol Hepatol 2001; 13(4):335–342.

73. Chojkier M, Conn HO. Esophageal tamponade in the treatment of bleeding varices. A decadel progress report. Dig Dis Sci 1980; 25(4):267–272.

74. Panes J, Teres J, Bosch J, Rodes J. Efficacy of balloon tamponade in treatment of bleeding gastric and esophageal varices. Results in 151 consecutive episodes. Dig Dis Sci 1988; 33(4):454–459.

75. Mandelstam P, Zeppa R. Endotracheal intubation should precede esophagogastric balloon tamponade for control of variceal bleeding. J Clin Gastroenterol 1983; 5:493–494.

76. Pasquale MD, Cerra FB. Sengstaken-Blakemore tube placement. Use of balloon tamponade to control bleeding varices. Crit Care Clin 1992; 8(4):743–753.

77. Zemel G, Katzen BT, Becker GJ, Benenati JF, Sallee DS. Percutaneous transjugular portosystemic shunt. JAMA 1991; 266(3):390–393.

78. LaBerge JM, Ring EJ, Gordon RL, Lake JR, Doherty MM, Somberg KA, Roberts JP, Ascher NL. Creation of transjugular intrahepatic portosystemic shunts with the wallstent endoprosthesis: results in 100 patients. Radiology 1993; 187(2):413–420.

79. Rossle M, Haag K, Ochs A, Sellinger M, Noldge G, Perarnau JM, Berger E, Blum U, Gabelmann A., Hauenstein K. The transjugular intrahepatic portosystemic stent-shunt procedure for variceal bleeding. N Engl J Med 1994; 330(3):165–171.

80. Ferral H, Foshager MC, Bjarnason H, Finlay DE, Hunter DW, Castaneda-Zuniga WR, Letourneau JG. Early sonographic evaluation of the transjugular intrahepatic portosystemic shunt (TIPS). Cardiovasc Intervent Radiol 1993; 16(5):275–279.

81. Sanyal AJ, Freedman AM, Luketic VA, Purdum PP, III, Shiffman ML, DeMeo J, Cole PE, Tisnado J. The natural history of portal hypertension after transjugular intrahepatic portosystemic shunts. Gastroenterology 1997; 112(3):889–898.

82. Ringe B, Lang H, Tusch G, Pichlmayr R. Role of liver transplantation in management of esophageal variceal hemorrhage. World J Surg 1994; 18(2): 233–239.

83. McGuire HH Jr. Bleeding colonic diverticula. A reappraisal of natural history and management. Ann Surg 1994; 220(5):653–656.

84. Zuckerman GR, Prakash C. Acute lower intestinal bleeding. Part II: etiology, therapy, and outcomes. Gastrointest Endosc 1999; 49(2):228–238.

85. Cheung O, Regueiro MD. Inflammatory bowel disease emergencies. Gastroenterol Clin North Am 2003; 32(4):1269–1288.

86. Robert JR, Sachar DB, Greenstein AJ. Severe gastrointestinal hemorrhage in Crohn's disease. Ann Surg 1991; 213(3):207–211.

87. Sorbi D, Norton I, Conio M, Balm R, Zinsmeister A, Gostout CJ. Postpolypectomy lower GI bleeding: descriptive analysis. Gastrointest Endosc 2000; 51(6):690–696.

88. Dusold R, Burke K, Carpentier W, Dyck WP. The accuracy of technetium-99 m-labeled red cell scintigraphy in localizing gastrointestinal bleeding. Am J Gastroenterol 1994; 89(3):345–348.

89. Zuckerman DA, Bocchini TP, Birnbaum EH. Massive hemorrhage in the lower gastrointestinal tract in adults: diagnostic imaging and intervention. AJR Am J Roentgenol 1993; 161(4):703–711.

90. Uden P, Jiborn H, Jonsson K. Influence of selective mesenteric arteriography on the outcome of emergency surgery for massive, lower gastrointestinal hemorrhage. A 15-year experience. Dis Colon Rectum 1986; 29(9):561–566.

91. Skillman JJ, Silen W. Stress ulceration in the acutely ill. Annu Rev Med 1976; 27:9–22.

92. Bowen JC, Fleming WH, Thompson JC. Increased gastrin release following penetrating central nervous system injury. Surgery 1974; 75(5):720–724.

93. Morgan D. Intravenous proton pump inhibitors in the critical care setting. Crit Care Med 2002; 30(6 suppl):S369–S372.

94. Mutlu GM, Mutlu EA, Factor P. Prevention and treatment of gastrointestinal complications in patients on mechanical ventilation. Am J Respir Med 2003; 2(5):395–411.

95. Peura DA, Johnson LF. Cimetidine for prevention and treatment of gastroduodenal mucosal lesions in patients in an intensive care unit. Ann Intern Med 1985; 103(2):173–177.

96. Terdiman JP, Ostroff JW. Gastrointestinal bleeding in the hospitalized patient: a case-control study to assess risk factors, causes, and outcome. Am J Med 1998; 104(4):349–354.

97. Cook D, Guyatt G, Marshall J, Leasa D, Fuller H, Hall R, Peters S, Rutledge F, Griffith L, McLellan A, Wood G, Kirby A. A comparison of sucralfate and ranitidine for the prevention of upper gastrointestinal bleeding in patients requiring mechanical ventilation. Canadian Critical Care Trials Group. N Engl J Med 1998; 338(12):791–797.

98. Cook DJ, Reeve BK, Guyatt GH, Heyland DK, Griffith LE, Buckingham L, Tryba M. Stress ulcer prophylaxis in critically ill patients. Resolving discordant meta-analyses. J Am Med Assoc 1996; 275(4):308–314.

99. Nicholson FB, Korman MG, Richardson MA. Percutaneous endoscopic gastrostomy: a review of indications, complications and outcome. J Gastroenterol Hepatol 2000; 15(1):21–25.

100. Cappell MS. The fetal safety and clinical efficacy of gastrointestinal endoscopy during pregnancy. Gastroenterol Clin North Am 2003; 32(1):123–179.

101. Kulier R, Gulmezoglu A, Hofmeyr G, Cheng L, Campana A. Medical methods for first trimester abortion. Cochrane Database Syst Rev 2004; 1:CD002855.

102. Prichard JA. Changes in blood volume during pregnancy and delivery. Anesthesiology 1965; 26:393–399.

103. Permutt RP, Cello JP. Duodenal ulcer disease in the hospitalized elderly patient. Dig Dis Sci 1982; 27:1–6.

104. Cooper BT, Weston CF, Neumann CS. Acute upper gastrointestinal haemorrhage in patients aged 80 years or more. Q J Med 1988; 68(258):765–774.

105. Cappell MS. A study of the syndrome of simultaneous acute upper gastrointestinal bleeding and myocardial infarction in 36 patients. Am J Gastroenterol 1995; 90(9):1444–1449.

106. Kupfer Y, Cappell MS, Tessler S. Acute gastrointestinal bleeding in the intensive care unit. The intensivist's perspective. Gastroenterol Clin North Am 2000; 29(2):275–307, v.

107. Gupta PK, Fleischer DE. Nonvariceal upper gastrointestinal bleeding. Med Clin North Am 1993; 77(5):973–992.

108. Silverstein FE, Gilbert DA, Tedesco FJ, Buenger NK, Persing J. The national ASGE survey on upper gastrointestinal bleeding. I. Study design and baseline data. Gastrointest Endosc 1981; 27(2):73–79.

109. Bramley PN, Masson JW, McKnight G, Herd K, Fraser A, Park K, Brunt PW, McKinlay A, Sinclair TS, Mowat NA. The role of an open-access bleeding unit in the management of colonic haemorrhage. A 2-year prospective study. Scand J Gastroenterol 1996; 31(8):764–769.

110. Colacchio TA, Forde KA, Patsos TJ, Nunez D. Impact of modern diagnostic methods on the management of active rectal bleeding. Ten year experience. Am J Surg 1982; 143(5):607–610.

111. Farrands PA, Taylor I. Management of acute lower gastrointestinal haemorrhage in a surgical unit over a 4-year period. J R Soc Med 1987; 80(2):79–82.

112. Jensen DM, Machicado GA. Diagnosis and treatment of severe hematochezia. The role of urgent colonoscopy after purge. Gastroenterology 1988; 95(6):1569–1574.

113. Jensen DM, Machicado GA. Colonoscopy for diagnosis and treatment of severe lower gastrointestinal bleeding. Routine outcomes and cost analysis. Gastrointest Endosc Clin N Am 1997; 7(3):477–498.

114. Richter JM, Christensen MR, Kaplan LM, Nishioka NS. Effectiveness of current technology in the diagnosis and management of lower gastrointestinal hemorrhage. Gastrointest Endosc 1995; 41(2):93–98.

115. Rossini FP, Ferrari A, Spandre M, Cavallero M, Gemme C, Loverci C, Bertone A, Pinna Pintor M. Emergency colonoscopy. World J Surg 1989; 13(2): 190–192.

12

Neurologic Emergencies in the Intensive Care Unit Setting

SCOTT SELCO

Stroke Program
Sunrise Hospital and Medical Center
Las Vegas, Nevada, U.S.A.

ANNA SOMERTO

Department of Medicine, Cedars–Sinai
  Medical Center
Los Angeles, California, U.S.A.

STANLEY N. COHEN

Stroke Prevention Program
Sunrise Hospital and Medical Center
Las Vegas, Nevada, U.S.A.

I. Introduction

Central nervous system (CNS) symptoms frequently arise in patients in an intensive care unit (ICU) setting. Many of these patients are eventually diagnosed with encephalopathy resulting from delirium, traumatic brain injury, CNS infection, CNS tumor, hepatic failure, uremia, and intoxications (1,2). For the most part, these are systemic illnesses that have neurologic manifestations. The approach to these neurologic problems is to treat the underlying systemic disease. In this chapter, we will focus on the clinical presentation, diagnostic work up, and treatment of the more common neurologic problems arising in the ICU that arise from disorders that primarily affect the CNS: ischemic stroke, hypoxic-ischemic injury, seizures, status epilepticus, and brain death.

II. Ischemic Stroke

A. Clinical Presentation

Ischemic stroke is traditionally defined as a focal impairment of cerebral circulation with symptoms lasting more than 24 hours. Transient ischemic attack is traditionally defined as focal ischemic symptoms that clear completely within 24 hours. Modern neuroimaging techniques frequently demonstrate evidence of subacute ischemic brain injury even when symptoms clear completely in under three hours, thereby blurring the distinction between these traditional definitions. The frequency of stroke occurring in hospitalized patients is not firmly established, but it has been estimated that between 6.5% and 15% of strokes occur during hospitalization for a different medical condition (3).

Stroke in the medical ICU is often discovered in the perioperative period. The exact incidence of perioperative stroke is not known due to underreporting and surveillance bias. Several evaluations of perioperative stroke have been reported (4–8). The most important risk factor associated with perioperative stroke is prior stroke (9). Stroke was studied most extensively in the setting of coronary artery bypass graft (CABG) surgery. In patients undergoing CABG, prior stroke is associated with about a four-fold increase in risk of perioperative stroke (10). Perioperative strokes were reported in one study to occur in up to 4.3% of cases following CABG surgery, two-thirds of which occurred by the end of the second postoperative day (6). Many of these studies relied on a single early postoperative computerized tomography (CT) scan, an approach that is insensitive to early ischemic changes. This method may result in an underestimation of the true incidence of this complication. Other more recent studies performed utilizing magnetic resonance imaging (MRI) with diffusion-weighted MR sequences (DWI), the most sensitive method to detect acute cerebral ischemia, demonstrated ischemic lesions following CABG in 31% of patients (11). There are many other conditions associated with an increased risk of stroke that are managed in the medical ICU. The most commonly encountered conditions are listed in Table 1.

A challenge facing medical intensivists is to determine which ICU patients with acute CNS deterioration need to undergo an emergent evaluation for acute ischemic stroke. History is critical. Obtaining the time the patient was last documented to be neurologically normal, rather than when symptoms are first observed, will help determine if the patient will be a candidate for thrombolytic therapy. For example, a patient waking in the morning with symptoms is almost never a candidate for treatment with intravenous (IV) recombinant tissue plasminogen (rt-PA) because they were last documented neurologically intact prior to going to sleep. It is important to recognize other neurologic syndromes that may mimic stroke. Seizures probably represent the most common stroke mimic. Although overt seizures may herald stroke onset, this occurs in a minority of patients. During an acute motor seizure, the gaze may deviate *toward* the involved hemibody owing to the positive stimulus in the contralateral hemisphere. In the immediate post-ictal period, a hemiparesis may be present on one side, and the gaze may deviate away from the paretic side, owing to a refractory neuronal state exhibited by the epileptogenic focus. This condition can

Table 1 Medical Problems Associated with Stroke in the ICU

Atrial fibrillation
Aortic atheromata
Aortic dissection
Cardiothoracic surgery involving the aorta
Neurosurgical procedures
Carotid endarterectomy
Coronary artery bypass grafting
Cardiac valvular surgery
Intraoperative hypotension
Perioperative cardioembolism
Low left ventricular ejection fraction (<20%)
Myocardial infarction
Septic embolism
Nonbacterial thrombotic endocarditis
Paradoxical embolism (e.g., atrial-septal defect, patent foramen ovale)
Hypercoagulability (postoperative, systemic malignancy, antiphospholipid syndrome)
Disseminated intravascular coagulation with circulatory collapse
Meningitis-associated secondary vasculitis
Cerebral venous thrombosis
Systemic vasculitides (Takayasu's arteritis, polyarteritis nodosa, Churg–Strauss)
Cerebral vasospasm following surgical repair of ruptured aneurysm

sometimes be confused with middle cerebral artery occlusion if the seizure was not witnessed. Fortunately, post-ictal hemiparesis generally resolves fairly rapidly, which helps to distinguish this presentation from that of acute middle cerebral artery occlusion. Of course, a history of epilepsy may also provide an important clue.

An acute alteration in mental status without focal neurologic findings on examination rarely represents acute stroke. This type of presentation more commonly represents delirium or encephalopathy from another cause. The hallmarks of delirium are waxing and waning consciousness, global inattention, and an altered sensorium. Finally, posterior cerebral artery territory ischemic strokes may present with aphasia, confusion, and amnesia without other clear focal neurologic findings and may be mistaken for delirium. Bedside language testing will generally help distinguish between aphasia and confusion.

A focused, rather than an exhaustive, examination is needed in this setting. A funduscopic examination, neck examination for rigidity, and a neurovascular examination, including cardiac examination, peripheral pulses and carotid pulses, are required. Neurologic evaluation of level of consciousness, orientation, volitional activity, speech and language function (intelligibility of speech, comprehension, naming, and repetition), visual fields, eye movements, strength and coordination, and sensation and testing for hemineglect provides indispensable clues regarding localization. Use of a quantified examination, such as the National Institute of Health Stroke Scale (NIHSS), is a fast and reproducible exam that allows comparison of the patient's deficit from examiner to examiner at points separated in time (Table 2).

(Text continues on p. 428)

Table 2 National Institutes of Health Stroke Scale

Item explanation	Response	Points
1a. Level of consciousness—measure of responsiveness assessed when patient first examined. Gently stimulate the patient (by patting or tapping). Occasionally, more noxious stimulation such as pinching is warranted	Alert—fully alert and keenly responsive	0
	Drowsy—not fully alert but arousable by minor stimulation. Able to obey, answer, and respond to commands	1
	Stuporous—lethargic, wakefulness waxes and wanes, and repeated stimulation (sometimes strong or noxious) is required to arouse patient and get them to respond or follow commands	2
	Coma—eyes closed and unresponsive, or only reflexive motor or automatic responses noted	3
1b. Level of consciousness—patient is asked to provide month of the year and his/her age. Both questions must be answered correctly on the initial attempt; no partial credit is granted. 1a. The presence of aphasia, dysarthria, or mutism limiting verbal responding counts as incorrect responses.	Answers both questions correctly	0
	Answers one question correctly	1
	Answers neither question correctly	2
1c. Level of consciousness—patient is asked to (a) open eyes and (b) grip and release nonparetic hand.	Performs both tasks correctly	0
	Performs one task correctly	1
	Performs neither task correctly	2
2. Gaze—spontaneous eye movements to the left and right should be noted. Only horizontal eye movements are directly tested. The patient is asked to move his/her eyes to the extremes of left and right lateral gaze.	Normal; looks fully to right and left	0
	Partial gaze palsy; gaze limitation in one or both eyes only but without forced gaze deviation or complete conjugate gaze paresis	1
	Forced gaze deviation or total gaze paresis not overcome by oculocephalic maneuvers	2

3. Visual—patient is asked to indicate how many of the examiners fingers are seen in each visual field. Assess each visual quadrant individually (left and right, upper and lower) and then the left and right upper visual fields simultaneously to assess for visual neglect.

No visual loss	0
Partial hemianopsia	1
Complete hemianopsia	2
Bilateral hemianopsia	3

4. Facial palsy—the face is observed at rest for asymmetry (e.g., flattening of the nasolabial fold), and then the two sides of the face are assessed during smiling, puckering, and/or cheek puffing.

Normal symmetric facial movement	0
Minimal unilateral weakness	1
Moderate unilateral weakness	2
Severe unilateral or bilateral weakness	3

5. Motor arm (right and left scored individually)—patient is asked to raise and extend the bilateral upper extremities for 10 sec. Each limb may be tested individually. In an awake, uncooperative (e.g., mute or aphasic) patient, the examiner may lift and extend the limb to the desired position and observe the response. In a comatose patient, an estimate of strength should be made based on observed responses to noxious stimulation. A partly amputated limb should be tested and scored. If a limb is missing or completely amputated, or a significant limitation in range of motion exists that limits testing (e.g., fused shoulder joint), a score of X (untestable) is registered.

Drift absent, arm extended (at 90° if sitting or 45° if supine) and maintained for 10 sec	0
Outstretched limb maintained for 10 sec, but fluttering or drift is noted	1
Outstretched limb is not maintained for 10 sec, but some antigravity effort is present	2
The patient is not able to bring the limb off the bed. The limb is raised to the correct position by the examiner, but the patient is unable to sustain the position	3
The patient is unable to move the limb	4
Untestable	X

(Continued)

Table 2 National Institutes of Health Stroke Scale (*Continued*)

Item explanation	Response	Points
6. Motor leg (right and left scored individually)—patient is asked to raise and extend the bilateral lower extremities 30° above the bed for 5 sec. Each limb may be tested individually. In an awake, uncooperative (e.g., mute or aphasic) patient, the examiner may lift and extend the limb to the desired position and observe the response. In a comatose patient, an estimate of strength should be made based on observed responses to noxious stimulation. A partly amputated limb should be tested and scored. If a limb is missing or completely amputated, or a significant limitation in range of motion exists that limits testing, a score of X (untestable) is registered.	Drift absent, leg extended (at 90° if sitting or 45° if supine) and maintained for 5 sec	0
	Outstretched limb maintained for 10 sec, but fluttering or drift is noted	1
	Outstretched limb is not maintained for 10 sec, but some antigravity effort is present	2
	The patient is not able to bring the limb off the bed. The limb is raised to the correct position by the examiner, but the patient is unable to sustain the position	3
	The patient is unable to move the limb	4
	Untestable	X
7. Limb ataxia—this item tests for evidence of a unilateral cerebellar lesion. It will also detect limb movement abnormalities related to sensory or motor dysfunction. Perform finger-to-nose testing in the bilateral upper extremities and heel-to-shin testing in the bilateral lower extremities.	Absent	0
	Present in one limb	1
	Present in both limbs	2
	Untestable	X

8. Sensory—test using a pin in the proximal portions of all four limbs. Only sensory loss that can be attributed to stroke (hemisensory loss) should be counted as abnormal; sensory loss owing to a neuropathy should not be graded as abnormal. In the comatose, aphasic, or mute patient, score this item based on non-verbal responses, such as facial grimace or withdrawal; observe for asymmetric responses.	Normal; no sensory loss 0 Partial sensory loss; touch is felt but pin feels dull 1 Dense sensory loss; stimulation is not felt, or no response to noxious stimuli is noted, on affected side of body 2
9. Best language—language is assessed through fluency, naming, repetition, reading, writing, and comprehension. Patients are asked to identify standard groups of objects and by reading a series of words and sentences. Only the first response is measured. Initial object misidentification or misreading of a sentence is scored incorrect. If visual loss precludes visual object identification or reading, object identification can be tested by placing an object in the patient's hands. An evaluation of writing should be attempted if the patient is mute or intubated.	No aphasia, normal language 0 Mild-to-moderate aphasia; the patient has some loss of fluency and/or comprehension, mild to moderate naming or word finding difficulty, or paraphasias 1 Severe aphasia; all communication is through fragmentary expression. Information exchange and meaningful communication between patient and examiner almost impossible 2 Mute 3

(Continued)

Table 2 National Institutes of Health Stroke Scale (*Continued*)

Item explanation	Response	Points
10. Dysarthria—patients are asked to read and pronounce a standard list of words. Alternatively, patients can be asked to name objects or repeat spoken words or a phrase. If the patient has severe aphasia, the clarity of articulation of spontaneous speech should be rated. If the patient is mute, comatose, or has an endotracheal tube, this item should be rated as X (untestable).	Normal; pronunciation is clear	0
	Mild-to-moderate dysarthria; speech is understandable despite difficulty with articulation	1
	Severe dysarthria; speech is unintelligible	2
	Intubation or other physical barrier present	X
11. Neglect (extinction and inattention)—this item is aimed at detecting lack of awareness of an acquired problem with an affected limb, hemibody, or with extrapersonal space opposite an injured hemisphere (typically the nondominant one). Inattention is commonly assessed by displaying a standard picture and asking patients to describe it. Patients should be encouraged to scan the picture and identify features on both the right and left sides of the picture and to compensate for any preexisting visual loss. Alternatively, patients can be asked to draw a clock face. The presence of extinction is examined by assessing patients' ability to detect simultaneously presented cutaneous sensory (with eyes closed) or visual stimuli to the right and left sides.	No abnormality	0
	Extinction or inattention is present in only one testing modality	1
	Profound inattention or extinction is present; patient fails to recognize own hand and orients to one side of space only	2

Table 3 Common Stroke Syndromes, Their Associated Vascular Supply, and Affected Brain Regions

Stroke syndrome	Vascular supply	Brain region
Aphasia, right hemiparesis, left gaze deviation	Left MCA	Left temporal and frontal lobes
Left hemiparesis and hemineglect, right gaze deviation	Right MCA	Right temporal and frontal lobes
Leg predominant weakness and lower extremity ataxia	Contralateral ACA	Contralateral medial frontal lobe
Right hemianopsia and hemisensory impairment, disordered visual perception, alexia, memory impairment, simultagnosia	Left PCA	Left temporal, occipital, and parietal lobes, thalamus
Left hemianopsia and hemisensory impairment, disordered visual perception, topographic disorientation, prosopagnosia	Right PCA	Right temporal, occipital, and parietal lobes, thalamus
Hemiplegia along with ipsilateral hemisensory impairment and hemianopsia	Contralateral anterior choroidal artery	Internal capsule, basal ganglia, temporal lobe, thalamus, optic tract
Pure motor hemiparesis (involving face, arm, and leg)	Deep penetrating end arteries from MCA or basilar artery	Contralateral internal capsule, pons, or corona radiata
Pure hemisensory impairment (involving face, arm, and leg)	Deep penetrating end arteries from MCA or basilar artery	Contralateral thalamus, pons, or corona radiata
Mixed hemiparesis and hemisensory impairment (involving face, arm, and leg)	Deep penetrating end arteries from MCA	Contralateral thalamus and internal capsule

(*Continued*)

Table 3 Common Stroke Syndromes, Their Associated Vascular Supply, and Affected Brain Regions (*Continued*)

Stroke syndrome	Vascular supply	Brain region
Ataxia hemiparesis	Deep penetrating end arteries from MCA or basilar artery	Contralateral internal capsule and thalamus or pons
Clumsy-hand dysarthria syndrome	Deep penetrating end arteries from MCA or basilar artery	Contralateral internal capsule, pons, or corona radiata
Vertigo, dysequilibrium, gait ataxia, and nystagmus	Vertebrobasilar system	Cerebellum or lateral medulla
Loss of consciousness and tetraplegia	Basilar artery	Pons along with bilateral midbrain, occipital lobes, and thalami

Abbreviations: MCA, middle cerebral artery; PCA, posterior cerebral artery; ACA, anterior cerebral artery.

A list of common ischemic stroke syndromes, the brain regions typically affected, and the associated vascular supply are shown in Table 3. Two examples that are most important to recognize are the middle cerebral artery syndromes. Left middle cerebral artery ischemic stroke commonly presents with aphasia and right hemiparesis, whereas right middle cerebral artery ischemic stroke presents with left hemiparesis and left-sided neglect. Each may exhibit gaze preference or fixed deviation towards the involved hemisphere, gaze paresis in the opposite direction, and hemianopsia.

If the clinical presentation raises a strong clinical suspicion of stroke, the major differential diagnosis is usually between acute ischemic and acute hemorrhagic stroke. Headache is approximately twice as common following hemorrhagic stroke as compared to ischemic stroke (two-thirds vs. one-third of cases, respectively) (12,13). However, because no single or composite clinical indicator exists that provides sufficient sensitivity and specificity to discriminate ischemic from hemorrhagic stroke, neuroimaging is mandatory to make the distinction.

B. Diagnostic Work-Up

Once an acute stroke is suspected, and after ensuring that the ABCs are adequately addressed, a stat blood draw should be ordered to obtain a complete blood cell (CBC) count, basic chemistry panel, prothrombin time (PT) and partial thromboplastin time (PTT). An immediate assessment of blood glucose is needed, because both hypoglycemia and hyperglycemia may mimic acute stroke. Determine the cardiac rhythm and obtain a 12-lead EKG. Initiate a workup for myocardial infarction if appropriate.

Due to the widespread accessibility of CT scanners, head CT images are used much more commonly than MRI to manage acute stroke in most hospitals. The ability of noncontrast cranial CT to detect acute intracerebral hemorrhage is excellent and is still considered to be the gold standard. When available and easily accessible, multimodal imaging should be considered in addition to basic imaging. Multimodal CT, including CT angiography (CTA) and CT perfusion (CTP), can be accomplished with an extra 10 minutes of scanning time in addition to the basic noncontrast head CT (14). CTA allows for visualization of the carotid and vertebral arteries in the neck as well as the circle of Willis and its major branches. Collateral channels of blood flow and a vasodilatory response mediated by cerebral autoregulation may provide important sources of compensatory blood flow to ischemic brain tissue. CTP imaging provides quantitative determinations of various blood flow parameters, from which tissue perfusion maps can be derived. For example, decreased cerebral blood volume (CBV) in an area of increased mean transit time (MTT) indicates little compensatory vasodilatation and suggests an area of damaged brain. In contrast, if the area of increased MTT is much greater than the area of decreased CBV, the mismatch indicates there is an area of ischemic brain tissue that remains "at-risk" and more aggressive therapy may be justified.

Multimodal brain MRI (15–18) includes basic imaging sequences plus MR angiography (MRA), gradient echo imaging (GRE), DWI, and perfusion weighted imaging (PWI). The MRA allows visualization of both intracranial and extracranial blood vessels. GRE is very sensitive to small amounts of hemosiderin, which is a marker for intraparenchymal blood. DWI visualizes cytotoxic edema and can identify an ischemic brain region within minutes of the stroke. PWI gives a picture of relative blood flow to the brain. A mismatch between the DWI and PWI scans may indicate ischemic brain that is at-risk but not yet infarcted.

The strength of noncontrast head CT scanning is that it is a ubiquitous, rapid, and easily accessible means of imaging the intracranial contents. It is an excellent imaging choice for patients who are critically ill, intubated, hemodynamically unstable, or extremely claustrophobic. In acute stroke, the major downside is the relative insensitivity to early ischemic changes. CT also does not provide adequate visualization of the contents of the posterior fossa (medulla, pons, cerebellum). In addition, CTP has not been completely validated in acute ischemic stroke. Because CTA and CTP imaging require the administration of intravenous contrast media, it may be contraindicated in patients with renal compromise. Impaired cardiac function or a suboptimal bolus inject of contrast can significantly interfere with the timely passage of contrast through the cerebral vessels, a problem that may limit acquisition and interpretation of CTA and CTP imaging data.

The strength of MRI scanning is that it permits several different image sequences to be obtained during one visit to the scanner. Brain imaging with gradient-echo, DWI, PWI, and intracranial MRA comprises a typical image set obtained during the evaluation of acute ischemic stroke. Spatial resolution is superior to CT, especially in the posterior fossa. Acquisition of the perfusion sequences requires the administration of an intravenous bolus of contrast (gadolinium) that does not depend on normal renal function. The cervical carotid arteries in the neck may also be visualized with MRA. The downsides to MRI imaging in acute stroke are the limited availability at many centers, the longer duration for acquisition of images (up to 30 minutes in some patients), the greater patient cooperation needed, and the difficulty to perform a study on an intubated patient. As is true of CT, MR perfusion has not been completely validated in acute ischemic stroke, and data acquisition may be hampered by impaired cardiac function.

C. Management

While there is a temptation to rush the acute stroke patient off for diagnostic testing, respiratory status, blood pressure, glucose, hydration, and temperature must be stable first. In the setting of acute stroke, upper airway compromise is not uncommon. If the oxygen saturation is less than 95% on room air, supplemental oxygen should be given. If the patient is having difficulty handling his secretions, intubation for airway protection should be considered.

Acute blood-pressure management is somewhat controversial. Current recommendations include avoiding giving antihypertensive medications unless the pressures exceed 220/120, there is evidence of other organ failure due to the hypertension, or the patient will be a candidate for IV-rt-PA (see preceeding text) (19). When antihypertensive therapy is needed acutely, intravenous labetolol or nicardipine are the drugs of choice. For diastolic pressures greater than 140, nitroprusside should be considered. If the pressure is lower than normal for the patient, the underlying cause should be investigated. Not uncommonly, stroke patients present with volume depletion. In this setting, blood pressure support by rehydrating with normal saline is reasonable. In patients with a mismatch between the area of completed infarction and the area of hypoperfusion, pharmacologically-induced blood pressure elevation may improve cerebral perfusion and improve outcome (20). Clinical trials employing this aggressive approach are underway.

Extreme hyperglycemia and hypoglycemia may cause symptoms that can mimic stroke and need to be diagnosed and treated on an urgent basis. Glucose reduction should be limited to 75 to 100 mg/dL per hour to avoid osmotic injury to the brain (21). Observational studies reported that clinical outcome is worse in patients who have hyperglycemia at the time of their stroke (22,23). A reasonable approach to glucose management is to avoid dextrose in IV fluids and write for an insulin sliding scale to keep the blood glucose below 200 mg/dL.

Hyperthermia following stroke is also associated with larger infarct volumes and worse outcomes (24,25). In acute stroke, hyperthermia should be treated with antipyretics and the cause of the fever treated. Induced hypothermia for acute stroke is being studied but has not yet been shown to be of benefit.

Stroke occurring in an ICU setting affords the ideal opportunity to initiate treatment as early as possible after symptom onset and optimize the opportunity for stroke reversal. The only treatment currently proven to reverse stroke is IV rt-PA. Patients should be considered for IV rt-PA if they have an acute ischemic stroke, were known neurologically normal within the last three hours, have ongoing measurable deficit that is not rapidly improving, and have a CT scan that is consistent with ischemic stroke. Blood pressures in excess of 185/110 that cannot be brought down consistently below that level with two doses of labetolol should not be given IV rt-PA. Caution should be used in giving rt-PA to patients who have CT changes indicating abnormality in greater than one-third of the middle cerebral artery (MCA) distribution. It may indicate that the stroke onset was earlier than originally thought and may indicate a patient less likely to have a good response to therapy. Detailed inclusion and exclusion criteria for IV rt-PA use are outlined in Table 4.

Table 4 Inclusion and Exclusion Criteria for Treatment of Acute Ischemic Stroke with IV rt-PA

Inclusion criteria
    Stroke onset <3 hr
    No hemorrhage visible on CT scan or MRI
    Measurable persistent deficit on the NIHSS
Exclusion criteria
    History
        Active bleeding
        Arterial puncture at a noncompressible site or lumbar puncture within previous seven days
        Major surgery or serious trauma within past 14 days
        Gastrointestinal or urinary tract hemorrhage within 21 days
        Stroke or serious head trauma within past 3 mo
        Myocardial infarction within 3 mo
        History of intracerebral hemorrhage
    Clinical
        Rapidly improving neurologic signs or minor symptoms
        Systolic BP >185 or diastolic BP >110 OR aggressive IV treatment required to lower blood pressure to specified limits
        Seizure at stroke onset
        Symptoms strongly suggestive of subarachnoid hemorrhage
    Laboratory
        INR >1.5 if anticoagulated
        PTT above normal if exposed to heparin in prior 48 hr
        Platelets <100,000/mm^3
        Glucose <50 or >400 mg/dL
        Positive pregnancy test
    Radiologic
        Exercise caution if CT shows multilobar infarction OR if MRI GRE sequence shows hemorrhage (see text)

Source: From Ref. 53.

It is important to initiate a discussion of the potential risks and benefits of rt-PA with the patient (or their decision makers if the patient cannot understand or communicate). The risk of intravenous administration of rt-PA can be summarized as an approximate 6% chance of symptomatic intracranial hemorrhage. However, the administration of rt-PA does not alter the risk of severe disability or death. The potential benefit is a 30% better chance of being neurologically normal or near-normal at 90 days. Written consent is not required to administer intravenous rt-PA. In circumstances in which the patient's wishes cannot be communicated (e.g., because of aphasia) and proxy consent cannot be obtained, and it is felt that withholding treatment would be unethical, rt-PA should be given. Whatever decision is made, documentation of clinical reasoning should be in the chart.

The dose for IV rt-PA (alteplase) is 0.9 mg/kg (up to 90 mg maximum). Ten percent is given as a bolus over one minute and the remaining 90% as an intravenous infusion over one hour. Because the chances of a good outcome with rt-PA decrease with every minute lost, for a patient who is otherwise a good candidate for the drug, rt-PA should be ordered prior to sending the patient to the scanner, so that it may be hung as soon as possible once the images are interpreted. Guidelines recommend that the following protocol should be adhered to for the 24 hours following rt-PA administration: (1) admit to an intensive care unit; (2) monitor blood pressure every 15 minutes for the first two hours, every 30 minutes for the next six hours, and then every hour after that until 24 hours post-treatment; (3) maintain blood pressure below 180/105 during and after rt-PA infusion; (4) perform neurologic monitoring every 15 minutes during rt-PA infusion and every 30 minutes for the next six hours and every hour after that until 24 hours post-treatment; (6) if symptoms improve significantly then return abruptly, worsen outright, or significant headache appears, order a stat noncontrast head CT to determine whether intracerebral hemorrhage has occurred; (7) no anticoagulant or antithrombotic therapy should be given for 24 hours; and (8) if indwelling catheters were not in place prior to rt-PA infusion, where possible, delay their placement for 24 hours.

There are no prospective randomized trial data to support the use of rt-PA beyond the three-hour window. While the rt-PA trials with five- and six-hour windows did not find a significant benefit, a meta-analysis of all rt-PA trials indicated that it may be effective up to 4.5 hours after stroke onset (T. Brott, personal communication, 2002). A European-based trial is currently testing the efficacy of rt-PA up to a four-hour window. Until more data are available, use of rt-PA beyond three hours is considered off-label. Intra-arterial (IA) administration of thrombolytic agents, though not approved by the FDA for treatment of acute stroke, is available at some centers in the context of a clinical trial or on a compassionate use basis. The window of opportunity for its use and the appropriate dosing are not established. Many centers consider IA rt-PA for patients seen within six hours after stroke onset who are not candidates for IV rt-PA. A trial combining IV rt-PA with IA rt-PA is currently underway. Another experimental interventional approach is the use of small microcatheter devices that permit IA mechanical clot retrieval up to eight hours after stroke onset in patients who are not candidates for standard IV rt-PA.

For patients who are not candidates for thrombolysis, the only agent proven to reduce the risk of recurrent stroke in the acute/subacute period is aspirin (26). While the risk reduction for aspirin use in this setting is statistically significant, the number needed to treat to prevent one stroke is approximately 100. A combination of two antiplatelet agents was shown to be more effective than aspirin alone for long-term stroke prevention, but no trials have looked at the safety and efficacy of combination therapy in the acute/subacute period (27).

The use of anticoagulation in the acute/subacute setting is controversial. There are no compelling data to show that anticoagulation decreases the risk of stroke recurrence or the degree of disability from the initial stroke. There are data to indicate that anticoagulation increases the risk of intracranial and systemic hemorrhage in acute stroke patients (28). For this reason, routine use of anticoagulation in acute stroke is not recommended (29). The so-called "stroke-in-progress" is another area of controversy and confusion. Increasing edema, hypoperfusion of the ischemic penumbra, hemorrhagic conversion of an ischemic infarct, or recurrent embolization from a dissection or cardioembolic source may cause progressive symptoms. The underlying mechanism of the progression needs to be identified before a specific therapy initiated. Anticoagulation for "stroke-in-progress" should be reserved for patients with progression due to an identified source of aseptic emboli when the infarct is not large and the blood pressure is controlled.

III. Hypoxic-Ischemic Encephalopathy

A. Clinical Presentation

In the ICU setting, hypoxic-ischemic encephalopathy (HIE) most commonly results from diffuse temporary global cerebral ischemia occuring during cardiac arrest, the third leading cause of coma after traumatic brain injury and intoxications (30). Much less is understood about HIE than acute ischemic stroke and no effective treatment exists.

Attempts at resuscitation are frequently unsuccessful, and when resuscitation efforts succeed in restoring normal spontaneous circulation, roughly two-thirds of patients die within seven days (31). For those surviving beyond the first week, 80–90% enter a persistent vegetative state or die (28,32–35). The majority of the remaining survivors are left severely disabled (31,32). Death during the subacute and chronic phases is commonly the result of heart failure, systemic thrombosis, or overwhelming infection. Most of these data were culled from studies published prior to the advent of more aggressive attempts at out-of-hospital treatment and may not apply to modern ICU resuscitation.

In survivors of cardiac arrest, the deep coma that may ensue can last for hours or persist indefinitely. Impaired brainstem function and a flaccid tetraparesis are commonly seen early. Decerebrate or decorticate posturing may be noted, and post-anoxic myoclonus and other overt seizures may manifest after several hours. Nonconvulsive status epilepticus (NCSE) may occur; repetitive eye blinking or tonic gaze deviation with nystagmoid eye movements may be the only manifestations. Isolated hemodynamic instability may occasionally reflect nonconvulsive seizure activity. Significant injury to the brain can lead to several different short- and long-term fates: locked-in state, coma, vegetative state, minimally conscious state, or brain death.

B. Diagnostic Work-Up

The main purpose of diagnostic testing in HIE is the prediction of poor outcome. The neurologic examination findings in combination with electrodiagnostic testing during the initial three days following cardiac arrest carry enormous prognostic value. Several observational studies reported that HIE patients with absent pupillary reactivity on initial exam or absent or extensor motor responses to pain on day 3 have no chance of a favorable outcome at one year (28,30,36). However, others reported HIE patients with absent pupillary reflexes on initial assessment regaining consciousness (37). Patients may also be encountered with intact brainstem reflexes who remain in a coma, presenting additional prognostic uncertainty. Thus, with the exception of the diagnosis of brain death (see below), the neurologic exam cannot be relied on in isolation for outcome prediction, as it appears to lack sufficient sensitivity and specificity.

Electroencephalography (EEG) and evoked potentials (EP) may improve on the accuracy of the neurologic exam (33,38,39). An EP test performed between days 2 and 4 with bilateral absence of cortical responses is a powerful marker for poor recovery. Any other abnormal EP result should be followed up with a repeat study three days later. In contrast, bilateral normal cortical responses portend a good outcome. Though not as specific as EP testing, the finding of a burst-suppression or isolectric EEG in the first week may also be useful. The electrodiagnostic results should be taken together with the clinical exam findings in developing prognostic considerations.

The predictive value of neuroimaging studies in HIE is unclear as this issue has not been systematically studied. Signal abnormalities are commonly seen bilaterally in cortical and subcortical tissue on CT and MRI. Positron emission tomography shows low resting blood flow rates are present diffusely in brain. However, due to small numbers of patients and the lack of validation of using neuroimaging to predict outcome, no recommendations can be made.

C. Management

Patients who have suffered significant injury to the CNS present unique clinical challenges. For individuals who survive the first 72 hours and do not demonstrate poor prognostic indicators, subsequent recovery of function is difficult to predict. With the return of consciousness, agitation, confusion, and hemodynamic lability are commonly observed. Paralytic, sedative, neuroleptic, or anxiolytic medication may be needed to smooth the transition out of coma. However, because they interfere with neurologic assessment, it is desirable to minimize their use. A reasonable approach is initiating therapy with a low dose of an atypical antipsychotic agent, such as quetiapine, risperidone, or olanzapine. These agents are preferred because of a relatively lower risk for sedation and induction of delirium. If parenteral therapy is necessitated, small doses of propofol are preferred over other agents because it can easily be titrated and turned off a few hours prior to a scheduled neurologic exam. Midazolam and dexmedetomidine, a potent selective α_2 agonist, are reasonable second-tier agents.

For patients demonstrating poor prognostic indicators, management focuses on end-of-life, withdrawal of care, and palliative care issues. During initial discussions with family and friends, it is important to be frank and prepare them for the worst in a sensitive way in order to set the stage for discussions that might be necessitated later. Firm predictions about outcome should not be made too early in the course. A lead spokesperson among family and a physician of record should be identified. Effective communication must take place between healthcare team members so that a unified front regarding the care plan and prognosis is conveyed to the patient's supportive cast. Healthcare team members should be instructed to defer questions regarding prognosis to the physician of record.

Managing patients at the end of life requires shifting the shared mindset from one in which supportive measures were actively being deployed to one in which they will be actively withdrawn (40). The healthcare team has an obligation to see to it that the patient and family and friends suffer as little as possible in the process. Five practices that define good end-of-life care include: adequate pain control and symptom management, avoidance of prolongation of dying, achieving a sense of control, relieving burden, and strengthening relationships with loved ones (41). Loved ones should be given the opportunity to be with the dying person if they wish. It is also useful to inquire as to whether the patient would like to have a special person of their faith present to provide stewardship through this difficult time. When the time comes to withdraw life support, distractions should be eliminated, monitors turned off, and leads and cables removed. Consideration should be given to discontinuing all superfluous treatments, medications, intravenous fluids, enteral or parenteral feedings, phlebotomy, radiographic examinations, and removing all intravascular catheters and indwelling tubes. Healthcare team members should attempt to leave family alone with the patient, if possible, yet avail themselves to the needs of family should they arise.

IV. Status Epilepticus

A. Clinical Presentation

Status epilepticus (SE) is a life-threatening medical emergency requiring early recognition and immediate, vigorous intervention in order to reduce morbidity and mortality. Most seizures last less than five minutes. Classically, SE is defined as a generalized tonic clonic (GTC) seizure lasting more than

30 minutes or two or more consecutive seizures without a recovery of consciousness in between. However, a current operational definition for GTC SE includes any seizure lasting for at least five minutes (42). The morbidity and mortality rates are closely correlated with a delayed or inappropriate treatment. Any patient having a seizure lasting longer than five to ten minutes should be treated as SE.

SE may be grouped into three types. GTC SE usually presents with bilateral abnormal involuntary tonic clonic movements. GTC SE induces the greatest metabolic and systemic stress, as well as neuronal damage, and thus carries a highest risk of complications.

Nonconvulsive SE (NCSE) may present with a continuous or fluctuating alteration of consciousness, also described as an epileptic "twilight state." It may also present as continuing subtle, rhythmical motor activity, such as facial, finger, or toe twitching, or rhythmical eye deviation or nystagmus. Clinically, the presentation may be deceivingly subtle, and is easily missed even by an experienced neurologist. Large, hospital-based studies have reported that NCSE is under recognized, and that it is the cause of coma in up to 8% of ICU patients (43). EEG should be part of the routine work-up for a comatose patient in the ICU, even if no apparent clinical seizure activity is noted.

Simple partial SE (also known as "epilepsia partialis continua" or "EPC") presents as focal abnormal involuntary movements with preserved consciousness. This has less potential for inducing neuronal damage, and can usually be treated more conservatively.

More than 30–50% of patients presenting in SE have no history of epilepsy. Having an established diagnosis of epilepsy does not affect the management of SE. In about two-thirds of SE cases, a precipitating factor or underlying cause can be identified. SE affects people of all ages but is more common and carries greater morbidity and mortality in the very young and the elderly. Age groups at highest risk for SE are children less than five and patients over 60-years old. Patients aged 15–40 years are at a lowest risk for SE (44).

The determination of the underlying cause is an important part of the initial evaluation in the management of SE. The most likely underlying cause varies with age of the patient (Table 5). In the very young, febrile seizures is the leading cause for SE. In the elderly, cerebrovascular disease is the most common culprit (45). In patients with pre-existent epilepsy, the most common cause for SE is noncompliance with anti-epileptic drugs (AEDs). In the ICU setting, toxic-metabolic, traumatic brain injury, hemorrhagic stroke (both intraparenchymal hemorrhage and subarachnoid hemorrhage), and hypoxic-ischemic etiologies are most common.

B. Diagnostic Work-Up

Because SE is an emergency, the diagnostic work-up has to take place simultaneously with the prompt initiation of treatment. Both the response to treatment

Table 5 Etiology of Status Epilepticus by Age

Children (%)	Diagnosis	Adults (%)
3	Stroke	25
20	Low AED level	20
10	Toxic-metabolic	10
5	Anoxia or hypoxia	10
35	Infection (systemic), fever	2
5	CNS infection	10
<1	Tumor	5
3.5	Trauma	5
2	Alcohol/drugs	15
10	Congenital	<1

Source: From Ref. 54.

and the long-term outcome correlate strongly with the duration of the seizure. Only after the acute management is initiated should the diagnostic work-up for a potential underlying pathology and precipitating factors be initiated. Certain underlying causes of SE are known to predispose the patient to fail to respond to anticonvulsant therapies ("refractory SE") unless corrected (e.g., electrolyte abnormalities).

Prior to initiating intravenous therapy to stop the SE, bloods should be drawn to look for an underlying toxic-metabolic cause and to measure pre-existing AED levels. Once the seizures have stopped, brain imaging can be ordered, unless there is a previously established structural abnormality known to be responsible for the SE (e.g., brain tumor). In patients with SE due to stroke, re-imaging is often appropriate because of the risk of change requiring adjustment in management of the underlying lesion. The threshold for obtaining CSF should be low in order to rule out CNS infection and subarachnoid hemorrhage.

In most cases of an obvious, generalized convulsive seizure, an immediate EEG is not necessary. Treatment of SE should never be delayed while awaiting the results of an EEG. However, if there is any suspicion of on-going subclinical seizure activity, such as failure to completely recover mental status, a stat EEG is appropriate. The purpose of EEG at this point is to assist the management (i.e., rule out ongoing seizure activity), as opposed to differential diagnostic (seizure or not).

Continuous EEG monitoring should be considered in the ICU patient with altered mental status of unknown origin in order to rule out NCSE. It should also be considered for any patient who is treated for status but fails to recover consciousness within one to two hours in order to ensure that the generalized status did not evolve into subtle status or NCSE.

C. Management

The main goals of the management of SE are to rapidly terminate the seizure activity and to prevent adverse neuronal and metabolic sequela. These can be achieved by (1) maintaining adequate vital functions (ABCs); (2) preventing systemic complications, such as hypotension, acidosis and hyperpyrexia; (3) promptly administering of AEDs intravenously; and (4) identifying and treating of the underlying cause.

Unless the underlying cause/abnormality is addressed, SE may be extremely resistant to any medical therapies. Up to 10–15% of SE cases are resistant to conventional therapies and may need the administration of intravenous anesthetics to induce a burst suppression pattern on continuous EEG monitoring (46).

A protocol for treating SE in adults is summarized in Table 6. Initial use of either lorazepam or diazepam will stop 79% of all SE (47). Due to its high lipid solubility, diazepam has the advantage of faster onset of action but the disadvantage of a shorter duration of action, 15–30 minutes. Compared to diazepam, lorazepam has a higher affinity binding to benzodiazepine receptor sites, and thus longer duration of action, 12–24 hours, but takes somewhat longer to stop the seizures. Each may cause respiratory depression with repeated doses and may require ventilatory support.

Phenytoin can be used as a second line agent to follow a benzodiazepam. The duration of action is >24 hours. It should be considered in addition to a benzodiazepam even when the SE stops with the first agent. Its major side effects include hypotension and cardiac arrythmias, especially in the elderly.

Fosphenytoin is a phosphate ester prodrug of phenytoin, which is dosed in phenytoin equivalents. It has identical pharmacological properties to phenytoin. However, it has multiple favorable qualities that are in favor for its use in an emergency situation. Unlike phenytoin, it is compatible with all intravenous

Table 6   Treatment of Status Epilepticus

Time (min)	Action
0–5	ABCs including nasal O_2, intravenous line with 0.9 NS, ECG, BP-monitor, blood draw for chemistry panel, CBC, Mg, Ca, AED-levels, ABG, toxicology screen
6–10	Thiamine 100 mg iv, 50 mL of D50 iv if indicated
10–20	Lorazepam 0.1 mg/kg (children: 0.05–0.5 mg/kg) @ 2 mg/min; repeat once in 8–10 min PRN, or diazepam 0.15–0.25 mg/kg (children 0.1–1.0 mg/kg) @ 5 mg/min
20–30	Phenytoin (or fosphenytoin) 18–20 mg/kg @ 0.3 mg/kg/min or 25 mg/min (or 50 mg/min), monitor BP and ECG closely; if SE persists, give additional 10 mg/kg (max of 30 mg/kg), Reassess, intubate, get stat EEG
30+	Phenobarbital: 20 mg/kg (max rate 100 mg/min)
ICU setting	Pentobarbital (5–15 mg/kg), maintain at 0.5–5.0 mg/kg/hr, Midazolam 0.2 mg/kg slow iv bolus, then 0.75–10 μgm/kg/min, or Propofol 1 mg/kg, then 2–10 mg/kg/hr for 12–24 hr

solutions in common use, it causes only minimal local irritation when extravesated, and has minimal risk for cardiovascular events, therefore allowing administration at much faster rates than phenytoin. The major disadvantage of fosphenytoin compared to phenytoin is cost.

When SE continues for >30 minutes, a third agent is needed. Phenobarbital can be given with an initial dose of 20 mg/kg (max rate 100 mg/min, duration of action >48 hours). In instances of a prolonged or refractory SE, it is customary to induce a burst suppression EEG pattern (with interburst intervals two to 30 seconds) with an intravenous anesthetic agent (e.g., propofol, midazolam, or pentobarbital) for at least 24–48 hours. The burst suppression presumably represents a disconnection between the gray and white matter. However, it is uncertain whether the burst suppression pattern actually improves the outcome of SE.

V. Brain Death, Persistent Vegetative State, and Minimally Conscious State

A. Clinical Presentation

Death can be determined reliably by either cardiopulmonary or neurological criteria. Brain death is the absence of clinical function of the brain, including the brain stem, where the proximate cause is known and irreversible and confounding factors have been eliminated (hypotension, electrolyte, acid-base, or endocrine disturbances, drug intoxication, poisoning, or neuromuscular blocking agents, and severe hypothermia with core temperature <32°C). Brain death in adults results most commonly from severe head injury and subarachnoid or intracerebral hemorrhage. However, in the ICUs, hypoxic-ischemic encephalopathy and fulminant liver failure are common culprits. In children, abuse is the most common cause, followed by motor vehicle accidents and asphyxia. Conditions that can mimic brain death include locked-in-syndrome, hypothermia, and drug intoxication.

The distinction between brain death and persistent vegetative state (PVS) is extremely important. PVS is a condition of complete unawareness of self or environment and an inability to interact with others, along with the absence of reproducible purposeful or voluntary behavioral responses to stimuli, language comprehension or expression, and bowel and bladder continence. However, there is preservation of sleep-wake cycles and sufficient hypothalamic and brain-stem autonomic functions to permit survival with medical care (48). The clinical course and outcome of PVS depends on its cause. Patients in non-traumatic PVS for three or six months have a ≤1% chance of improving to moderate disability or good recovery. The remainder has severe disability, ongoing PVS, or death. Non-traumatic PVS is considered permanent after three months.

A third category of impaired consciousness that should be distinguished from irreversible coma and PVS is the minimally conscious state (MCS). In MCS, there is severely altered consciousness in which minimal but definite behavioral evidence of self or environmental awareness is demonstrated (49). If the behavior is a simple response, it should be reproducible to be certain it is not a chance reflex action. Following commands, intelligible verbalization, purposeful behavior, or a verbal yes/no response are examples of behaviors demonstrating awareness. At one year, patients with MCS have significantly better outcomes than patients with PVS, especially after traumatic head injury (50).

B. Diagnostic Work-Up

The diagnoses of brain death, PVS, and MCS are primarily made on clinical grounds (see Table 7). Brain death requires documentation of coma or unresponsiveness, absence of brainstem reflexes, and apnea. Coma is documented by an absence of response to pain in all extremities with nailbed and supraorbital pressure. Absence of brainstem reflexes requires assessment of pupillary responsiveness, extraocular movements (oculocephalics or caloric testing), facial sensation or

Table 7 Clinical Characteristics of Impaired States of Responsiveness

State	Characteristics
Coma	Eyes closed, unresponsive, unarousable; perceptual awareness and intellectual capacity absent; brainstem function may be normal or abnormal; individuals in this state will awaken, transition to a vegetative state, or die
Brain death	Comatose, absence of motor responses, and complete absence of brain stem function, including apnea on two separate exams (time period between exams unspecified in individuals over 18 yr of age)
Vegetative state	Waking alternates with periods of diminished responsiveness; waking state associated with no or extremely limited interaction with the external environment; capacity for perceptual awareness and intellectual function not understood; brainstem and autonomic function generally preserved; doubly incontinent; preserved sleep–wake cycles; may transition to minimal response state
Minimally conscious state	Similar to vegetative state except perceptual awareness and primitive attempts at communication (motor, visual, or verbal) appear; in rehabilitation centers, one-third of patients misdiagnosed as being in vegetative state
Locked-in state	Consciousness preserved, eyes open; some eye movements and/or blinking are present; response repertoire limited by upper and lower brainstem dysfunction and quadriplegia

motor response, corneal reflex, and pharyngeal and tracheal reflexes. Testing for absence of respiratory drive at pCO_2 of 60 mmHg or 20 mmHg above a normal baseline should follow a protocol (51,52). Prior to testing, the following is required: core temperature $\geq 36.5°C$ (or 97°F), systolic blood pressure ≥ 90 mmHg, euvolemia, normal pCO_2 or arterial $pCO_2 \geq 40$ mmHg (levels may be higher in patients with chronic hypercapnia), and normal pO_2. To test for apnea, a pulse oximeter is connected and the ventilator disconnected; 100% O_2 (6 L/min) is delivered into the trachea (or cannula at the level of carina). The patient is observed closely for respiratory movements. Arterial pO_2, pCO_2, and pH are measured after approximately six to eight minutes and the patient reconnected to the ventilator. If there are no respiratory movements and the arterial pCO_2 is ≥ 60 mmHg, apnea is present (the tests support the diagnosis of brain death). If respiratory movements are observed, the apnea test result is negative (does not support the clinical diagnosis of brain death), and the test should be repeated at a later time. The ventilator is reconnected if, during testing, the systolic BP becomes ≤ 90 mmHg or the pulse oximeter indicates significant oxygen desaturation and cardiac arrythmias are present. An arterial blood sample is drawn. If pCO_2 is ≥ 60 mmHg (or pCO_2 increase ≥ 20 mmHg over the baseline), the apnea test result is positive; if pCO_2 is < 60 mmHg or pCO_2 increase is < 20 mmHg over baseline normal pCO_2, the test result is indeterminate, and additional confirmatory tests may be considered.

Some recommend a repeat clinical evaluation at an interval of several hours after the initial brain death examination. If components of the clinical exam cannot be performed reliably, confirmatory testing is recommended. These tests include contrast cerebral angiography, EEG for brain death, transcranial Doppler, nuclear brain scan, and somatosensory evoked potentials.

A physician comfortable with detailed neurologic examination and diagnosis must take appropriate steps to distinguish between PVS and MCS. Adequate stimulation on repeated examinations must be given to elicit behavioral responses that do not often occur on a reflex basis.

C. Treatment

Treatment decisions for MCS patients are difficult because so little is known about the prognosis. Early on, with good supportive care, improvement can be seen. Family and healthcare providers must be aware of the patient's potential for understanding and for feeling pain. After 12 months in MCS, the chances for good outcome or even minimal disability are small.

After diagnosing PVS, the physician should discuss with the family the prognosis and chances for meaningful recovery. Comfort, dignity, and hygiene must be maintained. Based on the family's ethical and religious beliefs, decisions need to be made about the appropriate level of care, including use of medications, antibiotics, supplemental oxygen, nutrition, hydration, and complex organ sustaining treatments, such as dialysis. A Do-Not-Resuscitate order is usually indicated.

Once a diagnosis of brain death is confirmed, no therapeutic measures are appropriate. Next of kin may be approached for organ donation. If organ donation is declined, terminating mechanical ventilation is appropriate. If mechanical ventilation and aggressive support are continued, cardiac arrest will occur within days to weeks.

References

1. Bleck TP, Smith MC, Pierre-Louis SJ, Jares JJ, Murray J, Hansen CA. Neurologic complications of critical medical illnesses. Crit Care Med 1993; 21:98–103.
2. Wijdicks EF, Scott JP. Stroke in the medical intensive-care unit. Mayo Clin Proc 1998; 73:642–646.
3. Blacker DJ. In-hospital stroke. Lancet Neurol 2003; 2:741–746.
4. Charlesworth DC, Likosky DS, Marrin CA, et al., for the Northern New England Cardiovascular Disease Study Group. Development and validation of a prediction model for strokes after coronary artery bypass grafting. Ann Thorac Surg 2003; 76:436–443.
5. Kelley RE. Postoperative medical complications: Stroke in the postoperative period. Med Clin North Am 2001; 85:1263–1276.
6. Likosky DS, Marrin CA, Caplan LR, et al., for the Northern New England Cardiovascular Disease Study Group. Determination of etiologic mechanisms of strokes secondary to coronary artery bypass graft surgery. Stroke 2003; 34:2830–2834.
7. Blossom GB, Fietsam R Jr, Bassett JS, et al. Characteristics of cerebrovascular accidents after coronary artery bypass grafting. Am Surg 1992; 58:584–589.
8. Dashe JF, Pessin MS, Murphy RE, Payne DD. Carotid occlusive disease and stroke risk in coronary artery bypass graft surgery. Neurology 1997; 49:678–686.
9. Limburg M, Wijdicks EF, Li H. Ischemic stroke after surgical procedures: clinical features, neuroimaging, and risk factors. Neurology 1998; 50:895–901.
10. Naylor AR, Mehta Z, Rothwell PM, Bell PR. Carotid artery disease and stroke during coronary artery bypass: a critical review of the literature. Eur J Vasc Endovasc Surg 2002; 23:283–294.
11. Restrepo L, Wityk RJ, Grega MA, et al. Diffusion- and perfusion-weighted magnetic resonance imaging of the brain before and after coronary artery bypass grafting surgery. Stroke 2002; 33:2909–2915.
12. Melo TP, Pinto AN, Ferro JM. Headache in intracerebral hematomas. Neurology 1996; 47:494–500.
13. Ferro JM, Melo TP, Oliveira V, et al. A multivariate study of headache associated with ischemic stroke. Headache 1995; 35:315–319.
14. Wintermark M, Reichhart M, Cuisenaire O, et al. Comparison of admission perfusion computed tomography and qualitative diffusion- and perfusion-weighted magnetic resonance imaging in acute stroke patients. Stroke 2002; 33:2025–2031.
15. Shih LC, Saver JL, Alger JR, et al. Perfusion-weighted magnetic resonance imaging thresholds identifying core, irreversibly infarcted tissue. Stroke 2003; 34:1425–1430.
16. Neumann-Haefelin T, Wittsack HJ, Wenserski F, et al. Diffusion- and perfusion-weighted MRI. The DWI/PWI mismatch region in acute stroke. Stroke 1999; 30:1591–1597.

17. Baird AE, Warach S. Magnetic resonance imaging of acute stroke. J Cereb Blood Flow Metab 1998; 18:583–609.
18. Schellinger PD, Fiebach JB, Jansen O, et al. Stroke magnetic resonance imaging within 6 hours after onset of hyperacute cerebral ischemia. Ann Neurol 2001; 49:460–469.
19. Adams HP Jr, Adams RJ, Brott T, et al., for the Stroke Council of the American Stroke Association. Guidelines for the early management of patients with ischemic stroke: a scientific statement from the Stroke Council of the American Stroke Association. Stroke 2003; 34:1056–1083.
20. Hillis AE, Ulatowski JA, Barker PB, Torbey M, Ziai W, Beauchamp NJ, Oh S, Wityk RJ. A pilot randomized trial of induced blood pressure elevation: effects on function and focal perfusion in acute and subacute stroke. Cerebrovas Dis 2003; 16:236–246.
21. Wass C, Lanier W. Glucose modulation of ischemic brain injury: review and clinic recommendations. Mayo Clin Proc 1996; 71:801.
22. Alvarez-Sabin J, Molina CA, Montaner J, et al. Effects of admission hyperglycemia on stroke outcome in reperfused tissue plasminogen activator—treated patients. Stroke 2003; 34:1235–1241.
23. Bruno A, Levine SR, Frankel MR, et al. Admission glucose level and clinical outcomes in the NINDS rt-PA Stroke Trial. Neurology 2002; 59:669–674.
24. Reith J, Jorgensen HS, Pedersen PM, et al. Body temperature in acute stroke: relation to stroke severity, infarct size, mortality, and outcome. Lancet 1996; 347:422–425.
25. Wang Y, Lira LL, Levi C, Heller RF, Fisher J. Influence of admission body temperature on stroke mortality. Stroke 2000; 31:404–409.
26. Chen ZM, Sandercock P, Pan HC, et al. Indications for early aspirin use in acute ischemic stroke: A combined analysis of 40 000 randomized patients from the chinese acute stroke trial and the international stroke trial. On behalf of the CAST and IST collaborative groups. Stroke 2000; 31:1240–1249.
27. Diener HC, Cunha L, Forbes C, et al. European Stroke Prevention Study. 2. Dipyridamole and acetylsalicylic acid in the secondary prevention of stroke. J Neurol Sci 1996; 143:1–13.
28. Berge E, Sandercock P. Anticoagulants versus antiplatelet agents for acute ischemic stroke. Stroke 2003; 34:1571–1572.
29. Coull BM, Williams LS, Goldstein LB, et al. Anticoagulants and antiplatelet agents in acute ischemic stroke. Stroke 2002; 33:1934–1942.
30. Shewmon DA, De Giorgio CM. Early prognosis in anoxic coma. Reliability and rationale. Neurol Clin 1989; 7:823–843.
31. Levy DE, Caronna JJ, Singer BH, et al. Predicting outcome from hypoxic-ischemic coma. J Am Med Assoc 1985; 253:1420–1426.
32. Bassetti C, Bomio F, Mathis J, Hess CW. Early prognosis in coma after cardiac arrest: a prospective clinical, electrophysiological, and biochemical study of 60 patients. J Neurol Neurosurg Psychiatry 1996; 61:610–615.
33. Chen R, Bolton CF, Young B. Prediction of outcome in patients with anoxic coma: a clinical and electrophysiologic study. Crit Care Med 1996; 24:672–678.
34. Longstreth WT Jr, Inui TS, Cobb LA, Copass MK. Neurologic recovery after out-of-hospital cardiac arrest. Ann Intern Med 1983; 98:588–592.
35. Medical aspects of the persistent vegetative state (2). The Multi-Society Task Force on PVS. N Engl J Med 1994; 330:1572–1579.

36. Zandbergen EG, de Haan RJ, Stoutenbeek CP, et al. Systematic review of early prediction of poor outcome in anoxic-ischaemic coma. Lancet 1998; 352:1808–1812.

37. Edgren E, Hedstrand U, Kelsey S, et al. Assessment of neurological prognosis in comatose survivors of cardiac arrest. BRCT I Study Group. Lancet 1994; 343:1055–1059.

38. Young GB. The EEG in coma. J Clin Neurophysiol 2000; 17:473–485.

39. Robinson LR, Micklesen PJ, Tirschwell DL, Lew HL. Predictive value of somato-sensory evoked potentials for awakening from coma. Crit Care Med 2003; 31:960–967.

40. Truog RD, Cist AF, Brackett SE, et al. Recommendations for end-of-life care in the intensive care unit: The Ethics Committee of the Society of Critical Care Medicine. Crit Care Med 2001; 29:2332–2348.

41. Singer PA, Martin DK, Kelner M. Quality end-of-life care: patients' perspectives. J Am Med Assoc 1999; 281:163–168.

42. Lowenstein DH. Status epilepticus: an overview of the clinical problem. Epilepsia 1999; 40:S3–S8.

43. Towne AR, Waterhouse EJ. Prevalence of nonconvulsive status epilepticus in coma-tose patient. Neurology 2000; 54:340–345.

44. Wu YW, et al. Incidence and mortality of generalized convulsive status epilepticus in California. Neurology 2002; 58:1070–1076.

45. Willmore LJ. Epilepsy emergencies: the first seizure and status epilepticus. Neurology 1998; 51(suppl 4):S34–S38.

46. Lowenstein DH, Alldredge BK. Status epilepticus. N Engl J Med 1998; 338:970–976.

47. Runge JW. Emergency treatment of status epilepticus. Neurology 1996; 46:S20–S23.

48. Quality Standards Subcommittee of the American Academy of Neurology. Practice parameters: assessment and management of patients in the persistent vegetative state. Neurology 1995; 1015–1018.

49. Giacino JT, Ashwal S, Childs N, Cranford R, Jennett B, Katz DI, Kelly JP, Rosenberg JH, Whyte J, Zafonte RD, Zasler ND. The minimally conscious state. Neurology 2002; 58:349–353.

50. Giacino JT, Kalmar K. The vegetative and minimally conscious states: a comparison of clinical features and functional oooutcome. J Head Trauma Rehabil 1997; 12:36–51.

51. Quality Standards Subcommittee of the American Academy of Neurology. Practice parameters for determining brain death. Neurology 1995; 45:1012–1014.

52. Wijdicks EFM. Determining brain death I adults. Neurology 1995; 45:1003–1011.

53. Kalafut MA, Saver JL. The acute stroke patient: the first 6 hours. In: Cohen SN, ed. Management of Ischemic Stroke. New York: McGraw-Hill, 2000:17–52.

54. Hauser W. Status epilepticus: Epidemiologic considerations. Neurology 1990; 40:S9–S13.

13

Evaluation and Treatment of Acute Renal Failure in the Intensive Care Unit

JEFFREY A. KRAUT, JOANNA DUFFNEY, and BEHRAN VAGHAIWALLA

VA Greater Los Angeles Healthcare System and Geffen School of Medicine at UCLA
Los Angeles, California, U.S.A.

I. Introduction

Acute renal failure (ARF) develops in approximately 5% of all hospitalized patients (1,2). When it is uncomplicated, ARF can usually be managed in a non-intensive care setting, and the mortality is low (less than 5%) (2).

ARF occurs in the Intensive Care Unit (ICU) far more frequently (5–17%) and is often associated with failure of other organs (1–3). ARF in this setting has a great influence on clinical outcome: mortality approaches 55–65% in individuals with ARF requiring renal replacement therapy (1). Given the importance of ARF to survival, it is essential that all physicians caring for these patients, including intensivists, are cognizant of the proper approach to the diagnosis and treatment of this disorder.

In the present chapter, we will summarize our approach to the diagnosis of ARF, the immediate treatment upon recognition of ARF, the conservative approach to treatment of established ARF, and the indications for and complications of renal replacement therapy.

II. Diagnosis of ARF

ARF is defined as an abrupt decline in glomerular filtration rate (GFR). It is associated with a rise in the concentrations of blood urea nitrogen (BUN) and serum creatinine, and in some cases, a change in urine output. With the exception of rhabdomyolysis, muscle release of creatinine is constant from day to day, so the serum creatinine concentration is generally examined to assess changes in GFR. Although any rise in serum creatinine is indicative of a fall in GFR, studies of the impact of treatment on the course of ARF have utilized specific criteria. Unfortunately, there is no consensus on the precise change in serum creatinine that denotes acute renal failure, as several different values have been proposed. We presently utilize the criteria of Solomon et al.: an increment in serum creatinine of 0.3–0.5 mg/dL above baseline or >25% rise in serum creatinine from baseline over 48 hours (5). However, the clinician should be aware that other definitions can be equally valid.

Recently, there has been an impetus to introduce the use of multidimensional criteria to categorize patients with acute renal failure so as to promote more individualization of treatment. In this schema, information from four domains is utilized to differentiate among patients, including: factors that predispose to injury, so-called susceptibility; the nature and timing of the insult producing renal failure; the biological responses to the insult, such as change in serum creatinine concentration; and changes in physiologic parameters, such as urine output (6). Patients are stratified based on different aspects of each domain being assigned a score from 1 to 4. In the future, this categorization of patients may be commonplace; however, until it becomes ingrained in clinical practice, the physician should continue to use well accepted definitions of acute renal failure. A reduction in urine output to less than 400–600 mL/24 h (the minimum quantity of urine in which the normal solute of 600 mOsm can be excreted each day at the maximum urine concentration of 1200 mOsm/L) is found in as many as 20% of patients with ARF (7). These patients are said to have oliguric renal failure. However, the majority of patients with ARF will have apparently adequate urine output, so-called nonoliguric renal failure (7,8). On the other hand, a low urine output does not always indicate ARF: if solute load is low, it can be excreted in urine volumes as low as a few hundred milliliters. A small minority of patients with ARF (<5%) will be anuric (urine output less than 100 mL/day). A urine volume this low has some diagnostic significance: it is most frequent in patients with obstruction of the collecting system or arterial supply to the kidney.

In addition to being of diagnostic value, examination of the quantity of urine excreted each day is of prognostic significance: patients with ARF who have normal urine volumes have a higher GFR than those who are oliguric or anuric (7). As a consequence, the requirement for dialytic therapy, the presence of significant derangements of fluid and electrolyte balance, and the morbidity and mortality are substantially greater in individuals who are anuric or oliguric than those in whom urine output remains unchanged (7).

For diagnostic purposes, ARF is usually divided into three categories based on the presumed location of the renal insult: pre-renal, parenchymal or intrarenal, and post-renal. The frequency of each type of ARF depends on whether the patient is hospitalized or not. In hospitalized patients, prerenal azotemia is the most common form of ARF, accounting for 40–60% of cases (8). Post-renal causes of ARF are present in 1–15% of hospitalized azotemic patients. The remaining cases of ARF are due to intrinsic or parenchymal disease, with the vast majority being due to acute tubular necrosis (ATN) (8).

With the exception of anatomical obstruction of the renal arteries, prerenal renal failure is a functional lesion in which there is a decrease in renal perfusion resulting from extracellular volume loss or decreased cardiac output. Operationally defined, prerenal renal failure is reversible, with renal function returning to baseline values within 48 hours after renal perfusion has been restored. As shown in Table 1, patients with prerenal azotemia often have an abnormal BUN/creatinine ratio of greater than 15 to 20 : 1, a bland or negative urinary sediment (that is, one without cellular elements), low fractional excretion of sodium (FeNa) (<1%), and a concentrated urine (Uosm > 600 mOsm). Since this disorder is completely reversible if recognized and treated early, all patients with ARF should have prerenal renal failure excluded. In some instances, this may require administration of a fluid challenge (500–1000 cc of isotonic saline over 30 minutes).

Postrenal renal failure due to obstruction of the collecting system is also often reversible. The extent of the reversibility will depend largely upon the prior level of renal function and the duration of the obstruction. In men, urinary tract obstruction is most frequently due to prostatic hypertrophy or prostate cancer. Symptoms of an enlarged prostate, such as decreased urinary stream, hesitancy, and dribbling, are prominent. By contrast, in women the obstruction is due to ureteral involvement from gynecological malignancy. These patients may also have a BUN/creatinine ratio of greater than 15 to 20:1 and a urine free of cellular elements. However, the FeNa and urine concentration may be variable depending upon the duration of obstruction. Thus, FeNa and other urinary indices can be similar to that of pre-renal renal failure (<1%) or to that of acute tubular necrosis (>3%). The diagnosis of urinary tract obstruction should be considered in all patients with acute renal failure and excluded by obtaining a renal ultrasound which is diagnostic in more than 90% of cases (9).

Finally, various intraparenchymal disorders affecting the interstitium (acute interstitial nephritis), glomerulus (acute glomerulonephritis), and tubules (acute tubular necrosis) can cause ARF. Acute interstitial nephritis occurs in the setting of exposure to various drugs that are allergens and is often characterized by eosinophilia and eosinophiluria (10). Acute glomerulonephritis may be idiopathic or can be or associated with various systemic diseases. It is characterized by proteinuria and an active urinary sediment (dysmorphic red blood cells and red blood cell casts).

ATN is observed in patients with hypotension or who are exposed to various nephrotoxic agents, such as drugs or radiocontrast material. With rare exceptions (burns, presence of liver failure or volume retaining states), FENa is high (>3%) (11). Examination of the urine will reveal pigmented granular

Table 1 Differential Diagnosis of Acute Renal Failure

	Prerenal	Renal			Post-renal
		AG	AIN	ATN	
History	↓ECF	Post-infection; systemic disease	Exposure to allergens	Hypotension, exposure to nephrotoxins	Obstructive symptoms
PE	Orthostatic BP changes	Signs of systemic disease e.g., arthritis in SLE	Skin rash	—	Increased prostate, increased bladder
Blood					
BUN	↑	↑	↑	↑	↑
Cr	↑	↑	↑	↑	↑
BUN/Cr	>20:1	10–15:1	10–15:1	10–15:1	Early, 10–15:1; late, >20:1
Urine					
Protein	—	++	+	—	—
Blood	—	++	+	—	+
Micro	—	Dysmorphic rbc, rbc casts	Eosinophils	Pigmented granular casts, rtc	—
Na (mEq/L)	<20	<20	>20	>20	Early, <30; late, >20
FENa %	<1	<1	>3%	>3	Early, <1; late, >3
Osmolality (mOsm)	>800	>800	300	300	Early, >800; late, 300
Renal ULTZ	—	—	—	—	Dilated collecting system
Renal Bx	NA	Glomerular inflamation	Interstitial infiltrates	Patchy tubular necrosis	NA

Abbreviations: AG, acute glomerulonephritis; AIN, acute interstitial nephritis; ATN, acute tubular necrosis; rtc, renal tubular cells.

casts and renal tubular cells in approximately 60–70% of patients (12). Furthermore, the urine is poorly concentrated: urine osmolality remains close to that of blood, approximately 300 mOsm (7,12).

Hepatorenal syndrome characterized by evidence of severe liver injury associated with highly concentrated urine, low fractional excretion of sodium, and urine free of protein and cellular elements is often a terminal event in patients with end-stage liver disease. This disorder may be difficult to distinguish from pre-renal, renal failure, and often a trial of volume expansion is necessary to exclude volume depletion. The mortality of this disorder is high and in many centers these patients will not receive dialysis once this diagnosis is made unless a liver transplant is imminent.

A careful history should be obtained with particular attention to the presence of hypotension, exposure to nephrotoxic or allergenic drugs, or sepsis and the presence of underlying systemic diseases. A complete physical examination should be performed with supine and upright blood pressure measurements. Examination of the skin for the presence of skin lesions and of the joints for evidence of arthritis should be done. The bladder area should be percussed and prostate examination done in males looking for signs of bladder obstruction. Renal function should be assessed by measurement of the BUN and serum creatinine concentrations. A urinalysis should be performed looking for proteinuria, or hematuria, and the urine should be perused to try to detect cellular elements. Sodium excretion should be assessed using the fractional excretion of sodium [(urine sodium/plasma sodium)/(urine creatinine/plasma creatinine) × 100], where U_{Na} and P_{Na} are urine and plasma sodium concentrations, and U_{Cr} and P_{Cr} are urine and plasma creatinine concentrations, respectively. Assessment of urine concentration by measurement of the specific gravity or osmolality can also be helpful. Other values, such as urine to plasma urea nitrogen, or creatinine ratios, have been obtained and can be useful in selected cases. All patients with renal failure should have a renal ultrasound to exclude urinary tract obstruction. In selected cases, we will also obtain a Doppler ultrasound to exclude renal arterial obstruction.

By obtaining a good history, performing a complete physical examination, and obtaining the blood and urine studies described above, the cause of ARF can be established in more than 90% of cases. Rarely, if these studies are unsuccessful in delineating the cause of the renal failure, a renal biopsy may be required, particularly in cases in which the clinical and laboratory information available points to glomerular or interstitial disease.

Recently, there has been an interest in the use of state-of-the-art magnetic resonance imaging (MRI) for the early and accurate detection of ARF, delineation of its etiology, and obtaining insight into possible mechanisms underlying its development. Animal studies have confirmed the utility of this technique to determine the exact site of injury within the kidney and to detect inflammatory changes that may be an important factor in its perpetuation (13). MRI in the future might be used to follow the course of patients with ARF to allow prediction of the outcome and thus aid in the designation of targeted therapies (13).

III. Clinical Course of Renal Failure

Since ARF due to ATN comprises the majority of patients with severe renal failure seen by the intensivist, we will restrict our comments to this group of patients. The clinical course of ATN is variable. Renal failure is generally present for an average of seven to 21 days. If patients are oliguric upon presentation, the period of oliguria can last for several hours to several weeks. The more severe the renal failure the more prolonged is the oliguria. The oliguric phase of ARF is distinguished by a low GFR and urine output, resulting in minimal excretion of sodium, potassium, hydrogen, water, and phosphorus. Clinically, serum creatinine will tend to rise by 1–2 mg/dL and BUN by 30 mg/dL per day (14). If patients are very catabolic or have a crush injury, the rate of rise of both parameters can increase dramatically to as much as 2–3 mg/dL and 60 mg/dL per day, respectively.

During the recovery phase of ATN (so-called polyuric phase), which usually lasts for several days, urine output will increase in a step-wise fashion. The rise in urine output is often associated with only minor improvement in GFR, however. As a consequence, serum creatinine may continue to rise. Eventually, a significant improvement in GFR is manifest; serum creatinine falls, eventually reaching baseline values in four to 10 days. Indeed, in greater than 55–60% of patients who survive, renal function will return to baseline levels, but as many as 5–11% of patients will eventually require maintenance dialysis (15). Improvements in tubular function lag behind that of GFR. Therefore, during the recovery phase, sodium and potassium handling and concentrating ability remain impaired. In this phase, patients can manifest significant degrees of sodium and potassium wasting. The clinician will have to carefully evaluate these patients during recovery so as to avoid development of volume depletion that might aggravate or further induce renal deterioration.

In patients who have suffered a prolonged course of ARF (greater than four weeks), bouts of hypotension and exposure to nephrotoxins may have contributed. A large percentage of these patients may actually recover sufficient renal function to discontinue dialysis (16). However, some degree of persistent renal function will be present.

In the vast majority of patients with ARF, urine output will remain unchanged (nonoliguric ARF). These patients have higher levels of GFR than those with oliguria. The increments in BUN, serum creatinine, and electrolyte abnormalities are substantially less than in oliguric patients, and recovery of renal function is more rapid. These individuals are less likely to require dialysis, and renal failure generally lasts for less than 10–14 days (7).

IV. Clinical and Electrolyte Abnormalities in ARF

The kidney is the prime site for excretion of all the solutes resulting from metabolism of protein, including urea and other poorly described end-products. It is also the site for excretion of the creatinine derived from muscle. The kidney is responsible for regulation of salt and water homeostasis and potassium and acid-base balance. It is integral to the maintenance of phosphate balance and bone metabolism through its excretion of phosphate and production of the active vitamin D sterol, 1, 25 hydroxy D. Finally, it is the main site of erythropoietin synthesis, which is necessary to maintain hemoglobin levels in the normal range. Since the kidney has a large functional reserve, it is usually capable, despite a significant decline in renal function, of preventing marked electrolyte derangements, the development of severe anemia, and disturbances in divalent ion metabolism. However, once GFR has fallen below 10–15% of normal (10–15 mL/min), significant derangements in electrolyte balance and divalent ion metabolism occur, and BUN and serum creatinine rise substantially (14). When the renal failure is prolonged for several days, anemia also usually supervenes. These derangements often lead to the syndrome termed uremia, which literally means "urine in blood." The development of severe renal failure causing the uremic syndrome can contribute substantially to the morbidity and mortality of individuals in the intensive care unit who have failure of other organs (1,17,18).

Most patients with severe acute renal failure will have, in addition to elevations in BUN and serum creatinine, metabolic acidosis, hyperphosphatemia, hypocalcemia, and hyperkalemia. If careful attention is not paid to fluid balance, they may also develop hyponatremia or hypernatremia and volume overload. These derangements are summarized in Table 2.

The magnitude of the metabolic acidosis, hyperkalemia, and hyperphosphatemia in patients with ARF will depend not only on the severity of the reduction in GFR, but also upon the catabolic state of the patient. The severity of these derangements is higher in catabolic patients. Patients with high catabolic rates may require initiation of dialysis earlier in the course of their disease, and the frequency and total duration of dialysis therapy may be greater.

Renal failure severe enough to require dialysis is most often due to ATN developing in the context of multiorgan failure. Although hypotension and nephrotoxic exposure are major etiological factors, ATN is often multifactorial in origin, and a single etiological event is difficult to identify (1,19).

V. Treatment of ARF

Patients with specific types of glomerular disease, such as rapidly progressive glomerulonephritis, may require use of plasmapheresis, administration of steroids, and cytotoxic agents, and those with interstitial nephritis may require administration of steroids (10,20). However, the intensivist will rarely have to

Table 2 Clinical and Laboratory Abnormalities in Acute Renal Failure

Parameter	Expected finding in oliguric ARF[a]	Magnitude of change[b]
BUN	Elevated	Rise of 20–30 mg/dL/day
Serum creatinine	Elevated	Rise of 1–2 mg/dL/day
Serum potassium	Elevated	Rise of 0.3–0.6 mEq/L/day
Serum HCO_3^-	Depressed	Fall of 1–2 mEq/L/day
Serum Na	Elevated or depressed	Variable depending on fluid balance
Serum phosphorus	Elevated	Variable
Serum calcium	Depressed or normal	Variable related in part to phosphorus level
Extracellular volume	Elevated, normal or depressed	Variable depending on cardiac status and intake
Hematocrit	Depressed or normal	Variable depending on co-morbid conditions

[a]Changes with nonoliguric renal failure generally less prominent and less predictable than in oliguric renal failure.
[b]Deviations in these parameters may be greater in the presence of crush injury of extremely catabolic patient.
Abbreviations: ARF, acute renal failure; BUN, blood urea nitrogen.

deal with treatment of these disorders. More frequently, they will have to deal with treatment of patients who have acute tubular necrosis, the most common cause of sustained severe ARF seen in the hospital (19).

Treatment of ATN can be divided into three phases: immediate therapy, conservative therapy, and renal replacement therapy. Immediate therapy of ARF includes measures geared to rapidly reverse or modify the course of the disease. Unfortunately, once injury is established, it is often too late. Conservative therapy of ARF is used for the treatment of patients without uremic symptoms, marked electrolyte disturbances, or severe volume overload. Renal replacement therapy is initiated in patients with severe renal failure who have marked electrolyte disturbances or show evidence of the uremic syndrome. It may also be initiated prophylatically to prevent the onset of the uremic syndrome.

VI. Immediate Treatment of Established ARF

The immediate treatment of ARF due to ATN generally has included the use of pharmacologic agents shown in Table 3, which are designed to reverse or attenuate the course of the disorder. These agents, which include diuretics, calcium channel blockers, atrial natriuretic peptides, and dopamine, remain popular in the intensive care setting, despite the dearth of evidence supporting their effectiveness (21–23).

Table 3 Agents Used in the Immediate Treatment of Acute Renal Failure

Agent	Comments
Diuretics	Dose start at 2–4 mg/kg/body wt.; if no response after two doses, discontinue
Dopamine renal dose ($<$5 ug/kg/bd wt./day)	Data do not demonstrate beneficial effects
Calcium channel blockers	Experimental data in animals show some benefit but no clinical evidence of beneficial effect in humans
Natriuretic peptides	Experimental studies in animals show beneficial effects, but controlled clinical studies in patients have not demonstrated effectiveness

Diuretics have been used by clinicians for many years with the expressed goal of converting oliguric to nonoliguric renal failure (24). Patients with non-oliguric renal failure have a more benign course than those with oliguric renal failure and are easier to manage (7). Since experimental studies have shown diuretics reduce renal oxygen demand in portions of the nephron injured in ATN and can also induce higher flow rates to prevent nephron obstruction (25), these agents have been conceived as potential therapies accelerating the rate of recovery of renal function. However, clinical studies have not borne out any significant benefit of the use of diuretics in the majority of patients. Although a detectable increment in urine output can be observed, there is no detectable rise in GFR (23). Moreover, although in some studies the need for dialysis may be reduced, there is no evidence that renal function recovers more rapidly or mortality is reduced (23). Indeed, mortality may even be increased (23). Thus, although this could potentially make management of fluid and electrolyte balance easier, we and others do not advocate the continual administration of diuretics. Rather we recommend administering furosemide 200–400 mg and repeating it again if urine output fails to rise. It should be emphasized that it is important that the patient be demonstrated to be euvolemic prior to diuretic use, as volume depletion can exacerbate nascent renal failure. Intermittent or continuous diuretic administration in a patient with established renal failure is not recommended and should be discouraged.

A. Calcium Antagonists

Experimental studies have supported the concept that changes in intracellular calcium play a role in the genesis of ARF (14,26). Moreover, administration of calcium channel inhibitors cause a rise in GFR. Studies in patients receiving renal transplants or radiocontrast material have shown both improvement and no benefit from administration of calcium channel blockers (26,27). The role of these agents in the treatment and prevention of ARF remains to be clarified. At present, we do not advocate the administration of calcium antagonists either to patients with established acute renal failure or to those who are to receive intravenous contrast.

B. Dopamine

The administration of dopamine in low doses, so-called renal dose dopamine (<5 ug/kg/min), has been popularized in the treatment of ARF, as it is commonly associated with an increase in urine output and has been thought to increase renal blood flow (22). In several controlled clinical trials in which renal dose dopamine was administered, there was no difference between the dopamine and placebo groups in peak serum creatinine concentrations during treatment, in the increase from baseline to highest value during treatment, in the numbers of patients whose serum creatinine concentration exceeded 300 μmol/L, or in who required renal replacement therapy (28). Durations of ICU and hospital stay and death rates were also similar in the groups (23). Moreover, administration of this agent can cause tachyarrhythmias, pulmonary shunting, and in rare cases, gut or digital necrosis. Thus, despite its popularity, at present we do not advocate the use of renal dose dopamine in the treatment of ARF.

VII. Natriuretic Peptides

Natriuretic peptides, such as atrial natriuretic peptide (ANP), are hormones secreted by many cells in the cardiac atria in response to plasma volume expansion. The renal effects of ANP are to directly increase GFR by altering pre- and post-glomerular resistances and to inhibit salt and water reabsorption by the collecting duct (29). Experimental studies in animals had suggested potential beneficial effects of ANP. The efficacy of ANP in established ATN in humans has been evaluated in several major trials. In a larger, multicenter trial in which 504 patients with ATN were randomized to a 24-hour infusion of placebo or a synthetic form of ANP (30), no overall difference between the two groups (43% vs. 47% dialysis-free survival with placebo) was found, although oliguric patients had a better dialysis-free survival (8% vs. 27%). Oliguric patients who subsequently became nonoliguric had the best dialysis-free survival.

Since it appeared that oliguric patients might benefit from the administration of this agent, a subsequent study was performed to evaluate the use of the drug alone in 222 patients with oliguric ARF. In contrast to the previous study, the 24 hour infusion of ANP provided no benefit (21). Thus administration of ANP in patients with established ARF at this time is not recommended. Further studies, however, are in progress.

Several other agents have been used in attempts to modify the course of experimental ARF. These include ATP-MgCl$_2$, amino acids and small oligopeptides (e.g., glutathione), growth factors, and thyroxine (31,32). Clinical data using these compounds are scanty or nonexistent.

In summary, once patients with established ARF have been demonstrated to be euvolemic, an attempt should be made to convert them from oliguric to nonoliguric renal failure by administration of diuretics. If this is not successful, no further diuretic should be administered. Administration of renal dose dopamine, ANP, or calcium channel blockers is not recommended at this time.

VIII. Conservative Therapy of ARF

Once a diagnosis of intrinsic renal failure has been made, potentially reversible causes have been identified and treated, and pharmacological interventions have been used without success, patients should be treated conservatively. The goals of conservative treatment include: prevention of severe electrolyte derangements, such as hyperkalemia or metabolic acidosis; prevention of severe volume overload; maintenance of nutrition; and prevention of uremic symptoms. During this and other phases of ARF, exposure to nephrotoxins and development of hypotension or volume depletion should be avoided. Avoiding the latter is particularly important since the kidney with ATN is very sensitive to diminished perfusion. Although the vessels of the normal kidney can dilate in response to ischemia, thereby preserving renal blood flow, the kidney with ATN has an impaired response, presumably because vascular endothelial injury reduces the release of vasodilating substances (25).

The patient should be monitored carefully with particular attention to blood pressure, volume status, and fluid and electrolyte balance, including measurement of daily intake and output, body weight, serum sodium, potassium, chloride, bicarbonate, calcium, phosphorus, BUN, creatinine, hemoglobin and hematocrit, and serum albumin. With the exception of hemoglobin, hematocrit, and serum albumin, these measurements should be obtained daily, but in some cases may have to be obtained more frequently. During the period of conservative therapy, the patient should also be observed for the development of neurological complications, infections, and pulmonary or cardiovascular disease that might cause the physician to initiate renal replacement therapy earlier than he/she had intended.

In some patients, clinical assessment of cardiovascular function is insufficient, and more invasive techniques to assess volume status, such as central venous pressure or Swan–Ganz catheterization, may be required. We tend to favor the aggressive use of these procedures given the difficulty of assessing volume status in critically ill patients. The use of these procedures, however, continue to be controversial (33).

Fluid intake should be reduced to match urine output and insensible losses. This will often require hyperconcentration of intravenous solutions in patients requiring antibiotics and vasopressor agents, a task that is often neglected. To maintain a euvolemic 'state', sodium intake should be adjusted to match urine excretion and gastrointestinal losses. Similarly, potassium intake should be carefully regulated. It is common to use the so-called renal diet, which includes 40 mEq per day of potassium and sodium intake of 2 g. A slight loss of weight each day is common, but one must be vigilant to avoid malnutrition, which can develop rapidly in the seriously ill septic patient. In this regard, serum albumin can fall precipitously in several days and contribute to increased mortality, besides making the dialysis procedure more difficult (34).

Nutritional management should be geared to slow the accumulation of nitrogen waste products and avoid severe electrolyte disturbances. Patients capable of being fed can receive 40 g high-quality protein to meet a minimum daily requirement of 0.6 g/kg/bd wt. Calories can be provided in the form of simple carbohydrates, such as jelly and sugar. An intake of 3000 kcal/day or more a day can be required to prevent hypercatabolism. If the patient cannot eat, a stomach tube should be inserted and tube feeding given by constant infusion or intermittent bolus. If the patient cannot tolerate tube feeding, total parenteral nutrition will be necessary.

Electrolyte derangements are not uncommon given the loss of the kidney's ability to regulate water excretion, potassium, acid-base, and divalent ion balance. Hyperkalemia, the most serious electrolyte disturbance since it can cause important cardiac rhythm disturbance, is inevitable. The combined effects of acidemia, cellular release of potassium, and a marked decrement in GFR are important contributing factors. This disturbance is far more severe in the oliguric or anuric patient, and the patient should be monitored carefully for the onset of this abnormality. Hyperkalemia may be manifest by electrocardiographic changes, but this is not invariable. Several studies have demonstrated the failure of routine EKG to detect changes in serum potassium (35). As noted below, if the hyperkalemia is mild, it can be treated with the potassium exchange resin, kayexelate. It is important to remember that the effectiveness of this agent requires an intact distal colon and a functional bowel. Also, use of this agent results in sodium input as each 1 g of kayexelate administered results in the exchange of 1 mEq of sodium for every mEq of potassium removed. Disorders of water balance are also common with hyponatremia, occurring more frequently than hypernatremia, but both electrolyte derangements should be avoided. Poor attention to fluid balance, including failure to take into account water produced from carbohydrate metabolism and that released from injured tissue, is an important factor in the production of hyponatremia.

A high anion gap metabolic acidosis is common. It is most frequently due to the impairment in renal acid excretion but can also be due to lactic acidosis occurring in patients with sepsis and hypotension. When associated with renal failure, the fall in plasma bicarbonate concentration is approximately 1–2 mEq/L per day, but it can be substantially greater in the face of muscle breakdown or a hypercatabolic state as seen in patients with crush injury or sepsis. Given the potential contribution of severe metabolic acidosis to impaired cardiovascular function and muscle breakdown, the acidosis is often treated with base to maintain plasma bicarbonate concentration above 20 mEq/L (36). Calculation of the total bicarbonate deficit and space of distribution of administered bicarbonate is essential for determining the quantity of base to be administered to individual patients as illustrated below:

Bicarbonate requirements (mEq)

= Bicarbonate deficit (desired plasma bicarbonate

− Actual plasma bicarbonate) × Bicarbonate space

The bicarbonate space can range from 50% to 200% body weight and is dependent in large part on the prevailing level of plasma bicarbonate (37). It is approximately 50% body weight with values above 10–15 mEq/L but is closer to 100% body weight when plasma bicarbonate falls below 5 to 6 mEq/L.

Patients with severe lactic acidosis can require large quantities of bicarbonate given the substantial production of organic acid. The accompanying sodium given with bicarbonate can exacerbate volume overload and should be considered in estimates of sodium balance.

An increased serum phosphorus concentration is inevitable once renal function is severely reduced, but its magnitude will depend in part on the catabolic state of the patient. Hyperphosphatemia has been traditionally treated by the oral administration of phosphate binders, such as calcium carbonate or calcium acetate. The recent recognition of vessel calcifications resulting from the increased calcium intake with these binders has caused some to recommend the use of noncalcium containing binders, such as Renagel, in patients with chronic renal failure. Similar recommendations have not been made for ARF.

Hypocalcemia due to the high serum phosphorus, low vitamin D levels, and bone resistance to the actions of parathyroid hormone is frequent. In cases of severe hyperphosphatemia observed in patients with rhabdomyolysis, serum calcium can be extremely low. Clinical complications, such as tetany or seizure, are infrequent, so hypocalcemia rarely requires specific treatment.

Uric acid levels usually rise but generally remain below 12–15 mg/dL; values higher than this often suggest tumor lysis syndrome or some variant of uric acid nephropathy (38). Gout is unusual and, for the most part, no specific treatment of the elevated uric acid levels is required.

Rarely, metabolic alkalosis rather than metabolic acidosis can be observed. The alkalosis can be due to the use of nasogastric suction with the generation of substantial quantities of bicarbonate or prior excessive use of diuretics. The gastric alkalosis can be prevented or ameliorated by the administration of H2 blockers or proton pump inhibitors. There is evidence that severe alkalemia (blood pH > 7.55) can contribute to increased morbidity and mortality in patients in the ICU (39). Therefore, if severe alkalemia develops, treatment with 0.1 N HCl or the use of a low bicarbonate dialysate might be required. If acid is administered, the quantity of acid necessary to lower plasma bicarbonate a desired

458 Kraut, Duffney, and Vaghaiwalla

amount can be calculated in a similar fashion to the method used for determining base requirements with metabolic acidosis.

The development of renal failure, particularly when it is severe, has a dramatic impact on the mortality of hospitalized patients. However, even among patients with ARF, mortality can vary greatly depending not only on the severity of renal dysfunction but also on the types of comorbid conditions (17–19). Uncomplicated ARF generally has a mortality of 7–20%. By contrast, the mortality of patients postoperatively or who are critically ill can be as high as 50–80% (19).

Prior to the advent of dialysis, the most frequent cause of death of patients with ARF included severe electrolyte disturbances, such as hyperkalemia and metabolic acidosis, gastrointestinal hemorrhage, and severe volume overload. Presently, infection is the most frequent cause of death, followed by gastrointestinal bleeding and cardiovascular disease (1,40).

Infection accounts for 50–70% of the mortality of ARF patients. The increased risk for infection is due, in part, to the impaired immune function associated with the uremic milieu, but also to the presence of important comorbid conditions. All patients with ARF should be monitored carefully for evidence of infection and treated aggressively with antibiotics if infection is detected.

Gastrointestinal hemorrhage due to stress ulceration was a frequent cause of death prior to the introduction of antacids and proton pump inhibitors or histamine H_2 blockers as prophylactic agents. Bleeding from the GI tract and other sites is favored by the abnormalities in platelet factor 3, which prolong the bleeding time characteristic of severe renal failure. Amelioration of the uremic milieu by dialysis can be effective in improving the bleeding time in approximately 50% of patients. However, administration of deamino-8-L-arginine vasopressin (DDAVP), cryoprecipitate, and conjugated estrogens are often more effective and should be considered should a rapid improvement in bleeding status be necessary. DDAVP is typically infused over 30 minutes in a dose of 0.3 ug/kg of body weight and is effective within minutes. Unfortunately, because of the short duration of action of this compound (one to four hours), frequent dosing may be required. Conjugated estrogens (0.6 mg/kg IV daily for five days) have a delayed onset of action (three to five days), but the duration of the therapeutic effect can be as long as 14 days.

IX. Renal Replacement Therapy

In patients with severe ARF, which lasts more than a few days, particularly if it is oliguric or anuric in nature, conservative therapy may be insufficient to prevent significant electrolyte derangements, marked volume overload, and/or the onset of the uremic syndrome. Therefore, renal replacement therapy will have to be started.

The absolute indications for immediate initiation of dialysis are shown in Table 4. The indications have changed little in the last 30 years. They include: severe

Table 4 Indications for Initiation of Dialysis in Acute Renal Failure

Indication	Comments
Hyperkalemia	Serum K > 6–6.5. If serum K > 7.0 mEq/L, aggressive measures to stabilize membrane and shift K into cells should be taken. Most frequent cause for immediate initiation of dialysis
Severe volume overload	Indicated in patients unresponsive to diuretics
Metabolic acidosis	Unresponsive to bicarbonate administration or base contraindicated because of risk of volume overload
Pericarditis	Can occur with BUN ≥60 mg/dL but unusual with BUN <100–150 mg/dL
Severe central nervous System abnormalities	Includes stupor or coma and seizures. Unusual with BUN <100–150 mg/dL
Presence of uremic symptoms	Nausea, vomiting, decreased mentation
Prophylatic dialysis[a]	Initiated before onset of uremic symptoms with BUN <100 mg/dL and serum creatinine <8 mg/dL (estimated GFR <10 mL/min)

[a]In older patients or those with reduced muscle mass may be initiated at lower level of BUN and serum creatinine.
Abbreviations: BUN, blood urea nitrogen; GFR, glomerular filteration rate.

hyperkalemia, severe volume overload and severe metabolic acidosis that are unresponsive to conservative treatment, acute pericarditis, and severe CNS disturbances.

Hyperkalemia is the most frequent reason for emergent initiation of dialysis. A serum potassium concentration higher than 6.5 mEq/L can induce heart block or cause severe rhythm disturbances. Treatment with agents meant to protect the myocardium, such as calcium, or cause uptake of potassium by cells, such as administration of bicarbonate, insulin, or β-adrenergic agents, are important, but temporizing measures. Eventually, potassium has to be removed from the body. The use of the cation-exchange resin, kayexelate requires intact colonic function and is associated with retention of sodium; therefore, it should only be used in stable patients with mild hyperkalemia, serum potassium concentrations less than 6 to 6.5 mEq/L. Thus, most patients with severe renal failure and hyperkalemia will require renal replacement therapy. Potassium removal is most rapid with intermittent haemodialysis and is least rapid with peritoneal dialysis. Clinicians should be aware of the rebound effect noted when potassium is rapidly removed with intermittent hemodialysis: serum potassium may fall during the treatment but, several hours after dialysis is discontinued, can rise close to pre-dialysis levels (41). Therefore, in some patients with marked hyperkalemia treated with intermittent haemodialysis, more frequent dialyses might be necessary. Slower but continual removal of potassium with continuous renal replacement therapies may avoid the rebound effect.

Volume overload is frequent in patients with sepsis and other disorders associated with ARF, particularly since cardiac function may be concomitantly impaired. Administration of antibiotics, blood products, and saline for the treatment of critically ill patients contributes to fluid excess. In this regard, Mukau et al. found that more than 95% of patients with postoperative ARF had a fluid excess of greater than 10 L prior to initiation of dialysis (42). Preventing volume overload and achieving negative fluid balance may have important implications for survival. Negative fluid balance in patients within the first three days of admission for septic shock was associated with improved survival (43). Given the presence of a marked reduction in GFR, diuretics are usually ineffective. Although all modes of dialysis can remove fluid, various forms of continuous renal replacement therapy described below are usually the safest and most effective means or removing large volumes.

Metabolic acidosis due to renal failure per se or lactic acidosis, seen in patients with impaired perfusion, can have deleterious effects on cardiac function and muscle metabolism (36). If administration of base is contraindicated because of impending or actual volume overload, dialysis can be used both to deliver bicarbonate rapidly and remove fluid concomitantly.

Pericarditis due to renal failure was not uncommon in the past because patients were not dialyzed till blood urea nitrogen levels were often substantially above 100 mg/dL (44). This complication is rare today as it is the convention to start dialysis, even in the absence of uremic symptoms, before this point is reached. Marked changes in mental status and/or seizures are also unusual manifestations of ARF since this complication is only observed with marked elevations in BUN. Gastrointestinal symptoms, such as nausea, vomiting, and a decrease in appetite, may be observed reflecting the onset of the uremic syndrome. Obviously, in the critically ill patient it may be difficult to attribute these symptoms to uremia per se, but if they should occur in the presence of BUN values approaching 100 mg/dL, they should be assumed to be related to the uremic syndrome.

Even in the absence of overt symptoms or the indications for initiation of dialysis described above, it is common practice to begin dialysis in noncachetic patients with normal muscle mass when the BUN value exceeds 100 mg/dL or the serum creatinine level exceeds 9 mg/dL, so called "prophylactic dialysis." In patients with cachexia or the elderly in whom the serum creatinine concentration may belie the true reduction in glomerular filtration rate, one may initiate dialysis at levels of BUN and serum creatinine substantially lower.

The practice of prophylactic dialysis was first introduced by the landmark studies of Teschan et al. (44). In this study, 15 patients with acute oliguric renal failure had dialysis begun before the BUN reached 100 mg/dL. Patients were dialyzed for approximately six hours, sufficient to maintain BUN less than

75 mg/dL. Mortality of these patients was 33%, substantially lower than the 50–65% observed in historic controls. Several other uncontrolled or retrospective studies have also confirmed the benefits of early or prophylactic dialysis, although the level of BUN at which dialysis was initiated varied greatly (46).

In 1975, one of the first prospective studies examining the impact of prophylactic dialysis was done by Conger (47). Eighteen patients with post-traumatic acute renal failure were randomized to an intensive dialysis regimen to keep BUN and serum creatinine concentrations less than 70 mg/dL and 5 mg/dL, respectively. In a nonintensive-regimen group, the BUN was allowed to rise to 150 mg/dL and serum creatinine to 10 mg/dL prior to dialysis. Survival in the intensive group was 65%, as compared to 20% in the nonintensive dialysis group. Other similar studies have, for the most part, supported the benefits of early initiation of dialysis (48). The mechanisms underlying the improvement in mortality with early dialysis have not been established. Improvement in the uremic milieu enhancing immune function, prevention of volume overload, correction of acid-base and electrolyte abnormalities, and removal of fluid to allow the administration of increased quantities of protein and volume necessary to ameliorate the catabolic state that attends ARF are strong candidates (43). Recently, noting the possible benefits of continuous renal replacement therapy (CRRT) in treating sepsis, some clinicians have advocated initiating this treatment early in the course of ARF (49). Given the high mortality of sepsis, this may present an additional reason for starting this form of renal replacement therapy.

Presently, we advocate initiating renal replacement therapy on a prophylactic basis in all patients with severe ARF. However, the clinician should be aware that the issue of the point at which dialysis should be initiated remains a point of contention.

X. Modalities of Dialysis Used in the Treatment of ARF

The different types of renal replacement therapy available for the treatment of ARF, with their advantages and disadvantages, are shown in Table 5. The forms of renal replacement therapy include: peritoneal dialysis, intermittent or daily hemodialysis, slow low-efficiency dialysis, slow arteriovenous or venovenous ultrafiltration, slow continuous venovenous or arteriovenous hemofiltration, and continuous arteriovenous or venvovenous haemodialysis-hemofiltration.

XI. Peritoneal Dialysis

Peritoneal dialysis was the first modality of renal replacement therapy to be utilized in the treatment of ARF. In peritoneal dialysis, a stiff Teflon catheter is placed at the bedside to access the peritoneal cavity. Fluid is instilled into the peritoneal cavity and solute removal is accomplished via diffusion through the peritoneal membrane. Solute removal with this technique depends on the

Table 5 Modalities of Renal Replacement Therapy Available for Treatment of Acute Renal Failure

Modality of therapy	Advantages	Disadvantages
Peritoneal dialysis	Slow rate of solute and fluid removal No need for systemic anticoagulation	Slow rate of solute and fluid removal Increased protein losses Adverse effect of glucose load
Intermittent hemodialysis	Rapid solute and fluid removal Short duration allowing patients to be available for studies	Rapid osmotic shifts Risk of hemodynamic instability Systemic anticoagulation usually required[a] Solute removal correlated with ultrafiltration rate
SCUF	Slow fluid removal Hypotension less common than IHD	
SLED	Slow solute and fluid removal Can be done at night Special dialysis machines not required Hypotension less common than IHD	Rate of solute removal slower than with IHD
CAVH	Slow solute and fluid removal Does not require blood pump Hypotension less common than IHD	Requires arterial cannulation. Systolic BP > 80
CVVH	Slow fluid removal Solute removal by convection Hypotension less common than IHD Hypotension uncommon	Special machines required
CVVHDF[b]	Slow and continuous fluid and solute removal Effective small and middle molecule removal Hypotension less common than IHD	Special machines required

[a] All forms of CRRT including SCUF, SLED, CAVH, CVVH, CVVHDF also require some form of anticoagulation.
[b] Most common form of continuous renal replacement therapy used in U.S.
Abbreviations: SCUF, slow continuous ultrafiltration; SLED, slow low efficiency dialysis; CAVH, continuous arteriovenous hemofiltration; CVVH, continuous venovenous hemofiltration; CVVHDF, continuous venovenous hemodiafiltration; IHD, intermittent hemodialysis.

dialysate volume and length of time dialysate is allowed to stay in the peritoneal space before drainage (dwell time). In many cases, 2-L exchanges are accomplished every hour. Since there is a 50% equilibration between serum and dialysate urea levels during the 30 minute dwell time, this schedule provides 24 L of urea clearance per day. Associated net filtration of approximately 2 L/day will add to these predicted values.

Fluid removal with peritoneal dialysis is directly dependent on the concentration of glucose in the dialysate and the dwell times allowed. With 1.5% dextrose solution, a 2-L exchange performed every hour can extract approximately 100–200 mL of fluid whereas a 4.25% solution can remove 500 mL per hour. Prolonging dwell times decreases net filtration rate because of an increasing equilibration of dialysate glucose with serum levels, thus decreasing the osmotic drive for fluid removal.

Potassium is generally not present in the peritoneal fluid facilitating its removal from the body. However, even assuming almost complete equilibration of peritoneal fluid with serum potassium, the quantity of potassium extracted with this method is relatively small: approximately 8 mEq/hr. Thus, peritoneal dialysis is not a favored therapy for this purpose.

Theoretical advantages of peritoneal dialysis include slow rates of solute and fluid removal and the absence of the need for anticoagulation. The former, of course, can also be a liability in patients in whom large volumes or solute loads have to be removed. Despite the theoretical advantages, this mode of dialysis is not widely used in the U.S. for the treatment of ARF. Reasons given to explain its infrequent use include: the greater severity of renal failure and hypercatabolism of patients treated today, which requires more rapid solute removal than in the past; the presence of ARF in patients with intrabdominal surgery preventing the use of a peritoneal catheter; the increased intra-abdominal pressure accompanying PD, which can compromise lung function; the relatively large protein losses that can ensue during the procedure, contributing to protein malnutrition; and the possible deleterious effects of dextrose absorption from the peritoneal cavity (50) on the course of ARF. Moreover, several serious complications have been reported with this technique, including: perforation of intrabdominal viscuses, hemorrhage, and peritonitis.

A recent study comparing peritoneal dialysis to hemofiltration in the treatment of infection-associated ARF highlights the relative ineffectiveness of this modality of therapy. In this study of patients with sepsis-induced ARF, the rate of resolution of metabolic acidosis and the rate of decline in serum creatinine concentration were much lower in patients treated with PD than those treated with hemofiltration. More importantly, the mortality rate (15% vs. 47%) and duration of renal replacement therapy required was much less in patients treated with hemofiltration (51). Thus, although peritoneal dialysis can be used for the treatment of ARF, for the most part it is not a first line therapy. However, there continues to be a group of supporters for this mode of dialysis, particularly in countries with limited resources.

XII. Intermittent Hemodialysis

Intermittent hemodialysis (IHD) is presently the most widely utilized renal replacement therapy for the treatment of ARF in the U.S., with as many as 70% of
patients with renal failure requiring renal replacement therapy being treated
with IHD (52). Surveys of U.S.-based physicians confirmed their preference of
IHD. In the survey, the decision to use IHD was not based on controlled observations, but rather was made because intermittent hemodialysis was considered
easy to use, the practitioners had considerable experience with this modality of
treatment, and it had proved to be effective (52). By contrast, CRRT, the
second most popular method of renal replacement therapy, was usually restricted
to patients who were hemodynamically compromised, required significant nutritional support, or were considerably volume overloaded.

Intermittent hemodialysis is routinely administered for four hours three
times per week (53). Dialysis for a longer period of time or more frequently
has generally been restricted to patients who are very catabolic with high rates
of nitrogenous waste production or who are volume overloaded. On the other
hand, patients with significant residual renal function have often required
fewer treatments per week, especially when the renal failure is nonoliguric.
The major advantage of intermittent hemodialysis has been its highly efficient
solute and fluid removal, thus limiting treatment time, making the patient available for other procedures and treatments.

Paradoxically, the rapid fluid and solute removal can also be a disadvantage
as it may be poorly tolerated in critically ill hemodynamically-unstable patients.
Other disadvantages of this modality of therapy are the need for large-bore
hemoaccess, prolonged contact between blood and dialyzer membrane resulting
in the generation of various cytokines and other factors, and the requirement for
anticoagulation.

Although placement of a double-lumen catheter in the femoral vein was
first utilized to gain access to the circulation, this is less frequently used today
because the catheter can not remain in place for more than a few days. Catheterization of the subclavian vein was the next site chosen as it can be left in place for
prolonged periods. The procedure is rarely complicated by hemothorax or pneumothorax. These complications can occur even after previously successful treatments. Cardiac arrhythmias, thrombophlebitis, sepsis, air embolism, and access
site infection are other complications. It has also been shown that prolonged cannulation of the subclavian vein can lead to significant subclavian vein stenosis
(54). Given the risk and importance of catheter infection, careful attention to
sterile technique during placement and meticulous care of the access site are
essential.

Because of the latter complication of subclavian vein usage, the right
internal jugular vein is now more frequently used. The one advantage of this
method is that the catheter's route is relatively straight, thus avoiding the sharp
angulations associated with the subclavian route. Nonetheless, retrograde

cannulation of the subclavian vein is possible, and radiological evaluation of placement is required. A drawback to this technique is the relatively awkward placement and the difficulty of access site care. In patients in whom it is anticipated that renal failure might last for a prolonged period, a tunneled access to the internal jugular is becoming more popular and allows for much easier access site care. The need for anticoagulation is one of the most significant disadvantages associated with haemodialysis as it can contribute to bleeding in seriously ill patients. Several methods have been proposed for reducing hemorrhagic risks. Regional heparinization is performed by infusing heparin into the blood before it reaches the filter and infusion of protamine into the blood after the filter, but this procedure has fallen out of favor because of the "heparin rebound" effect, which may appear up to 10 hours after treatment.

Low-dose heparin (10–20 units/kg/hr) and bedside monitoring of coagulation status have been shown to be superior to regional heparinization in controlling hemorrhagic risks. Low-molecular-weight heparin has been proposed because of its limited effect on platelet function. Unfortunately, these low-molecular-weight fragments have a prolonged half-life (18 hours) and are not neutralized by protamine. Citrate anticoagulation has been used successfully but requires careful attention to dialysate calcium concentration and may require substantial amounts of sodium and fluid infusions.

Because of their short half-life, prostacyclin and its derivatives have been used. Although successfully employed in stable patients, prostacyclin may be inappropriate for the critically ill. Aside from a considerable list of potentially troublesome secondary effects, including flushing, nausea, headache, and abdominal pain, the antiplatelet action of prostacyclin is still demonstrable up to two hours after cessation of infusion, and there is no known method for reversing the effect.

An increasingly popular approach is to completely avoid anticoagulation by using high blood flows and frequent saline flushes of the filter. The quantity of saline used varies, but ranges between 100 and 200 mL every 30 minutes. The new, more porous dialyzers have ultrafiltration capabilities that will easily remove the excess fluid administered. In patients receiving anticoagulants to facilitate dialysis, the risk of hemorrhage is always present. If bleeding occurs during the dialysis procedure, previously administered heparin should be neutralized by protamine.

The solute clearance and ultrafiltration rate with intermittent dialysis depends upon the blood flow and the characteristic of the artificial dialyzer chosen. With a blood flow of 200 to 300 mL/min and dialysate flow of 500 to 800 mL/min, most dialyzers will produce 150–250 mL/min of urea clearance and an ultrafiltrate of 1 L–3 L/hr. The limiting factors in achieving effective clearance during the treatment are often the failure to maintain high blood flow using a temporary access and episodes of hypotension that cause a reduction in dialysis time and clotting of the dialyzer. In addition, the use of double-lumen catheters may allow a certain percentage of dialyzed blood leaving the efferent lumen to reenter the afferent lumen (recirculation of approximately 8–10%), which can hinder the effectiveness of the dialysis treatment.

Urea removal during hemodialysis follows first-order kinetics with a urea distribution equivalent to that of total body water. A typical four-hour dialysis will lower pretreatment urea levels by approximately 50–70%. With the newer computerized dialysis machines, solute and volume removal can be carefully controlled so as to limit the problems arising from the procedure. Sequential isolated ultrafiltration, in which diffusion of solute is stopped, has proved to be an especially effective means of removing large volumes rapidly (1–2 L/h) without inducing hypotension.

Determining the adequacy of dialysis has proved to be important in treatment of patients with chronic renal failure. Surprisingly, the adequacy of dialysis is not routinely monitored in patients with acute renal failure. This may be important as recent studies have indicated that many patients do not receive the prescribed dose of dialysis (55,56). Furthermore, some studies have suggested that more intensive dialysis can contribute to improved outcomes (57). The impact of intensive dialysis as compared to conventional treatment is presently being examined in a large prospective study sponsored by the NIH and Veterans Administration.

Complications of the dialysis procedure can occur and contribute to the morbidity and mortality of the underlying illness, including hypotension, cardiac arrhythmias, hypoxemia, hemorrhage, air embolism, pyrogenic reactions, and dysequilibrium syndromes.

Rapid fluid removal may not be well tolerated in seriously ill patients and is the most obvious cause of hypotension. Vasopressors are often utilized in IHD as well as other forms of dialysis to maintain blood pressure. Use of pressor agents can enable the physician to remove fluid without reducing blood pressure substantially. Logically, the physician should try to utilize as low a dose of pressor agents as possible so as not to promote regional ischemia or promote lactic acid production.

If a cuprophane- or cellulose-based membrane is used, it can, in rare cases, cause enhanced activation of complement and the acute onset of severe respiratory distress and hypotension resistant to volume replacement, sometimes referred to as the "first-use syndrome." This can be managed with intravenous or subcutaneous epinephrine, methylprednisolone, and diphenhydramine. This syndrome can largely be avoided by switching to a more biocompatible membrane.

More recently, a similar anaphylactoid type syndrome has been described involving the use of polyacrylonitrile dialyzers (AN-69) in patients treated with angiotensin-converting enzyme inhibitors (58). Regardless of the cause, symptomatic hypotension during dialysis should be initially treated by lowering the transmembrane pressure, decreasing the blood flow, evaluating for cardiogenic causes, and administering normal saline, albumin, or hypertonic glucose. If significant wheezing is present, the first-use syndrome should be suspected.

Cardiac arrhythmias may occur as a result of hypotension or due to rapid lowering of serum potassium concentration, even if serum potassium remains within the normal range. Of course, this can be a particular problem in patients receiving digitalis, and this can be avoided by raising the dialysate potassium concentration from 2 mEq/L to 3 or even 4 mEq/L.

The removal of lung fluid with the dialysis procedure can promote the transfer of fluid from the alveolar space, thereby improving pulmonary function and reducing the level of hypoxemia. Rarely, the dialysis procedure, per se, can actually induce hypoxemia as a result of rapid activation of complement leading to leukoagglutination in the lung and severe bronchospasm (59). This complication is uncommon with the utilization of biocompatible membranes.

A constellation of signs and symptoms, including headache, nausea, muscle irritability, obtundation, and delirium or seizures, may be associated with rapid correction of severe uremia, a syndrome termed dialysis disequilibrium (60). This syndrome is most frequent when the BUN values are above 150 mg/dL prior to starting dialysis but can be observed with lower values. To decrease the risk for this complication, short treatments (two to three hours) with a low blood flow (<200 mL/min) are generally utilized when dialysis is first started.

Although IHD is often required for the treatment of established ARF, there is some concern that the procedure itself might prolong the course of ARF. IHD usually leads to a reduction in urine output initially, the impact of which is unknown. Furthermore, during the procedure the patient can be subject to episodes of hypotension that might potentially exacerbate ARF. Finally, some clinical and animals studies had indicated contact of blood with the dialysis membrane induced generation of cytokines, with activation of platelets and white blood cells, induction of humoral factors, and activation of complement and coagulation pathways (61) that could prolong the course or delay recovery from ARF. This effect was attributed to dialysis with cuprophane membrane (62,63). To examine whether a more biocompatible membrane might affect the course of renal failure, Hakim et al. (64) compared the effects of biocompatible versus cuprophane membrane on mortality and recovery of renal function in 153 patients with ARF. In these studies, there was a higher rate of survival and rate of recovery of renal function in those patients treated with biocompatible membrane. On the other hand, other studies did not confirm these results (65). However, given that the cost of the biocompatible membranes is not dramatically greater than that of cuprophane-based dialyzers, and there may be some theoretical advantages to the use of these membranes, we favor the use of biocompatible membranes for the treatment of all patients with ARF.

XIII. Continuous Forms of Renal Replacement Therapy

Although peritoneal dialysis is in a sense a continuous form of renal replacement therapy, the term continuous renal replacement therapy (CRRT) has traditionally been restricted to procedures in which dialysis is carried out throughout the day, utilizing an extracorporeal circuit containing membranes that are highly permeable to water and low molecular weight solutes. This mode of dialysis was first introduced for the treatment of ARF approximately 20 years ago (66,67). Although clinical surveys have revealed it has remained less frequently used than IHD in the U.S., it is the preferred mode of treatment of ARF in Europe and Australia (68–70). Indeed, in some centers, such as the St Bartolo Hospital in Vincenza, Italy, CVVH was the sole renal replacement therapy given to over 400 patients with ARF since 1980 (71). More recently, large hospitals in the U.S. are utilizing CRRT more frequently; for example, at Massachusetts General Hospital, it accounts for more than 70% of patients with ARF (personal communication). Some of the more commonly used types of CRRT are schematically depicted in Figure 1. CRRT differs from intermittent hemodialysis in several ways. The blood flow (100–200 mL/min) is lower, and if hemodiafiltration is performed, the countercurrent dialysate flow (17–34 mL/min) is also substantially lower. As a consequence, the rate of small solute removal (such as urea) is lower in CRRT than in IHD. On the other hand, since there can be a significant component of convective transport, middle molecule clearance is higher than in IHD. Also, since there is considerable ultrafiltration, replacement fluids are often necessary. Most importantly, the procedures are performed continuously over a 24-hour span. CRRT is similar to IHD in that all modalities require some form of anticoagulation, and thus can be complicated by bleeding problems. Even when the quantity of anticoagulation utilized is restricted by use of frequent saline flushes, it still results in some degree of anticoagulation that could predispose to bleeding.

The individual procedures differ among themselves in how the vasculature is accessed and the way solute clearance is achieved. The initial technique described, continuous arteriovenous hemofiltration (CAVH), was a simple method of filtration, the force provided by the patient's blood pressure. This technique was inadequate to eliminate the large quantity of solute found in the catabolic patient with ARF. To improve the efficiency of solute removal, modifications were first made to add a diffusive component to solute removal, so-called continuous arteriovenous haemodialysis. To avoid cannulation of the arterial tree and to pump blood independently of the patient's blood pressure, various forms of continuous venovenous hemofiltration and diafiltration were developed. The latter procedures appear to be the most frequently performed.

XIV. CAVH and Slow Continuous Ultrafiltration

CAVH was one of the first continuous therapies introduced (66,67). In this treatment, blood flow through a highly permeable dialyzer is driven by the patient's blood pressure. A protein-free filtrate results at a rate of several hundred milliliters per hour. This filtrate is collected in a bag connected to the ultrafiltrate

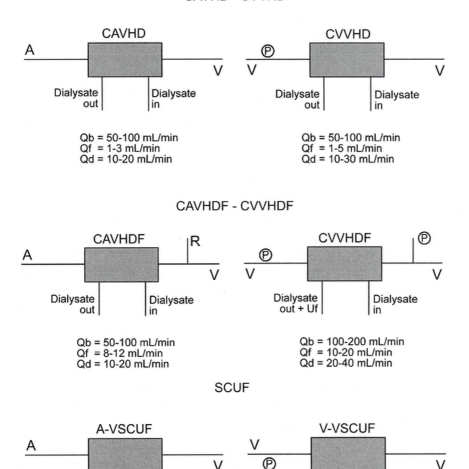

Figure 1 Schematic depicting commonly used modalities of continuous renal replacement therapy (CRRT): Continuous arteriovenous or venovenous hemodialysis (CAVHD/CVVHD); Continuous arteriovenous/venovenous hemodiafiltration (CAVHDF/CVVHDF) therapy; Continuous arteriovenous or venovenous slow ultrafiltration (SCUF). *Abbreviations*: A, artery; V, vein; Qb, blood flow; Qf, ultrafiltrate; Qd, dialysate flow; P, peristaltic pump; in, dialyzer inlet; out, dialyzer outlet. The venovenous forms of treatment have supplanted the arteriovenous forms since the former does not require cannulation of the arterial circulation.

port of the filter. Any ultrafiltrate produced can be replaced with individually prescribed solutions to achieve solute removal and volume control. In the postdilu-
tion mode, the replacement fluid is infused into the venous tubing. Continuous
anticoagulation is administered through a prefilter tubing connection. This
mode of dialysis is rarely used today because of the need for an indwelling arterial catheter and because of the relatively low solute removal rate.

Slow continuous ultrafiltration (SCUF) is a modification of CAVH in
which no fluid replacement is given (72). It is most commonly used for the management of refractory edema, both in the presence and absence of renal failure.

XV. Slow Low Efficiency Dialysis

This is a hybrid technique combining the benefits of traditional CRRT with those
of IHD (73). It utilizes standard hemodialysis machines, but dialysate flow is
reduced to only 100 mL/min for periods ranging from eight to 24 hours per day.
Blood flow is similar to CRRT of 200 mL/min. Advantages with this technique
include a high hemodynamic tolerance and an unsurpassed solute removal
capability. In some centers, the procedure is performed during the nighttime
allowing for patient availability for procedures during the day. Furthermore,
the nurse to patient ratio may be lower than in traditional CRRT.

XVI. Continuous Arteriovenous Hemodialysis and Hemodiafiltration

In continuous arteriovenous hemodialysis (CAVHD), the extracorporeal circuit
includes slow countercurrent dialysate flow into the ultrafiltrate compartment of
the filter. Because of the slow blood flow, complete blood to dialysate equilibrium
of urea is achieved, and thus clearance rates increase linearly with dialysate flow
rates up to 33.3 mL/min (2 L/hr). If dialysate flow is raised to 4 L/hr, urea clear-
ances can approach 50 mL/min. However, for the most part, dialysate flow rate is
set at only 1 L/hr, producing an urea clearance of approximately 17 mL/min.
The addition of this diffusive component of solute clearance is a major advantage
over pure hemofiltration and increases solute clearance substantially. In continuous
arteriovenous hemodiafiltration (CAVHDF), a slow countercurrent dialysate flow is
added into the ultrafiltrate dialysate compartment of the hemofilter. Fluid replacement is administered to replace fluid losses and to enhance effectiveness of dialysis
by predilution. Again this procedure is used less frequently than the venovenous-
based procedures because of the requirement for cannulation of the arterial
circulation.

XVII. Continuous Venovenous Hemofiltration

This form of dialysis uses a circuit similar to routine haemodialysis (68). Since
blood is pumped via a blood pump, an air detector and arterial and venous

pressure monitors are present. The use of this technique avoids arterial access and can provide substantial convection-dependent solute clearance. Ultrafiltrate can range from 1 L to 2 L per hour. Blood flow rates between 100 and 150 mL/min allow for a decreased tendency of filter clotting and limit the dosage requirements for anticoagulants. Small and middle molecule clearance can be substantial, but is limited by the rate of ultrafiltration. In patients in whom volume removal is pre-eminent, this might be preferable over hemodiafiltration.

XVIII. Continuous Venovenous Hemodialysis or Hemodiafiltration

The same basic circuit as continuous venovenous hemofiltration (CVVH) is used, but variable quantities of dialysate are allowed to flow past the filtrate component as in CAVHD. The resulting addition of a diffusive component enhances clearance of small molecular weight solutes, but is not effective in the removal of middle or large molecular weight solutes, including mediators of sepsis. When both convective and diffusive transport are performed, the procedure is called venovenous hemodiafiltration. This procedure maximizes diffusive and convective solute removal, facilitating removal of both small and middle molecular weight solutes, and is the most popular mode of CRRT used today, at least in the U.S.

In all CRRT, replacement fluid can be delivered into the prefilter tubing segment, so-called predilution of the circuit, or after the dialyzer, so-called post-dilution. Predilution reduces the plasma urea concentration and promotes the transfer of erythrocyte urea into the plasma compartment where it is available for removal in the filtrate, enhancing urea clearance. Predilution technique also limits the hemoconcentration that occurs at the venous side of the hemofilter. The potential advantages of the predilution mode include enhanced urea clearance and the possibility of increasing filter patency by the prefilter dilution of hematocrit, clotting factors, and platelets.

Issues that arise when considering the application of CRRT include the amount of solute clearance required, the type of replacement fluid or dialysate to administer, the type of anticoagulation to be employed, the amount of nutrition to be infused, the amount of nutrients lost in the filtrate or dialysate, and the impact of the treatment on drug dosing and the complications likely to be encountered. Furthermore, the personnel who are supervising the treatment are important, as experienced nurses are required. Each of these issues may have a substantial impact on outcome.

As with IHD, the delivered dose of CRRT may differ considerably from the prescribed dose of this treatment. Decreased delivery of CRRT could result from low blood flow and clotting of the circuit with resultant temporary discontinuation of dialysis. Similar to IHD, the appropriate dose of CRRT to deliver to patients with ARF remains unclear. A recent study demonstrated that patients receiving filtration rates of 35 mL/kg/hr (approximately 2.5 L/hr) had a significantly increased survival when compared with patients receiving filtration rates of 20 mL/kg/hr (approximately 1 L/hr) (74). A large prospective study to examine the impact of intensive versus conventional dialysis on morbidity, mortality, and cost of CRRT in the U.S. is presently in progress. However, the results of these studies will not be available for several years.

XIX.   Intermittent Hemodialysis vs. CRRT in Treatment of ARF

Although, the use of CRRT in the U.S. has lagged behind the use of IHD in the treatment of ARF, its popularity has risen in the last few years. Table 5 demonstrates some of the benefits and liabilities of various forms of CRRT and IHD that have been proposed. There are both practical and medical reasons for the increased popularity of CRRT. Practically, CRRT does not require the services of a dialysis nurse or technician but can be performed by well-trained intensive care nurses. This avoids the need for use of specialized nursing services. Medically, there are several reasons to use CRRT. Solute and fluid removal is substantially slower in CRRT than intermittent hemodialysis and accomplished over 24 hours. The seriously ill, often hypotensive patients, requiring dialysis may not tolerate the rapid solute shifts accompanying the high blood flow utilized in IHD nor the large volumes removed over short periods of time (74–76). Indeed, approximately 10% of patients with ARF are unable to be treated with intermittent hemodialysis because of hemodynamic instability and require CRRT (76). Fluid balance can be more finely regulated, since it can be managed on an hour to hour basis. This is extremely important because patients with acute renal failure are often hypercatabolic and require administration of TPN solutions. In this regard, with intermittent hemodialysis, nutritional management is often not optimal because of the requirement to restrict fluid intake (77). The rapid fluid and electrolyte shifts observed with intermittent hemodialysis can not only induce hypotension but also can be associated with cerebral edema (60).

Clearance of middle and high molecular weight solutes that have been implicated in the development of the uremic syndrome (78) are more efficiently removed with CRRT than hemodialysis. Moreover, recently it has been suggested that mediators of sepsis, which are largely middle molecules, are removed more efficiently with CRRT (79,80). Although it might be assumed that CRRT would be less expensive than IHD because it is less labor intensive, the few studies evaluating this issue have actually shown there is not a dramatic difference in cost (81). Future studies evaluating the cost of this therapy are in progress.

To further examine the benefits and liabilities of the two modes of treatment, several observational and randomized controlled studies comparing IHD to CRRT in the treatment of ARF have been carried out in the last few years. Mehta et al. (82) performed a randomized controlled study of 165 patients in the ICU with ARF requiring dialysis. Of interest, CRRT was actually associated with an increase in both ICU (59.5% vs. 41.5%) and in hospital mortality (65.5% vs. 47.6%). Some of the differences were attributed to less severe comorbid conditions as determined by APACHE score. Paradoxically, patients treated with CRRT had higher rates of recovery of renal function than patients treated with intermittent hemodialysis.

Kellum et al. (83) did a meta-analysis of the 13 randomized or observational studies available in which CRRT was compared to IHD in the treatment of ARF. One-thousand four-hundred patients were studied. When compared as an aggregate, there was no significant difference in mortality, although many of the studies were not randomized. Although there are theoretical reasons to prefer CRRT to IHD, at present there is insufficient evidence to support one modality of therapy over another. However, clearly there are certain situations in which one of the modalities is preferred. For example, when patients are hemodynamically compromised and markedly volume overloaded, CRRT is often utilized. On the other hand, in a hemodynamically stable patient in whom hyperkalemia is prominent, IHD is most effective in removing potassium and is the preferred mode of therapy. It has been recommended that CRRT be preferentially used for the treatment of septic patients with ARF because of the potential benefits of removal of inflammatory mediators (49,80). Since a large percentage of patients with ARF in the ICU have sepsis, this mode of therapy may be increasingly utilized in the U.S. as it is in Europe.

XX. Discontinuation of Renal Replacement Therapy

Although guidelines for the initiation of renal replacement therapy have been established, similar guidelines for discontinuation of therapy are not as clear. Most clinicians will discontinue dialysis once renal function is sufficient to prevent continual rises in plasma creatinine and BUN and to maintain volume, acid-base, and electrolyte balance.

Bellomo and Ronco have suggested guidelines for discontinuation of CRRT that may also be applicable to other forms of renal replacement therapy (76). These include the presence of a urine output of at least 1 mL/kg/hr, the ability to maintain neutral fluid balance, and the absence of laboratory abnormalities that would traditionally cause the clinician to initiate dialysis therapy. It should be understood that there may be variability in this regard among clinicians. Moreover, these authors suggest that a trial of weaning from renal replacement therapy for 12–24 hours be undertaken and the patient observed carefully. Only when the clinician is confident that the patient can be treated conservatively should the catheter be removed.

ARF in the ICU remains an important and challenging problem as it clearly dramatically increases the morbidity, mortality, and cost of therapy. Considerable resources are being expended to try to determine means of preventing this complication, rapidly reversing it should it occur, and determining when renal replacement therapy should be initiated and what form it should take. Prevention and aggressive treatment of ARF remain high priorities for all clinicians treating patients in the intensive care setting.

Acknowledgments

This work was supported by research funds from the Veterans Administration Healthcare System.

References

1. Levy EM, Viscoli CM, Horwitz RI. The effect of acute renal failure on mortality—a cohort analysis. J Am Med Assoc 1996; 275:1489–1494.
2. Hou SH, Bushinsky DA, Wish JB, Cohen JJ, Harrington JT. Hospital-acquired renal insufficiency—a prospective study. Am J Med 1983; 74:243–248.
3. Avasthi G, Sandhu JS, Mohindra K. Acute renal failure in medical and surgical intensive care units—a one year prospective study. Renal Failure 2003; 25: 105–113.
4. Morgera S, Kraft AK, Siebert G, Luft FC, Neumayer HH. Long-term outcomes in acute renal failure patients treated with continuous renal replacement therapies. Am J Kidney Dis 2002; 40:275–279.
5. Solomon R, Werner C, Mann D, Delia J, Silva P. Effects of saline, mannitol, and furosemide on acute decreases in renal-function induced by radiocontrast agents. N Engl J Med 1994; 331:1416–1420.
6. Mehta R, Chertow GM. Acute renal failure definitions and classification: time for change? J Am Soc Nephrol 2003; 2178–2187.
7. Klahr S, Miller SB. Acute oliguria. N Engl J Med 1998; 338:671–675.
8. Dixon B, Anderson R. Nonoliguric acute renal failure. Am J Kidney Dis 1985; 6:71–80.
9. O'Neill C. Sonographic evaluation of renal failure. Am J Kidney Dis 2000; 35:1021–1035.
10. Rossert J. Drug-induced acute interstitial nephritis. Kidney Int 2001; 60:804–817.
11. Carvounis CP, Nisar S, Guro-Razuman S. Significance of the fractional excretion of urea in the differential diagnosis of acute renal failure. Kidney Int 2002; 62:2223–2229.
12. Esson ML, Schrier RW. Diagnosis and treatment of acute tubular necrosis. Ann Int Med 2002; 137:744–752.
13. Dagher PC, Herget-Rosenthal S, Ruehm SG, Jo SK, Star RA, Agarwal R, Molitoris BA. Newly developed techniques to study and diagnose acute renal failure. J Am Soc Neph 2003; 14:2188–2198.
14. Singri N, Ahya SN, Levin ML. Acute renal failure. J Am Med Assoc 2003; 289:747–751.
15. Bonomini V, Stefoni S, Vangelista A. Long-term patient and renal prognosis in acute-renal-failure. Nephron 1984; 36:169–172.

16. Spurney RF, Fulkerson WJ, Schwab SJ. Acute-renal-failure in critically ill patients—prognosis for recovery of kidney-function after prolonged dialysis support. Crit Care Med 1991; 19:8–11.

17. Fort J, Camps J, Martin M, Bartolome J, Rodriguez JA, Segarra A, Roca R, Borrellas X, Ruiz P, Olmos A, Piera L. Predictive factors of mortality in acute-renal-failure patients. Kidney Int 1994; 46:564.

18. Mehta R, Farkas A, Pascual M, Fowler W. Effect of serial APACHE and organ failure scores on prediction of mortality in acute-renal-failure. J Am Soc Nephrol 1995; 6:550.

19. Nash K, Hafeez A, Hou S. Hospital acquired renal insufficiency. Am J Kidney Dis 2002; 39:930–936.

20. Vinen CS, Oliveira DB. Acute glomerulonephritis. Postgraduate Med 2003; 79:206–213.

21. Lewis J, Salem MM, Chertow GM, Weisberg LS, McGrew F, Marbury TC, Allgren RL. Atrial natriuretic factor in oliguric acute renal failure. Anaritide Acute Renal Failure Study Group. Am J Kidney Dis 2000; 36:767–774.

22. Bellomo R, Chapman M, Finfer S, Hickling K, Myburgh J. Low-dose dopamine in patients with early renal dysfunction: a placebo-controlled randomised trial. Lancet 2000; 356:2139–2143.

23. Mehta RL, Pascual MT, Soroko S, Chertow GM. Diuretics, mortality, and nonrecovery of renal function in acute renal failure. J Am Med Assoc 2002; 288:2547–2553.

24. Heyman SN, Rosen S, Epstein FH, Spokes K, Brezis ML. Loop diuretics reduce hypoxic damage to proximal tubules of the isolated perfused rat kidney. Kidney Int 1994; 45:981–985.

25. Conger JD, Robinette JB, Schrier RW. Smooth muscle calcium and endothelium-derived relaxing factor in the abnormal vascular responses of acute renal failure. J Clin Invest 1988; 82:532–542.

26. Wagner K, Albrecht S, Neumayer HH. Prevention of posttransplant acute tubular-necrosis by the calcium-antagonist diltiazem—a prospective randomized study. Am J Nephrol 1987; 7:287–291.

27. Cacoub P, Deray G, Baumelou A, Jacobs C. No evidence for protective effects of nifedipine against radiocontrast-induced acute renal-failure. Clinical Nephrology 1988; 29:215–216.

28. Kellum JA, Decker JM. Use of dopamine in acute renal failure: a meta-analysis. Crit Care Med 2001; 29:1526–1531.

29. Vesely DL. Natriuretic peptides and acute renal failure. Am J Physiol 2003; 285:F167–F177.

30. Allgren RL, Marbury TC, Rahman SN, Weisberg LS, Fenves AZ, Lafayette RA, Sweet RM, Genter FC, Kurnik BRC, Conger JD, Sayegh MH. Anaritide in acute tubular necrosis. N Engl J Med 1997; 336:828–834.

31. Lytton B, Vaisbort VR, Glazier WB, Chaudry IH, Baue AE. Improved renal-function using adenosine triphosphate-magnesium chloride in preservation of canine kidneys subjected to warm ischemia. Transplantation 1981; 31:187–189.

32. Sutter PM, Thulin G, Stromski M, Ardito T, Gaudio KM, Kashgarian M, Siegel NJ. Beneficial effect of thyroxine in the treatment of ischemic acute renal-failure. Ped Nephrol 1988; 2:1–7.

33. Richard C, Warszawski J, Anguel N, Deye N, Combes A, Barnoud D, Boulain T, Lefort Y, Fartoukh M, Baud F, Boyer A, Brochard L, Teboul JL. Early use of the pulmonary artery catheter and outcomes in patients with shock and acute respiratory distress syndrome—a randomized controlled trial. J Am Med Assoc 2003; 290: 2713–2720.

34. Obialo CI, Okonofua EC, Nzerue MC, Tayade AS, Riley LJ. Role of hypoalbumine-mia and hypocholesterolemia as copredictors of mortality in acute renal failure. Kidney Int 1999; 56:1058–1063.

35. Moulik PK, Nethaji C, Khaleeli AA. Lesson of the week—misleading electrocardio-graphic results in patient with hyperkalaemia and diabetic ketoacidosis. Brit Med J 2002; 325:1346–1347.

36. Mitch WE. Mechanisms causing loss of muscle in acute uremia. Renal Failure 1996; 18:389–394.

37. Adrogue HJ, Brensilver J, Cohen JJ, Madias NE. Influence of steady-state alterations in acid-base equilibrium on the fate of administered bicarbonate in the dog. J Clin Invest. 1983 Apr; 71(4):867–883.

38. Haas M, Ohler L, Watzke H, Bohmig G, Prokesch R, Druml W. The spectrum of acute renal failure in tumour lysis syndrome. Nephrol Dial Transplant 1999; 14:776–779.

39. Anderson LE, Henrich WL. Alkalemia-associated morbidity and mortality in medical and surgical patients. So Med J 1987; 80:729–733.

40. Metnitz PGH, Krenn CG, Steltzer H, Lang T, Ploder J, Lenz K, Le Gall JR, Druml W. Effect of acute renal failure requiring renal replacement therapy on outcome in critically ill patients. Crit Care Med 2002; 30:2051–2058.

41. Blumberg A, Roser HW, Zehnder C, MullerBrand J. Plasma potassium in patients with terminal renal failure during and after haemodialysis; relationship with dialytic potassium removal and total body potassium. Nephrol Dial Transplant 1997; 12:1629–1634.

42. Mukau L, Lattimer RG. Acute hemodialysis in the surgical intensive care unit. Am J Surg 1988; 54:548–552.

43. Weiss L, Danielson B, Wikstrom BM, Hedstrand U, Wahlberg J. Continuous arteriove-nous hemofiltration in the treatment of 100 critically ill patients with acute renal failure: report on clinical outcome and nutritional aspects. Clin Nephrol 1989; 31:184–189.

44. Wood JE, Mahnensmith RL. Pericarditis associated with renal failure: evolution and management. Sem Dial 2001; 14:61–66.

45. Teschan PE, Baxter CR, O'Brien TF, Freyhof JN, Hall WH. Prophylactic hemodia-lysis in the treatment of acute renal failure. Ann Int Med 1960; 53:992–1016.

46. Fisher RP, Griffen WOJ, Reiser M, Clark DS. Early dialysis in the treatment of acute renal failure. Surg Gynecol Obster 1996; 123:1019–1023.

47. Conger JD. A controlled evaluation of prophylatic dialysis in post traumatic acute renal failure. J Trauma 1975; 15:1056–1063.

48. Gettings LG, Reynolds HN, Scalea T. Outcome in post-traumatic acute renal failure when continuous renal replacement therapy is applied early vs. late. Inten Care Med 1999; 25:805–813.

49. Ronco C, Bellomo R, Lonneman G. Sepsis—theory and therapies. N Engl J Med 2003; 348:1600–1602.

50. Van de Noortgate N, Verbeke F, Dhondt A, Colardijn F, Van Biesen W, Vanholder R, Lameire N. The dialytic management of acute renal failure in the elderly. Sem in Dial 2002; 15:127–132.

51. Phu NH, Hien TT, Mai NTH, Chau TTH, Chuong LV, Loc PP, Winearls C, Farar J, White N, Day N. Hemofiltration and peritoneal dialysis in infection-associated acute renal failure in Vietnam. N Engl J Med 2002; 347:895–902.

52. Mehta RL, Letteri JM. Current status of renal replacement therapy for acute renal failure. A survey of US Nephrologists. Am J Nephrol 1999; 19:377–382.

53. Evanson JA, Himmelfarb J, Wingard R, Knights S, Shyr Y. Prescribed versus delivered dialysis in acute renal failure patients. Am J Kidney Dis 1998; 32:731–738.

54. Hernandez D, Diaz F, Rufino M, Lorenzo V, Perez T, Rodriguez A, De Bonis E, Losada M, Gonzalez-Posada JM, Torres A. Subclavian vascular access stenosis in dialysis patients: natural history and risk factors. J Am Soc Nephrol 1998; 9:1507–1510.

55. Kanagasundaram NS, Greene T, Larive AB, Daugirdas JT, Depner TA, Garcia M, Paganini EP. Prescribing an equilibrated intermittent hemodialysis dose in intensive care unit acute renal failure. Kidney Int 2003; 64:2298–2310.

56. Evanson JA, Ikizler TA, Wingard R, Knights S, Shyr Y, Schulman G, Himmelfarb J, Hakim RM. Measurement of the delivery of dialysis in acute renal failure. Kidney Int 1999; 55:1501–1508.

57. Tapolyai M, Fedak S, Chaff C, Paganini EP. Delivered dialysis dose may influence acute-renal-failure outcome in ICU patients. J Am Soc Nephrol 1994; 5:530.

58. Kammerl MC, Schaefer RM, Schweda F, Schreiber M, Riegger GAJ, Kramer BK. Extracorporal therapy with AN69 membranes in combination with ACE inhibition causing severe anaphylactoid reactions: still a current problem? Clin Nephrol 2000; 53:486–488.

59. Ing TS, Wong FKM, Cheng YL, Potempa LD. The 'first-use syndrome' revisited: a dialysis centre's perspective. Nephrol Dial Transplant 1995; 10:39–44.

60. Mahoney CA, Arieff AI. Uremic encephalopathies: clinical, biochemical, and experimental features. Am J Kidney Dis 1982; 2:324–336.

61. Schulman G, Fogo A, Gung A, Badr K, Hakim R. Complement activation retards resolution of acute ischemic renal-failure in the rat. Kidney Int 1991; 40:1069–1074.

62. Hakim RM. Clinical implications of hemodialysis membrane biocompatibility kidney int 1993; 44:484–494.

63. Zaoui P, Hakim RM. Natural-killer-cell function in hemodialysis-patients—effect of the dialysis membrane. Kidney Int 1993; 43:1298–1305.

64. Hakim RM, Wingard RL, Parker RA. Effect of the dialysis membrane in the treatment of patients with acute-renal-failure. N Engl J Med 1994; 331:1338–1342.

65. Jorres A, Gahl GM, Dobis C, Polenakovic MH, Cakalaroski K, Rutkowski B, Kisielnicka E, Krieter DH, Rumpf KW, Guenther C, Gaus W, Hoegel J. Haemodialysis-membrane biocompatibility and mortality of patients with dialysis-dependent acute renal failure: a prospective randomised multicentre trial. Lancet 1999; 354:1337–1341.

66. Burchardi H. History and development of continuous renal replacement techniques. Kidney Int 1998; 53:S120–S124.

67. Kellum JA, Mehta RL, Angus DC, Palevsky P, Ronco C. The first international consensus conference on continuous renal replacement therapy. Kidney Int 2002; 62:1855–1863.

68. Abdeen O, Mehta RL. Dialysis modalities in the intensive care unit. Crit Care Clinics 2002; 18:223–243.

69. Maxvold NJ, Bunchman TE. Renal failure and renal replacement therapy. Crit Care Clinics 2003; 19:563–575.

70. Guerin C, Girard R, Selli JM, Ayzac L. Intermittent versus continuous renal replacement therapy for acute renal failure in intensive care units: results from a multicenter prospective epidemiological survey. Intensive Care Med 2002; 28:1411–1418.

71. Ronco C, Bellomo R, Homel P, Brendolan A, Dan M, Piccinni P, LaGreca G. Effects of different doses in continuous veno-venous haemofiltration on outcomes of acute renal failure: a prospective randomised trial. Lancet 2000; 356:26–30.

72. Paganini E, O'Hara P, Nakamoto S. Slow continuous ultrafiltration in hemodialysis resistant oliguric acute renal failure patients. Trans Am Soc Artif Intern Organs 1984; 30:173–178.

73. Marshall MR, Golper TA, Shaver MJ, Alam MG, Chatoth DK. Sustained low-efficiency dialysis for critically ill patients requiring renal replacement therapy. Kidney Int 2001; 60:777–785.

74. Bellomo R, Parkin G, Love J, Boyce N. Use of continuous hemodiafiltration—an approach to the management of acute-renal-failure in the critically ill. Am J Nephrol 1992; 12:240–245.

75. John S, Griesbach D, Baumgartel M, Weihprecht H, Schmieder RE, Geiger H. Effects of continuous haemofiltration vs. intermittent haemodialysis on systemic haemodynamics and splanchnic regional perfusion in septic shock patients: a prospective, randomized clinical trial. Nephrol Dial Transplan 2001; 16:320–327.

76. Bellomo R, Ronco C. Continuous renal replacement therapy in the intensive care unit. Intensive Care Med 1999; 25:781–789.

77. Monson P, Mehta RL. Nutrition in acute renal failure: a reappraisal for the 1990s. J Ren Nutr 1994; 4:58–77.

78. Clark W, Mueller B, Kraus AM. Extracorporeal therapy requirements for patients with acute renal failure. J Am Soc Nephrol 1997; 8:804–812.

79. Tetta C, Bellomo R, Ronco C. Artificial organ treatment for multiple organ failure, acute renal failure, and sepsis: recent new trends. Artificial Organs 2003; 27:202–213.

80. Kellum JA. Blood purification in sepsis: an idea whose time has come? Crit Care Med 2002; 30:1387–1388.

81. Silvester W. Outcome studies of continuous renal replacement therapy in the intensive care unit. Kidney Int 1998; 53:S138–S141.

82. Mehta RL, McDonald B, Gabbai FB, Pahl M, Pascual MT, Farkas A, Kaplan RM. A randomized clinical trial of continuous versus intermittent dialysis for acute renal failure. Kidney Int 2001; 603:1154–1163.

83. Kellum JA, Angus DC, Johnson JP, Leblanc M, Griffin M, Ramakrishnan N, Linde-Zwirble WT. Continuous versus intermittent renal replacement therapy: a meta-analysis. Intensive Care Med 2002; 28:29–37.

14

Nutritional Support of the Critically Ill Patient

PAUL E. MARIK

Division of Pulmonary/Critical Care Medicine, Thomas Jefferson
  University Hospital and Jefferson Medical College
Philadelphia, Pennsylvania, U.S.A.

> Do it enterally, do it early, do it slowly. Just do it!
>
> —Markus Shem, M.D.

I. Introduction

Critically ill patients have a characteristic metabolic response to injury whether their illness is secondary to trauma, burns, systemic infection, severe head injury, or sterile inflammatory processes. This response is associated with an increase in metabolic rate and rapid loss of fat and muscle mass; if prolonged, it has several adverse effects, including immunosuppression, decreased or delayed wound healing, loss of muscle strength, and diminished activity. Nutrition support in the early stages of critical illness may be necessary to mitigate these potential adverse effects. Of note, the metabolic response to critical illness is very different from simple or uncomplicated starvation in which loss of muscle is much slower and visceral proteins may be spared for a long period. This is because individuals who suffer from simple starvation are hypometabolic and, therefore, have decreased caloric demands compared with normal individuals. This is in contrast to critically ill patients, who typically are hypermetabolic and have increased caloric demands compared with normal individuals. In addition, starved individuals have adaptive responses that lead to decreased glucose utilization, decreased gluconeogenesis, and consequently a slower rate of protein loss. These adaptive responses do not occur or are limited in severe illness and, therefore, net protein loss can be high and compromise host defense mechanisms if nutrition support is not initiated early in the disease process.

479

Stress-induced hyperglycemia is common in the critically ill. A combination of several factors, including the presence of excessive counter regulatory hormones, such as glucagon, growth hormone, catecholamines, glucocorticoids, and cytokines [such as interleukin-1 (IL-1), IL-6, and tumor necrosis factor-α (TNF-α)], combined with exogenous administration of catecholamines, dextrose and nutritional support, together with relative insulin deficiency play an important role (1). Gluconeogenic substrates released during stress include lactate, alanine, and glycerol, with exogenous glucose failing to suppress gluconeogenesis (2,3). Increased gluconeogenesis combined with hepatic insulin resistance are the major factors leading to hyperglycemia (4). Stress-induced hyperglycemia has important implications when considering nutritional support in the critically ill. Specifically, recent provocative data suggests that tight glycemic control with insulin may restore the balance between pro-inflammatory and anti-inflammatory mediators and improve the outcome of critically ill patients (5,6).

It has become increasingly recognized that nutritional compounds have specific biological properties that can alter cellular, tissue, and organ function and thereby modulate many disease processes. Once considered an afterthought, nutrient pharmacology currently plays an integral role in the multimodality management of critically ill patients. The key elements when considering nutritional support include the route of feeding, the timing, the nutrient composition, and the quantity. Each of these elements will be reviewed as they apply to the critically ill patient. In addition, nutritional support in a number of specific disease states/circumstances will be briefly reviewed.

II. Route of Feeding

A. Parenteral vs. Enteral Nutrition

The origins of "modern" parenteral nutrition can be traced to the publication in 1937 by Robert Elman of his successful studies in humans of intravenous amino acid infusion in the form of protein hydrolysates (7). However, even at this time there were sceptics who argued that the infusion of amino acids that circumvented the liver was "unphysiologic" and probably "toxic to the brain and other organs" (8). Undoubtedly, the introduction of total parenteral nutrition (TPN) to clinical medicine in 1968 was life saving for those patients with short gut syndrome in whom enteral nutrition was not possible. However, the availability of this new therapeutic intervention led to its indiscriminate use in many disease processes without an appropriate evaluation of its impact on clinical outcome. It soon became clear that TPN was associated with a myriad of complications and was not the panacea first imagined. Nonetheless, unlike other therapeutic interventions that disappeared once their ineffectiveness and complications were established by controlled clinical trials, TPN has managed to survive to this day.

The adverse sequela associated with TPN result from the "double effect" of not directly feeding the bowel and the metabolic, immunologic, endocrine and infective complications associated with infusing a synthetic nutritional formula into a patient's systemic venous system (Tables 1 and 2). The mucosa of the gastrointestinal tract is highly metabolically active; enteral nutrition increases mucosal blood flow and provides a direct source of nutrients. Lack of enteral feeding results in gastrointestinal mucosal atrophy, bacterial overgrowth, increased intestinal permeability, and translocation of bacteria and/or bacterial products (9–17). Enteral nutrition has a major effect on the gut-associated lymphoid tissue (GALT), which is the source of most mucosal immunity in humans. Experimental data has demonstrated that the small intestine GALT is preserved by enteral nutrition; however, TPN (starvation) results in rapid and severe atrophy of this tissue (18–21). Kundsk et al. have demonstrated that atrophy of the GALT in animals receiving parenteral nutrition is associated with decreased IgA in the upper respiratory tract and that this is associated with a reduced resistance to infection (18–20). Enteral feeding during or after parenteral nutrition is associated with rapid repletion of GALT cellularity (19).

In addition, to its effects on the GALT, TPN impairs humoral and cellular immunologic defenses (22–25). TPN is associated with impaired leucocyte chemotaxis, impaired phagocytosis, impaired bacterial and fungal killing, and an attenuated inflammatory response (22,26–29). Experimental sepsis models have demonstrated a significantly higher mortality in animals receiving parenteral as compared to enteral nutrition (30–33). In a murine intraperitoneal sepsis model, Lin et al. (33) have demonstrated that TPN as compared to

Table 1 Composition of Enteral as Compared to Parental Nutrition

Nutrient	Parenteral	Enteral
Protein		
Intact	No	Yes
Peptides	No	Yes
Amino acids	Yes	Yes
Glutamine	No	Yes
Cysteine	No	Yes
Arginine	Low	Yes
Lipid	High 0–6	Balanced
MCT	No	Yes
CHO		
Simple	Yes	Yes
Complex	No	Yes

Abbreviation: MCT, medium chain triglycerides.

Table 2 Contrasting Effects of Parenteral and Enteral Nutrition on Organ Function

	Parenteral	Enteral
Gastrointestinal tract		
GI blood flow	Decreased	Increased
GI mucosal	Atrophy	Prevents atrophy
GI lymphoid tissue	Atrophy	Prevents atrophy
Bacterial translocation	Increased	Decreased
GI flora virulence	Increased	Decreased
Hepatic		
Hepatis steatosis	++	−
Hepatic atrophy	++	−
Hepatocellular dysfunction	++	−
Depletion of antioxidants	++	−
Renal and metabolic		
Recovery following ATN	Delayed	Enhanced ˙
Hyperglycemia	++	+
Hypomagnesemia	++	+
Hypophosphatemia	++	+
Hypertriglyceridemia	++	−
Immunologic		
Neutrophil function	Impaired	Preserved
Mononuclear phagocyte function	Impaired	Preserved
Mucosal IgA	Decreased	Preserved
Blood stream infections	Increased	−
Pro-inflammatory response	Increased	−

enteral nutrition was associated with decreased mobilization of inflammatory cells with decreased bacterial clearance.

Clinical studies have consistently demonstrated a higher risk of infection in patients receiving TPN (34–40). The risk of infection may be particularly increased in malnourished patients receiving TPN (34,39). In the Veterans Affairs Total Parental Nutrition Study, 395 malnourished patients who required noncardiac surgery were randomly assigned to receive perioperative TPN (seven to 10 days before and three days after surgery) or to a control group who received no nutritional support (34). There were significantly more infectious complications in the TPN group than in the control group (14.1% vs. 6.4%, $p = 0.01$), with a trend toward a higher 90-day mortality in the TPN group (13.4% vs. 10.5%). Kudsk (36) demonstrated a significantly lower risk of septic morbidity in patients fed enterally after blunt and penetrating trauma, with the most significant changes occurring in the more severely injured patients. In a large multicenter study, patients with gastrointestinal cancer undergoing elective surgery were randomized to receive early enteral nutrition ($n = 159$) or parenteral nutrition ($n = 158$) (41). Postoperative complications occurred in 34% of patients fed enterally versus 49% fed parenterally.

While TPN as compared to enteral nutrition is associated with impaired innate and acquired immunity, predisposing patients to infection, TPN is associated with a more pronounced pro-inflammatory response. Clinical and experimental studies have consistently demonstrated higher levels of both local and systemic pro-inflammatory mediators with parenteral as compared to enteral nutrition (33,42). Lin et al. (43) demonstrated higher levels of IL-6 and IL-8 after colorectal surgery in patients receiving TPN as compared to those fed enterally. Similarly, Gianotti (40) found higher levels of IL-6 in patients undergoing major abdominal surgery for malignant neoplasms who received TPN as compared to enteral nutrition. In a remarkable study, Fong et al. (44) challenged healthy volunteers with endotoxin after having received enteral feedings or TPN (without oral intake) for seven days. In this study, circulating levels of TNF and C-reactive protein (CRP) were significantly higher in the TPN as compared to the enteral nutrition group. Due to the pro-inflammatory and immunoparetic effects of parenteral nutrition, this mode of nutritional support may be particularly harmful in patients with pancreatitis. This contention is supported by clinical studies that have demonstrated a higher risk of infective and noninfective complications in patients with severe pancreatitis who were receiving TPN as compared to patients fed enterally (proximal jejunal feeding) (37,38,42,45–49).

In addition to its effects on the immune system, TPN is associated with an impressive array of metabolic and endocrine complications, including hyperglycemia, hypertriglyceridemia, azotemia, metabolic acidosis, an exaggerated stress response, and numerous electrolyte abnormalities (17,43,50–52). In addition, TPN is associated with increased free radical formation (53,54); this complication may be of considerable importance in critically ill patients.

TPN is associated with significant hepatobiliary complications, including liver atrophy, hepatosteatosis, and hepatocellular injury leading to liver failure (55). In addition, the absence of enteral nutrition causes rapid depletion of the liver's antioxidant enzyme systems (56). The effect of TPN on hepatic function may be a consequence of the fact that nutrients supplied by parenteral nutrition largely bypass the liver, whereas enteral nutrients are delivered directly to the liver via the portal circulation. Enteral nutrition therefore results in a higher concentration of nutrients and trophic gastrointestinal hormones in the portal circulation (57,58).

It is well established that the route of feeding affects wound healing. Enteral as compared to parenteral nutrition is associated with greater wound strength, enhanced wound hydroxyproline and collagen accumulation, and grater expression of the gene for type 1 collagen (59–61). This finding may partly explain the lower risk of anatomic leaks and fistula is patients who have had bowel surgery and received enteral nutrition as compared to delayed feeding or parenteral nutrition (46,62).

The deleterious effects of TPN may be most evident in critically ill and inured patients who are at a particularly high risk for nosocomial infections and developing multisystem organ failure. While there are few randomized studies in this patient population, the available data supports this contention. Heyland et al. (63) performed a meta-analysis of TPN (compared to no nutritional support) in critically ill patients. These authors demonstrated that, in critically ill patients, TPN almost doubles the risk of dying (RR 1.78; 95% CI: 1.11–2.85). Similarly, using a risk-adjusted mortality ratio, we have demonstrated that, in critically ill ICU patients, TPN as compared to enteral nutrition doubles the risk of dying (64). Furthermore, we have demonstrated that the toxicity of TPN can be reduced by the addition of "trickle" enteral nutrition (64,65).

Enteral nutritional support may not be possible in patients with short gut syndromes (or no gut) and in those with high output small bowel fistulas; however, these patients are uncommon in clinical practice. In a landmark study, Ochoa et al. (66) demonstrated a 78% reduction in the use of TPN with the introduction of a nutrition support service. In this study, the reduction in the use of TPN was associated with a dramatic increase in the number of patients who were fed enterally. The study by Ochoa et al. supports the contention that most patients who receive TPN can be fed enterally.

A number of studies have been reported that have not demonstrated an increased risk of infectious complications, length of hospital stay, or mortality in patients receiving TPN (67,68). It is, however, important to point out that these studies were not performed in critically ill patients; in critically ill patients, TPN likely increases morbidity and mortality. There is compelling scientific and clinical rationale to support the use of enteral rather than parenteral nutrition in critically ill intensive care unit (ICU) patients as well as non-ICU patients with pancreatitis or polytrauma and patients who have undergone abdominal surgery.

B. Gastric vs. Jejunal Feeding

Many clinicians advocate postpyloric as compared to gastric feeding on the basis that critically ill patients frequently have gastroparesis and that gastric feeding may predispose to emesis and aspiration. While Mentec et al. (69) demonstrated some degree of upper digestive intolerance in 79% of nasogastrically fed patients, only 4.5% were unable to tolerate gastric feeding. In a meta-analysis of nine published studies, Marik and Zaloga demonstrated no significant difference in the incidence of pneumonia (OR 1.44; 95% CI: 0.84–2.46), percentage of caloric goal achieved (−5.2%; 95% CI: −18.0–7.5%), mean total caloric intake (−169 calories; 95% CI: −320–34 calories), ICU length of stay (−1.4 days, 95% CI: −3.7–0.85), or mortality (OR 1.08; 95% CI: 0.69–1.68) between those patients fed gastrically as compared to those patients who received postpyloric tube feeding (70). However, the time to the initiation of enteral nutrition was significantly shorter in those patients randomized to receive nutrition by the gastric route (−16.0; 95% CI: −19.5 to −12.6 hr, $p < 0.00001$). Based on this data, critically ill patients who are not at a high risk for aspiration should have a naso/orogastric tube placed on admission to the ICU for the early initiation of enteral nutrition. Promotility agents should be considered in patients with high gastric residual volumes (>300 mL) (71). Diabetes mellitus, head injury, burn injury, abdominal surgery, sepsis, narcotics, the recumbent position, and use of catecholamines contribute to gastroparesis. It is important to realize that over 6000 mL of secretions are produced by the upper gastrointestinal tract each day, with the stomach producing approximately 1500 mL. In a normal healthy individual, a nasogastric tube placed on free drainage can therefore be expected to drain up to 2000 mL/day. It is thus a serious error to conclude that a patient has a gastroparesis or small bowel obstruction (ileus) on the basis of the drainage from a nasogastric tube on free drainage. It is important that the nasogastric tube should be clamped and the gastric residual checked every six hours. A gastric residual in excess of 400 mL over six hours is suggests gastroparesis or gastric outlet obstruction.

The use of prokinetic agents to improve gastric emptying may avert the need for placement of a small-bowel feeding tube (72). Patients who remain intolerant of gastric tube feeding despite the use of promotility agents, patients with clinically significant reflux, and patients with documented aspiration should have a small intestinal feeding tube inserted for continuation of enteral nutritional support. Patients undergoing major intra-abdominal surgery are at a high risk for postoperative gastroparesis and should have a small bowel feeding tube placed intraoperatively. This will facilitate the initiation of early enteral nutritional support (see Timing of Nutritional Support).

While some authors recommend the use of a promotility agent in all gastrically fed patients (73), others have recommended promotility agents only in those patients with increased gastric residual volumes (72,74–76). For economic reasons, as well as to avoid potential side-effects, it could be argued that only those patients who are intolerant of nasogastric feedings (residual >300 mls– 250 mL) should receive a prokinetic agent. Which promotility agent should we use? Erythromycin and metoclopramide are currently the only promotility agents available in the U.S. Metoclopramide stimulates gut motility by antagonizing the gut inhibitory neurotransmitter dopamine and sensitizes the gut to acetylcholine, while erythromycin acts on motilin receptors. Since these agents act via different mechanisms, the combination may have an additive effect on promoting gastric emptying in refractory cases. Using acetaminophen absorption, Jooste et al. (77) demonstrated improved gastric emptying after intravenous administration of metoclopramide in a heterogeneous group of critically ill patients. The side-effects of metoclopramide include dystonic and dyskinetic movements, tremors, restless, agitation, and cardiac dysrhythmias (78). Erythromycin is a macrolide antibiotic that increases gastric motility by acting on motilin receptors in the gut (79). Motilin is a 22-amino acid peptide produced by enterochromaffin cells of the proximal small intestine. Most motilin receptors are found on cholinergic nerves, and motilin receptor activation mediates its motility effects via activation of cholinergic pathways (enteric nervous system, vagus nerve). Motilin receptors may also be present on smooth muscle in the stomach and small intestine. In addition, erythromycin increases lower esophageal sphincter tone and esophageal peristalsis but has little effect on colonic motility. Some have suggested that motilin release is inhibited in critically ill patients, causing gastroparesis. Erythromycin improves gastric emptying in diabetics with delayed gastric emptying, patients after vagotomy, patients with chronic intestinal pseudo-obstruction, and unselected critically ill patients (72,80–82). In addition, erythromycin also has been shown to facilitate passage of feeding tubes in critically ill patients. It is important to note the erythromycin should be given intravenously at least until gastric emptying has been achieved; the recommended dose is 70 mg iv q eight hourly. Induction of antibiotic resistance is a concern with the prolonged use of erythromycin (83).

Placement of small bowel feeding tubes by the blind naso-enteric approach is technically challenging. Zaloga (84) described the "cork-screw" method of achieving post-pyloric placement of feeding tubes with a success rate of 92%. This method entails placing the patient on his/her right side. The tip of the feeding tube stillete is bent at a 45° angle. The feeding tube is advanced into the stomach, and then with a rotating action (like a cork-screw), the tube is advanced into the small bowel. Although success rates as high as 90% have been claimed by others for placing post-pyloric feeding tubes at the bedside (85–87), most studies report a success rate of 15–30% (88–90). Success with bedside placement of small bowel feeding tubes is influenced by the technique and degree of expertise of the clinician. Furthermore, unlike a naso/orogastric tube, which can be passed in less than a minute, it can take an experienced operator up to 30 minutes to achieve postpyloric placement of a small bowel feeding tube. In order to improve the success at postpyloric placement, modifications have been made to the feeding tubes, including lengthening the tube, altering the configuration and profile of the tip, and adding various types of weights (88,91). Innovative methods of placement have also been described, which include using industrial magnets, bedside sonography, fiberoptics through the tube, gastric insufflation, and electrocardiogram-guided placement (33,37–40). Prokinetic agents have also been used to improve the likelihood of trans-pyloric passage of the feeding tube (89,92–95). The number of variations and modifications of the blind bedside technique attest to the fact that none are ideal. Furthermore, misplacement of the small bore feeding tube into the lung with resultant pneumothorax is not a rare complication (96–100).

In order to improve the success rate of the blind bedside technique, small bore feeding tubes may be placed endoscopically or radiographically. Hillard (90) compared the success rate and time to placement of small bowel feeding tubes placed by fluoroscopy as compared with placement at the bedside. Ninety-one percent of fluoroscopic procedures were successful compared to a success rate of 17% with bedside placement. The average time delay before initiation of feeding was 28.1 hours for the bedside method and 7.5 hours for fluoroscopy. Although both fluoroscopy and endoscopy are highly effective for placement of small bowel feeding tubes, they require expertise that is not readily available 24 hours per day and seven days per week. These techniques frequently require patient transfer to specialized areas of the hospital where the procedures are performed. In addition, both techniques are expensive.

C. Enteral Nutrition in Patients on Vasopressor Support

Many clinicians mistakenly believe that patients receiving vasopressors agents should not receive enteral nutrition. This assumption is based on the premise that enteral nutrition may cause bowel ischemia or infarction in these patients. Consequently, enteral nutritional support is often withheld until the vasopressor agents are discontinued or, alternatively, TPN is initiated. Clinical and experimental data, however, strongly support the concept that enteral nutrition increases splanchnic blood flow and nutrient utilization and may prevent bowel ischemia in patients receiving vasopressor agents. In a lung-injury canine model, Purcell et al. (101) demonstrated that continuous enteral nutrition restores depressed splanchnic blood flow and increases splanchnic oxygen utilization. Kazamias et al. (102) studied the effects of enteral nutrition in an *Escherichia coli* canine endotoxin model. In this study, enteral nutrition restored depressed hepatic and superior mesenteric arterial and portal venous blood flow with normalization of intestinal mucosal and hepatic microcirculation and restoration of tissue oxygenation and hepatic ATP stores. Revelly et al. (103) confirmed these findings in postoperative cardiac surgery patients who were receiving vasopressor agents. In this study, continuous enteral nutrition increased cardiac index, splanchnic blood flow, insulin secretion, and glucose utilization. The blood flow redistribution noted with enteral nutrition may be affected by the nutrient composition of the diet. Immune enhancing nutritional formulations have been demonstrated to increase splanchnic blood flow to a greater degree than standard formulations (104,105). While these data suggest that enteral nutrition may restore splanchnic blood flow and tissue oxygenation in patients with shock, it is probably prudent to delay the initiation of feeding until the patient has been volume resuscitated and an adequate mean arterial blood pressure has been achieved (this goal should be attained within six hours of presentation to hospital) (106,107). This approach does not apply to patients who have obstructive splanchnic vascular disease in whom enteral nutrition may cause further bowel ischemia.

III. Timing of Feeding

As many critically ill patients have a gastroparesis, and many of these patients have diminished or absent bowel sounds, enteral nutrition is frequently withheld for five to seven days until the return of gastric emptying and bowel sounds. In addition, many clinicians mistakenly believe that patients can tolerate five to seven days of starvation without detrimental clinical effects. Furthermore, it is standard surgical practice to withhold enteral nutrition until the return of bowel sounds and the passage of flatus. This thesis, however, is unsupported, and available evidence suggests that it is both safe and desirable to initiate enteral feeding (via a small bowel feeding tube) in the immediate postoperative period (108). Furthermore, many surgeons delay the initiation of enteral nutrition following bowel surgery on the basis that the "large" volume of feed will disrupt the surgical anastomoses. This assertion is incorrect, as experimental studies have demonstrated that the early initiation of enteral nutrition enhances anastomotic strength (60,61), and clinical studies have demonstrated a reduction in the incidence of anastomotic dehiscence with early enteral feeding (62). It is important to note that the gastrointestinal tract normally produces in excess of 6 L of fluid per day, and that an additional volume of 500 mL/day (by initiating a tube feed at 20 cc/hr) is hardly likely to have a significant mechanical effect.

Early enteral nutrition (as opposed to delayed enteral nutrition) has been demonstrated to improve nitrogen balance, wound healing, and host immune function, augment cellular antioxidant systems, decrease the hypermetabolic response to tissue injury, and preserve intestinal mucosal integrity (9,56,109–119). A meta-analysis of 15 prospective, randomized clinical trials that compared early versus delayed enteral nutritional support in critically ill surgical patients demonstrated that early feeding decreases infectious complications and ICU length of stay (108). Based on the results of this meta-analysis and the experimental data presented above, it is recommended that enteral nutrition should be initiated within 12 hours of admission to the ICU in all critically ill patients. There can be no benefit from delaying the initiation of nutritional support.

IV. Nutrient Composition

A variety of enteral nutritional formulas are currently available; these are best classified as standard polymeric enteral formulas, immunomodulating diets, elemental formulas, and disease specific formulas (Table 3). Elemental formulas are reserved for patients with enteric fistulae and short gut syndrome. The role of immunomodulating and disease specific formulas will be reviewed further.

A. The Role of Immunomodulating Diets in Critically Ill Patients

It has recently been recognized that a number of specific nutritional supplements are able to modulate the biologic response to injury, inflammation, and infection. The addition of these specific nutrients to standard enteral formulations has resulted in a new generation of enteral nutritional formulas and the concept of immuno-modulating nutritional support. In general, these immunomodulating nutritional formulas contain supplemented glutamine, arginine, ω-3 fatty acids, and antioxidants. Experimental data has demonstrated that each of these nutritional supplements have favorable biological and clinical effects (120–126). Glutamine is a nonessential amino acid that is synthesized and released from

Table 3 Composition of the Commonly Used Enteral Formulas

	Impact[a]	Crucial[a,d]	Perative[d]	Traumacal[f]	Jevity[b,c]	Osmolyte[b]	Nepro[g]	Peptinex DT[d]	Peptamen[d]	Vivonex Plus[e]
Kcal/mL	1	1.5	1.3	1.5	1.2	1	2	1	1	1
Protein g/L	56	94	67	82	55	37	70	50	40	45
Sodium meq/L	48	51	45	51	58	26	36	74	24	27
Potassium meq/L	36	48	44	36	47	26	27	21	38.5	27
Osmolarity mosmol/L	375	490	385	560	450	300	665	460	270	650
Arginine g/L	12.5	15	8	—	—	—	—	—	—	—
Glutamine g/L	0	7.2	0	—	—	—	—	—	6.8	—
Fat g/L	28	67.6[i]	37	68[h]	39.3	34.7	95.6	17.4	39[j]	6.7
EPA/DHA g/L	1.7	2.8	—	—	—	—	—	—	—	—
n6:n3 fatty acids	1.4:1	2:1	4.8:1	—	—	—	—	—	—	—
Omega-3 (%)	1.6	6.9	—	—	—	—	—	—	—	—

[a]Immunomodulating formula.
[b]"Standard" polymeric formula.
[c]"Renal formula."
[d]Semi-elemental formula (peptides and amino acids).
[e]Elemental formula (100% amino acids).
[f]"Other" formula.
[g]Fiber containing.
[h]30% medium chain triglyceride.
[i]50% medium chain triglyceride.
[j]70% medium chain triglyceride.

skeletal muscle into the circulation, where it acts as an interorgan nitrogen and carbon transporter for intracellular glutamate (122,123). It is a precursor for the synthesis of the major antioxidant glutathione. Most importantly glutamine is a primary nutrient for enterocytes and the gut associated lymphoid tissue. In the critically ill, glutamine synthesis may be unable to keep pace with demand, and a deficiency state ensures (123). This may have profound effects on the integrity of the gastrointestinal tract and lymphoid tissue. Arginine is traditionally regarded as a nonessential amino-acid. In the critically ill, however, arginine may become essential. Arginine has diverse biological actions, including the stimulation of growth hormone, prolactin, and insulin-like growth factor; it is the precursor of nitric oxide (NO), is required for the synthesis of hydroxy-proline, and is required for lymphocyte function (121,125,127). The ω-3 fatty acids eicosapentaenoic acid and docosahexaenoic acid, which are derived from fish oil, are usually added to immuno-modulating nutritional formulas (128). An increase in the proportion of ω-3 as opposed to ω-6 fatty acids has numerous biological effects; however, in the critically ill, its effects on leukotriene and prostaglandin production may be most important. Overall, inflammatory mediators derived from ω-3 fatty acids are less inflammatory and less immunosuppressive (124,128,129).

To date, over 20 randomized clinical trials have been performed that have evaluated the role of immunomodulating enteral formulas in critically ill patients. While the results of these studies have been widely debated, most have demonstrated a clinical benefit in terms of reduced infectious complications and reduced ICU and hospital length of stay (130–132). The effect of these formulations on organ failure and mortality is less clear. As the composition of many of these formulas differ, it is likely that they do not have equivalent biological and clinical effects. Indeed in the meta-analysis reported by Heyland et al. (131), formulas with a high arginine content were associated with a significant reduction in infectious complications and a trend towards a lower mortality rate, compared to immuno-modulating formulas with little to no supplemented arginine.

The use of arginine supplemented immunomodulating diets in patients with sepsis is controversial. It has been suggested that arginine is an "immuno-stimulating nutrient" that increases the pro-inflammatory response in patients with sepsis and "adds fuel to the fire" (133–135). This argument is based on the fact that arginine is the precursor for NO synthesis and that the generation of NO appears to be a fundamental finding in sepsis. In addition to mediating vasodilation, NO has been implicated in the causation of the myocardial depression of sepsis (136–138).

Arginine supplementation increase NO generation in sepsis (139), while arginine depletion reduces NO production (140). It has therefore been suggested that arginine supplementation will increase NO mediated tissue damage in sepsis (133,134). The notion that arginine is pro-inflammatory and increases tissue inflammation and injury in patients with sepsis may be incorrect. Emerging data suggests that NO may be an important anti-inflammatory mediator and regulator of microvascular blood flow in sepsis. NO has been demonstrated to down-regulate the expression of endothelial cell adhesion molecules (ECAMs) as well as the pro-inflammatory cytokines (141–145). In addition, NO decreases tissue factor expression and inhibits platelet adhesion and aggregation to the endothelium, actions that may prevent microvascular thrombosis in sepsis (146–150). While the anti-inflammatory effects of NO have not been fully delineated, it is thought that NO inhibits the activation of nuclear transcription factor kappa-B (NF-κB).

The most persuasive evidence to support the notion that L-arginine may be anti-inflammatory is the effect of arginine supplementation on the microvascular reperfusion injury and allograft survival in both experimental transplantation models and in transplant patients. Numerous experimental studies have demonstrated that L-arginine reduces the reperfusion injury in transplanted organs with attenuation of leukocyte infiltration, tissue injury, and improved microvascular perfusion (151–154). In a prospective, randomized clinical trial in patients undergoing renal transplant Alexander and colleagues demonstrated a reduction in the number of rejection episodes from 37% in the control group to 7% in the group of patients receiving a nutritional supplement containing arginine and canola oil (155).

The effect of arginine supplementation and nitric oxide synthase (NOS) inhibition has been investigated in a number of experimental sepsis models. L-arginine has been demonstrated to increase cardiac output in endotoxic shock models, whereas NOS inhibition decreases cardiac output, contractility, oxygen delivery, and oxygen utilization (156,157). In a porcine model, inhalation of NO prevented endotoxin-induced left ventricular impairment (158). Price et al. (159) have demonstrated that L-arginine reverses the myocardial depression seen in endotoxic shock. Madden et al. (160) demonstrated that arginine supplementation increased the survival times of rats with peritonitis induced by cecal ligation and puncture (CLP). Similarly, Gianotti et al. (161) and colleagues demonstrated a survival rate of 56% following CLP in arginine-supplemented mice, compared to 20% in those receiving standard nutrition. This survival advantage was reversed with the arginine inhibitor NMA. Minard et al. (162) demonstrated that inhibition of NO synthesis decreased survival in a murine endotoxin model. Similarly, in an awake canine endotoxin model, Cobb et al. (163) demonstrated that inhibition of NOS decreased cardiac index and oxygen consumption and increased mortality. In a murine endotoxin model, Park et al. (164) demonstrated an increased mortality with NOS inhibition, which was associated with an increase in tissue damage in the lung, liver, and kidney.

The benefits of L-arginine (and NO) supplementation in critically ill septic patients can be inferred from two complementary clinical studies; the first investigated the "impact" of supplemental L-arginine, while the second studied the outcome of a NOS inhibitor in patients with sepsis. Galban et al. (165) demonstrated a significant reduction in all-cause mortality in septic ICU patients fed an enteral formula enriched with arginine. Recently, a randomized, placebo-controlled, clinical trial of a nonselective NOS inhibitor in patients with sepsis was stopped prematurely due to a significantly higher mortality in the treatment arm (166).

In summary, this data suggests that L-arginine supplementation may be beneficial in patients with sepsis. The importance of L-arginine supplementation is underscored by the fact that sepsis may be an L-arginine deficient state. L-arginine levels may become critically reduced in septic patients due to deceased intake, increased metabolism, and diversion of L-arginine through the urea cycle as a consequence of increased arginase expression (167–171).

B.   The Role of "Nutritional" Antioxidants

The release of free radicals with damage to host cell membranes and other cell components plays an important role in tissue damage in critically ill patients. Endogenous antioxidants are rapidly depleted in critically ill patients, and low levels of antioxidants are associated with organ dysfunction and increased mortality (172–174). One of the main scavenger systems responsible for cleavage of free radicals is the selenium-dependent glutathione peroxidase (174). In a small randomized controlled trial in patients with sepsis, Angstwurm et al. (175) demonstrated that selenium replacement reduced organ dysfunction and improved clinical outcome.

Flavonoids are a large group of naturally occurring antioxidants ubiquitously distributed in the plant kingdom. Flavonols, such as quercetin, are predominantly found in onions, broccoli, apples, tea, and red wine (176,177). Multiple biological effects of the flavonoids have been described in addition to their antioxidant properties, including anti-inflammatory, antiallergic, and antimutagenic (178–181). The anti-inflammatory action is mediated in part by inhibition of cytokine action (182). In addition, flavonoids have been reported to inhibit the catalytic activities of a variety of enzymes involved in the inflammatory cascade, including phospholipase C, cyclooxygenase, lipoxygenase, and myeloperoxidase (178–181). Peng et al. (183) demonstrated a lower mortality with a reduction in the serum levels of TNF-α and CRP in patients with SIRS treated with rhubarb (high concentration of flavonoids). The clinical benefit of flavonoids in the treatment of sepsis and SIRS requires further study.

V.   Disease Specific Nutritional Formulations

Many patients with chronic renal failure, cirrhosis, atherosclerotic and degenerative neurological diseases, and chronic respiratory failure are malnourished prior to admission to the ICU, and nutritional support is particularly important in these patients. In general, the principles outlined above apply to these patients, that is, the early initiation of enteral nutrition. However, specific issues apply to certain disease states, and these will be outlined below.

A.   Chronic Respiratory Failure

Nutritional hypercapnia may become a problem in patients with chronic lung disease and CO_2 retention and may interfere with attempts at weaning. Limiting total caloric intake to 20–25 kcal/kg/day may avert this problem. As the respiratory quotient is lower for fats than carbohydrates, a formula with a higher fat content may further limit CO_2 production.

B. Liver Failure

The use of protein restriction in hepatic encephalopathy/liver failure is controversial. No controlled studies have been performed. Intolerance of dietary protein should be balanced against the increasing evidence that adequate nutrition, including fair amounts of protein, can improve clinical outcome in patients with hepatic encephalopathy. Therefore, in patients with liver cirrhosis and hepatic encephalopathy, one should initially restrict daily protein intake to 0.5 g/kg/day and slowly increase the intake to 1.0 g/kg/day. In patients with alcoholic hepatitis who can be treated with standard anti-encephalopathy medications (e.g., lactulose), low protein intake may be associated with worsening hepatic encephalopathy, while a higher protein intake correlates with improvement in hepatic encephalopathy (184). Enteral formulations supplemented with ornithine-aspartate reduce ammonia levels and have useful therapeutic effects in patients with mild encephalopathy. L-ornithine-L-aspartate can be administered three times daily in a total dose of 18 g/day. Zinc deficiency is common in patients with cirrhosis. Zinc is required for the metabolism of ammonia to urea. Zinc supplementation (600 mg zinc sulphate daily) should be considered.

Specific enteral formulas that contain relative large amounts of the branched chain amino acids valine, leucine, and isoleuicne with low quantities of aromatic amino acids have been developed for patients with liver failure. The rationale for these formulas is that the infusion of branched chain amino acids corrects the imbalance between aromatic and branched chain amino acids in plasma and the central nervous system, thereby improving nitrogen balance and lessening encephalopathy (185). The clinical benefit of these formulas has yet to be demonstrated.

The role/benefit of immune-modulating diets with added arginine and glutamine has not been established in patients with liver disease. Arginine supplementation will increase NO production; since NO plays a pivotal role in the pathophysiology of both the hepatorenal and hepatopulmonary syndromes, arginine may adversely effect the outcome in patients with liver failure. Similarly, glutamine supplementation should be used with great caution in patients with liver failure. Owing to the extra nitrogen molecule on this amino acid, it may worsen hepatic encephalopathy (186).

C. Renal Failure

Most patients with acute renal failure are hypercatabolic and require increased quantities of nutrients. Patients with ARF should receive a minimum of 1 g protein/kg/day and optimal nonprotein calories. Protein intake in critically patients should not be limited in an attempt to avoid initiation of dialysis. In patients who are not undergoing dialysis, specialized "renal enteral formulas" are available, which are more concentrated (less volume) with lower sodium and potassium content. These formulas, however, have no advantage in patients who are being dialyzed. In patients with chronic renal failure, keto-analogs may be useful in patients with decreased protein intake for greater than one week. In an experimental model of ischemic acute renal failure, enteral as compared to parental nutrition was associated with a more rapid recovery of renal function (187), thus reinforcing the advantages of enteral versus parenteral nutrition in the critically ill patient.

D. Acute Pancreatitis

Acute pancreatitis results is a hypermetabolic, hyperdynamic, systemic inflammatory response syndrome (SIRS) that creates a highly catabolic stress state. Despite the lack of prospective data, gut rest (prohibiting enteral intake), with or without the provision of parental nutrition, has become regarded as the "standard of care" in patients with acute pancreatitis (188). However, recent evidence suggests that enteral nutrition may be feasible (and desirable) in patients with acute pancreatitis. Animal studies have demonstrated that the site in the gastrointestinal tract to which feedings are delivered determines whether the pancreas is simulated and that jejunal feedings result in negligible increases in enzyme, bicarbonate, and volume output from the pancreas (189,190). This observation has been confirmed in humans (191). Five randomized studies have been reported that compared early jejunal enteral feeding with TPN in patients with pancreatitis (38,42,45,49,192). In all of these studies, enteral nutrition was associated with a lower risk of infections, fewer surgical interventions were required to control the pancreatitis, and this was associated with a shorter hospital length of stay. Based on these data, patients with moderate and severe pancreatitis (greater than three Ranson or Imrie criteria) should have a jejunal feeding tube placed soon after admission to hospital with the early initiation of enteral feed. Most cases of acute pancreatitis, however, are mild and self-limiting, with serum enzyme levels returning toward normal within two to four days. Specific nutritional support interventions may not be required in these patients. Indeed, Abou-Assi et al. (38) reported that 75% of patients with pancreatitis could resume oral feeding within 48 hours of admission.

E. Oral Intake Postendotracheal Extubation

After tracheal extubation, patients are especially at risk of aspiration because of the residual effects of sedative drugs, the presence of nasogastric tubes, and swallowing dysfunction related to alterations of upper airway sensitivity, glottic injury, and laryngeal muscular dysfunction (193–195). Alteration in the swallow reflex can be detected in patients who have been intubated for as short as 24 hours. This abnormality usually recovers within 48 hours (193). However, 25% of elderly patients will still have residual swallow dysfunction two weeks postextubation (196). Oral feeding should be withheld for at least six hours after extubation (in case reintubation is required), followed by a pureed and then soft diet for at least 48 hours. A formal swallow evaluation by a speech–language pathologist is suggested in cases of traumatic intubations, in patients who have difficultly swallowing a pureed/soft diet, in patients with a history of a cerebovascular accident, and in patients with anatomical or functional abnormalities of the upper airway (197).

F. Patients on High Dose Propofol

Propofol emulsion contains approximately 0.1 g of fat (1.1 kcal) for every milliliter. An infusion of propofol may therefore provide a significant caloric load. In patients receiving high-dose propofol infusions, the enteral feeds need to be adjusted to take into account the added caloric load. A low-fat enteral formulation, such as Peptinex™, may be used.

VI. Nutrient Quantity

A caloric intake of 25–30 kcal/kg/day and a protein intake of 1–1.5 g/kg/day is the nutrient intake currently recommended in critically ill patients based on estimated energy expenditure (Table 4). There are no data to suggest that matching caloric intake to energy expenditure measured by indirect calorimetry is beneficial. Indeed, experimental studies suggest that administration of nutrients at metabolic expenditure can exacerbate inflammation and increase mortality (198).

Anorexia is a component of the stress response. Animals and humans decrease nutrient intake during illness and following injury. There is debate regarding the significance of decreased nutrient intake following injury. Clearly, long-term starvation leads to loss of lean body mass, cellular and organ dysfunction, and increased mortality. However, there are no data available to suggest that short term underfeeding (as opposed to complete starvation) has any detrimental effects on recovery from critical illness. Although full nutrient intake may optimally support protein synthesis and growth, it may also stimulate detrimental processes such as bacterial

Table 4 The Recommended Average Daily Nutritional Requirements

Nonprotein calories	20–25 kcals/kg/day
CHO	Max 4 mg/kg/day ($\pm$1600 cals)
Lipid	4–12 kcals/kg/day
Protein	1–1.5 g/kg/day
Other	Water soluble vitamins, fat soluble vitamins and trace elements

virulence, autoimmune processes, cytokine release, inflammation, and energy consumption (198). This has led to the concept of "permissive underfeeding" (198).

Animal studies clearly indicate that overfeeding (administering nutrients at levels which exceed energy consumption) is detrimental. Yamazaki et al. (199) randomized rats to receive a normal diet or a high calorie/protein diet. After six days of feeding, the animals were subjected to cecal ligation and perforation. Although the high calorie/protein diet resulted in better nitrogen balance, four-day mortality was increased from 14% to 53%. Alexander et al. induced peritonitis in guinea pigs by infusing *Escherichia coli* and *Staphylococcus aureus* (200). Overfeeding decreased survival rates (10% vs. 38%).

Many animal studies of critical illness suggest that moderate underfeeding (administering nutrients at less than metabolic expenditure) improves outcome. Alexander et al. (200) reported improved survival with underfeeding in a model of *E. coli/S. aureus* sepsis (57% vs. 38%). Survival was improved despite greater weight loss. Peck et al. (201) studied calorie and protein restriction in mice with *Salmonella peritonitis*. Calorie restriction (50% of normal) improved survival. On the other hand, severe protein restriction decreased survival. These authors further studied dietary restriction during guinea pig peritonitis produced with *E. coli/S. aureus* infection (202). Moderate protein restriction improved survival despite worsening of nitrogen balance. Other studies have demonstrated improved survival with restricted diets in mice infected with *Salmonella typhimurium* and in rats following endotoxin administration (203,204). In experimental models of sepsis, severe dietary restriction (as opposed to moderate restriction) has been reported to increase mortality (205). Overall, these studies suggest that severe dietary restriction is associated with increased mortality during infection. However, moderate restriction may improve survival following infection.

Overfeeding critically ill septic patients is associated with increased morbidity. The role of permissive underfeeding requires further study. However, until additional data is available, it may be reasonable to limit the caloric intake of critically ill patients to approximately 20 kcal/kg/day and protein to 1 g/kg/day. Permissive underfeeding may not be appropriate in burn patients and patients with severe malnutrition.

VII. Conclusion

The current published scientific data clearly and unambiguously demonstrates that enteral nutrition is the preferred route of nutritional support in critically ill patients. Furthermore, the earlier enteral nutritional support is initiated, the better the outcome. An accumulating body of evidence suggests that enteral formulas supplemented with glutamine, arginine, and ω-3-fatty acids improve immune function and reduce the complication rate (specifically infections) in critically ill patients. Based on this data we recommend placement of an oro/nasogastric tube or a small bowel feeding tube (following abdominal surgery) and the initiation of enteral feeding with an immunomodulating formula within 12 hours of admission to the ICU. Enteral feeding should commence at a rate of 20 cc/hr, with the rate advanced by 20 cc every six hours in patients with a gastric residual of less than 300 mL. The rate of increase should be slower in patients with risk factors for gastroparesis and/or ileus. A promotility agent should be considered in patients with high gastric residuals.

References

1. McCowen KC, Malhotra A, Bistrian BR. Stress-induced hyperglycemia. Crit Care Clin 2001; 17:107–124.
2. Cerra FB. Hypermetabolism, organ failure, and metabolic support. Surgery 1987; 101:1–14.
3. Siegel JH, Cerra FB, Coleman B, Giovannini I, Shetye M, Border JR, McMenamy RH. Physiological and metabolic correlations in human sepsis. Invited commentary. Surgery 1979; 86:163–193.
4. Mizock BA. Alterations in fuel metabolism in critical illness. Hyperglycemia. In: Ober KP, ed. Endocrinology of Critical Disease. Totawa, NJ: Humana Press, 1997:197–297.
5. van den Berghe G, Wouters P, Weekers F, Verwaest C, Bruyninckx F, Schetz M, Vlasselaers D, Ferdinande P, Lauwers P, Bouillon R. Intensive insulin therapy in critically ill patients. N Engl J Med 2001; 345:1359–1367.
6. van den Berghe G, Wouters PJ, Bouillon R, Weekers F, Verwaest C, Schetz M, Vlasselaers D, Ferdinande P, Lauwers P. Outcome benefit of intensive insulin therapy in the critically ill: Insulin dose versus glycemic control. Crit Care Med 2003; 31:359–366.
7. Elman R. Amino acid content of the blood following intravenous injection of hydrolyzed casein. Proc Soc Exp Biol Med 1937; 37:437–440.
8. Wretlind A. Recollections of pioneers in nutrition: landmarks in the development of parenteral nutrition. J Am Coll Nutr 1992; 11:366–373.
9. Hadfield RJ, Sinclair DG, Houldsworth PE, Evans TW. Effects of enteral and parenteral nutrition on gut mucosal permeability in the critically ill. Am J Respir Crit Care Med 1995; 152:1545–1548.
10. Nakasaki H, Mitomi T, Tajima T, Ohnishi N, Fujii K. Gut bacterial translocation during total parenteral nutrition in experimental rats and its countermeasure. Am J Surg 1998; 175:38–43.
11. Shou J, Lappin J, Minnard EA, Daly JM. Total parenteral nutrition, bacterial translocation, and host immune function. Am J Surg 1994; 167:145–150.
12. Qiu JG, Delany HM, Teh EL, Freundlich L, Gliedman ML, Steinberg JJ, Chang CJ, Levenson SM. Contrasting effects of identical nutrients given parenterally or enterally after 70% hepatectomy: bacterial translocation. Nutrition 1997; 13:431–437.
13. Levine GM, Deren JJ, Steiger E, Zinno R. Role of oral intake in maintenance of gut mass and disaccharide activity. Gastroenterology 1974; 67:975–982.
14. Deitch EA. Bacterial translocation of the gut flora. J Trauma 1990; 30:S184–S189.
15. Langkamp-Henken B, Donovan TB, Pate LM, Maull CD, Kudsk KA. Increased intestinal permeability following blunt and penetrating trauma. Crit Care Med 1995; 23:660–664.

16. Deitch EA, Winterton J, Li M, Berg R. The gut as a portal of entry for bacteremia. Role of protein malnutrition. Ann Surg 1987; 205:681–692.

17. Sugiura T, Tashiro T, Yamamori H, Takagi K, Hayashi N, Itabashi T, Toyoda Y, Sano W, Nitta H, Hirano J, Nakajima N, Ito I. Effects of total parenteral nutrition on endotoxin translocation and extent of the stress response in burned rats. Nutrition 1999; 15:570–575.

18. Kudsk KA, Li J, Renegar KB. Loss of upper respiratory tract immunity with parenteral feeding. Ann Surg 1996; 223:629–635.

19. Janu P, Li J, Renegar KB, Kudsk KA. Recovery of gut-associated lymphoid tissue and upper respiratory tract immunity after parenteral nutrition. Ann Surg 1997; 225:707–715.

20. King BK, Li J, Kudsk KA. A temporal study of TPN-induced changes in gut-associated lymphoid tissue and mucosal immunity. Arch Surg 1997; 132:1303–1309.

21. Li J, Kudsk KA, Gocinski B, et al. Effects of parenteral and enteral nutrition on gut-associated lymphoid tissue. J Trauma 1995; 39:44–51.

22. Alverdy JC, Burke D. Total parenteral nutrition: iatrogenic immunosuppression. Nutrition 1992; 8:359–365.

23. Gogos CA, Kalfarentzos F. Total parenteral nutrition and immune system activity: a review. Nutrition 1995; 11:339–344.

24. Gogos CA, Kalfarentzos FE, Zoumbos NC. Effect of different types of total parenteral nutrition on T-lymphocyte subpopulations and NK cells. Am J Clin Nutr 1990; 51:119–122.

25. Sedman PC, Somers SS, Ramsden CW, Brennan TG, Guillou PJ. Effects of different lipid emulsions on lymphocyte function during total parenteral nutrition. Br J Surg 1991; 78:1396–1399.

26. Waitzberg DL, Lotierzo PH, Logullo AF, Torrinhas RS, Pereira CC, Meier R. Parenteral lipid emulsions and phagocytic systems. Br J Nutr 2002; 87(suppl 1): S49–S57.

27. Maderazo EG, Woronick CL, Quercia RA, Hickingbotham N, Drezner AD. The inhibitory effect of parenteral nutrition on recovery of neutrophil locomotory function in blunt trauma. Ann Surg 1988; 208:221–226.

28. Granato D, Blum S, Rossle C, et al. Effects of parenteral lipid emulsions with different fatty acid composition on immune cell functions in vitro. JPEN 2000; 24:113–118.

29. Okada Y, Papp E, Klein NJ, Pierro A. Total parenteral nutrition directly impairs cytokine production after bacterial challenge. J Pediatr Surg 1999; 34: 277–280.

30. Petersen SR, Kudsk KA, Carpenter G, Sheldon GE. Malnutrition and immunocompetence: increased mortality following an infectious challenge during hyperalimentation. J Trauma 1981; 21:528–533.

31. Kudsk KA, Carpenter G, Petersen S, Sheldon GF. Effect of enteral and parenteral feeding in malnourished rats with *E. coli*-hemoglobin adjuvant peritonitis. J Surg Res 1981; 31:105–110.

32. Kudsk KA, Stone JM, Carpenter G, Sheldon GF. Enteral and parenteral feeding influences mortality after hemoglobin-*E. coli* peritonitis in normal rats. J Trauma 1983; 23:605–609.

33. Lin MT, Saito H, Fukushima R, Inaba T, Fukatsu K, Inoue T, Furukawa S, Han I, Muto T. Route of nutritional supply influences local, systemic, and remote organ responses to intraperitoneal bacterial challenge. Ann Surg 1996; 223:84–93.

34. Perioperative total parenteral nutrition in surgical patients. The Veterans Affairs Total Parenteral Nutrition Cooperative Study Group. N Engl J Med 1991; 325:525–532.

35. Parenteral nutrition in patients receiving cancer chemotherapy. Ann Intern Med 1989; 110:734–736.

36. Kudsk KA, Croce MA, Fabian TC, Minard G, Tolley EA, Poret HA, Kuhl MR, Brown RO. Enteral versus parenteral feeding. Effects on septic morbidity after blunt and penetrating abdominal trauma. Ann Surg 1992; 215:503–511.

37. Moore FA, Feliciano DV, Andrassy RJ, McArdle AH, Booth FV, Morgenstein-Wagner TB, Kellum JM, Jr., Welling RE, Moore EE. Early enteral feeding, compared with parenteral, reduces postoperative septic complications. The results of a meta-analysis. Ann Surg 1992; 216:172–183.

38. Abou-Assi S, Craig K, O'Keefe SJ. Hypocaloric jejunal feeding is better than total parenteral nutrition in acute pancreatitis: results of a randomized comparative study. Am J Gastroenterol 2002; 97:2255–2262.

39. Braga M, Gianotti L, Vignali A, Cestari A, Bisagni P, Di C, V. Artificial nutrition after major abdominal surgery: impact of route of administration and composition of the diet. Crit Care Med 1998; 26:24–30.

40. Gianotti L, Braga M, Vignali A, Balzano G, Zerbi A, Bisagni P, Di C, V. Effect of route of delivery and formulation of postoperative nutritional support in patients undergoing major operations for malignant neoplasms. Arch Surg 1997; 132:1222–1229.

41. Bozzetti F, Braga M, Gianotti L, Gavazzi C, Mariani L. Postoperative enteral versus parenteral nutrition in malnourished patients with gastrointestinal cancer: a randomized multicenter trial. Lancet 2001; 358:1487–1492.

42. Windsor AC, Kanwar S, Li AG, Barnes E, Guthrie JA, Spark JI, Welsh F, Guillou PJ, Reynolds JV. Compared with parenteral nutrition, enteral feeding attenuates the acute phase response and improves disease severity in acute pancreatitis. Gut 1998; 42:431–435.

43. Lin MT, Saito H, Fukushima R, Inaba T, Fukatsu K, Inoue T, Furukawa S, Han I, Matsuda T, Muto T. Preoperative total parenteral nutrition influences postoperative systemic cytokine responses after colorectal surgery. Nutrition 1997; 13:8–12.

44. Fong YM, Marano MA, Barber A, et al. Total parenteral nutrition and bowel rest modify the metabolic response to endotoxin in humans. Ann Surg 1989; 210:449–456.

45. Kalfarentzos F, Kehagias J, Mead N, Kokkinis K, Gogos CA. Enteral nutrition is superior to parenteral nutrition in severe acute pancreatitis: results of a randomized prospective trial. Br J Surg 1997; 84:1665–1669.

46. Pupelis G, Selga G, Austrums E, Kaminski A. Jejunal feeding, even when instituted late improves outcomes in patiens with severe pancreatitis and peritonitis. Nutrition 2001; 17:91–94.

47. Sax HC, Warner BW, Talamini MA, Hamilton FN, Bell RH, Fischer JE, Bower RH. Early total parenteral nutrition in acute pancreatitis: LAck of beneficial effects. Am J Surg 1987; 153:117–124.

48. Dejong HH, Greve JW, Soeters PB. Nutrition in patients with acute pancreatitis. Curr Opin Crit Care 2001; 7:251–256.

49. Olah A, Pardavi G, Belagyi T, Nagy A, Issekutz A, Mohamed GE. Early nasojejunal feeding in acute pancreatitis is associated with a lower complication rate. Nutrition 2002; 18:259–262.

50. Lyman B. Metabolic complications associated with parenteral nutrition. J Infusion Nurs 2002; 25:36–44.

51. Meadows N. Monitoring and complications of parenteral nutrition. Nutrition 1998; 14:806–808.

52. Klein CJ, Stanek GS, Wiles CE III. Overfeeding macronutrients to critically ill adults: metabolic complications. J Am Diet Assoc 1998; 98:795–806.

53. Basu R, Muller DP, Papp E, et al. Free radical formation in infants: the effect of critical illness, parenteral nutrition, and enteral feeding. J Pediatr Surg 1999; 34:1091–1095.

54. Pitkanen O, Hallman M, Andersson S. Generation of free radicals in lipid emulsion used in parenteral nutrition. Pediatr Res 1991; 29:56–59.

55. Sandhu IS, Jarvis C, Everson GT. Total parenteral nutrition and cholestasis. Clinics in Liver Disease 1999; 3:489–508.

56. Strubelt O, Dost-Kempf E, Siegers CP, Younes M, Volpel M, Preuss U, Dreckmann JG. The influence of fasting on the susceptibility of mice to hepatotoxic injury. Toxicol Appl Pharmacol 1981; 60:66–77.

57. Gimmon Z, Murphy RF, Chen MH, Nachbauer CA, Fischer JE, Joffe SN. The effect of parenteral and enteral nutrition on portal and systemic immunoreactivities of gastrin, glucagon and vasoactive intestinal polypeptide (VIP). Ann Surg 1982; 196:571–575.

58. Bozzetti F, Baticci F, Cozzaglio L, Biasi S, Facchetti G. Metabolic effects of intra-portal nutrition in humans. Nutrition 2001; 17:292–299.

59. Kiyama T, Witte MB, Thornton FJ, Barbul A. The route of nutrition support affects the early phase of wound healing. JPEN 1998; 22:276–279.

60. Khalili T, Navarro RA, Middleton YM, Margulies DR. Early postoperative enteral feeding increases anastomotic strength in a peritonitis model. Am J Surg 2001; 182:621–624.

61. Kiyama T, Efron DT, Tantry U, Barbul A. Effect of nutritional route on colonic ana-stomotic healing in the rat. J Gastrointestinal Surg 1999; 3:441–446.

62. Lewis SJ, Egger M, Sylvester PA, Thomas S. Early enteral feeding versus "nil by mouth" after gastrointestinal surgery: systematic review and meta-analysis of con-trolled trials. Br Med J 2001; 323:773–776.

63. Heyland DK, MacDonald S, Keefe L, Drover JW. Total parenteral nutrition in the critically ill patient: a meta-analysis. J Am Med Assoc 1998; 280: 2013–2019.

64. Marik PE, Karnack C. The effect of enteral nutrition, parenteral nutrition and par-enteral nutrition together with "trickle" feeds on mortality in Critically Ill ICU patients. Crit Care Med 2001; 29(suppl):A126.

65. Marik PE, Karnack C, Varon J. The addition of trickle feeds reduces the complications associated with parenteral nutrition. Crit Care Shock 2002; 5:165–169.

66. Ochoa JB, Magnuson B, Swintowsky M, et al. Long term reduction in the cost of nutritional intervention achieved by a nutrition support service. Nutrition in Clinical Practice 2000; 15:174–180.

67. Braga M, Gianotti L, Gentilini O, Parisi V, Salis C, Carlo V. Early postoperative enteral nutrition improves gut oxygenation and reduces costs compared with total parenteral nutrition. Crit Care Med 2001; 29:242–248.

68. Pacelli F, Bossola M, Papa V, Malerba M, Modesti C, Sgadari A, Bellantone R, Doglietto GB, Modesti C, EN-TPN Study Group. Enteral vs parenteral nutrition after major abdominal surgery: an even match. Arch Surg 2001; 136:933–936.

69. Mentec H, Dupont H, Bocchetti M, et al. Upper digestive intolerance during enteral nutrition in critically ill patients: frequency, risk factors, and complications. Crit Care Med 2001; 29:1955–1961.

70. Marik PE, Zaloga G. Gastric vs Post-Pyloric Feeding? A systematic Review. Critical Care 2003; 7:R46–R51.

71. Zaloga GP, Marik P. Promotility agents in the intensive care unit. Crit Care Med 2000; 28:2657–2659.

72. Chapman MJ, Fraser RJ, Kluger MT, Buist MD, De Nichilo DJ. Erythromycin improves gastric emptying in critically ill patients intolerant of nasogastric feeding. Crit Care Med 2000; 28:2334–2337.

73. Boivin MA, Levy H. Gastric feeding with erythromycin is equivalent to transpyloric feeding in the critically ill. Crit Care Med 2001; 29:1916–1919.

74. Kortbeek JB, Haigh PI, Doig C. Duodenal versus gastric feeding in ventilated blunt trauma patients: a randomized controlled trial. J Trauma 1999; 46: 992–998.

75. Esparza J, Boivin MA, Hartshorne MF, Levy H. Equal aspiration rates in gastrically and transpylorically fed critically ill patients. Intensive Care Med 2001; 27: 660–664.

76. Heyland DK, Drover JW, MacDonald S, Novak F, Lam M. Effect of postpyloric feeding on gastroesophageal regurgitation and pulmonary microaspiration: results of a randomized controlled trial. Crit Care Med 2001; 29:1495–1501.

77. Jooste CA, Mustoe J, Collee G. Metoclopramide improves gastric motility in critically ill patients. Intensive Care Med 1999; 25:464–468.

78. Withington DE. Dysrhythmias following intravenous metoclopramide. Intensive Care Med 1986; 12:378–379.

79. Weber FH Jr, Richards RD, McCallum RW. Erythromycin: a motilin agonist and gastrointestinal prokinetic agent. Am J Gastroenterol 1993; 88:485–490.

80. Janssens J, Peeters TL, Vantrappen G, Tack J, Urbain JL, De Roo M, Muls E, Bouillon R. Improvement of gastric emptying in diabetic gastroparesis by erythromycin. Preliminary studies. N Engl J Med 1990; 322:1028–1031.

81. Urbain JL, Vantrappen G, Janssens J, Van Cutsem E, Peeters T, De Roo M. Intravenous erythromycin dramatically accelerates gastric emptying in gastroparesis diabeticorum and normals and abolishes the emptying discrimination between solids and liquids. J Nuclear Med 1990; 31:1490–1493.

82. Mozwecz H, Pavel D, Pitrak D, Orellana P, Schlesinger PK, Layden TJ. Erythromycin stearate as prokinetic agent in postvagotomy gastroparesis. Dig Dis Sci 1990; 35:902–905.

83. Seppala H, Klaukka T, Vuopio-Varkila J, Muotiala A, Helenius H, Lager K, Huovinen P. The effect of changes in the consumption of macrolide antibiotics on erythromycin resistance in group A streptococci in Finland. Finnish Study Group for Antimicrobial Resistance. N Engl J Med 1997; 337:441–446.

84. Zaloga GP. Bedside method for placing small bowel feeding tubes in critically ill patients. A prospective study. Chest 1991; 100:1643–1646.

85. Smith HG, Orlando R, III. Enteral nutrition: should we feed the stomach? Crit Care Med 1999; 27:1652–1653.

86. Davis TJ, Sun D, Dalton ML. A modified technique for bedside placement of naso-duodenal feeding tubes. J Am Coll Surg 1994; 178:407–409.

87. Thurlow PM. Bedside enteral feeding tube placement into duodenum and jejunum. JPEN 1986; 10:104–105.

88. Rees RG, Payne-James JJ, King C, Silk DB. Spontaneous transpyloric passage and performance of 'fine bore' polyurethrane feeding tubes: a controlled clinical trial. JPEN 1988; 12:469–472.

89. Hernandez-Socorro CR, Marin J, Ruiz-Santana S, Santana L, Manzano JL. Bedside sonographic-guided versus blind nasoenteric feeding tube placement in critically ill patients. Crit Care Med 1996; 24:1690–1694.

90. Hillard AE, Waddell JJ, Metzler MH, McAlpin D. Fluoroscopically guided naso-enteric feeding tube placement versus bedside placement. South Med J 1995; 88:425–428.

91. Lord LM, Weiser-Maimone A, Pulhamus M, Sax HC. Comparison of weighted vs unweighted enteral feeding tubes for efficacy of transpyloric intubation. JPEN 1993; 17:271–273.

92. Gabriel SA, Ackermann RJ, Castresana MR. A new technique for placement of nasoenteral feeding tubes using external magnetic guidance. Crit Care Med 1997; 25:641–645.

93. Grathwohl KW, Gibbons RV, Dillard TA, Horwhat JD, Roth BJ, Thompson JW, Cambier PA. Bedside videoscopic placement of feeding tubes: development of fiberoptics through the tube. Crit Care Med 1997; 25:629–634.

94. Spalding HK, Sullivan KJ, Soremi O, Gonzalez F, Goodwin SR. Bedside placement of transpyloric feeding tubes in the pediatric intensive care unit using gastric insufflation. Crit Care Med 2000; 28:2041–2044.

95. Keidan I, Gallagher TJ. Electrocardiogram-guided placement of enteral feeding tubes. Crit Care Med 2000; 28:2631–2633.

96. Kaufman JP, Hughes WB, Kerstein MD. Pneumothorax after nasoenteral feeding tube placement. Am Surg 2001; 67:772–773.

97. Wendell GD, Lenchner GS, Promisloff RA. Pneumothorax complicating small-bore feeding tube placement. Arch Intern Med 1991; 151:599–602.

98. Arsura EL, Munoz AD. Pneumothorax following feeding tube placement. Arch Intern Med 2476; 151:2473.

99. Kools AM, Snyder LS, Cass OW. Pneumothorax: complication of enteral feeding tube placement. Dig Dis Sci 1987; 32:1212–1213.

100. Khan MS, Gross JS. Pneumothorax complicating small-bore nasogastric feeding tube insertion. J Am Geriatr Soc 1987; 35:1130–1131.

101. Purcell PN, Davis K Jr, Branson RD, Johnson DJ. Continuous duodenal feeding restores gut blood flow and increases gut oxygen utilization during PEEP ventilation for lung injury. Am J Surg 1993; 165:188–193.

102. Kazamias P, Kotzampassi K, Koufogiannis D, Eleftheriadis E. Influence of enteral nutrition-induced splanchnic hyperemia on the septic origin of splanchnic ischemia. World J Surg 1998; 22:6–11.

103. Revelly JP, Tappy L, Berger MM, Gersbach P, Cayeux C, Chiolero R. Early metabolic and splanchnic responses to enteral nutrition in postoperative cardiac surgery patients with circulatory compromise. Intensive Care Med 2001; 27:540–547.
104. Rhoden D, Matheson PJ, Carricato ND, Spain DA, Garrison RN. Immune-enhancing enteral diet selectively augments ileal blood flow in the rat. J Surg Res 2002; 106:25–30.
105. Houdijk AP, van Leeuwen PA, Boermeester MA, Van Lambalgen T, Teerlink T, Flinkerbusch EL, Sauerwein HP, Wesdorp RI. Glutamine-enriched enteral diet increases splanchnic blood flow in the rat. Am J Physiol 1994; 267:G1035–G1040.
106. Marik PE, Varon J. Sepsis: state of the art. Dis Mon 2001; 47:463–532.
107. Rivers E, Nguyen B, Havstad S, Ressler J, Muzzin A, Knoblich B, Peterson E, Tomlanovich M. Early goal-directed therapy in the treatment of severe sepsis and septic shock. N Engl J Med 2001; 345:1368–1377.
108. Marik PE, Zaloga GP. Early enteral nutrition in acutely ill patients: a systematic review. Crit Care Med 2001; 29:2264–2270.
109. Gianotti L, Alexander JW, Nelson JL, Fukushima R, Pyles T, Chalk CL. Role of early enteral feeding and acute starvation on postburn bacterial translocation and host defense: prospective, randomized trials. Crit Care Med 1994; 22:265–272.
110. Minard G, Kudsk KA. Is early feeding beneficial? How early is early? New Horiz 1994; 2:156–163.
111. Chuntrasakul C, Siltharm S, Chinswangwatanakul V, Pongprasobchai T, Chockvivatanavanit S, Bunnak A. Early nutritional support in severe traumatic patients. J Med Assoc Thailand 1996; 79:21–26.
112. Tanigawa K, Kim YM, Lancaster JR Jr, Zar HA. Fasting augments lipid peroxidation during reperfusion after ischemia in the perfused rat liver. Crit Care Med 1999; 27:401–406.
113. Bortenschlager L, Roberts PR, Black KW, Zaloga GP. Enteral feeding minimizes liver injury during hemorrhagic shock. Shock 1994; 2:351–354.
114. Beier-Holgersen R, Brandstrup B. Influence of early postoperative enteral nutrition versus placebo on cell-mediated immunity, as measured with the Multitest CMI. Scand J Gastroenterol 1999; 34:98–102.
115. Kompan L, Kremzar B, Gadzijev E, Prosek M. Effects of early enteral nutrition on intestinal permeability and the development of multiple organ failure after multiple injury. Intensive Care Med 1999; 25:157–161.
116. Gaal T, Mezes M, Miskucza O, Ribiczey-Szabo P. Effect of fasting on blood lipid peroxidation parameters of sheep. Res Vet Sci 1993; 55:104–107.
117. Wohaieb SA, Godin DV. Starvation-related alterations in free radical tissue defense mechanisms in rats. Diabetes 1987; 36:169–173.
118. Brass CA, Narciso J, Gollan JL. Enhanced activity of the free radical producing enzyme xanthine oxidase in hypoxic rat liver. Regulation and pathophysiologic significance. J Clin Invest 1991; 87:424–431.
119. Maruyama E, Kojima K, Higashi T, Sakamoto Y. Effect of diet on liver glutathione and glutathione reductase. J Biochem 1968; 63:398–399.
120. Houdijk AP, Rijnsburger ER, Emmy R, Jansen J, Wesdorp RI, Weiss KK, McCamish MA, Teerlink T, Meuwissen SG, Haarman HJ, Thijs LG, van Leeuwen PA. Randomized trial of glutamine-enriched enteral nutrition on infectious morbidity in patients with mutliple trauma. Lancet 1998; 352:772–776.

121. Efron D, Barbul A. Role of arginine in immunonutrition. J Gastroenterol 2000; 35(suppl 12):20–23.

122. Novak F, Heyland DK, Avenell A, Drover JW, Su X. Glutamine supplementation in serious illness: a systematic review of the evidence. Crit Care Med 2002; 30: 2022–2029.

123. Andrews FJ, Griffiths RD. Glutamine: essential for immune nutrition in the critically ill. Br J Nutr 2002; 87(suppl 1):S3–S8.

124. Alexander JW. Immunonutrition: the role of omega-3 fatty acids. Nutrition 1998; 14:627–633.

125. Evoy D, Lieberman MD, Fahey TJ III, Daly JM. Immunonutrition: the role of arginine. Nutrition 1998; 14:611–617.

126. Efron DT, Barbul A. Modulation of inflammation and immunity by arginine supplements. Curr Opin Clin Nutr Metab Care 1998; 1:531–538.

127. Kirk SJ, Barbul A. Role of arginine in trauma, sepsis, and immunity. JPEN 1990; 14:226S–229S.

128. Zaloga G, Marik P. Lipid modulation and systemic inflammation. Crit Care Clin 2001; 17:201–218.

129. Grimm H, Mayer K, Mayser P, Eigenbrodt E. Regulatory potential of n-3 fatty acids in immunological and inflammatory processes. [Review.] [83 refs]. Br J Nutr 2002; 87(suppl 1):S59–S67.

130. Beale RJ, Bryg DJ, Bihari DJ. Immunonutrition in the critically ill: a systematic review of clinical outcome. Crit Care Med 1999; 27:2799–2805.

131. Heyland DK, Novak F, Drover JW, Jain M, Su X, Suchner U. Should immunonutrition become routine in critically ill patients? A systematic review of the evidence. JAMA 2001; 286:944–953.

132. Zaloga GP. Immune-enhancing enteral diets: where's the beef? Crit Care Med 1998; 26:1143–1146.

133. Heyland DK. Immunonutrition in the critically ill: putting the cart before the horse? Nutr Clin Pract 2002; 17:267–272.

134. Suchner U, Heyland DK, Peter K. Immune-modulatory actions of arginine in the critically ill. Br J Nutr 2002; 87(suppl 1):S121–S132.

135. Marik PE. The cardiovascular dysfunction of sepsis: a NO and L-arginine deficient state? Crit Care Med 2003; 31:971–973.

136. Kumar A, Haery C, Parrillo JE. Myocardial dysfunction in septic shock. Crit Care Clin 2000; 16:251–287.

137. Kumar A, Brar R, Wang P, Dee L, Skorupa G, Khadour F, Schulz R, Parrillo JE. Role of nitric oxide and cGMP in human septic serum-induced depression of cardiac myocyte contractility. Am J Physiol 1999; 276:R265–R276.

138. Rangel-Frusto MS, Pittet D, Costigan M, Hwang T, Davis CS, Wenzel RP. The natural history of the systemic inflammatory response syndrome (SIRS): A prospective study. JAMA 1995; 273:117–123.

139. Bruins MJ, Soeters PB, Lamers WH, Meijer AJ, Deutz NE. L-arginine supplementation in hyperdynamic endotoxemic pigs: effect on nitric oxide synthesis by the different organs. Crit Care Med 2002; 30:508–517.

140. Bune AJ, Shergill JK, Cammack R, Cook HT. L-arginine depletion by arginase reduces nitric oxide production in endotoxic shock: an electron paramagnetic resonance study. FEBS Letters 1995; 366:127–130.

141. Peng HB, Spiecker M, Liao JK. Inducible nitric oxide: an autoregulatory feedback inhibitor of vascular inflammation. J Immunol 1998; 161:1970–1976.

142. Spiecker M, Darius H, Kaboth K, Hubner F, Liao JK. Differential regulation of endothelial cell adhesion molecule expression by nitric oxide donors and antioxidants. J Leukoc Biol 1998; 63:732–739.

143. Spiecker M, Peng HB, Liao JK. Inhibition of endothelial vascular cell adhesion molecule-1 expression by nitric oxide involves the induction and nuclear translocation of IkappaBalpha. J Biol Chem 1997; 272:30969–30974.

144. Meldrum DR, McIntyre RC, Sheridan BC, Cleveland JC, Jr., Fullerton DA, Harken AH. L-arginine decreases alveolar macrophage proinflammatory monokine production during acute lung injury by a nitric oxide synthase-dependent mechanism. J Trauma 1997; 43:888–893.

145. Laroux FS, Lefer DJ, Kawachi S, Scalia R, Cockrell AS, Gray L, van der Heyde H, Hoffman JM, Grisham MB. Role of nitric oxide in the regulation of acute and chronic inflammation. Antioxidants & Redox Signaling 2000; 2: 391–396.

146. Gerlach M, Keh D, Bezold G, Spielmann S, Kurer I, Peter RU, Falke KJ, Gerlach H. Nitric oxide inhibits tissue factor synthesis, expression and activity in human monocytes by prior formation of peroxynitrite. Intensive Care Med 1998; 24:1199–1208.

147. Yang Y, Loscalzo J. Regulation of tissue factor expression in human microvascular endothelial cells by nitric oxide. Circulation 2000; 101:2144–2148.

148. Radomski MW, Moncada S. Regulation of vascular homeostasis by nitric oxide. Thromb Haemost 1993; 70:36–41.

149. Radomski MW, Vallance P, Whitley G, Foxwell N, Moncada S. Platelet adhesion to human vascular endothelium is modulated by constitutive and cytokine induced nitric oxide. Cardiovasc Res 1993; 27:1380–1382.

150. Yao SK, Ober JC, Krishnaswami A, Ferguson JJ, Anderson HV, Golino P, Buja LM, Willerson JT. Endogenous nitric oxide protects against platelet aggregation and cyclic flow variations in stenosed and endothelium-injured arteries. Circulation 1992; 86:1302–1309.

151. Vollmar B, Janata J, Yamauchi JI, Menger MD. Attenuation of microvascular reperfusion injury in rat pancreas transplantation by L-arginine. Transplantation 1999; 67:950–955.

152. Mueller AR, Platz KP, Heckert C, Hausler M, Radke C, Neuhaus P. L-arginine application improves mucosal structure after small bowel transplantation. Transplantation Proceedings 1998; 30:2336–2338.

153. Lau JY, Sung JJ, Lee KK, Yung MY, Wong SK, Wu JC, Chan FK, Ng EK, You JH, Lee CW, Chan AC, Chung SC. Effect of intravenous omeprazole on recurrent bleeding after endoscopic treatment of bleeding peptic ulcers. N Engl J Med 2000; 343:310–316.

154. Mueller AR, Platz KP, Schirmeier A, Nussler NC, Seehofer D, Schmitz V, Nussler AK, Radke C, Neuhaus P. L-arginine application improves graft morphology and mucosal barrier function after small bowel transplantation. Transplantation Proceedings 2000; 32:1275–1277.

155. Alexander JW. Role of immunonutrition in reducing complications following organ transplantation. Transplantation Proceedings 2000; 32:574–575.

156. Pastor C, Teisseire B, Vicaut E, Payen D. Effects of L-arginine and L-nitro-arginine treatment on blood pressure and cardiac output in a rabbit endotoxin shock model [see comments]. Crit Care Med 1994; 22:465–469.

157. Statman R, Cheng W, Cunningham JN, Henderson JL, Damiani P, Siconolfi A, Rogers D, Horovitz JH. Nitric oxide inhibition in the treatment of the sepsis syndrome is detrimental to tissue oxygenation. J Surg Res 1994; 57:93–98.

158. Ishihara S, Ward JA, Tasaki O, Pruitt BA, Jr., Goodwin CW, Jr., Mozingo DW, Cioffi WG, Jr. Inhaled nitric oxide prevents left ventricular impairment during endotoxemia. J Appl Physiol 1998; 85:2018–2024.

159. Price S, Evans T, Mitchell JA. Atrial dysfunction induced by endotoxin is modulated by L-arginine: role of nitric oxide [Abstr]. Br J Pharmacol 1999; 126:77P.

160. Madden HP, Breslin RJ, Wasserkrug HL, Efron G, Barbul A. Stimulation of T cell immunity by arginine enhances survival in peritonitis. J Surg Res 1988; 44: 658–663.

161. Gianotti L, Alexander JW, Pyles T, Fukushima R. Arginine-supplemented diets improve survival in gut-derived sepsis and peritonitis by modulating bacterial clearance. The role of nitric oxide. Ann Surg 1993; 217:644–653.

162. Minnard EA, Shou J, Naama H, Cech A, Gallagher H, Daly JM. Inhibition of nitric oxide synthesis is detrimental during endotoxemia. Arch Surg 1994; 129:142–147.

163. Cobb JP, Natanson C, Hoffman WD, Lodato RF, Banks S, Koev CA, Solomon MA, Elin RJ, Hosseini JM, Danner RL. N omega-amino-L-arginine, an inhibitor of nitric oxide synthase, raises vascular resistance but increases mortality rates in awake canines challenged with endotoxin. J Exp Med 1992; 176:1175–1182.

164. Park JH, Chang SH, Lee KM, Shin SH. Protective effect of nitric oxide in an endotoxin-induced septic shock. Am J Surg 1996; 171:340–345.

165. Galban C, Montejo JC, Mesejo A, Marco P, Celaya S, Sanchez-Segura JM, Farre M, Bryg DJ. An immune-enhancing enteral diet reduces mortality rate and episodes of bacteremia in septic intensive care unit patients. Crit Care Med 2000; 28:643–648.

166. Grover R, Lopez A, Lorente J, Steingrub J, Bakker J, Willatts A, McLuckie A, Takala J. Multicenter, randomized, placebo-controlled, double blind study of the nitric oxide synthase inhibitor 546C88: effect on survival in patients with septic shock [Abstract] Crit Care Med 1999; 27(suppl):A33.

167. Klasen S, Hammermann R, Fuhrmann M, Lindemann D, Beck KF, Pfeilschifter J, Racke K. Glucocorticoids inhibit lipopolysaccharide-induced up-regulation of arginase in rat alveolar macrophages. Br J Pharmacol 2001; 132:1349–1357.

168. Bernard AC, Mistry SK, Morris SM, Jr., O'Brien WE, Tsuei BJ, Maley ME, Shirley LA, Kearney PA, Boulanger BR, Ochoa JB. Alterations in arginine metabolic enzymes in trauma. Shock 2001; 15:215–219.

169. Ochoa JB, Bernard AC, O'Brien WE, Griffen MM, Maley ME, Rockich AK, Tsuei BJ, Boulanger BR, Kearney PA, Morris JS, Jr. Arginase I expression and activity in human mononuclear cells after injury. Ann Surg 2001; 233:393–399.

170. Tsuei BJ, Bernard AC, Shane MD, Shirley LA, Maley ME, Boulanger BR, Kearney PA, Ochoa JB. Surgery induces human mononuclear cell arginase I expression. J Trauma 2001; 51:497–502.

171. Ochoa JB, Bernard AC, Mistry SK, Morris SM, Jr., Figert PL, Maley ME, Tsuei BJ, Boulanger BR, Kearney PA. Trauma increases extrahepatic arginase activity. Surgery 2000; 127:419–426.

172. Cowley HC, Bacon PJ, Goode HF, Webster NR, Jones JG, Menon DK. Plasma antioxidant potential in severe sepsis: a comparison of survivors and nonsurvivors. Crit Care Med 1996; 24:1179–1183.

173. Goode HF, Cowley HC, Walker BE, Howdle PD, Webster NR. Decreased antioxidant status and increased lipid peroxidation in patients with septic shock and secondary organ dysfunction. Crit Care Med 1995; 23:646–651.

174. Goode HF, Webster NR. Free radicals and antioxidants in sepsis. Crit Care Med 1993; 21:1770–1775.

175. Angstwurm MW, Schottdorf J, Schopohl J, Gaertner R. Selenium replacement in patients with severe systemic inflammatory response syndrome improves clinical outcome. Crit Care Med 1999; 27:1807–1813.

176. Hertog MG, Hollman PC, Katan MB. Content of potentially anticarcinogenic flavonoids of 28 vegetables and 9 fruits commonly consumed in The Netherlands. Journal of Agriculture and Food Chemistry 1992; 40:2379–2383.

177. Hertog MG, Hollman PC, van de Putte B. Content of potentially anticarcinogenic flavonoids in tea infusions, wines and fruit juices. Journal of Agriculture and Food Chemistry 1993; 41:1242–1246.

178. Cotelle N, Bernier JL, Catteau JP, et al. Antioxidant properties of hydroxy-flavones. Free Radic Biol Med 1996; 20:35–43.

179. Husain SR, Cillard J, Cillard P. Hydroxyl radical scavengng activity of flavonoids. Phytochemistry 1987; 26:2489–2492.

180. Kandaswami C, Middleton E Jr. Free radical scavenging and antioxidant activity of plant flavonoids. Adv Exp Med Biol 1994; 366:351–376.

181. Panes J, Gerritsen ME, Anderson DC, Miyasaka M, Granger DN. Apigenin inhibits tumor necrosis factor-induced intercellular adhesion molecule-1 upregulation in vivo. Microcirculation 1996; 3:279–286.

182. Gerritsen ME. Flavonoids: inhibitors of cytokine induced gene expression. Adv Exp Med Biol 1998; 439:183–190.

183. Peng SM, Wang SZ, Zhao JP. Effect of rhubarb on inflammatory cytokines and complements in patients with systemic inflammation reaction syndrome and its significance. Zhongguo Zhong Xi Yi Jie He Za Zhi Zhongguo Zhongxiyi Jiehe Zazhi 2002; 22:264–266.

184. Kearns PJ, Young H, Garcia G, Blaschke T, O'Hanlon G, Rinki M, Sucher K, Gregory P. Accelerated improvement of alcoholic liver disease with enteral nutrition. Gastroenterology 1992; 102:200–205.

185. Maddrey WC. Branched chain amino acid therapy in liver disease. J Am Coll Nutr 1985; 4:639–650.

186. Oppong KN, Al Mardini H, Thick M, Record CO. Oral glutamine challenge in cirrhotics pre- and post-liver transplantation: a psychometric and analyzed EEG study. Hepatology 1997; 26:870–876.

187. Mouser JF, Hak EB, Kuhl DA, Dickerson RN, Gaber LW, Hak LJ. Recovery from ischemic acute renal failure is improved with enteral compared with parenteral nutrition. Crit Care Med 1997; 25:1748–1754.

188. Yeo CJ, Cameron JL. The pancreas. In: Sabiston DC, Lyerly HK, eds. Textbook of Surgery. The Biological Basis of Modern Surgical Practice. Philadelphia: W.B. Saunders Company, 1997:1151–1186.

189. Ragins H, Levenson SM, Signer R, Stamford W, Seifter E. Intrajejunal administration of an elemental diet at neutral pH avoids pancreatic stimulation. Studies in dog and man. Am J Surg 1973; 126:606–614.

190. Cassim MM, Allardyce DB. Pancreatic secretion in response to jejunal feeding of elemental diet. Ann Surg 1974; 180:228–231.

191. Vu MK, van der Veek PP, Frolich M, Souverijn JH, Biemond I, Lamers CB, Masclee AA. Does jejunal feeding activate exocrine pancreatic secretion? Eur J Clin Invest 1999; 29:1053–1059.

192. McClave SA, Greene LM, Snider HL, et al. Comparison of the safety of early enteral vs parenteral nutrition in mild acute pancreatitis. JPEN 1997; 21:14–20.

193. de Larminat V, Montravers P, Dureuil B, Desmonts JM. Alteration in swallowing reflex after extubation in intensive care unit patients. Crit Care Med 1995; 23:486–490.

194. Tolep K, Getch CL, Criner GJ. Swallowing dysfunction in patients receiving prolonged mechanical ventilation. Chest 1996; 109:167–172.

195. Leder SB, Cohn SM, Moller BA. Fiberoptic endoscopic documentation of the high incidence of aspiration following extubation in critically ill trauma patients. Dysphagia 1998; 13:208–212.

196. El-Sohl A, Okada M, Bhat A, Pietrantoni C. Swallowing disorders post orotracheal intubation in the elderly. Intensive Care Med 2003; 29:1451–1455.

197. Marik PE, Kaplan D. Aspiration pneumonia and dysphagia in the elderly. Chest 2003; 124:328–336.

198. Zaloga GP, Roberts P. Permissive underfeeding. New Horiz 1994; 2:257–263.

199. Yamazaki K, Maiz A, Moldawer LL, Bistrian BR, Blackburn GL. Complications associated with the overfeeding of infected animals. J Surg Res 1986; 40:152–158.

200. Alexander JW, Gonce SJ, Miskell PW, Peck MD, Sax H. A new model for studying nutrition in peritonitis. The adverse effect of overfeeding. Ann Surg 1989; 209:334–340.

201. Peck MD, Babcock GF, Alexander JW. The role of protein and calorie restriction in outcome from Salmonella infection in mice. JPEN 1992; 16:561–565.

202. Peck MD, Alexander JW, Gonce SJ, Miskell PW. Low protein diets improve survival from peritonitis in guinea pigs. Ann Surg 1989; 209:448–454.

203. Gauthier Y, Isoard P. Increased resistance to Salmonella infection of hypoferremic mice fed a low-protein diet. Microbiol Immunol 1986; 30:425–435.

204. Yelch MR. Effects of naloxone on glucose and insulin regulation during endotoxicosis in fed and fasted rats. Circ Shock 1988; 26:273–285.

205. Bhuyan UN, Ramalingaswami V. Responses of the protein-deficient rabbit to staphylococcal bacteremia. Am J Pathol 1972; 69:359–368.

15

Assessment and Management of Sedation in the Intensive Care Unit

D. KYLE HOGARTH and JESSE HALL

Department of Medicine, Section of Pulmonary and Critical Care
University of Chicago Hospitals
Chicago, Illinois, U.S.A.

I. Introduction

Patients admitted to an intensive care unit (ICU) in the U.S. will likely receive life support measures, which often include intubation and mechanical ventilation (MV). Whether a patient is intubated simply to secure an airway or requires additional positive pressure support to correct life-threatening hypoxemia or provide adequate alveolar ventilation, it is likely that one or more analgesic and/or sedative medications will be administered (1,2). This chapter will review the indications, goals, complications, specific agents, and monitoring that encompass sedation in the course of mechanical ventilatory support.

II. The Stress Response

The bodily response to injury, including trauma, surgery, and sepsis, is loosely referred to as the Stress Response (3). The normal physiologic stress response results in central, autonomic, and peripheral nervous system activation, as well as release of humoral factors, such as catacholamines, cortisol, glucagon, leukotrienes, and prostaglandins. Activation of these diverse systems results in elevation of heart rate, blood pressure, and oxygen consumption and enhances myocardial contractility (3). When activation of these systems occurs in the pathophysiologic state of various diseases, and in individuals with underlying chronic illnesses and compromised cardiopulmonary function, the result may

509

be worsening of an already precarious circumstance. For example, take a 70-year old male patient undergoing an open cholycystectomy. Unknown to the primary medical and surgical team, the man has a fixed stenotic lesion of the left anterior descending coronary artery that will limit any increase in blood flow in response to the extra demand that will come from the systemic effects of the stress response. He undergoes the procedure successfully, but has poor pain control in the postoperative recovery phase. The "physiologic insult" to his body from the surgery combined with the lack of adequate pain control will initiate a stress response, predominately manifested through the release of cortisol and epinephrine. The increase in afterload and subsequent increased demand on his heart will ultimately require increased myocardial oxygen consumption, a need that may not be met because of his limited coronary artery reserve. Furthermore, due to the large incision and the proximity to the diaphragm, he will likely splint and develop atelectasis, potentially compromising oxygenation and increasing the work of breathing and the demands placed upon his circulatory system. This patient would be at an increased risk of coronary ischemia from any physiologic stress, and this risk can be quite magnified in this perioperative setting. The rate of perioperative myocardial infarction for noncardiac surgery is 0.0–0.7% but increases to 1.1–1.8% in patients with coronary disease (3). Mortality from a perioperative infarction ranges from 36% to 70%. Clearly, recognizing and limiting adverse effects of the stress response has important implications in cardiac critical care and, more broadly, in the realm of surgical and medical critical illness.

III. Pain and Analgesia

Any discussion of sedation of a mechanically ventilated patient in the ICU needs to begin by focusing on the role pain plays in their care. Pain is defined by the Subcommittee on Taxonomy of the International Association for the Study of Pain as "an unpleasant sensory and emotional experience associated with actual or potential tissue damage, or described in terms of such damage" (4). By this very definition, pain is subjective, and therefore can be very difficult to measure and quantify. Furthermore, patients receiving MV are often unable to adequately communicate their needs, including their need for pain control. The agitated patient who is combative and not synchronous with the ventilator may be behaving so due to unrelieved pain. Post-ICU survivor interviews have demonstrated that many patients in the ICU recall significant unrelieved pain, ranging from 45% to 82% in some studies (5–8).

Pain may come from obvious sources such as trauma, a surgical incision, or an invasive procedure, but many patients recall significant pain simply from the presence of the endotracheal tube and airway suctioning (9). Furthermore, pain has been rated by patients as one of the main sources of anxiety they experienced during their ICU stay (9,10). In one study, endotracheal suctioning was given a pain score of 4.9 on a 1 (no pain) to 10 (worst pain ever) scale (11). Chest tube removal was scored at 6.6 (11). Acknowledging the prior history of poor pain control for patients, The Joint Commission for Accreditation of Health Care Organizations (JCAHO) (12) in the U.S. has mandated the monitoring of pain in all patients.

Given this context—that pain is common, if not nearly universal, amongst patients undergoing MV for significant periods of time, that their ability to communicate the precise nature of their pain is impaired, and that agitation can be a final common pathway for pain, anxiety, physiologic stress, and other neuro-psychiatric states—the clinician must begin all assessments of agitation and need for sedation with a consideration of the adequacy of pain control. In very rare patients, minor analgesics, such as acetaminophen or nonsteroidal anti-inflammatories, can control pain. In most patients, an opioid analgesic will be required, but the possibility of this agent achieving both analgesia and tranquility should be considered, and additional sedative agents should not be given as a matter of routine, but rather because agitation appears present above and beyond that associated with pain. Medications for analgesia and sedation can be given intermittently or through continuous infusion, and many hospitals will use a combination of both strategies. Often the recently intubated patient receives multiple intermittent doses to achieve early tranquility and is then transitioned to a continuous infusion. Data are lacking to indicate the superiority of one agent over another, but the specific strategy of analgesic and sedation management that is employed is more important than the actual medication selected (13,14). In the large number of patients who will require both an analgesic and sedative, it should be noted that opioid medications have significant synergistic effects with sedative drugs, particularly benzodiazepines, and combined use of an analgesic and sedative often results in lesser doses of each (13,15). Figure 1 offers an approach to assessing and managing an agitated patient receiving mechanical ventilation. This figure stresses the importance of addressing all areas of patient care that may provide discomfort before the addition of sedative medications.

A. Pain Assessment

No matter which agents are being employed to provide analgesia, the use of a pain scale to quantify pain and titrate the medication should be routine (16–19). The Visual Analog Scale (VAS) is often employed to measure level of pain. The VAS is a horizontal nongraded scale ranging from 0 (no pain) to 100 (worst pain imaginable) (20). Patients indicate their pain level somewhere on the scale. Studies have demonstrated that a score of 30 or greater is defined as moderate to severe pain (21). In cases where the patient is unable to indicate his/her pain score, a behavioral system can be employed. This scoring system rates pain by observing facial expression, compliance with ventilation, and upper limb behavior (16).

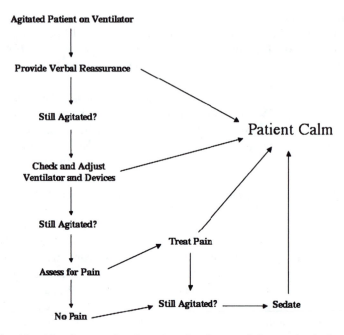

Figure 1   Algorithm for assessing the agitated patient receiving mechanical ventilation.

Studies of many different patient populations indicate physicians and nurses often do not provide adequate pain control (22–27). Fear of complications, concern about tolerance and addiction, and improper assessment of pain seem to be leading reasons for why inadequate analgesia is prescribed. In one well-done study, the rate of addiction to opioids was documented to occur in only four out of 11,882 patients (28). Other research has shown that tolerance to these medications may arise during ICU stay, as indicated by a small but steady increase in dose administered during prolonged ICU times (29). However, this may only reflect a down-regulation of opiate receptors and not necessarily indicate the development of a physical addiction once the medication is later discontinued. As this chapter discussion focuses on the use of sedatives and analgesics in the patient undergoing MV, serious complications of opioid administration (i.e., respiratory depression) are relatively negligible. In a small study of patients on assisted modes of ventilation, the use of continuous sufentanil versus nothing was shown to increase the average P_aCO_2 to 42.7 mmHg versus 39.5 mmHg in the control group (30). Though the results were statistically significant, there is probably little to no clinical significance of hypercapnea of this magnitude. The most important data regarding pain control are seen in studies of ICU survivors that indicate a high recall of unrelieved pain (9,10,31,32). While physician and nurse concerns about adverse effects from drugs employed in patient management are generally to be applauded, current data suggest that serious complications from opioids in the ICU are rare and poor pain control is common, suggesting we readjust our thinking about the risk–benefit relationship of these agents and our current practices. Table 1 compares the commonly used opioid drugs employed in the ICU.

B. Benefits of Pain Control

While the merits of adequate pain control in regard to the development of long-term sequelae such as post-traumatic stress disorder have been debated in the medical literature, there is strong clinical evidence that adequate pain control will minimize pulmonary and cardiac complications in the critically ill. A recent study of neonates demonstrated improved outcomes in the group receiving opioids (33). Infants who received morphine had improved neurologic outcomes compared to those receiving either midazolam or placebo. A meta-analysis of the effects of various pain control methods on the development of postoperative atelectasis favored pain management with epidural anesthesia compared to intra-venous delivery of analgesics (34). While this study did not evaluate the patients' pain scores to allow adequate comparison between the two methods, it seems intuitive that an epidural block of pain from a thoracotomy procedure would minimize splinting and subsequently diminish the likelihood of atelectasis. Further studies demonstrated improved pain relief with epidural compared to systemic analgesia and again demonstrated decreased rates of atelectasis (35,36). It therefore seems that the reduction in complications is not an effect of the medication per se, but the effect of preventing the reduction in functional residual capacity that is associated with surgery of the chest and the upper abdomen.

As discussed in the prior patient example, cardiac complications may arise in the context of the postoperative period or during critical illness related to the activation of the stress response. Poor management of the stress response and pain can make the physiologic management of the patients even more difficult.

Table 1 Comparison of Commonly Used Intravenous Opioid Medications in the ICU

Drug	Peak effect	Elimination half-life	Minimal suggested dose
Morphine	30 min	2–4 hr	1–4 mg bolus 1–10 mg/hr infusion
Fentanyl	3 min	1–2 hr	25–100 μg bolus 25–200 μg/hr infusion
Hydromorphone	20 min	2–4 hr	0.2–1 mg bolus 0.2–2 mg/hr infusion
Pentazocine	3 min	2–3 hr	30 mg bolus, no infusion
Butorphanol	5 min	3–4 hr	1 mg bolus, no infusion
Ketorolac (NSAID)	2 hr	6–8 hr	30 mg bolus, no infusion

Source: From Ref. 45.

In a meta-analysis of over 500 postoperative patients, thoracic epidural anesthesia versus the systemic administration of analgesia was associated with a reduction of postoperative myocardial infarction to 2.6% compared to 5.5% (37). In a randomized controlled trial in patients undergoing abdominal aortic surgery, a similar reduction in rate of myocardial infarction was noted, along with diminished time on the ventilator postoperatively, improved pain scores, and a decrease in ICU length of stay (38).

There is some indirect evidence that inadequate pain control in the postoperative period is associated with poor wound healing and increased rates of wound infection (39,40). There is diminished oxygen tension in the subcutaneous tissue in patients with poor analgesia, likely related to the vasoconstrictive effect of epinephrine as a result of the stress response (39). Decreased oxygen tension has been associated with increased rates of surgical wound infection (40).

Inadequate pain control increases the rate of patient agitation and increases the risk of unintended self-extubation and loss of intravascular catheters. The sudden interruption of life-sustaining therapies can obviously have catastrophic effects and put the patient at risk for further complications during re-establishment of an airway or central venous catheter. Patients in pain are often treated with further sedative drugs and ultimately may require physical restraining. Physical restraints have a negative impact on family's satisfaction with the level of care and have been demonstrated to be a large source of anxiety to patients in post-ICU surveys (41–43).

C. Methods of Pain Control

Most pain management in the ICU will be in the form of systemically delivered parenteral opioids or regionally administered anesthesia and analgesia. Both strategies have strengths and weaknesses, such as ease of use in systemic administration versus the need for an epidural catheter, or avoidance of systemic effects by regional techniques. A comprehensive approach to pain management should consider the use of all forms of pain control to provide the best degree of analgesia with the least amount of medication (44). Where available, the consultation of a pain management team would be advisable for complicated ICU patients, especially those receiving post-surgical care. Also, depending on the nature of the pain, the use of nonsteroidal anti-inflammatory drugs (NSAIDs) may offer distinct advantages (e.g., pericarditis, pleuritis, etc.).

D. Medications for Pain Management

The parenteral administration of opioid drugs (morphine, methadone, hydromorphone, fentanyl) is the mainstay of pain control for most critically ill patients. All analgesic medications have a minimal effective analgesic concentration (MEAC), with serum levels below this value ineffective in providing analgesia (3). The MEAC can be different for each individual patient, depending on the patient's genetics as well as prior exposure to opioids, both prescribed and nonprescribed. The response curve has a steep incline once the MEAC is reached, and small increases in plasma drug levels can have large effects on perception of pain. There is also a plateau to the effect of opioids, a point at which the addition of more drug may provide little analgesic benefit but may increase the incidence and magnitude of side effects. The concept of the plateau is important to consider when a patient has received large doses of opioids parenterally and is still complaining of pain. This may be a circumstance in which another approach to pain control needs to be entertained, such as a regional block or the use of nonsteroidal anti-inflammatory drugs.

Opioid medications bind to μ and κ receptors in the peripheral tissue and the central nervous system. The μ receptors have two subtypes; μ-1 is responsible for analgesia and μ-2 mediates respiratory depression, nausea, vomiting, constipation, and euphoria (3). The effect of activation of the μ-2 receptor in the medulla is to decrease the respiratory rate with a preserved tidal volume. With the administration of opioids, the CO_2 response curve is shifted to the right, resulting in increased CO_2 levels from the diminished minute ventilation. The normal response to hypoxia is obliterated. These effects make opioids the best drugs to attenuate the subjective sense of dyspnea many ICU patients experience, especially patients with hypercapnea. Patients undergoing a strategy of permissive hypercapnea who are not being treated with opioid agents will often exhibit dysynchrony with the ventilator, in part as a result of their high respiratory drive. Inadequate administration of opioids in this setting often results in inappropriately large doses of sedatives being given, or even the unnecessary use of muscle relaxants. The κ receptor is responsible for sedation, miosis, and spinal analgesia. Opioids do not have any amnestic properties.

Morphine

Morphine has low lipid solubility, which results in a moderately slow onset of action of approximately five to 10 minutes and a peak effect at approximately 30 minutes. The duration of action is dose dependent but is approximately four hours on average. Morphine is metabolized in the liver via conjugation to a glucuronide, and morphine-6-glucuronide is an active metabolite. The kidney eliminates both morphine and the metabolites, so the duration of action of morphine is increased in renal insufficiency. Prolonged administration of morphine can lead to increased duration of action. Morphine administration can lead to hypotension via vasodilation and decreased heart rate through sympatholysis and direct effects on the sinoatrial node of the heart (45). These cardiovascular effects can be amplified in the hypovolemic patient.

Fentanyl

Fentanyl is highly lipid soluble, resulting in a rapid onset of action (two to four minutes) but also a short duration of action of one hour. The drug rapidly redistributes to peripheral tissue, resulting in the short half-life from a single administration. Continuous infusion of fentanyl can result in prolonged mechanism of action as the drug accumulates in the peripheral tissue and then redistributes into the vascular space upon stopping the infusion (46). It is metabolized in the liver into inactive forms that are eliminated by the kidney. Unlike other opioid drugs, fentanyl does not cause histamine release, which may result in less nausea and cardiovascular effects, though this has not been definitively shown (45). Fentanyl does not affect the hemodynamics as significantly as does morphine.

Hydromorphone

Hydromorphone is very similar to morphine in time to onset and duration of effect. None of the metabolites from the liver are metabolically active, and this may result in shorter duration of effects during prolonged administration of hydromorphone.

Meperidine

Meperidine has a short onset of action (three to five minutes) due to greater lipid solubility than morphine. Duration of action is also shorter due to redistribution, much like fentanyl. It undergoes metabolism in the liver and excretion by the kidney, similar to the other opioid medications. Normeperidine is the active metabolite of meperidine and is a central nervous system stimulant (46). Normeperidine toxicity manifests as delirium, myoclonus, and seizures. As some degree of renal dysfunction is prevalent in the critically ill, and other suitable agents exist, meperidine should not be routinely used in the ICU.

Pentazocine

Pentazocine has a rapid onset of action, providing potent analgesia quickly. It is cleared renally after metabolism in the liver, so dosing needs to be adjusted for renal or liver impairment. In patients prone to seizures, pentazocine may lower the seizure threshold. As the drug is a mixed agonist–antagonist, it can precipitate withdrawal symptoms in opioid dependent patients. Furthermore, pentazocine has the potential to diminish the therapeutic effects of μ agonists, such as morphine. Thus, this agent has limited usefulness in the ICU setting.

Butorphanol

Butorphanol is a mixed agonist–antagonist with a rapid onset of action. It is metabolized in the liver and eliminated in the urine, so dosing adjustment is necessary for liver or kidney disease. It has been primarily used for acute pain management, especially in the outpatient management of migraine headaches. Butorphanol has an "analgesic ceiling," a point where increased dosing will provide not extra benefit beyond that already obtained. As it can also block the effect of potent μ agonists, butorphanol has limited use in the ICU.

Ketorolac

Ketorolac is a NSAID medication that may have some use in the ICU, as it can be delivered intravenously. Onset of action is usually with in thirty minutes and will deliver peak analgesia at two hours. As with all NSAIDS, caution needs to be taken in patients with renal disease and gastric ulceration. Ketorolac should not be used as the primary analgesic for mechanically ventilated patients, but it may provide supplemental analgesia for certain clinical conditions (e.g., pericarditis, pleuritis, etc.).

E. Complications of Opioid Administration

Pruritis, nausea, and vomiting are well described complications of opioids and are related to activation of the μ-2 receptor (2,45). In the postoperative patient who is not prophylactically treated with an anti-emetic medication, the incidence of emesis following opioid administration is 30% (47). Besides the uncomfortable feeling of nausea and vomiting the patient may experience, the act of emesis increases the risk of aspiration, even in patients with an endotracheal tube. Enteral feeding can be complicated by the diminished gut motility caused by opioids and can further increase the risk of emesis and aspiration (48). Though patient gastric residuals are often monitored, there have been no definitive studies showing that monitoring of gastric residuals diminishes the rate of aspiration or ventilator-associated pneumonia. A recent trial in chronic ambulatory opioid users of the peripheral opioid antagonist methylnaltrexone demonstrated improved oral-cecal transit times and increased laxation without inducing central opioid withdrawal (49). Though not studied in the critically ill, this drug holds great promise for the management of opioid induced constipation in the ICU.

Opioid medications cause a systemic vasodilation, with a decline in systemic vascular resistance and diminished venous return and a reflex increase in heart rate (3). In the euvolemic patient, this is of little hemodynamic significance. However, in the hypovolemic patient or patient with co-existent sepsis, drug-related venodilation might produce unacceptable degrees of hypotension. This hemodynamic effect of opioids highlights the need for assessment of the adequacy of intravascular volume in all patients being considered for opioid analgesia.

The continuous infusion of opioids raises the possibility of a patient developing a physical tolerance or even addiction to these medications. The agitation and restlessness of a ventilated patient during liberation from mechanical ventilation may be manifestations of some degree of withdrawal. The problem of tolerance affects patient populations of all ages (50–53). Though almost all studies on this subject are retrospective, no precise correlation between quantity and duration of drug exposure predicts dependency. The majority of patients exhibiting withdrawal from opioids will either have had significant exposure prior to their critical illness or will have received high doses of drugs for more than three to five days during their ICU management (52). In one prospective study of infants, higher total dose and duration of fentanyl administration was associated with the development of withdrawal symptoms (54). The incidence of withdrawal symptoms has been shown to increase with concurrent use of neuromuscular blockade, but this may be a consequence of the generally increased levels of opioids and sedatives used in this patient population (55).

IV. Indications for Sedation

A critically ill patient often realizes (s)he has a life-threatening disease or event, is often in some degree of pain, and has a feeling of loss of control as life-support therapies are put in place and tethering to mechanical devices ensues (6,56). After ensuring adequate analgesia, providing anxiolysis in order to facilitate respiratory support and ventilator synchrony is a central goal of sedation management. The indication for MV sometimes dictates the requirement for sedation, as not all people receiving MV will require much sedation, if any. For example, the end-stage emphysema patient with ventilatory failure may be quite comfortable on the ventilator with only a minimal amount of intermittent analgesia and may not require any sedation. This is contrasted to the mechanically ventilated asthmatic who is undergoing a strategy of permissive hypercapnea while being ventilated. This patient would require deep sedation and analgesia to overcome the ventilatory drive to breathe from a climbing P_aCO_2 (57,58).

Sedation is often administered to facilitate care by the nursing team. Critically ill patients are frequently confused, delirious, and sometimes combative (59). Struggling patients may compromise their care by the traumatic removal of the endotracheal tube or vascular access devices (60). The unplanned abrupt removal of the endotracheal tube can damage vocal cords, cause airway edema and bleeding, cause aspiration, and will interrupt the needed mechanical ventilation. Emergent re-intubation increases the risk for further airway damage and for a ventilator-associated pneumonia. In two combined studies of over 700 ventilated patients, the self-removal of the endotracheal tube occurred in 14% of the patients (61,62). In 60% of these patients, confusion and agitation was present prior to the self-extubation. The traumatic removal of a vascular access device places the patient at risk for bleeding, interruption of possibly life-sustaining therapy, and the risk of undergoing another invasive procedure when the device is re-inserted.

Frequently, a patient on MV will be physically restrained if inadequate sedation is being provided. Retrospective interviews of patients requiring MV indicate that the feeling of helplessness from being restrained is a significant cause of anxiety (42,43). For family members, seeing their loved one critically ill is difficult enough, and the addition of physical restraints only adds to this feeling of fear and helplessness (41). In general, if a patient is requiring physical restraint in the ICU, then not enough analgesia or sedation is being provided.

A. Goals of Sedation

Ideally, the goal of sedation is provide adequate anxiolysis to facilitate the care of the patient while minimizing the side effects of the medications used. However, this raises the questions of how we define "adequate anxiolysis" and to what extent we accept side effects. To answer these questions, it is helpful to first ask how we would define the ideal sedative.

The ideal sedative medication and strategy would provide quick, complete analgesia and anxiolysis and yet allow the patient to awaken instantly. The medication would have no negative cardiovascular effects and would not accumulate and cause continued central nervous system depression, respiratory depression, and altered gut motility. It would not interact with other medications, and the drug's pharmacodynamics and pharmacokinetics would not change with liver or renal disease. It would also be simple to store, inexpensive, and easy to deliver to the patient.

Defining adequate anxiolysis and sedation is difficult because these concepts are inherently subjective. Some physicians have advocated defining adequate sedation as sedation intense enough to provide complete amnesia of the ICU stay. In some ICU experiences, amnesia may be desirable (i.e., receiving neuromuscular blockade) (15). It seems intuitive that a lack of memory of any painful, frightening experience would be an admirable goal. Indeed, many ICU survivors have a strong recollection of pain and anxiety from their ICU stay. This high recall of pain simply redemonstrates the importance of ensuring adequate analgesia. Some contrasting research indicates that an absence of memories from the time in the ICU may increase the risk of depression and post-traumatic stress disorder (42,43). Because it is not clear if amnesia should be a goal for sedation, another definition needs to be used.

Objective observer scales have attempted to assess sedation by a scale that describes level of consciousness and comfort along a continuum. Scales such as the Ramsay Sedation Scale (RSS) and the Richmond Agitation–Sedation Scale (RASS) provide the bedside clinician with such scales that facilitate description of inadequate sedation, adequate control of anxiety, and over-sedation (Tables 2 and 3) (63,64). Though these scales provide some help in defining a goal of sedation (i.e., a RSS score of 3 or a RASS score of 0), they do not provide a strategy for the

Table 2 Ramsay Sedation Score

---

1. Patient anxious and agitated or restless or both
2. Patient cooperative, oriented, and tranquil
3. Patient responds to commands only
4. Patient asleep, shows brisk response to light glabellar tap or loud auditory stimulus
5. Patient asleep, shows sluggish response to light glabellar tap or loud auditory stimulus
6. Patient asleep, shows no response to light glabellar tap or loud auditory stimulus

---

Source: From Ref. 64.

Table 3 Richmond Agitation–Sedation Scale

Score	Term	Description
+4	Combative	Overtly combative/violent. Danger to staff
+3	Very agitated	Pulls/removes tubes or catheters. Aggressive
+2	Agitated	Non-purposeful movement. Not synchronous with ventilator
+1	Restless	Anxious, but movements not aggressive/violent
0	Alert and Calm	
−1	Drowsy	Sustained awakening (>10 sec) with eye contact, to voice
−2	Light Sedation	Briefly awakens (<10 sec) with eye contact, to voice
−3	Moderate Sedation	Movement to voice, but no eye contact
−4	Deep Sedation	No response to voice. Movement to physical stimulation
−5	Unarousable	No response to voice or physical stimulation

Procedure:
(1) Observe patient. Calm? (score zero) Does patient have restless or agitated behavior? (1 to 4)
(2) If not alert, speak name in loud clear voice, and direct patient to look at speaker. Repeat once if necessary. Gauge response (−1 to −3)
(3) If no response to voice, then physically stimulate patient. Gauge response (−4 to −5)

Source: From Ref. 63.

choice of medication or the manner in which it is administered. As there can be a wide variety of opinion amongst caregivers on how to define adequate sedation, a numerical value to represent a goal of sedation can provide unity of care for a patient whose care is assumed by various members of the provider team (65).

Studies have clearly demonstrated that a protocol-driven approach to mechanical ventilation and spontaneous breathing trials leads to reduced time on the ventilator and that excessive sedation can be a principle reason for failure to implement a ventilator weaning (66–69). In Europe, a survey of the rate of use of a protocol driven assessment of sedation demonstrated that only 16% of Danish ICUs and 67% of British ICUs had established policies for the use of sedation evaluation scores (2,70). Nursing studies have also shown that ICUs that are understaffed with RNs use larger quantities of sedatives, increasing the chance of prolonged sedation and MV (71,72).

A few published professional organization guidelines exist to aid the ICU physician in achieving the goals of sedation. The American College of Critical Care Medicine, under the auspices of the Society of Critical Care Medicine, published practice parameters in 1995 for the optimal use of sedatives and analgesics in the critically ill patient (73). These were updated in 2002 (44). Despite these recommended goals, there is little standardization regarding the management of ICU sedation (1,74,75). Within the same hospital, different sedation strategies are often implemented, with a wide range of physician and nurse views of how best to identify and approach adequate and excessive sedation (76). Often the principles and goals of sedation in an ICU are governed by historical or institutional biases and not adequately informed by evidence.

In the end, the difficulty in defining the goal and adequacy of sedation reminds the ICU physician that sedation management, like all therapies in the ICU, is a dynamic process that requires continuous attention and adjustment.

B. Monitoring of Sedation

Early use of a spontaneous breathing trial (SBT) will reduce the total time spent on a ventilator (77). However, in order to effectively perform a SBT, the patient should be awake and interactive with care providers. Patients often receive continuous infusions of sedative medications in the ICU, but this has been shown to lead to prolonged intubation and mechanical ventilation (78). Various scales to assess level of sedation have been developed, all with the goal of permitting the bedside clinician to adjust sedative dose to achieve adequate, but not excessive, sedation.

The use of objective scales to measure sedation would have multiple benefits for the mechanically ventilated patient. Aside from allowing for easy communication among those caring for the patient, it would also control for differing opinions among the health care team regarding the level of sedation: an agreed upon number on the sedation scale would become the goal of care.

Several bedside measurement scales have been developed to assess a patient's level of sedation. The majority of the ICU literature regarding sedation has used the relatively simple Ramsay Sedation Scale (Table 2), developed in 1974 (64). Though easy to perform, the Ramsay scale was not originally intended to be used as a tool for clinical monitoring and has not been rigorously tested for reliability and validity in diverse ICU populations.

The recently introduced RASS has proven to be a useful bedside tool in the management of sedation (Table 3) (63). This scale was developed by a multidisciplinary team using a 10-point scale that is scored using three well-defined, simple steps. Performing the assessment and assigning a score is a straightforward process and can be done after minimal training, allowing the scale to be an extremely useful clinical and research tool. In addition to being easy to learn and perform, the RASS has components of consciousness assessed that are not present in other published sedation scales. In the nonagitated patient, the RASS assessment follows length of eye contact by the patient upon receiving a verbal command. Two components of consciousness are arousal and content of thought, and by measuring degree of eye contact, the RASS more effectively allows the measurement of consciousness in the sedated patient. The RASS has undergone many studies of reliability and has consistently demonstrated excellent inter-rater correlations (63,79). The RASS has also proven to be reliable across a variety of different patient ages and populations (63,79). Unfortunately, most of the sedation research done in the past used Ramsay for monitoring of sedation. Based upon its more careful validation and its use of a more expanded scale to describe ideal sedation as well as the extremes of under- and over-sedation, it is likely that RASS will find increasing application to sedation during MV and will be the preferred instrument for conducting research on ICU sedation in the future.

The inherent problem with all scoring systems is the observer-dependent nature of the measurements, making them inherently subjective. An objective tool that could accurately measure a level of sedation would provide the ICU physician a valuable instrument to deliver the correct amount of sedative medications. One such tool that has been studied is the Bispectral Index Score (BIS). The BIS is a numeric value from 0 (deep sedation) to 100 (awake) derived from complex mathematical analysis of the electroencephalographic (EEG) signals (80). BIS recording is achieved by modified electrodes placed on the scalp and feeding into a small bedside monitor. Original devices were stand-alone machines, but current BIS systems are integrated into the patient's other monitoring systems. A challenge for any such monitoring system, apart from the proper interpretation of the complex EEG signal, is to provide for "filtering" of artifact from muscle electrical activity and from the general "noise" of electronic equipment in the ICU.

The BIS number and scale have been derived from an EEG database of normal volunteers who were given one or more sedative drugs. These studies, in a noncritically ill population, have shown that a BIS of 45–60 correlates to a low probability of response to verbal stimulation. To date, small studies of the critically ill have shown moderate to good correlation of the BIS with traditional bedside scoring systems, such as Ramsay in adults and the COMFORT scale (a scale that rates sedation using eight factors such as alertness, blood pressure, heart rate, facial expressions, and others) in children, but randomized trials demonstrating improved outcomes with routine BIS monitoring have not been performed (81,82). Other studies have not demonstrated a good correlation of BIS to other measures of level of sedation, especially in a heterogeneous surgical population (83). Much additional study will be required to determine if BIS monitoring is beneficial for titration of sedatives in the ICU.

C. Medications for Sedation Management

Benzodiazepines

Benzodiazepines (diazepam, lorazepam, midazolam) are frequently used to provide anxiolysis and are the most commonly used sedatives in the ICU (1). They mediate their effect via the gamma amino-butyric acid receptor-complex. This complex regulates a chloride channel on the cell membrane. Activation of this complex will cause increased permeability of the membrane with an intracellular increase of chloride ions, resulting in hyperpolarization of the neurons. This results in depression of the central nervous system as the neurons now have a higher threshold for excitability. These drugs provide amnesia, with lorazepam producing the longest duration of antegrade amnesia (84,85).

Benzodiazepines provide no pain relief; therefore, a patient's level of pain should always be assessed before sedatives are administered. Furthermore, opioids and benzodiazepines have synergistic effects when co-administered, allowing for lower doses of both drugs to be used (86,87). Benzodiazepines have large volumes of distribution, owing to their high lipid solubility. The kinetics of drug metabolism and the volume of distribution of benzodiazepine drugs change during critical illness, especially in patients with impaired renal and hepatic function. The implication of the altered kinetics and dynamics of benzodiazepines in the critically ill is that even drugs considered "ultra-short acting" when given as a single bolus (such as midazolam) may accumulate when given by continuous infusion or repeated bolus in the critically ill patient (88). A paradoxical reaction to benzodiazepines, resulting in a state of agitation that worsens with higher doses, is sometimes seen in the elderly and alcohol abusers. Table 4 compares the commonly used medications for sedation.

Midazolam

Midazolam has a rapid onset of action (30 seconds to five minutes), and the duration of action from a single intravenous dose is only two hours. The duration of action is dependent on how quickly the drug redistributes to the peripheral tissue, where it has no activity. Midazolam undergoes hepatic metabolism and renal excretion. In patients with impaired hepatic metabolism, the half-life of midazolam can increase to four to 12 hours. There is an active metabolite of midazolam, 1-hydroxy-midazolam, but it has a half-life of only one hour in a patient with normal renal function. When midazolam is given via continuous infusion for at least 24 hours, the drug accumulates in the peripheral tissues rather than being metabolized. As the infusion is stopped, the drug redistributes to the plasma and continues to have clinical effect. Full recovery from a continuous infusion

Table 4 Comparison of Commonly Used Medications for Sedation in the ICU

Drug	Peak effect	Elimination half-life	Minimal suggested dose
Diazepam	3–5 min	20–40 hr	5–10 mg bolus Infusion not recommended
Midazolam	2–5 min	3–5 hr	1–2 mg bolus 0.5–10 mg/hr infusion
Lorazepam	2–20 min	10–20 hr	1–2 mg bolus 0.5–10 mg/hr infusion
Propofol	90 sec	20–30 hr	Bolus not recommended 25–100 μg/kg/min infusion
Dexmedetomidine	60 sec	2 hr	1 μg/kg bolus over 10 min 0.2–0.7 μg/kg/min infusion

Source: From Ref. 45.

can take days. Obese patients with larger volumes of distribution or chronically ill patients with altered hepatic and renal function can have even longer clinical effects from continuous infusion.

Lorazepam

The onset of action of lorazepam is five minutes due to the lower lipid solubility compared to midazolam. Consequently, the duration of action is longer, lasting from six to 10 hours. Little is known of the effects of critical illness and continuous infusion on the kinetics and dynamics of lorazepam metabolism. Lorazepam is diluted in propylene glycol, and high cumulative doses of lorazepam have been associated with lactic acidosis, acute tubular necrosis, and hyperosmolar states from propylene glycol toxicity (89–92). This toxicity occurs when the propylene glycol levels reach 2.4 mmol/L (18 mg/dL) (93). A specific dose of lorazepam at which this occurs has not been noted, but in a patient receiving high doses of lorazepam with an ongoing acidosis and osmolal gap, propylene glycol toxicity should be considered.

Diazepam

Diazepam has a short onset of action of one to three minutes. The duration of a single administered dose is short (30–60 minutes), but continuous infusion of the drug results in a prolonged termination half-life. The drug can easily saturate peripheral tissues, leading to the prolonged effect even once the infusion is stopped. Diazepam is metabolized in the liver and has several active metabolites that also have prolonged half-lives.

Propofol

Propofol is an alkylphenol anesthetic that provides no analgesia and, when used concurrently with opioids, may require higher analgesic dosing than do the benzodiazepines (13). The exact method of action of propofol is not clear, but it appears to work through the gamma-aminobutyric acid (GABA) receptor. It has a short half-life and a rapid onset of action, but it has not been shown to be superior to other sedating agents (94–96). As the drug is extremely lipophilic, it has a large volume of distribution (97). The continuous infusion of propofol can lead to prolonged sedation, even with discontinuation of the drug (46,98). Propofol is metabolized in the liver, and an undescribed extra-hepatic form of clearance and the non-active metabolites are excreted in the urine (97).

Ventilatory depression from propofol can be sudden and profound, and propofol should only be administered to a patient with a secured airway or with staff immediately available to intubate. Propofol is insoluble in water, so it is delivered in a lipid emulsion, which can lead to elevated triglyceride levels (99–101). Patients on parenteral nutrition must have their lipid infusion adjusted if receiving propofol. All patients receiving propofol should have baseline, 72 hours, and then weekly triglyceride levels measured, and if significant elevations occur, the infusion should be stopped. The lipid medium in which propofol is delivered to the patient is an excellent growth media for bacteria and fungi, and strict aseptic technique must be used when handling and administering the drug (102). A dose of 75 mcg/kg/min is a recommended maximum to minimize the possibility of a Propofol Infusion Syndrome (97). First described in a pediatric population, but also seen in adults, the syndrome involves profound myocardial failure and severe lactic acidosis and has significant mortality (97,103,104).

Ketamine

Ketamine is structurally related to phencyclidine (the illicit drug PCP) and causes a profound dissociative state in the patient. Patients can appear awake with their eyes open and protect their airway with an intact cough/gag reflex but appear unaware of their surrounding environment (46). The drug provides analgesia via μ-1 and has some amnestic qualities. It is metabolized by the liver and has a less potent active metabolite. There is minimal respiratory suppression when the drug is administered slowly over 60 seconds. Hemodynamic effects include tachycardia, increased cardiac output, and hypertension. Some instances of hypotension have also been described. As the drug can induce hallucinations and emergence delirium, the usefulness in the ICU setting is limited. It has traditionally been utilized for short painful procedures, such as dressing changes in the burn unit, though fentanyl has been replacing ketamine use.

Haloperidol

Haloperidol is a butyrophenone antipsychotic drug and has no analgesic or amnesic properties. Given this profile and its long half-life, it is not a very attractive medication for use as a standard ICU sedative. It can be very useful in the management of acute delirium and in patients with underlying or newly acquired psychosis. An optimal dose and regimen for haloperidol administration has not been defined, but it is usually administered intravenously in the ICU. Of note, haloperidol is not FDA approved for parenteral use. Patients receiving haloperidol demonstrate indifference to their surrounding environment, and may even have cataleptic immobility, making it difficult to perform pain and sedation assessment. Major concerns with the use of haloperidol are extrapyramidal effects, neuroleptic-malignant syndrome, hypotension, and prolongation of the QT-interval. A case-controlled study of critically ill patients, using historical controls, suggested an incidence of torsades de pointes of 3.6% (105). Haloperidol is useful for acute agitation and treating patients with psychotic behavior, but it should not be used as a primary agent for sedation.

Dexmedetomidine

Dexmedetomidine is a relatively new agent for sedation, recently approved for use in the United States. It is a lipophilic derivative of imidazole, with high affinity for α_2-adrenoreceptors. Dexmedetomidine has sedative, analgesic, and sympatholytic effects (106,107). In early studies in the ICU and the operating room, it has been shown to reduce the quantity of IV sedation, inhalation anesthesia, and intravenous opioid administered (108–111). Dexmedetomidine also provides anxiolysis, improved perioperative hemodynamic stability, and no suppression of respiratory drive (108–111). In normal volunteers, the drug has allowed easy arousal from a sedated state as well as a quick return to their previous sedation level. This effect has also been demonstrated in post-operative patients and the critically ill (112,113). Though the drug holds great promise, the studies to date are limited by size of the patient populations studied and length of administration of the drug. In a randomized double-blinded study in patients who spent less than 24 hours on the ventilator, dexmedetomidine was associated with less use of propofol and morphine (109). Trials demonstrating decreased mechanical ventilation time from using dexmedetomidine, presumably due to increased opportunities to perform spontaneous breathing trials, have not been performed to date. Therefore, until further study demonstrates a superior outcome to current less expensive therapy, dexmedetomidine is not recommended for routine use in the ICU.

Barbiturates

Barbiturates are very potent agents that cause amnesia and profound sedation. They frequently lead to hemodynamic instability and accumulate in peripheral tissue, leading to prolonged effect after discontinuation of the continuous infusion. They are not frequently used for sedation because of these effects.

Inhalational Anesthetics

Inhalational anesthetics, such as isoflurane, have been shown to be safe and effective in the critically ill (114,115). They have analgesic, amnestic, and hypnotic properties, making them an almost near-perfect agent for sedation. Isoflurane undergoes only minimal metabolism and is almost completely eliminated by the lungs. Technical limitations delivering the drug safely through the ventilator at accurate concentrations and collecting all exhaled gas have limited the use of these agents in the ICUs of the U.S.

D. Complications of Sedation

Administration of analgesic and sedative medications have many beneficial effects, but these come with some significant risk and complications. In the short-term, these medications can cause vasodilation with hypotension and reflexive tachycardia, something many patients in the ICU may already be experiencing. In the euvolemic patient, these effects should be minimal. With adequate intravenous access, most patients can be managed when these hemodynamics appear with judicious use of additional fluid infusions and, on occasion, vasoactive drugs. By their inherent sedating qualities, the medications used for sedation in the ICU cause central nervous system depression and an inability to protect the airway as well as decreased respiratory drive. Having an experienced airway manager ready to assist in the intubation of the trachea is essential if sedatives are being administered in the absence of an endotracheal tube.

As a majority of studies on medications commonly used in the ICU are extrapolated from the operating room, the precise nature of action of a sedative in the altered physiology of the critically ill is only beginning to be appreciated and understood. Furthermore, the use of sedatives in the operating room is for short periods of time, such as hours, whereas sedatives may be administered in the ICU for days and even weeks (116,117). Thus the published pharmacodynamics and pharmacokinetics of the medication may be different in the critically ill (88,118–120). The medications commonly used for sedation in the ICU have many drug–drug interactions and have a wide range of half lives (118). Often, their metabolism is impaired, usually related to the frequent organ failures associated with critical illness (i.e., acute renal failure and hepatic insufficiency) (121,122). A common complication of the prolonged administration of sedation is drug accumulation (78). There are many complications associated with "over-sedation." The accumulation of sedatives and analgesics can cause prolonged depression of central nervous system function (15). This often results in patients receiving extra diagnostic tests and procedures to determine why they are not "waking up" once the medication has been stopped. Besides increased utilization of diagnostic procedures and imaging modalities, continuous infusion of sedation has been associated with prolonged time on the ventilator, prolonged ICU stays, prolonged hospital stays, and difficulty in adequately monitoring a patient's neurologic function (14,78). Patients who spend more time on the ventilator are also at further risk of nosocomial infections from urinary and intravenous catheters, as well as ventilator-associated pneumonias. Management and prevention of "over-sedation" has led to the development of different strategies for sedation and different scales and tools to monitor a level of sedation.

The continuous infusion of opioids and benzodiazepines for prolonged periods of time raises the possibility of a patient developing a physical tolerance or addiction to these medications. The agitation and restlessness of a ventilated patient whose sedation has been lifted in order to undergo a spontaneous breathing trial may relate in large part to withdrawal symptoms. Development of addiction to sedatives and analgesics in the ICU affects patient populations of all ages (50–53). Though almost all studies on this subject are retrospective, no precise correlation between quantity and duration of drug exposure predicts the development of dependency. The majority of patients exhibiting withdrawal from benzodiazepines will either have had significant exposure prior to their critical illness or will have received high doses of drugs for more than three to five days during their ICU stay (52). Options for management of dependence include the use of medications like clonidine to control withdrawal symptoms, switching the patient to longer-acting medications such as diazepam, utilizing the expertise of a behavioral psychologist, and on occasion employing antidepressants and antipsychotics.

As discussed earlier, amnesia for some ICU experiences may be a reasonable goal of sedation. Many patients have memory of being uncomfortable while in the ICU, but this may in part relate to inadequate analgesia (9). Complete amnesia for the duration of critical illness may carry adverse consequences (123). There is some evidence that lack of memory of a critical illness may predispose patients to long-term psychological problems (123–126). Many groups approach the management of sedation to ensure adequate analgesia and sedation but do not focus on a need for amnesia.

E. Sedation Strategies

Ely et al. (77) demonstrated that performing early SBT decreased the time patients spent on the ventilator, while Kollef et al. (78) observed that the continuous infusion of sedatives increased the time spent on the ventilator. In attempting to improve the rate of patient's liberation from the ventilator, it was demonstrated that a protocol driven approach to mechanical ventilation and SBTs leads to reduced time on the ventilator (66–69). However, over-sedation remains a principle reason for failure to implement a ventilator weaning. Sedating a patient receiving MV is the ultimate ICU balancing act: on one side, the goal is to provide adequate analgesia and sedation to ensure comfort and ease of care. On the competing side is the goal to liberate the patient from the ventilator as soon as possible, which requires an alert and interactive patient. In the background of this discussion is the effect of continuous infusion of these medications on medical cost and the demand on medical staff. How do we reconcile these competing goals?

Daily Interruption of Sedation

Kress et al. (14) demonstrated that the daily interruption of continuous sedation decreased the length of time on the ventilator (Fig. 2) and the time in the ICU, and it also diminished the number of diagnostic tests performed to evaluate why a patient was not waking up once sedatives had been discontinued. The protocol involved the daily stopping of the continuous drug infusion (including opiates) and monitoring the patient until he/she started to show signs of awakening. The drugs were then restarted at half the previous dose and were titrated at the discretion of the bedside nurse to achieve a Ramsay sedation score of 3 to 4. In comparison to routine management, the daily cessation of drug infusions significantly reduced time on the ventilator and in the ICU and provided a valuable window of opportunity for assessment of the patient's neurologic function. Interestingly when the data in this trial were analyzed by drug used (Fig. 3), little difference was noted between midazolam and propofol, making the point that the particular agent used might be less important than the protocol used to titrate drug administration. Though a concern has been raised that daily interruption of sedation may increase the risk of a stress response and possible myocardial ischemia, early follow-up data have not demonstrated any such findings (Dr. Kress,

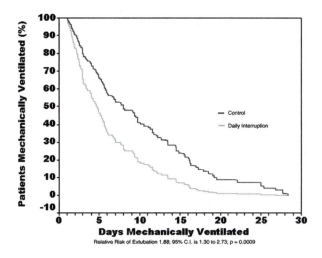

Figure 2   Daily interruption of sedation. *Source*: From Ref. 14.

personal communication). Patients receiving neuromuscular blockade (NMB) should never undergo a strategy of sedation interruption unless the NMB agent has first been stopped and spontaneous muscle movement has returned (14). Early data has not indicated any long-term psychological effects from a strategy of daily awakening from sedation (127).

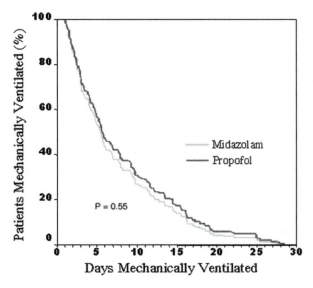

Figure 3   Daily awakening strategy: Midazolam versus propofol. *Source*: JP Kress, personal communication.

Intermittent Administration of Sedation

Kollef et al.'s observation that the continuous intravenous infusion of sedative medication prolonged mechanical ventilation and increased the length of stay in the ICU provided the rationale to give sedation through intermittent infusions. However, no studies to date demonstrate an improved length of stay in the ICU using this strategy of sedation. Furthermore, the potential for drug levels to fall below the minimal threshold to provide effect raises the possibility of the patient experiencing increased pain, anxiety, or agitation without a real proven benefit to this mode of sedation. Given budget limitations of today, a strategy that is dependent on a potentially understaffed ICU having the time to acquire more medication to deliver just as the patient is starting to experience pain or anxiety seems impractical. It should also be noted that in ICUs that are understaffed, the amount of sedation that is administered is greater than ICUs with adequate nursing staff, possibly increasing the chance of prolonged time on the ventilator (71).

F.   Delirium

Delirium is a frequent problem in the ICU (128). It is defined as an acute, potentially reversible change in level of consciousness and cognitive function. Delirium can fluctuate in severity and is usually associated with impaired memory, abnormal perception, and disorientation. These changes can be difficult to distinguish from the agitation accompanying poorly controlled pain or anxiety. A variety of conditions can produce delirium, including renal failure, sepsis, hepatic failure, cerebral edema, drug withdrawal, and medications (128). Delirium is associated with increased length of stay and increased six-month mortality (129). Delirium has historically been difficult to diagnose in the sedated ICU patient.

The Confusion Assessment Method for the ICU (CAM-ICU), a recently validated bedside scering system, is a valuable bedside tool that can be used to diagnose delirium in the ICU (128). Traditional methods to diagnose delirium require a patient that is able to verbalize, but this tool is useful in that it can quickly measure delirium in the mechanically ventilated patient and can be performed by the bedside nurse in two minutes. In a series of four steps, the operator assesses the onset of mental status change, level of attention, presence of disorganized thinking, and level of consciousness. If the first two tests are failed and either of the last two is failed as well, then the patient is diagnosed with delirium. This test had excellent inter-rater reliability (128).

As delirium is a predictor of poor outcomes, it is very important to recognize it and try to remove the underlying cause (129). One common cause of delirium is medications used in the ICU for sedation and analgesia. The study by Ely and colleagues demonstrating increased mortality with delirium provides further support that the attentive management of sedation through bedside scoring systems and daily sedation interruption can minimize the amount of medication the patient receives and possibly decrease the rate of delirium. Furthermore, it is also important to distinguish delirium from anxiety or pain in the critically ill as the management is different. Delirium should first be managed by attempting to fix the underlying cause (e.g., substance withdrawal, uremia). Only after that fails should medication be used to manage the delirium. The drug most commonly used to manage delirium in the ICU is haloperidol.

V. Neuromuscular Blockade

Neuromuscular blockade is a unique situation in the ICU. The chemical induction of paralysis is extremely anxiety-provoking and should never be done to the conscious patient. Therefore, in all patients receiving NMB, complete and deep sedation is mandatory (130,131). Strategies of daily awakening or intermittent dosing in order to minimize over-sedation effects should not be employed unless they are linked to prior cessation of NMB. Interactive scoring systems obviously can not be employed in patients receiving NMB, but paralysis level should be followed by electrophysiologic assessment with a nerve stimulator (132).

VI. Conclusion

Patients may require MV for a multitude of reasons, but the principles of management remain constant. An assessment and management of all sources of pain should be undertaken and corrected. The need for assessment of pain is not only mandated by JCAHO, but is demonstrated by ICU survivors' high incidence of significant recall of pain. Optimal pain management with intravenous opioids, NSAIDs, and epidural/regional blocks should be assessed for each individual patient on a continuous basis, and the use of pain scales needs to be routine in every ICU.

Once optimal pain management is achieved, then the still agitated patient should be sedated with either midazolam or propofol. A strategy of the daily interruption of the opioid and sedative medications should be employed in the ICU to ensure maximum effect with minimal complications and to promote the early liberation from the ventilator. The sedated patient should have his/her level of sedation monitored with a bedside scoring system such as Ramsay or the more recent RASS. Once a patient is undergoing a SBT and liberation from the ventilator, assessment for possible withdrawal symptoms should be considered in the agitated patient.

References

1. Hansen-Flaschen JH, Brazinsky S, Basile C, Lanken PN. Use of sedating drugs and neuromuscular blocking agents in patients requiring mechanical ventilation for respiratory failure. A national survey. J Am Med Assoc 1991; 266:2870–2875.
2. Christensen BV, Thunedborg LP. Use of sedatives, analgesics and neuromuscular blocking agents in Danish ICUs 1996/97. A national survey. Intensive Care Med 1999; 25:186–191.

3.   Hall JB, Schmidt G, Wood LDH. Principles of Critical Care. New York: McGraw-Hill, USA, 1998:1767.
4.   Merskey H. Pain terms: a list with definitions and notes on usage. Recommended by the International Association for the Study of Pain Subcommittee on Taxonomy. Pain 1979; 6:249–252.
5.   Walder B, Frick S, Guegueniat S, Diby M, Romand JA. Pain following cardiac surgery is present for at least one month. Intensive Care Med 2002; 28:S109.
6.   Novaes MA, Knobel E, Bork AM, Pavao OF, Nogueira-Martins LA, Ferraz MB. Stressors in ICU: perception of the patient, relatives and health care team. Intensive Care Med 1999; 25:1421–1426.
7.   Carroll KC, Atkins PJ, Herold GR, Mlcek CA, Shively M, Clopton P, Glaser DN. Pain assessment and management in critically ill postoperative and trauma patients: a multisite study. Am J Crit Care 1999; 8:105–117.
8.   Ferguson J, Gilroy D, Puntillo K. Dimensions of pain and analgesic administration associated with coronary artery bypass grafting in an Australian intensive care unit. J Adv Nurs 1997; 26:1065–1072.
9.   Rotondi AJ, Chelluri L, Sirio C, Mendelsohn A, Schulz R, Belle S, Im K, Donahoe M, Pinsky MR. Patients' recollections of stressful experiences while receiving prolonged mechanical ventilation in an intensive care unit. Crit Care Med 2002; 30:746–752.
10. Szokol JW, Vender JS. Anxiety, delirium, and pain in the intensive care unit. Crit Care Clin 2001; 17:821–842.
11. Puntillo K. Dimensions of procedural pain and its analgesic management in critically ill surgical patients. Am J Crit Care 1994; 3:116–122.
12. http://www.jcaho.org/. May 04, 2004.
13. Kress JP, O'Connor MF, Pohlman AS, Olson D, Lavoie A, Toledano A, Hall JB. Sedation of critically ill patients during mechanical ventilation. A comparison of propofol and midazolam. Am J Respir Crit Care Med 1996; 153:1012–1018.
14. Kress JP, Pohlman AS, O'Connor MF, Hall JB. Daily interruption of sedative infusions in critically ill patients undergoing mechanical ventilation. N Engl J Med 2000; 342:1471–1477.
15. Kress JP, Pohlman AS, Hall JB. Sedation and analgesia in the intensive care unit. Am J Respir Crit Care Med 2002; 166:1024–1028.
16. Payen JF, Bru O, Bosson JL, Lagrasta A, Novel E, Deschaux I, Lavagne P, Jacquot C. Assessing pain in critically ill sedated patients by using a behavioral pain scale. Crit Care Med 2001; 29:2258–2263.
17. McCaffery M. The patient's report of pain. Am J Nurs 2001; 101:73–74.
18. Phillips DM. JCAHO pain management standards are unveiled. Joint Commission on Accreditation of Healthcare Organizations. J Am Med Assoc 2000; 284:428–429.
19. Acello B. Meeting JCAHO standards for pain control. Nursing 2000; 30:52–54.
20. Pilowsky I, Kaufman A. An experimental study of atypical phantom pain. Br J Psychiat 1965; 111:1185–1187.
21. Collins SL, Moore RA, McQuay HJ. The visual analogue pain intensity scale: what is moderate pain in millimetres? Pain 1997; 72:95–97.
22. Harden N, Cohen M. Unmet needs in the management of neuropathic pain. J Pain Symptom Manage 2003; 25:S12–S17.

23. Reyes-Gibby CC, McCrory LL, Cleeland CS. Variations in patients' self-report of pain by treatment setting. J Pain Symptom Manage 2003; 25:444–448.

24. Blengini C, Joranson DE, Ryan KM. Italy reforms national policy for cancer pain relief and opioids. Eur J Cancer Care (Engl) 2003; 12:28–34.

25. Potter VT, Wiseman CE, Dunn SM, Boyle FM. Patient barriers to optimal cancer pain control. Psychooncology 2003; 12:153–160.

26. Pederson C, Matthies D, McDonald S. A survey of pediatric critical care nurses' knowledge of pain management. Am J Crit Care 1997; 6:289–295.

27. Cascinu S, Giordani P, Agostinelli R, Gasparini G, Barni S, Beretta GD, Pulita F, Iacorossi L, Gattuso D, Mare M, Munao S, Labianca R, Todeschini R, Camisa R, Cellerino R, Catalano G. Pain and its treatment in hospitalized patients with metastatic cancer. Support Care Cancer 2003 Sep; 11(9):587–592. Epub 2003 Aug 5.

28. Porter J, Jick H. Addiction rare in patients treated with narcotics. N Engl J Med 1980; 302:123.

29. Hofbauer R, Tesinsky P, Hammerschmidt V, Kofler J, Staudinger T, Kordova H. No reduction in the sufentanil requirement of elderly patients undergoing ventilatory support in the medical intensive care unit. Eur J Anaesthesiol 1999; 16:702–707.

30. Prause A, Wappler F, Scholz J, Bause H, Schulte am Esch J. Respiratory depression under long-term sedation with sufentanil, midazolam and clonidine has no clinical significance. Intensive Care Med 2000; 26:1454–1461.

31. Schelling G, Stoll C, Haller M, Briegel J, Manert W, Hummel T, Lenhart A, Heyduck M, Polasek J, Meier M, Preuss U, Bullinger M, Schuffel W, Peter K. Health-related quality of life and posttraumatic stress disorder in survivors of the acute respiratory distress syndrome. Crit Care Med 1998; 26:651–659.

32. Mendelsohn AB, Chelluri L. Interviews with intensive care unit survivors: assessing post-intensive care quality of life and patients' preferences regarding intensive care and mechanical ventilation. Crit Care Med 2003; 31:S400–S406.

33. Anand K, Barton B, McIntosh N. Analgesia and sedation in preterm neonates who require ventilatory support: results from the NOPAIN trial. Neonatal Outcome and Prolonged Analgesia in Neonates. Arch Pediatr Adolesc 1999; 153:331–338.

34. Ballantyne JC, Carr DB, deFerranti S, Suarez T, Lau J, Chalmers TC, Angelillo IF, Mosteller F. The comparative effects of postoperative analgesic therapies on pulmonary outcome: cumulative meta-analyses of randomized, controlled trials. Anesth Analg 1998; 86:598–612.

35. Rigg JR, Jamrozik K, Myles PS, Silbert BS, Peyton PJ, Parsons RW, Collins KS. Epidural anaesthesia and analgesia and outcome of major surgery: a randomised trial. Lancet 2002; 359:1276–1282.

36. Walder B, Schafer M, Henzi I, Tramer MR. Efficacy and safety of patient-controlled opioid analgesia for acute postoperative pain. A quantitative systematic review. Acta Anaesthesiol Scand 2001; 45:795–804.

37. Beattie WS, Badner NH, Choi P. Epidural analgesia reduces postoperative myocardial infarction: a meta-analysis. Anesth Analg 2001; 93:853–858.

38. Park WY, Thompson JS, Lee KK. Effect of epidural anesthesia and analgesia on perioperative outcome: a randomized, controlled Veterans Affairs cooperative study. Ann Surg 2001; 234:560–569; discussion 569–571.

39. Akca O, Melischek M, Scheck T, Hellwagner K, Arkilic CF, Kurz A, Kapral S, Heinz T, Lackner FX, Sessler DI. Postoperative pain and subcutaneous oxygen tension. Lancet 1999; 354:41–42.

40. Hopf HW, Hunt TK, West JM, Blomquist P, Goodson WH, 3rd, Jensen JA, Jonsson K, Paty PB, Rabkin JM, Upton RA, von Smitten K, Whitney JD. Wound tissue oxygen tension predicts the risk of wound infection in surgical patients. Arch Surg 1997; 132:997–1004; discussion 1005.

41. Kanski GW, Janelli LM, Jones HM, Kennedy MC. Family reactions to restraints in an acute care setting. J Gerontol Nurs 1996; 22:17–22.

42. Jones C, Griffiths RD, Humphris G. Disturbed memory and amnesia related to intensive care. Memory 2000; 8:79–94.

43. Jones C, Griffiths RD, Humphris G, Skirrow PM. Memory, delusions, and the development of acute posttraumatic stress disorder-related symptoms after intensive care. Crit Care Med 2001; 29:573–580.

44. Jacobi J., Fraser GL, Coursin DB, Riker RR, Fontaine D, Wittbrodt ET, Chalfin DB, Masica MF, Bjerke HS, Coplin WM, Crippen DW, Fuchs BD, Kelleher RM, Marik PE, Nasraway SA, Jr., Murray MJ, Peruzzi WT, Lumb PD. Clinical practice guidelines for the sustained use of sedatives and analgesics in the critically ill adult. Crit Care Med 2002; 30:119–141.

45. Liu LL, Gropper MA. Postoperative analgesia and sedation in the adult intensive care unit: a guide to drug selection. Drugs 2003; 63:755–767.

46. Gehlbach BK, Kress JP. Sedation in the intensive care unit. Curr Opin Crit Care 2002; 8:290–298.

47. Tramer MR. A rational approach to the control of postoperative nausea and vomiting: evidence from systematic reviews. Part II. Recommendations for prevention and treatment, and research agenda. Acta Anaesthesiol Scand 2001; 45:14–19.

48. Marik PE, Zaloga GP. Early enteral nutrition in acutely ill patients: a systematic review. Crit Care Med 2001; 29:2264–2270.

49. Yuan C, Foss JF, O'Connor MF, Osinski J, Karrison T, Moss J, Roizen MF. Methylnaltrexone for reversal of constipation due to chronic methadone use: a randomized controlled trial. J Am Med Assoc 2000; 283:367–372.

50. Fonsmark L, Rasmussen YH, Carl P. Occurrence of withdrawal in critically ill sedated children. Crit Care Med 1999; 27:196–199.

51. French JP, Nocera M. Drug withdrawal symptoms in children after continuous infusions of fentanyl. J Pediatr Nurs 1994; 9:107–113.

52. Brown C, Albrecht R, Pettit H, McFadden T, Schermer C. Opioid and benzodiazepine withdrawal syndrome in adult burn patients. Am Surg 2000; 66:367–370; discussion 370–371.

53. Tobias JD. Tolerance, withdrawal, and physical dependency after long-term sedation and analgesia of children in the pediatric intensive care unit. Crit Care Med 2000; 28:2122–2132.

54. Katz R, Kelly HW, Hsi A. Prospective study on the occurrence of withdrawal in critically ill children who receive fentanyl by continuous infusion. Crit Care Med 1994; 22:763–767.

55. Cammarano WB, Pittet JF, Weitz S, Schlobohm RM, Marks JD. Acute withdrawal syndrome related to the administration of analgesic and sedative medications in adult intensive care unit patients. Crit Care Med 1998; 26:676–684.

56. Westcott C. The sedation of patients in intensive care units: a nursing review. Intensive Crit Care Nurs 1995; 11:26–31.

57. Vinayak AKJ, Gehlbach B, Pohlman A, Hall J. The relationship between sedative infusion requirements and permissive hypercapnia in critically ill, mechanically ventilated patients. ATS Abstract 2003 [Poster: 904], 2003.

58. Bidani A, Tzouanakis AE, Cardenas VJ Jr, Zwischenberger JB. Permissive hypercapnia in acute respiratory failure. J Am Med Assoc 1994; 272:957–962.

59. Fraser GL, Prato BS, Riker RR, Berthiaume D, Wilkins ML. Frequency, severity, and treatment of agitation in young versus elderly patients in the ICU. Pharmacotherapy 2000; 20:75–82.

60. Fraser GL, Riker RR, Prato BS, Wilkins ML. The frequency and cost of patient-initiated device removal in the ICU. Pharmacotherapy 2001; 21:1–6.

61. Chevron V, Menard JF, Richard JC, Girault C, Leroy J, Bonmarchand G. Unplanned extubation: risk factors of development and predictive criteria for reintubation. Crit Care Med 1998; 26:1049–1053.

62. Boulain T. Unplanned extubations in the adult intensive care unit: a prospective multicenter study. Association des Reanimateurs du Centre-Ouest. Am J Respir Crit Care Med 1998; 157:1131–1137.

63. Sessler CN, Gosnell MS, Grap MJ, Brophy GM, O'Neal PV, Keane KA, Tesoro EP, Elswick RK. The Richmond Agitation-Sedation Scale: validity and reliability in adult intensive care unit patients. Am J Respir Crit Care Med 2002; 166:1338–1344.

64. Ramsay MA, Savege TM, Simpson BR, Goodwin R. Controlled sedation with alphaxalone-alphadolone. Br Med J 1974; 2:656–659.

65. Egerod I. Uncertain terms of sedation in ICU. How nurses and physicians manage and describe sedation for mechanically ventilated patients. J Clin Nurs 2002; 11:831–840.

66. Crocker C. Nurse led weaning from ventilatory and respiratory support. Intensive Crit Care Nurs 2002; 18:272–279.

67. Ely EW, Bennett PA, Bowton DL, Murphy SM, Florance AM, Haponik EF. Large scale implementation of a respiratory therapist-driven protocol for ventilator weaning. Am J Respir Crit Care Med 1999; 159:439–446.

68. Ely EW. The utility of weaning protocols to expedite liberation from mechanical ventilation. Respir Care Clin N Am 2000; 6:303–319,vi.

69. Ely EW, Meade MO, Haponik EF, Kollef MH, Cook DJ, Guyatt GH, Stoller JK. Mechanical ventilator weaning protocols driven by nonphysician health-care professionals: evidence-based clinical practice guidelines. Chest 2001; 120:454S–463S.

70. Murdoch S, Cohen A. Intensive care sedation: a review of current British practice. Intensive Care Med 2000; 26:922–928.

71. Burns AM, Shelly MP, Park GR. The use of sedative agents in critically ill patients. Drugs 1992; 43:507–515.

72. Thorens JB, Kaelin RM, Jolliet P, Chevrolet JC. Influence of the quality of nursing on the duration of weaning from mechanical ventilation in patients with chronic obstructive pulmonary disease. Crit Care Med 1995; 23:1807–1815.

73. Shapiro BA, Warren J, Egol AB, Greenbaum DM, Jacobi J, Nasraway SA, Schein RM, Spevetz A, Stone JR. Practice parameters for intravenous analgesia

and sedation for adult patients in the intensive care unit: an executive summary. Society of Critical Care Medicine. Crit Care Med 1995; 23:1596–1600.

74. Reeve W, Wallace P. A survey of sedation in intensive care. Care Critically Ill 1991; 7:238.

75. Dasta J, Furhman T, McCandles C. Patterns of prescribing and administering drugs for agitation and pain in patients in a surgical intensive care unit. Crit Care Med 1994; 22:974–980.

76. Rhoney D, Murry K. A national survey of the use of sedating and neuromuscular blocking agents in the intensive care unit [abstract]. Crit Care Med 1998; 26:A24.

77. Ely EW, Baker AM, Evans GW, Haponik EF. The prognostic significance of passing a daily screen of weaning parameters. Intensive Care Med 1999; 25:581–587.

78. Kollef MH, Levy NT, Ahrens TS, Schaiff R, Prentice D, Sherman G. The use of continuous i.v. sedation is associated with prolongation of mechanical ventilation. Chest 1998; 114:541–548.

79. Ely EW, Truman B, Shintani A, Thomason JW, Wheeler AP, Gordon S, Francis J, Speroff T, Gautam S, Margolin R, Sessler CN, Dittus RS, Bernard G R. Monitoring sedation status over time in ICU patients: reliability and validity of the Richmond Agitation-Sedation Scale (RASS). J Am Med Assoc 2003; 289:2983–2991.

80. Mondello E, Siliotti R, Noto G, Cuzzocrea E, Scollo G, Trimarchi G, Venuti FS. Bispectral Index in ICU: correlation with Ramsay Score on assessment of sedation level. J Clin Monit Comput 2002; 17:271–277.

81. Crain N, Slonim A, Pollack MM. Assessing sedation in the pediatric intensive care unit by using BIS and the COMFORT scale. Pediatr Crit Care Med 2002; 3:11–14.

82. Ambuel B, Hammlett K, Marx C. Assessing distress in pediatric intensive care environments: the COMFORT scale. J Pediatr Psychol. 1992 Feb; 17(1):95–109.

83. Frenzel D, Greim CA, Sommer C, Bauerle K, Roewer N. Is the bispectral index appropriate for monitoring the sedation level of mechanically ventilated surgical ICU patients? Intensive Care Med 2002; 28:178–183.

84. Dundee J, Wilson D. Amnestic action of midazolam. Anaesthesia 1980; 35: 459–461.

85. George K, Dundee J. Relative amnesiac actions of diazepam, flunitrazepam and lorazepam in man. Br J Clin Pharm 1977; 4:45–50.

86. Kissin I, Vinik HR, Castillo R, Bradley EL Jr. Alfentanil potentiates midazolam-induced unconsciousness in subanalgesic doses. Anesth Analg 1990; 71:65–69.

87. Ben-Shlomo I, abd-el-Khalim H, Ezry J, Zohar S, Tverskoy M. Midazolam acts synergistically with fentanyl for induction of anaesthesia. Br J Anaesth 1990; 64:45–47.

88. Byatt CM, Lewis LD, Dawling S, Cochrane GM. Accumulation of midazolam after repeated dosage in patients receiving mechanical ventilation in an intensive care unit. Br Med J (Clin Res Ed) 1984; 289:799–800.

89. Tayar J, Jabbour G, Saggi S. Severe hyperosmolar metabolic acidosis due to a large dose of intravenous lorazepam. N Engl J Med 2002; 346:1253–1254.

90. Tayar J, Jabbour G, Saggi SJ. Severe hyperosmolar metabolic acidosis due to a large dose of intravenous lorazepam. N Engl J Med 2002; 346:1253–1254.

91. Tuohy KA, Nicholson WJ, Schiffman F. Agitation by sedation. Lancet 2003; 361:308.

92. Laine GA, Hossain SM, Solis RT, Adams SC. Polyethylene glycol nephrotoxicity secondary to prolonged high-dose intravenous lorazepam. Ann Pharmacother 1995; 29:1110–1114.

93. Arbour R, Esparis B. Osmolar gap metabolic acidosis in a 60-year-old man treated for hypoxemic respiratory failure. Chest 2000; 118:545–546.

94. Weinbroum AA, Halpern P, Rudick V, Sorkine P, Freedman M, Geller E. Midazolam versus propofol for long-term sedation in the ICU: a randomized prospective comparison. Intensive Care Med 1997; 23:1258–1263.

95. Walder B, Elia N, Henzi I, Romand JR, Tramer MR. A lack of evidence of superiority of propofol versus midazolam for sedation in mechanically ventilated critically ill patients: a qualitative and quantitative systematic review. Anesth Analg 2001; 92:975–983.

96. Hall RI, Sandham D, Cardinal P, Tweeddale M, Moher D, Wang X, Anis AH. Propofol vs midazolam for ICU sedation: a Canadian multicenter randomized trial. Chest 2001; 119:1151–1159.

97. McKeage K, Perry CM. Propofol: a review of its use in intensive care sedation of adults. CNS Drugs 2003; 17:235–272.

98. Bailie G, Cockshott I, Douglas E. Pharmacokinetics of propofol during and after long-term continuous infusion for maintenance of sedation on ICU patients. Br J Anaesth 1992; 68:486–491.

99. Gottardis M, Khuenl-Brady K, Koller W. Effect of prolonged sedation with propofol on serum triglyceride and cholesterol concentrations. Br J Anaesth. 1989 Apr; 62(4):393–396.

100. Theilen HJ, Adam S, Albrecht MD, Ragaller M. Propofol in a medium- and long-chain triglyceride emulsion: pharmacological characteristics and potential beneficial effects. Anesth Analg 2002; 95:923–929, table of contents.

101. Sanchez-Izquierdo-Riera JA, Caballero-Cubedo RE, Perez-Vela JL, Ambros-Checa A, Cantalapiedra-Santiago JA, Alted-Lopez E. Propofol versus midazolam: safety and efficacy for sedating the severe trauma patient. Anesth Analg 1998; 86:1219–1224.

102. Bennett SN, McNeil MM, Bland LA, Arduino MJ, Villarino ME, Perrotta DM, Burwen DR, Welbel SF, Pegues DA, Stroud L, Zeitz PS, Jarvis WR. Postoperative infections traced to contamination of an intravenous anesthetic, propofol. N Engl J Med 1995; 333:147–54.

103. Cremer OL, Moons KG, Bouman EA, Kruijswijk JE, de Smet AM, Kalkman CJ. Long-term propofol infusion and cardiac failure in adult head-injured patients. Lancet 2001; 357:117–118.

104. Cray S, Robinson B, Cox P. Lactic acidemia and bradyarrhythmia in a child sedated with propofol. Crit Care Med 1998; 26:2087–2092.

105. Sharma ND, Rosman HS, Padhi ID, Tisdale JE. Torsades de Pointes associated with intravenous haloperidol in critically ill patients. Am J Cardiol 1998; 81:238–240.

106. Scheinin H, Virtanen R, MacDonald E, Lammintausta R, Scheinin M. Medetomidine—a novel alpha 2-adrenoceptor agonist: a review of its pharmacodynamic effects. Prog Neuropsychopharmacol Biol Psychiatry 1989; 13:635–651.

107. Ebert T, Hall J, Barney J. The effects of increasing plasma concentrations of dexmedetomidine in humans. Anesthesiology 2000; 93:382–394.

108. Venn RM, Bradshaw CJ, Spencer R, Brealey D, Caudwell E, Naughton C, Vedio A, Singer M, Feneck R, Treacher D, Willatts SM, Grounds RM. Preliminary UK experience of dexmedetomidine, a novel agent for postoperative sedation in the intensive care unit. Anaesthesia 1999; 54:1136–1142.

109. Triltsch AE, Welte M, von Homeyer P, Grosse J, Genahr A, Moshirzadeh M, Sidiropoulos A, Konertz W, Kox WJ, Spies CD. Bispectral index-guided sedation with dexmedetomidine in intensive care: a prospective, randomized, double blind, placebo-controlled phase II study. Crit Care Med 2002; 30:1007–1014.

110. Ben-Abraham R, Ogorek D, Weinbroum AA. Dexmedetomidine: a promising agent for anesthesia and perioperative care. Isr Med Assoc J 2000; 2:793–796.

111. Arain SR, Ebert TJ. The efficacy, side effects, and recovery characteristics of dexmedetomidine versus propofol when used for intraoperative sedation. Anesth Analg 2002; 95:461–466, table of contents.

112. Venn RM, Grounds RM. Comparison between dexmedetomidine and propofol for sedation in the intensive care unit: patient and clinician perceptions. Br J Anaesth 2001; 87:684–690.

113. Venn RM, Karol MD, Grounds RM. Pharmacokinetics of dexmedetomidine infusions for sedation of postoperative patients requiring intensive care. Br J Anaesth 2002; 88:669–675.

114. Spencer E, Wilatts S. Isoflurane for prolonged sedation in the intensive care unit: efficacy and safety. Intensive Care Med 1992; 18:415–421.

115. Meiser A, Sirtl C, Bellgardt M, Lohmann S, Garthoff A, Kaiser J, Hugler P, Laubenthal HJ. Desflurane compared with propofol for postoperative sedation in the intensive care unit. Br J Anaesth 2003; 90:273–280.

116. Dundee J, Samuel I, Toner W, Howard P. Midazolam, a water soluble benzodiazepine: studies in volunteers. Anaesthesia 1980; 35:454–458.

117. Wagner BK, O'Hara DA. Pharmacokinetics and pharmacodynamics of sedatives and analgesics in the treatment of agitated critically ill patients. Clin Pharmacokinet 1997; 33:426–453.

118. Bodenham A, Shelly MP, Park GR. The altered pharmacokinetics and pharmacodynamics of drugs commonly used in critically ill patients. Clin Pharmacokinet 1988; 14:347–373.

119. Shelly MP, Mendel L, Park GR. Failure of critically ill patients to metabolise midazolam. Anaesthesia 1987; 42:619–626.

120. Malacrida R, Fritz ME, Suter PM, Crevoisier C. Pharmacokinetics of midazolam administered by continuous intravenous infusion to intensive care patients. Crit Care Med 1992; 20:1123–1126.

121. Driessen JJ, Vree TB, Guelen PJ. The effects of acute changes in renal function on the pharmacokinetics of midazolam during long-term infusion in ICU patients. Acta Anaesthesiol Belg 1991; 42:149–155.

122. Bertz R, Granneman G. Use of in vitro and in vivo data to estimate the likelihood of metabolic pharmacokinetic interactions. Clin Pharmacokinet 1997; 32:210–258.

123. Jones C. 'Take me away from all this' ... can reminiscence be therapeutic in an intensive care unit? Intensive Crit Care Nurs 1995; 11:341–343.

124. Rundshagen I, Schnabel K, Wegner C, am Esch S. Incidence of recall, nightmares, and hallucinations during analgosedation in intensive care. Intensive Care Med 2002; 28:38–43.

125. Scragg P, Jones A, Fauvel N. Psychological problems following ICU treatment. Anaesthesia 2001; 56:9–14.

126. Jones C, O'Donnell C. After intensive care—what then? Intensive Crit Care Nurs 1994; 10:89–92.

127. Kress JPLM, Pliskin N, Pohlman A, Hall J. The long term psychological effects of daily sedative interruption in critically ill patients. Abstract: ATS 2001.

128. Ely EW, Margolin R, Francis J, May L, Truman B, Dittus R, Speroff T, Gautam S, Bernard GR, Inouye SK. Evaluation of delirium in critically ill patients: validation of the Confusion Assessment Method for the Intensive Care Unit (CAM-ICU). Crit Care Med 2001; 29:1370–1379.

129. Ely EW, Shintani A, Truman B, et al. Delirium as a predictor of mortality in mechanically ventilated patients in the intensive care unit. J Am Med Assoc 2004; 291: 1753–1762.

130. Shapiro BA, Warren J, Egol AB, Greenbaum DM, Jacobi J, Nasraway SA, Schein RM, Spevetz A, Stone JR. Practice parameters for sustained neuromuscular blockade in the adult critically ill patient: an executive summary. Society of Critical Care Medicine. Crit Care Med 1995; 23:1601–1605.

131. Nasraway SA Jr, Jacobi J, Murray MJ, Lumb PD. Sedation, analgesia, and neuro-muscular blockade of the critically ill adult: revised clinical practice guidelines for 2002. Crit Care Med 2002; 30:117–118.

132. Murray MJ, Cowen J, DeBlock H, Erstad B, Gray AW, Jr, Tescher AN, McGee WT, Prielipp RC, Susla G, Jacobi J, Nasraway SA, Jr., Lumb PD. Clinical practice guidelines for sustained neuromuscular blockade in the adult critically ill patient. Crit Care Med 2002; 30:142–156.

16

Infection Control Issues in the Intensive Care Unit

REKHA MURTHY

Hospital Epidemiology
Cedars–Sinai Medical Center and
  Geffen School of Medicine at UCLA
Los Angeles, California, U.S.A.

MATTHEW BIDWELL GOETZ

VA Greater Los Angeles Healthcare System
  and Geffen School of Medicine at UCLA
Los Angeles, California, U.S.A.

I. Introduction

Nosocomial infections (NIs) are an unfortunately common and important complication in intensive care unit (ICU) patients. The overall risk of acquiring nosocomial infections for patients admitted to ICUs is estimated to be five to 10-fold higher than that of other hospitalized patients. Altogether, ICU-acquired infections account for more than 20% of all hospital acquired infections, although admissions to ICUs represent only 8–15% of hospital admissions (1–3).

The impact of NI on morbidity, mortality, and costs has been well demonstrated (4,5). For example, the increased cost of nosocomial blood stream infection (BSI) in ICU patients was estimated at an average of $34,508 per patient (6). Overall, NIs result in as many as 3.5 million additional hospital days per year in the U.S., with an estimated (based on 1989 dollars) additional annual hospital cost of over $3.5 billion (7). Mortality rates associated with NI vary from 12% to 80% (8) and are exacerbated in patients with NI due to antibiotic-resistant micro-organisms, especially in patients who initially receive ineffective antimicrobial therapy (9,10).

Numerous studies indicate that the actions of healthcare providers and the development of appropriate systems of care can reduce the rate of NIs (1,11–18). Not only are such programs effective in reducing NIs, but they are important requirements for accreditation of healthcare facilities (19).

541

This chapter reviews the epidemiology of major ICU acquired infections and current strategies for prevention and control of ICU acquired infections. Particular attention is paid to the most common causes of nosocomial infections, namely ventilator-associated pneumonia (VAP), catheter-associated urinary tract infection (UTI), and central venous catheter-associated BSI.

II. Epidemiology of NI

In the European Prevalence of Infection Study (EPIC), which assessed NIs in 10,038 patients from 1417 ICUs, 21% of ICU patients had an ICU-acquired NI; of these NIs, pneumonia (47%) and other lower respiratory tract infections (18%) were most common, followed by UTIs (18%) and BSIs (12%) (8). In contrast, in U.S. medical ICUs that participate in the National Nosocomial Infection Surveillance (NNIS) System, UTIs were the most frequent nosocomial infections, followed by pneumonia and BSIs (Fig. 1). Together these three infections accounted for up 77% of all NIs (20). Other types of nosocomial infection include those of surgical sites, the gastrointestinal tract, the lower respiratory tract without pneumonia, the cardiovascular system (primarily phlebitis without bacteremia), ear, nose and throat (mainly sinusitis), skin and soft tissues, and rarely endocarditis and meningitis (20).

Table 1 outlines the most recent NNIS data for device-related NI rates in ICUs (21). The three most common infections (i.e., UTI, nosocomial pneumonia,

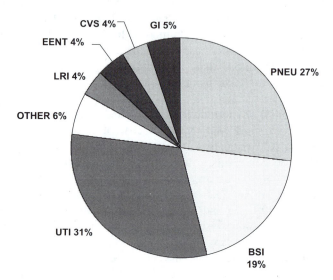

Figure 1 Site distribution of nosocomial infections in adult medical intensive care unit patients, 1992–1997. *Abbreviations*: BSI, primary bloodstream infections; PNEU, pneumonia; UTI, urinary tract infections; other: GI, gastrointestinal infections; CVS, cardiovascular system; EENT, eye, ear, nose, throat infections; LRI, lower respiratory tract infections other than pneumonia.

Table 1 Rates of Device: Associated Nosocomial Infections in ICUs

Type of ICU	Urinary catheter-associated UTI (Mean: 10–90%)	Central line-associated BSI (Mean: 10–90%)	Ventilator-associated pneumonia (Mean: 10–90%)
Burn	8.5 (0.3–11.6)	8.5 (0–18.1)	9.6
Coronary	5.4 (0.7–10.7)	4.2 (0–8.4)	4.2 (0–11.2)
Cardiothoracic	3.1 (0.6–5.5)	2.9 (0.4–4.9)	7.9 (0 –15.6)
Medical	6.2 (2.4–9.8)	5.7 (2.1–9.6)	5.0 (0–9.6)
Med/surg (major teaching)	5.3 (1.7–9.2)	5.0 (2.2–7.7)	6.0 (0–12.1)
Med/surg (other)	3.8 (0.7–7.0)	3.7 (0–6.8)	6.0 (0–11.2)
Neurosurgical	7.7 (2.1–12.9)	4.8 (0–9.0)	12.9 (1.7–19.4)
Pediatric	4.7 (0–7.9)	7.3 (0.7–11.5)	2.9 (0–9.0)
Surgical	5.1 (1.2–9.0)	5.2 (1.1–9.3)	9.9 (2.2–18.4)
Trauma	6.4 (3.7–9.3)	7.8 (2.5–12.3)	15.1
Respiratory	5.5	3.4	4.2

Pooled means and percentiles of the distribution of device-associated infection rates, by type of ICU, January 1995–June 2003. Rates are defined as: number of catheter-associated UTIs/number of urinary catheter-days × 1000; number of central line-associated BSIs/number of central line-days × 1000; number of ventilator-associated pneumonias/number of ventilator-days × 1000.
Abbreviations: BSI, blood stream infection; UTI, urinary tract infection.
Source: From Ref. 21.

and BSI) are almost always associated with the use of an invasive device. In the NNIS analysis of medical ICU patients, 87% of BSIs were associated with a central line, 86% of nosocomial pneumonia occurred in patients undergoing mechanical ventilation, and 95% of UTIs were in catheterized patients (20).

In addition to medical devices, the risk of NI is also determined by host factors (i.e., underlying co-morbid conditions), length of ICU stay, prior surgical procedures, and processes of care (e.g., infection control techniques). Thus, it is not surprising that the incidence of NI, VAP, BSI and UTI as well as the infection rate per device day differs substantially by type of ICU (Table 1) (21). For example, surgical ICUs demonstrate a very high use rate of central venous catheters (CVC) but a low infection rate, whereas burn ICUs report a low-use rate and high infection rate. This reflects differences in the duration of ICU care in these patient populations as well as the severe skin breakdown and consequent heavy bacterial colonization of devitalized tissue that compromises catheter sterility in burn patients. Similarly, relatively high rates of VAP in neurosurgical ICUs and burn ICUs may reflect the long duration of endotracheal intubation in these patients and, in burn patients, potential thermal damage of airways.

Both gram-negative bacilli (GNB) and gram-positive bacteria (GPB) are important causes of NI (21). The relative frequency of different nosocomial pathogens varies by site of infection (Table 2). For example, there is over-representation of infections due to *Candida* spp. with UTIs or BSIs, coagulase-negative staphylococci

Table 2 Commonly Reported Pathogens from Patients in Adult Medical Intensive Care Units

Pathogen	Blood stream infection (%) ($n = 2971$)	Pneumonia infection (%) ($n = 4389$)	Urinary tract infection (%) ($n = 4956$)
Coagulase negative Staphylococci	36	1	2
Enterococci	16	2	14
Staphylococcus aureus	13	20	2
Candida albicans	6	5	21
Klebsiella pneumoniae	4	8	6
Pseudomonas aeruginosa	3	21	10
Enterobacter spp.	3	9	5
Other *Candida* spp.	3	1	5
Escherichia coli	3	4	14
Candida glabrata	2	0.2	5
Acinetobacter spp.	2	6	1
Serratia marcescens	1	4	0.7
Other fungi	0.8	1	8
Citrobacter spp.	0.5	2	1
Proteus spp.	0.5	2	2
Aspergillus	0	0.6	0

Source: From Ref. 20.

with BSIs, and *P. aeruginosa* and *Acinetobacter* spp. with VAP (20). These associations may be explained by tissue-specific bacterial adherence properties, catheter-specific development of biofilms, and environmental factors, such as water condensation in endotracheal tubes (20).

Infections due to organisms with increased antimicrobial resistance are a special concern in ICU patients. The prevalent antibiotic-resistance organisms (ARO) in ICU acquired infections include methicillin-resistant *S. aureus* (MRSA), vancomycin-resistant Enterococci (VRE), third generation cephalosporin-resistant GNB, fluoroquinolone- and imipenem-resistant *P. aeruginosa*, and fluconazole-resistant *Candida* spp. (8,21). Of great concern is the steady and dramatic increase in antibiotic resistance of these pathogens over the past two decades (8,22–24). Compared with 1997–2001 data, results from NNIS surveys in 2002 show that the rate of vancomycin resistance among clinical isolates of enterococci in the ICU setting has increased from 10.4% to 27.5% and that the rate of methicillin-resistance among *Staphylococcus aureus* has increased from 35.9% to 57.1% (Table 3) (21). For *P. aeruginosa*, rates of resistance in 2002 compared with the preceding five-year period (1997–2001) represented a 37% increase in quinolone resistance, 32% increase in imipenem resistance, and 22% increase in resistance to third generation cephalosporins (3GC). Indeed, in many ICUs, rates of quinolone resistance in *P. aeruginosa* have risen to over 40% (21). Even more

Table 3 Resistance Rates of Selected Nosocomial ICU Pathogens: 2002 Versus 1997–2001

Antibiotic/organism	N	% of Resistant isolates	% Increase[a]
Vancomycin/enterococci	2253	27	11
Methicillin/*S. aureus*	4303	57	13
Methicillin/coag (−) staphylococci	3675	89	1
Third ceph/*E. coli*	1439	6	14
Third ceph/*K. pneumoniae*	990	14	−2
Imipenem/*P. aeruginosa*	1569	22	32
Quinolone/*P. aeruginosa*	2064	33	37
Third ceph/*P. aeruginosa*	2383	30	22
Third ceph/*Enterobacter* spp.	1485	32	−5

Third Ceph = 3rd generation cephalosporins (either ceftriaxone, cefotaxime, or ceftazidime).
Quinolone = either ciprofloxacin or ofloxacin.
[a]Percent (%) increase in resistance rate of year January–December 2002 compared with mean rate of resistance over previous five years (1997–2001).
Source: From CDC, Ref. 21.

ominous are recent reports of infections due to *S. aureus* strains with high level resistance to vancomycin (VRSA), acquired due to genetic transfer of the vanA resistance gene from vancomycin-resistant *E. faecalis* (25–27), and of GNB that manifest resistance to most or all classes of currently available antibiotics [e.g., those that produce extended-spectrum beta-lactamases (ESBL)]. The increasing prevalence of infections with ARO in critically ill patients is likely due to several factors, including increasing antibiotic selective pressure from frequent use of broad-spectrum antibiotics, which promotes the emergence and persistence of these organisms, prolonged hospitalization of chronically and acutely ill patients who serve as a reservoir of ARO, and factors that increase the patient-to-patient transmission of AROs, such as crowding of patients and increased workload of ICU personnel (28,29). Several studies have shown that a lower nurse-to-patient ratio is significantly associated with the relative risk of nosocomial infections among patients in ICUs (30,31).

Infections caused by ARO are more likely to result in prolonged hospitalization, death, especially when the infecting micro-organism is resistant to empiric antimicrobial therapy (5), and the use of more toxic or expensive antibiotics when compared with those caused by infections due to susceptible organisms (9). In 1989, the overall annual costs of control and treatment of infections caused by ARO were estimated to be between $100 million and $300 million (32); these costs are likely far greater now as a result of inflation of healthcare costs. Both the rise in antimicrobial resistance and the increasingly limited therapeutic options available to treat infections arising from AROs underscore the need for effective strategies for limiting the spread of drug-resistant bacteria and reducing the risk of NIs, especially within the critical care setting (33).

III. Prevention and Control of NI

Over 20 years ago, the Study on the Efficacy of Nosocomial Infection Control showed that infection control measures can significantly decrease NI rates (11). The key elements of such programs are epidemiologic surveillance and intervention; reporting of NI rates to stake-holders; administrative controls for medical equipment, health-care personnel, and patients; and engineering controls (Table 4). Recent consensus recommendations outline the optimal infrastructure and essential activities of hospital infection control and epidemiology programs (34). The NNIS system, which uses standardized methodology and criteria for

Table 4   Elements of an Effective ICU Nosocomial Infection Plan

Program element	Specific items
Epidemiologic surveillance and intervention	Epidemiologic surveillance for NI rates • Total surveillance • Surveillance by objective (targeted to selected units, infections, or pathogens) • Outbreak surveillance and control • Computerized surveillance of laboratory data (targeted on resistance, device use) Provision of rates of key infection to key stakeholders
Engineering controls	Adequate space around beds Individualized cubicles (provided optimal nurse-to-patient staffing ratio is allocated) Adequate sink/hand hygiene facilities' location Isolation rooms in each ICU Identified traffic circuits for clean and dirty equipment and/or activities
Administrative controls for medical equipment	Procedures for introduction of new materials/devices Written cleansing protocols for multiple-use material Routine application of guidelines for the appropriate use of medical devices
Administrative controls for health-care personnel	Continuous postgraduate medical education to learn new technologies and the proper use of new medical devices and procedures Maintain the presence of highly skilled HCWs by extensive training of replacement workers. In-depth training on infection control procedures Recommendations for nurse/patient staffing ratio Monitoring quality of patient care using defined indicators
Administrative controls for patients	Guidelines for ICU admission Guidelines for patient isolation

Abbreviation: NI, nosocomial infection.

NI, publishes regular reports on the rate of various ICU infections that can be used as a benchmark by individual institutions (21).

Consensus conferences and expert panels have established numerous guidelines (1,12–18,35,36) that address three main approaches for the prevention and control of NI. First, prevention and control of cross-contamination and of potential sources of pathogens that could be transmitted from patient to patient, from health care worker (HCW) to patient, or from device to patient is paramount; these methods and techniques include hand hygiene, protocols for the handling of medical devices, and appropriate cleansing and disinfection of equipment. Second, guidelines call for the appropriate use of surgical antibiotic prophylaxis and of empirical antimicrobial therapy to improve treatment outcomes and to reduce the risk of emergence of antimicrobial resistance. Finally, measures to prevent specific NIs and the transmission of highly antibiotic-resistant micro-organisms, such as vancomycin-resistant enterococci, MRSA, and highly resist-ant GNB (e.g., ESBL-producing or amikacin-resistant isolates), have also been developed.

General infection control strategies are reviewed below. Detailed infor-mation can be found in the Centers for Disease Control and Prevention (CDC) guidelines referenced in the respective discussions in this chapter. Infection control measures aimed at specific devices or procedures (e.g., ventilators, intra-vascular catheters, urinary catheters) are discussed in greater detail in the respect-ive sections in this chapter.

A. Prevention of Cross-Transmission

Pathogens causing nosocomial infections, such as GNB and *S. aureus*, are perva-sive in intensive care areas. Transmission of these micro-organisms to patients frequently occurs via hands of healthcare personnel that become contaminated or transiently colonized with the micro-organisms (16). The risk of cross-contamination can be reduced by using aseptic technique, appropriately steriliz-ing or disinfecting equipment when appropriate, and eliminating pathogens from the hands of personnel.

Hand Disinfection

Hand hygiene by healthcare workers is the single most important measure for the prevention of NI and remains the cornerstone of infection control (12,16,37,38). Improving hand hygiene compliance from 60% to 100% reduces the rate of nosocomial infection by 25% to 50% (16,39). Conversely, failure to perform appropriate hand hygiene is considered the leading cause of both health-care-associated infections and transmission of multi-resistant organisms (16).

Unfortunately, HCW adherence to recommended handwashing procedures ranges from 5% to 81% (overall average: 40%) (16). Rates in ICUs have been reported to be lower, especially during procedures that carry a high risk of bacterial contamination or when intensity of patient care is high (33,40). This is not surprising as 100% compliance with handwashing recommendations may require upto 16 hours of ICU personnel time over the course of an eight-hour shift (41). Thus full adherence to previous CDC guidelines for handwashing with soap and water may be unrealistic. In contrast, use of antiseptic alcohol-based hand rub solutions, which require less time and more effectively reduce hand contamination, may facilitate adherence with hand hygiene protocols, particularly in busy ICUs (16,42). However, use of alcohol-based handrubs may be insufficient during outbreaks of *C. difficile*-related infections as these agents are not reliably sporicidal (16). Details regarding the role of hand hygiene in infection prevention can be found in the recently published CDC guidelines (16).

Isolation Precautions

The CDC has published guidelines on isolation precautions to minimize the risk of patient-to-patient or patient-to-HCW transmission of infectious agents (12). Further details regarding infection control issues for ICU patients can be found in several excellent recent reviews and guidelines, (12–18,43). For isolation practices to be successful, the majority of, if not all, carriers of particular bacteria must be identified and isolated to prevent occult transmission. Depending on the pathogen of concern, isolation strategies may include geographic isolation of an infected or colonized patient, cohorting of patients and staff, and barrier isolation using gloves and/or gowns when in contact with the patient or potentially contaminated secretions (Table 5).

The use of barrier isolation with gloves and gowns when caring for colonized or infected patients has been associated with decreased spread of resistant organisms in the ICU (16,33). Gloves serve both to prevent the patient from acquiring organisms during routine care and to protect the provider from potential exposures to bloodborne pathogens. However, pathogens can colonize gloves (16,18), and gloved hands may get contaminated via leaks in the gloves. Thus, personnel should use gloves properly (i.e., change gloves after contact with each patient) and decontaminate their hands after gloves are removed (16,18). Although the role that gowns play in preventing transmission of nosocomial resistance in ICUs is not fully resolved (44,45), use of disposable gowns in conjunction with gloves has been associated with the termination of several outbreaks (33). Combined use of gowns or gloves is recommended as part of strict contact isolation, for example, when entering the room of a VRE-infected or -colonized patient if substantial contact with the patient or environmental surfaces is anticipated.

Specific recommendations for the management of patients with highly resistant pathogens [e.g., vancomycin-intermediate *S. aureus* (VISA), VRSA and VRE] have been issued by the CDC (46–48). In the event of VISA, for example, these recommendations include private room isolation, strict contact isolation, dedicated healthcare workers to provide one-on-one care, obtaining

Table 5 Standard Isolation Precautions

Hand hygiene	After direct contact with blood, body fluid, secretion, excretions, and contaminated items.
	Immediately before gloving and after glove removal
	Between patient contacts and between dirty and clean body site contact in the same patient
Gloves	For anticipated contact with blood, body fluid, secretion, excretions, and contaminated items
	For anticipated contact with mucous membranes and nonintact skin
Mask, eye protection, face shield	To protect mucous membranes of the eyes, nose, and mouth during procedures and patient-care activities likely to generate splashes or sprays of blood, body fluid secretions, or excretions
Gowns	To protect skin and prevent soiling of clothing during procedures and patient-care activities likely to generate splashes or spray of blood, body fluid secretions, or excretions
Patient-care equipment	Soiled devices, linen, or clothing should be handled to prevent skin and mucous membrane exposure and transfer of micro-organisms to the environment
	Reusable devices should be cleaned and reprocessed according to hospital policy
Sharp objects	Avoid recapping used needles
	Avoid removing used needles from disposable syringes by hand
	Avoid bending, breaking, or manipulating used needles by hand
	Place used sharp objects and needles in puncture-resistant containers

baseline cultures for VISA from the anterior nares and hands of all healthcare personnel, roommates, and visitors who may come in direct contact with the patient, and re-enforcement of infection control measures with the healthcare staff. The effectiveness of such measures is as yet untested.

Patients who are infected or colonized with the same microorganism may share a room if private rooms are not available for individual isolation precautions (an unlikely situation in most modern U.S. ICUs). This approach, referred to as cohorting, can also be used to manage staffing to minimize cross-transmission between patients and is most utilized during outbreak settings or in geographic separation of patients with multidrug-resistant organisms isolated (49).

Recently published guidelines regarding environmental infection control in healthcare facilities outline specific recommendations for cleaning and disinfection, including for antibiotic-resistant organisms and other emerging pathogens (17).

B. Control of Antimicrobial Resistance

Antimicrobial use generally falls into one of three categories: empirical therapy for suspicion of infection, definitive therapy for proven infections, and prophylaxis for surgical infections. In many ICUs, empiric therapy accounts for the majority of antibiotic use. Due to concerns about the considerable mortality and morbidity associated with inadequately treated NIs, early empirical therapy often utilizes very broad-spectrum agents. Antimicrobial pressure due to such practices increases the likelihood of emergence of antimicrobial resistance.

In an effort to reduce the impact of AROs, consensus guidelines not only recommend implementing infection control strategies (Table 6) to minimize transmission of ARO but also antibiotic control strategies (Table 7) to optimize therapy and thus prevent or reduce the emergence of resistance (35,36). In addition, guidelines for the systematic evaluation of potential infection in critically ill patients have been developed in an effort to decrease the need for empirical therapy (50).

One particularly effective intervention for optimizing antimicrobial therapy has been the use of computerized decision support tools at the time that physicians select antimicrobial therapy. Use of this system has been associated with reduction in costs, improvement of the quality of patient care, and the exposure of patients to lower amounts of antibiotics (51). Antimicrobial cycling, that is, the scheduled change of preferred empiric therapy, is another strategy that has been advocated to limit the trend of increasing antimicrobial resistance among nosocomial pathogens (35,52). One study reported that scheduled monthly rotation of preferred empiric therapy for VAP was followed by a significant decrease in the rate of VAP as well as of resistant GNB (53). However, nothing replaces a good knowledge of the local epidemiology and the resistance profile of the prevailing in-hospital and out-of-hospital pathogens. A multidisciplinary approach, including the microbiology laboratory and experts in infectious disease and infection control, is required to address institution-specific antimicrobial resistance issues.

Recent Society for Healthcare Epidemiology of America (SHEA) guidelines (49) recommend the use of surveillance strategies for patients admitted to

Table 6 Strategies to Optimize the Use of Antimicrobials

1.	Optimize antimicrobial prophylaxis for operative procedures
2.	Optimize choice and duration of empiric antimicrobial therapy
3.	Improve antimicrobial prescribing practices by educational and administrative means
4.	Establish a system to monitor and provide feedback on occurrence and impact of antibiotic resistance
5.	Define and implement institutional or health care delivery system guidelines for important types of antimicrobial use

Source: From Ref. 35.

Table 7 Strategies for Detecting, Reporting and Preventing Transmission of Antimicrobial-Resistant Micro-organisms

---

1. Develop a system to recognize and promptly report significant changes and trends in antimicrobial resistance
2. Develop a system for rapid detection and reporting of micro-organisms in individual patients to caregivers and infection control staff
3. Increase adherence to Infection Control policies and procedures
4. Incorporate the detection, prevention, and control of antimicrobial resistance into institutional strategic goals and provide required resources
5. Develop a plan for identifying, transferring, discharging, and readmitting patients colonized with specified antimicrobial-resistant micro-organisms

---

Source: From Ref. 35.

hospitals to facilitate early recognition and isolation of patients potentially colonized with resistant organisms. However, implementation of such strategies is complicated by their potential costs and difficulty in implementation.

IV. VAP

Hospital-acquired pneumonia (HAP) is defined as pneumonia occurring ≥ 48 hours after admission to the hospital (54). VAP is a subset of HAP and is defined as pneumonia in a mechanically ventilated patient that occurs >48 hours after intubation. Most cases of HAP are due to aspiration of oropharyngeal contents or, less commonly, inhalation of micro-organisms into the lower airways that may occur due to the receipt of aerosols produced by contaminated respiratory therapy equipment (13).

A. Epidemiology and Risk Factors

The incidence of HAP ranges from four to eight cases per 1000 hospitalized patients (13). Within the ICU, VAP occurs at a rate of three to 13 infections/1000 ventilator days (21) and contributes to as many as 60% of all deaths due to nosocomial infections (13). Nosocomial pneumonia prolongs ICU stay by an average of 4.3 days (55).

B. Pathogenesis

In intubated patients, the presence of an endotracheal tube circumvents host defenses and causes local trauma and inflammation. Despite adequate inflation, micro-organisms in oropharyngeal secretion commonly reach the lower respiratory tract by leaking around the endotracheal cuff (56). In addition, bacterial colonization of the extraluminal or intraluminal surface of the endotracheal tube commonly results in the formation of a biofilm that is resistant to the action of antimicrobials and host immune defenses (57).

C. Microbiology

HAP that occurs during the first five days of hospitalization is usually caused by "community" flora, including *S. pneumoniae*, methicillin-sensitive *S. aureus, H. influenzae*, and anaerobes. By contrast, cases of HAP that develop later during hospitalization are much more likely to be caused by "hospital" flora, such as enteric GNB (e.g., *Escherichia, Klebsiella*, and *Enterobacter* spp.), *P. aeruginosa*, and MRSA (13,57,58). Gram-negative isolates in general and organisms such as *P. aeruginosa, S. maltophilia, Burkholderia cepacia*, and *Acinetobacter baumanii* in particular often colonize respiratory equipment, are highly resistant to antimicrobials, and have been shown to be transmitted from person-to-person (59). *Legionella pneumophila* may contaminate potable water systems, ultrasonic mist devices, whirlpool baths, and air-conditioning condensate (60).

D. Specific Preventive Measures

Detailed guidelines and reviews of measures for the prevention of nosocomial pneumonia have been published (10,18,58,61). Recommended interventions are directed at reducing the concentration of micro-organisms within oropharyngeal secretions, limiting the risk of aspiration, and decreasing the risks of microbial contamination of nebulized medications or ventilatory equipment (Table 8).

The best validated patient-level measures for the prevention of VAP are elevation of the head of the bed and aspiration of subglottic secretions (18,61). Other once-promising measures have been shown to be ineffective or remain to be fully validated. These include use of sucralfate to reduce gastric acidity and measures designed to maintain aspiration, including the use of flexible, small-bore nasogastric tubes, intermittent rather than continuous enteral feeding, or small intestinal feeding (18,58,61,62).

Several studies have demonstrated that the prophylactic use of systemic and local (i.e., mucosal) antimicrobials reduces oropharyngeal colonization and decreases both the incidence of VAP and consequent mortality due to respiratory tract disease (64). However, the methodological quality of many of these studies is poor (63). Finally, there are concerns about the long-term societal impact of such regimens given their likely detrimental effect on overall antimicrobial

Table 8   Recommended Measures for the Prevention of Nosocomial Pneumonia

---

Monitor intestinal motility and enteral feedings to avoid regurgitation and aspiration
Avoid use of large-volume room air humidifiers
Clean and sterilize or disinfect all reusable equipment/devices and medication nebulizers
   between patients and at recommended intervals
Use only sterile fluids for nebulization and dispense aseptically
Provide analgesia to avoid compromise of respiratory excursions and cough reflex
Elevate the head of the bed

---

resistance, which has not been adequately evaluated (64). Thus this strategy is not recommended (18,61). In contrast, reduction of the bacterial burden in oropharyngeal secretions by using nonspecific measures to provide good oral hygiene and hypopharyngeal suctioning has been shown in several studies to decrease rates of HAP (10,56,65,66).

Not surprisingly, avoidance of intubation altogether reduces the risk of pneumonia. Specifically, the incidence of pneumonia is significantly lower in patients who receive noninvasive positive pressure ventilation through a face mask than in those who are intubated and receive mechanically-assisted ventilation. Furthermore, such patients have significantly shorter periods of ventilation and shorter stays in the ICU (67,68).

For those patients who do require intubation, orotracheal intubation is preferable to nasotracheal intubation (18). One specific advantage is that the risk of sinusitis is decreased. Furthermore, the rate of VAP is lowered by the use of high-volume, low-pressure cuffs (57). The role of early tracheotomy in VAP prevention is controversial (57).

Minimization of the risk of VAP requires that attention also be paid to the use of respiratory therapy devices (e.g., nebulizers), diagnostic equipment (e.g., bronchoscopes and spirometers), ventilator circuits, and humidifiers (18,57). Detailed recommendations regarding the selection, frequency of replacement, sterilization, and disinfection of elements of ventilatory circuit have been published elsewhere (18). Because tap or distilled water may harbor micro-organisms that can cause pneumonia, the use of sterile or pasteurized water is necessary when items require rinsing to remove disinfectants (e.g., glutaraldehyde) (17,18). There is no demonstrable advantage to routinely changing ventilator circuits at fixed interval unless there is visual and/or known contamination or mechanical malfunction of the circuit (10,18,57). Several studies demonstrate that this results in substantial cost savings without there being any increase in the incidence of VAP (18).

Equipment choices include the use of open single-use versus closed multi-use catheter systems for tracheal suctioning. Use of closed-suction systems results in decreased environmental contamination and lower costs, as the closed system catheter can remain unchanged for an indefinite period without increasing the patient's risk of healthcare-associated pneumonia (10). Although some studies have shown that the use of the closed system is also associated with decreased rates of VAP, further studies are required to confirm these findings (10,18,57).

Condensate in the tubing of ventilator circuits is a potential risk factor for VAP because this liquid can rapidly become contaminated with bacteria that usually originate from the patient's oropharynx. Poor management can result in such fluid refluxing through the tubing directly into the lower respiratory tract (57). Although heat–moisture exchangers successfully eliminate condensate formation, these devices have not been conclusively demonstrated to reduce the rate of VAP (18,57,69). Furthermore, they increase dead space and resistance to breathing.

Finally, patients with community-acquired pneumonia due to *S. pyogenes* and *S. aureus* pneumonia should be placed on respiratory droplet isolation during the first 24 hours of therapy (12). In addition, as with infection at other sites, isolation is recommended for patients with infections due to pathogens such as MRSA or highly-resistant GNB (e.g., ESBL-producing *E. coli*, or *K. pneumoniae*, and organisms resistant to amikacin or carbapenems). There is no evidence to suggest person-to-person transmission of *Legionella*.

E. Diagnosis and Management of Ventilator-Associated Pneumonia

The clinical manifestations of VAP and the utility of differing diagnostic strategies is discussed in the separate ventilator-associated pneumonia chapter of this book.

V. Sinusitis

The lack of specific diagnostic criteria has led to reports of nosocomial sinusitis among ICU patients that range from 38.5% to 100%. In contrast, studies that use more restrictive criteria have found rates of sinusitis to be 5% to 35% (43). The risk for these infections is increased by nasotracheal (rather than orotracheal) intubation and the presence of nasogastric tubes (13,43). In one randomized study, a systematic approach to the diagnosis and treatment of maxillary sinusitis among mechanically ventilated patients with a nasotracheal tube decreased the incidence of VAP and 60-day mortality (70). This study defined nosocomial sinusitis as the presence of fever ($\geq 38°C$), CT evidence of air–fluid level or opacification in the maxillary sinus, and presence of purulent aspirate from the involved sinus puncture with $\geq 10^3$ CFU of bacteria/mL. Using this systemic approach, sinusitis was diagnosed in 80 of 199 study patients versus none of 200 control patients.

VI. UTIs

A. Epidemiology and Risk Factors

UTIs account for more than 40% of NIs and affect an estimated 600,000 patients per year (21). In medical ICUs, UTIs represent approximately 30% of NIs and occur at the rate of 3.1–8.5 per 1000 urinary catheter-days (20,21). Although most catheter associated (CA) UTIs are asymptomatic (71), rarely extend hospitalization, and add only $500 to $1000 to the direct costs of acute-care hospitalization (72), asymptomatic UTIs commonly precipitate unnecessary antimicrobial therapy. Additionally, CA UTIs likely comprise the largest reservoir of nosocomial antibiotic-resistant pathogens (73), due to the rapid colonization of the catheter with nosocomial flora.

The single most important risk factor for UTI is the presence of an indwelling bladder catheter; 95% of UTIs from medical ICUs have been associated with use of urinary catheters (20). Other risk factors include the duration of catheterization (with the rate of bacteriuria increasing 5% per catheter day) (74), the method of catheterization, the quality of catheter care, and host risk factors (i.e., increased risk in female patients, persons with diabetes, and individuals with rectal and meatal colonization by uropathogens) (75).

B. Pathogenesis and Complications

After the insertion of an indwelling catheter, micro-organisms enter the urinary tract by either an intraluminal or extraluminal route. Extraluminal contamination may occur early, by direct inoculation when the catheter is inserted, or later, by organisms ascending from the perineum by capillary action in the thin mucous film contiguous to the external catheter surface (75,76). Intraluminal contamination occurs by reflux of micro-organisms gaining access to the catheter lumen from violation of closed drainage or contamination of urine in the collection bag. Microbial adherence to the catheter surface is likely important in the pathogenesis of many CA UTIs (73). Ultimately, most infected urinary catheters are covered by a thick biofilm containing the infecting micro-organisms embedded in a matrix of host proteins and microbial exoglycocalyx (73).

CA UTIs in otherwise healthy patients are often asymptomatic and likely to resolve spontaneously with the removal of the catheter. Complications of CA UTIs include prostatitis, epididymitis, cystitis, pyelonephritis, and bacteremia (77). Bacteremia may occur immediately upon catheter insertion or withdrawal as the result of mucosal trauma, as a consequence of catheter obstruction, or as a complication of mucosal ulcerations in patients undergoing prolonged catheterization (78). Although symptomatic bacteremia occurs in less than 1% of CA UTIs, the mortality rate may reach 30% (79).

C. Microbiology

The micro-organisms responsible for CA UTIs usually originate in the endogenous fecal flora of the patient, but they can also be acquired by cross-contamination from other patients or hospital personnel, or by exposure to contaminated solutions or nonsterile equipment. From 1992–1999, about 70% of CA UTI pathogens in the U.S. were caused by *E. coli* (17.5%), *Candida* (15.8%), *Enterococcus* (13.8%), *Pseudomonas* (11%), *Klebsiella* (6.2%), and *Enterobacter* spp. (5.1%) (80). Because of increasing antimicrobial use, these pathogens often demonstrate resistance to multiple antimicrobials. Unusual pathogens, such as *Serratia marcescens* and *Pseudomonas cepacia*, have special epidemiologic significance; since these micro-organisms do not commonly reside in the gastrointestinal tract, their isolation from catheterized patients suggests acquisition from an exogenous source (81). The incidence of nosocomial UTIs caused by *Candida* spp. and other yeasts has been increasing over the last decade (82). Risk factors for candiduria include duration of catheterization, duration of hospitalization, and antibiotic use. Notably, nonalbicans

Candida and other yeasts other than *Candida* spp. are steadily increasing as the etiologic agents of fungal UTI.

D. Specific Preventive Measures

Many CA UTIs can be prevented by proper catheter management. Aside from the avoidance of catheterization, the most important, potentially modifiable, risk factor is removal of the catheter as soon as possible (83); by the 30th day of catheterization, bacteriuria is almost-universal (73). General principles for prevention or delay of onset of CA UTI have been developed and are outlined below (73,84,85). Unfortunately, few of these practices have been explicitly proven to be effective by randomized controlled trials.

If the use of an indwelling urethral catheter is required, insertion should be done by trained personnel using aseptic technique, including sterile gloves, a fenestrated sterile drape, and an effective cutaneous antiseptic, such as 10% povidone-iodine or 1–2% aqueous chlorhexidine (73,81). The use of a condom catheter or suprapubic catheter may be associated with lower risks of CA UTI than occurs with indwelling urethral catheters (73,84). After a catheter is inserted, uncompromising maintenance of closed drainage is of the highest priority and can keep the overall risk of CA UTI under 25% for up to two weeks of catheterization (85,86). It is important to ensure dependent drainage, minimize manipulation of the system, and use good infection control technique when handling catheters (84,85). Although antimicrobial-drug therapy does protect against CA UTI in persons undergoing short-term catheterization, this approach clearly selects for risk of infection caused by multidrug-resistant micro-organisms, such as resistant GNB, enterococci, and yeasts, and is therefore not recommended (73,87). Intermittent catheterization is rarely appropriate in ICU patients in whom urinary catheterization is being considered.

The first major advance for preventing CA UTI since the wide-scale adoption of closed drainage more than three decades ago is the development of catheters with anti-infective surfaces (73). Impregnation of indwelling urinary catheters with silver alloy-hydrogel both inhibits microbial adherence to the catheter surface and significantly reduces the risk of extraluminal CA UTI caused by gram-positive organisms (73). However, since use of the silver alloy-hydrogel catheter does not confer protection against CA UTI caused by GNB, which most often gain access intraluminally, use of these catheters is of limited value in chronically catheterized patients (88). Two other small randomized trials have shown decreased rates of bacterial CA UTI with the use of catheters impregnated with either a urinary antiseptic (nitrofurazone) or the combination of minocycline and rifampin. However, these results remain to be replicated (73).

Other technologic innovations for the prevention of CA UTIs have not proven to be beneficial (73). Among these are use of anti-infective lubricants when inserting the catheter, regular metal cleansing, application of topical anti-infectives to the meatus, continuous bladder irrigation anti-infective solutions and or periodic instillation of an anti-infective solution into the urine collection system (73).

E. Diagnosis and Treatment

In noncatheterized patients, the presence of $>10^5$ bacteria per mL of clean-voided urine is often used as the criterion for "significant" bacteriuria (i.e., consistent with the presence of true infection) (85). However, in catheterized patients, unless suppressive antimicrobial-drug therapy is being administered, concentrations of bacteria in the urine rapidly and predictably increase to $>10^5$ CFU/mL within 72 hours (89). Thus, concentrations $>10^2$ or 10^3 CFU/mL in urine collected with a needle from the sampling port of the catheter are considered by most authorities to be indicative of true CA UTI (73). Treatment of bacteriuria with appropriate systemic antibiotics and/or removal or replacement of the urethral catheter is indicated for patients with symptoms of infection attributable to a CA UTI.

In comparison to bacterial UTI, the diagnostic criteria of significant funguria and fungal UTI are not well established. Management of asymptomatic catheter-associated candiduria is unclear since removal of the catheter results in resolution of the candiduria in approximately one-third of patients. Furthermore, candiduria is rarely the cause of candidemia. Indeed, when candidemia occurs in the context of candiduria, urinary tract infection is usually the consequence rather than the cause of bloodstream infection. In the setting of an obstructive uropathy, candiduria is also occasionally complicated by the development of fungal balls in the bladder or renal pelvis, renal or perirenal abscess, and disseminated candidiasis. Treatment of asymptomatic candiduria should be limited to adults who are neutropenic, have renal allografts or an obstructive uropathy, or will undergo urologic manipulations (90).

VII. BSI and Vascular Catheter Management

A. Epidemiology and Risk Factors

BSIs, usually due to contaminated vascular catheters, are the third leading cause of NIs among ICU patients. These infections prolong hospitalization, cost an additional \$34,508–\$56,000 per infection, and increase mortality by 35% (15,91). Up to 75% of intravascular device-related BSIs are associated with use of CVCs (92). Given that in US ICUs the use of CVC amounts to 15 million patient days/year (93) and that CVC-associated BSIs occur at an average rate of 4.9 infections per 1000 catheter-days (21), approximately 74,000 CVC-associated BSIs/year occur in American ICUs. The overall risk of BSI by type of vascular device is shown in Table 9.

Table 9   Risks of Bloodstream Infection by Type of Vascular Device

	Rates of bloodstream infection			
	Per 100 devices		Per 1000 device days	
Device	Mean	95% CI	Mean	95% CI
Peripheral IV	0.2	0.1–0.3	0.6	0.3–1.2
Arterial line	1.5	0.9–2.4	2.9	1.8–4.5
Central line	3.3	3.3–4.0	2.3	2.0–2.4
Tunneled/cuffed central line	20.9	18.2–21.9	1.2	1.0–1.3
PICC line	1.2	0.5–2.2	0.4	0.2–0.7
Subcutaneous port	5.1	4.0–6.3	0.2	0.1–0.2
Hemodialysis (noncuffed)	16.2	13.5–18.3	2.8	2.3–3.1
Hemodialysis (cuffed)	6.3	4.2–9.2	1.1	0.7–1.6

Abbreviation: PICC, peripherally inserted central catheters.
Source: From Ref. 93a.

B.   Pathogenesis

The major source for catheter-related BSIs (CRBSI) is colonization of the extra-
or intraluminal surface of the device. Rarely, there may be contamination of the
fluid administered through the device. Micro-organisms may gain access to the
extraluminal surface by invading the percutaneous tract by which the device
was inserted or by contaminating the intraluminal surface when the catheter is
inserted over a percutaneous guidewire or during manipulation of the catheter
hub and/or other components of the IV tubing (94,95). Less commonly, extraluminal or intraluminal colonization may occur due to bacteremia originating
at a remote site of infection (92).

   The extraluminal route is the major mechanism of infection for nearly two-
thirds of noncuffed, short-term, CVC-related BSIs, especially during the first
seven to 10 days of catheterization (96). The same is true for peripheral intravenous and arterial catheters. In contrast, contamination of the catheter hub and
lumen is the predominant route of BSI for long-term peripherally inserted
central catheters (PICC lines) as well as for cuffed and/or tunnelled Hickman-
and Broviac-type catheters, hemodialysis catheters, and catheters with subcutaneous ports (14,15,92).

   Pathogen characteristics determine the likelihood of catheter colonization and subsequent infection. The formation of a biofilm allows for sustained
microbial colonization that decreases local antimicrobial activity. For example,
S. aureus can adhere to host proteins (e.g., fibronectin) commonly present
on catheters (97,98). Additionally, adherent coagulase-negative staphylococci
may produce an extracellular polysaccharide often referred to as "slime"
(99,100).

C. Microbiology

The organisms that most commonly cause CRBSIs in ICU patients are shown in Table 10. Staphylococci (especially coagulase-negative Staphylococci), enterococci and *Candida* are the leading pathogens (15). These organisms are noteworthy not only because of their frequency but also because of their antimicrobial resistance. Overall, CVCs pose the highest risk for nosocomial candidemia (92).

Contaminated infusate is the cause of epidemic BSIs due to *Klebsiella*, *Enterobacter*, *Citrobacter*, *Serratia*, and *P. cepacia* (15,101,102). Use of intralipid has been associated with infection by unusual lipophilic micro-organisms, such as *Malassezia furfur* (103).

D. Preventive Measures

Modifiable factors that affect the risk of CRBSI include the method of preparing the site, the experience of the person inserting the catheter, the choice of vascular access site, the size of sterile drapes, duration of catheter use, catheter size, and catheter purpose (e.g., for hemodynamic monitoring or parenteral nutrition) (15,104). In patients receiving hyperalimentation, one catheter (or one port of a multilumen catheter) should be designated exclusively for this purpose (15). The importance of well-structured training programs to ensure appropriate practices and thereby reduce infection rates has been repeatedly demonstrated (105,106). Finally, although many ICU patients have absolute requirements for CVCs, the use of midline catheters and PICC lines results in lower rates of infection than does CVC use (107). The CDC recommends the use of these catheters (rather than peripheral short IV lines) when the duration of IV therapy will likely exceed six days (15).

Table 10 Microbiology of Catheter-Related Bloodstream Infections in the United States (1992–1999)

Organism	Proportion of all infections
S. aureus	13%
Coagulase-negative Staphylococci	37%
Enterococci	13%
Enterobacter	5%
P. aeruginosa	4%
E. coli	5%
Klebsiella pneumoniae	3%
Candida	8%
Other	27%

Source: From Ref. 15.

Site Preparation and Selection

Lower CRBSI rates follow site preparation with 2% aqueous chlorhexidine gluconate in place of 10% povidone-iodine or 70% alcohol (108). In contrast, a 0.5% tincture of chlorhexidine gluconate is no better than 10% povidone iodine (109). Although otherwise well-tolerated, the safety of chlorhexidine in infants aged <2 months has not been determined (15). Defatting of the insertion site with acetone or ether is not recommended; natural skin lipids have antimicrobial activity (15,110). Hair removal is rarely necessary for vascular catheter placement; when required, this should involve hair-cutting rather than shaving (105,111).

No randomized trial has satisfactorily compared infection rates for catheters placed in jugular, subclavian, and femoral sites (15). However, available evidence suggests that the subclavian site is associated with the lowest rate of CRBSI in adults. Catheters inserted into an internal jugular vein have a higher risk for infection than those inserted into a subclavian or femoral vein (94). Furthermore, although well tolerated in pediatric populations, the use of femoral catheters in adults is associated with higher rates of both microbial colonization of the catheter and deep venous thrombosis than occur with use of internal jugular or subclavian catheters (15,104,112,113). A trend towards increased rates of sepsis with use of femoral as opposed to subclavian catheters was found in one randomized controlled study (113).

Catheter Insertion

Use of maximal sterile barrier precautions (e.g., cap, mask, sterile gown, sterile gloves, and large sterile drape) during the insertion of CVCs or PICC lines substantially reduces CRBSI incidence and reduces total catheter-related costs compared with standard precautions (i.e., use of only sterile gloves and small drapes) (15,94,114). Tunneled short-term, jugular, or femoral CVCs that are not also used for drawing blood (a process that increases the rate of IV hub contamination) have been associated with a decreased rate of CR infection (93,115,116). Although there is no impact on infection, use of bedside ultrasound for the placement of CVCs substantially reduces the rate of mechanical complications (117).

Catheter-Selection

For patients undergoing short-term catheterization with a non-cuffed device (<30 days), use of catheters impregnated with either chlorhexidine and silver sulfadiazine or minocycline and rifampin decreases the incidence of CRBSI (15,94,95,118,119). Perhaps because of more prolonged antimicrobial elution and coating of both luminal surfaces rather than of only the extraluminal surface, the benefit of minocycline/rifampin-coated catheters was greater than that of first-generation chlorhexidine/silver sulfadiazine-coated catheters (118,120). A second-generation chlorhexidine/silver sulfadiazine-coated catheter is now available with three times the amount of chlorhexidine and coating of both the internal and external luminal surfaces. However, no comparative studies have been published using this device. Of potential concern is the possibility that minocycline/rifampin-impregnated catheters could increase antimicrobial resistance.

Other catheter modifications include the addition of a subcutaneous collagen cuff that is impregnated with ionic silver (121). However, placement of these devices requires greater technical skill, and the devices do no not protect against intraluminal infection (15,121). Regardless, if >3 weeks of temporary access is needed for hemodialysis, use of a cuffed catheter is preferable to a non-cuffed catheter, even in the ICU setting (15,104,122). A combination platinum/silver-impregnated catheter has recently been approved for use in the U.S.A., but no published clinical studies have as yet been presented to support the use of these devices. Because of increased rates of infectious complications, the majority of catheters sold in the U.S.A. are no longer made of polyvinyl chloride or polyethylene (123,124).

Finally, randomized clinical trials demonstrate that use of needleless connectors rather than standard hub connectors can reduce the risk of intravascular CRBSI if the devices are used correctly (92,125,126). Surgically-implanted subcutaneous central venous ports, which can be accessed intermittently with a steel needle, are associated with particularly low rates of CRBSI (Table 9) (127). The number of catheter lumens does not directly affect the rate of CRBSI (128).

Catheter Management

The use of topical antibiotic ointment or creams on insertion sites is not recommended, except for dialysis catheters, because of potential increases in the rates of fungal infections and of antimicrobial resistance (15). Although application of mupirocin ointment to the catheter site may reduce the risk for CRBSI (129), use of this ointment has been associated with mupirocin resistance and may adversely affect the integrity of polyurethane catheters (130). Intranasal mupirocin ointment has been used to decrease nasal carriage of *S. aureus* and lessen the risk for CRBSI (131). However, resistance to mupirocin develops in both *S. aureus* and coagulase-negative staphylococci soon after routine use of mupirocin is instituted (15). The full results of a multicenter trial that showed a chlorhexidine-impregnated sponge placed over the site of short-term arterial catheters and CVCs reduced the risk for catheter colonization and CRBSIs (132) have not yet been published.

Antibiotic lock prophylaxis, that is, flushing and filling the lumen of the catheter with an vancomycin-containing solution, has been shown to decrease the rate of CRBSI in neutropenic patients with long-term catheters. However, this practice is not recommended for routine use due to concerns about the potential effect on acquisition of VRE, VISA, or VRSA (15,46). Systemic antibiotic prophylaxis for the prevention of CRBSI is specifically not recommended (15).

The risk of CRBSI is similar regardless whether the site is covered by a semi-permeable transparent dressing or gauze dressing (133). A single small study found that the rate of CRBSI was reduced in patients whose PICC lines were secured by a sutureless device rather than by sutures (134). Because of increased risk of infection due to microbial growth in the infusate, tubing used to administer propofol should be changed every six to 12 hours (15,135). Similarly, tubing used to administer blood, blood products, or lipid emulsions should be replaced within 24 hours of initiating the infusion (15). Otherwise, administration sets do not need to be changed more frequently than every 72 hours (15). While the use of in-line vascular filters reduces rates of sterile phlebitis, these devices are not compatible with hemodynamic monitoring (e.g., pulmonary artery catheterization) or the administration of blood products, lipid emulsions, or amphotericin B, and they have not been shown to clearly reduce the incidence of BSI. Consequently, routine use of in-line vascular filters is not recommended (15).

Catheter Replacement

For any catheter inserted under emergency basis, a new catheter should be inserted at a different site within 48 hours (15). Otherwise, short peripheral venous catheters should be replaced every 72–96 hours (124,136,137). In contrast, no advantage has been found for using a strategy of replacing nontunneled CVCs every three to seven days as opposed to on an as-needed basis (Table 11) (138–140). Catheter replacement over a guidewire has become an accepted technique for replacing a malfunctioning catheter or exchanging a pulmonary artery catheter for a CVC when invasive monitoring no longer is needed. Although guidewire exchange is associated with nonsignificant trends toward a higher rate of catheter colonization, catheter exit-site infection, and CRBSI, this procedure is also associated with a trend towards fewer mechanical complications relative to replacement at a new site (141).

Table 11 Recommendations for Replacement of Intravascular Catheter Management in Adults

Catheter	Replacement and relocation of device
Peripheral venous catheters	Replace catheter and rotate site every 72–96 hr
Midline catheters	No recommendation
Peripheral arterial catheters	Do not replace catheters routinely to prevent catheter-related infection
Central venous catheters including PICC lines	Do not routinely replace catheters

Source: From Ref. 15.

If the CVC is exchanged over a guidewire and there is subsequent evidence of catheter infection as per the results of blood or catheter cultures, the replacement catheter should be removed and a new catheter should be placed in a new site (14). Similarly, replacement of a vascular catheter over a guidewire in the presence of bacteremia is not an acceptable replacement strategy because the source of infection is often at the percutaneous insertion site (15,94,140).

E. Considerations with Specific Intravascular Devices

Arterial Catheters

Arterial catheters used for hemodynamic monitoring pose a risk of CRBSI comparable to that of short-term CVCs (104). The CDC recommends replacement of disposable or reusable transducers every four days. Other components, including the tubing, continuous-flush device, and flush solution, should be changed at the same time (114,142). The CDC makes no specific recommendation regarding replacement of catheters that need to be in place for more than five days (15). Arterial lines should not be routinely used to obtain blood samples that do not require arterial blood.

Pulmonary Artery Catheters

Although the risk of CRBSI increases after five to seven days of pulmonary artery catheterization (143,144), no studies indicate that catheter replacement at scheduled time intervals is an effective method to reduce CRBSI (138,140). Nevertheless, the CDC recommends that pulmonary artery catheters be changed after seven days in patients who require continued hemodynamic monitoring (15). Use of the attached sleeve decreases the risk of CRBSI (143).

Unique complications of pulmonary artery catheterization include catheter-induced endothelial damage that increases the likelihood of secondary cardiac infection should bacteremia occur (145). In one study, up to 40% of patients with bacteremia while a pulmonary artery catheter was in place developed tricuspid or pulmonic valve endocarditis (146).

F. Diagnosis of Vascular Catheter Infection

Although nonspecific, blood culture results that are positive for *S. aureus*, coagulase-negative staphylococci, or *Candida* species should raise the suspicion for CRBSI (14). Unfortunately, more specific signs, such as the presence of localized embolic disease distal to a cannulated vein or artery and local phlebitis or inflammation at the catheter insertion site, have very poor sensitivity. The most sensitive clinical finding, that is, fever, has very poor specificity.

Patients with suspected CRBSI should have two sets of blood samples drawn for culture, with at least one set drawn percutaneously (14,128). The positive predictive value (i.e., rate of true bacteremia) of blood cultures obtained from an indwelling CVC is 58–64% versus 67–78% for peripheral blood cultures, whereas the negative predictive value is 98% versus 96–97% (147,148). The poor predictive value of a positive culture of blood drawn through a central vascular catheter is such that the secure diagnosis of BSI requires confirmatory peripheral blood cultures. This is especially important if a potential contaminant is isolated from the catheter culture (14).

Unless there are obvious signs of local infection at the catheter site, determination that a BSI is due to catheter infection requires specialized techniques for catheter or blood culture. These include semi-quantitative and quantitative catheter cultures, quantitative blood cultures, and measurement of the time required for the detection of microbial growth in blood cultures.

Catheter culture techniques report the presence or absence of bacteria on a 2-inch segment of the subcutaneous portion or the tip of the device. For suspected pulmonary artery catheter infection, culture of the introducer tip has a better diagnostic yield than does culture of the pulmonary artery catheter tip (14). For semiquantitative cultures the catheter segment is rolled over the surface of an agar plate; this allows identification of bacteria on the extraluminal surface only. A positive result is defined by the presence of ≥ 15 colony forming units (CFU) per catheter segment of the same organism (species and antibiogram) that is isolated from a catheter segment and a peripheral blood sample (96,104). Quantitative cultures rely upon vortexing or sonicating broth containing the catheter segment and enumerating the recovered CFU; a positive result is the detection of $\geq 10^2$ CFU. This technique samples intraluminal and extraluminal bacteria (149,150). The overall sensitivity and specificity are 85% and 85% for semiquantitative cultures versus 94% and 92% for quantitative cultures (151). The results of any of these cultures should be used only to diagnose the source of otherwise unexplained bacteremia or to provide microbiologic etiology of clinically evident infection at the catheter site. Patients should not be routinely treated solely on the basis of positive catheter cultures. Qualitative cultures, wherein the number of CFU on the catheter is not determined, are not recommended because of their poor specificity (14). These criteria are summarized in Table 12.

When catheter removal is not practical, analysis of blood cultures obtained simultaneously from the catheter and a peripheral site may be used to confirm CRBSI. In one method, a positive result is defined by a ratio of ≥ 5 to $10:1$ of CFU/mL found in quantitative cultures of blood obtained from the catheter versus from a peripheral source (14,152). Alternatively, CRBSI may be diagnosed based on differences in the time to culture positivity, that is, blood drawn through the catheter becomes positive for microbial growth at least two hours more rapidly than does blood obtained from a peripheral site (153,154). These techniques do not sample extraluminal bacteria and have been validated primarily in patients whose intravascular catheters were present for more than 30 days (152). In contrast, most central catheters in ICU settings are left in place for less than 10 days (140), and CRBSI are thus more likely to be due extraluminal catheter infection (152).

Table 12 Criteria for Diagnosis of Intravascular Catheter-Related Infection

Method	Criteria	Type of infection	Comment
Semiquantitative catheter culture obtained by rolling catheter segment on agar plate	≥ 15 CFU	Extraluminal	
Quantitative catheter culture obtained by vortexing or sonicating broth containing the catheter segment and enumerating the recovered CFU of catheter	$\geq 10^2$ CFU	Extraluminal and intraluminal	
Comparison of quantitative cultures of blood obtained percutaneously and through catheter	$\geq 5-10$ times greater recovery of micro-organisms through the catheter	Intraluminal	
Comparison of time to positive culture of blood obtained percutaneously and through catheter	Culture of catheter blood positive for growth >2 hr before percutaneous blood	Intraluminal	Requires continuous blood culture monitoring

These criteria should be used only to diagnose the source of otherwise unexplained bacteremia or to provide microbiologic etiology of clinically evident infection at the catheter site.
Abbreviation: CFU, colony forming unit.

G. Management of Vascular Catheter Infection

CVCs should not routinely be removed in febrile patients with fever as the vast majority of catheters from patients with suspected CRBSIs are sterile (14). Nevertheless, the cornerstone of management of confirmed CRBSI is removal of the infected catheter (14). In this regard, tunneled or surgically implanted CVCs, although less often present in ICU patients, offer special challenges due to the difficulty of removal and the limited vascular access often present in the patients who require these devices. Nevertheless, critically ill patients or persons with tunnel infection, abscesses at the site of subcutaneous ports, septic thrombosis, endocarditis, or other metastatic infections require removal of the catheter as well as appropriate antibiotic therapy.

In noncritically ill patients without local or metastatic complications, intra-luminal CRBSI due to *S. aureus*, coagulase-negative staphylococci, and gram-negative bacteria may be amenable to medical treatment without removal of the catheters if there is no evidence of tunnel or pocket infection. There has been extensive interest in antibiotic lock therapy of active infection; this is often used in combination with systemic antimicrobial therapy. However, catheters that have been in place for <2 weeks are most often infected extraluminally; such infections are not amenable to treatment with intraluminal therapy as is provided by the antibiotic lock technique (14). Antibiotic lock therapy relies upon administration of a small 2–5 mL volume (sufficient to fill the catheter lumen) of antimicrobial active against the infection pathogen mixed with either 50–100 U of heparin or normal saline during period of time when the catheter is not being used; the antimicrobial is thus "locked" into place. In published reports, vancomycin has been used at a final concentration of 1–5 mg/mL; gentamicin and amikacin at 1–2 mg/mL; and ciprofloxacin at 1–2 mg/mL. The volume of installed antibiotic is removed before the catheter is next used. Although the duration of antibiotic lock therapy has varied among different studies, it most often is two weeks (14).

A more extensive discussion of antibiotic lock therapy and further details regarding the management of vascular catheter infections is beyond the scope of this review. This topic has been covered in great depth by several recent reviews to which the reader is referred for more information (14,155).

VIII. Conclusions

More than one-third of NIs are acquired in ICUs and are associated with substantial excess length of stay and additional hospital costs. The prevention and control of NI in the ICU hinges primarily on reducing the transmissions of organisms. Clearly, antimicrobial resistance in the hospital setting has emerged as an important variable that influences patient outcomes and overall resource utilization, even more so in ICUs. Meticulous adherence to infection control measures, such as hand hygiene, remains the cornerstone of infection prevention; however, newer technologies have contributed to significant advances in further reducing the risks of nosocomial infection, particularly in individuals at high risk from device-related infections.

Acknowledgment

We would like to acknowledge the editorial contributions of Theodore Katsivas, M.D. to this chapter.

References

1. Fridkin SK, Welbel SF, Weinstein RA. Magnitude and prevention of nosocomial infections in the intensive care unit. Inf Dis Clin N Am 1997; 11(2): 479–496.
2. Brown RB, Hosmer D, Chen HC, Teres D, Sands M, Bradley S, Opitz E, Szwedzinski D, Opalenik D. A comparison of infections in different ICUs within the same hospital. Crit Care Med 1985; 13:472–476.

3. Weinstein RA. Epidemiology and control of nosocomial infections in adult intensive care units. Am J Med 1991; 91(suppl 3B):179S–184S.
4. Vincent JL. Nosocomial infections in adult intensive care units. Lancet 2003; 361:2068–2077.
5. Kollef MH, Fraser VJ. Antibiotic resistance in the intensive care unit. Ann Int Med 2001; 134(4):298–314.
6. Digiovine B, Chenoweth C, Watts C, Higgins M. The attributable mortality and costs of primary nosocomial bloodstream infections in the intensive care unit. Am J Respir Crit Care Med 1999; 160:976–981.
7. Correa L, Pittet D. Problems and solutions in hospital-acquired bacteraemia. J Hosp Inf 2000; 46(2):89–95.
8. Vincent JL, Bihari DJ, Suter PM, Bruining HA, White J, Nicolas-Chanoin MH, Wolff M, Spencer RC, Hemmer M. The prevalence of nosocomial infection in intensive care units in Europe. Results of the European Prevalence of Infection in Intensive Care (EPIC) study. J Am Med Assoc 1995; 274:639–644.
9. Holmberg SD, Solomon SL, Blake PA. Health and economic impacts of antimicrobial resistance. Rev Inf Dis 1987; 9:1065–1078.
10. Kollef MH, Sherman G, Ward S, Fraser VJ. Inadequate antimicrobial treatment of infections: a risk factor for hospital mortality among critically ill patients. Chest 1999; 115:462–474.
11. Haley RW, Culver DH, White JW, Morgan WM, Emori TG, Munn VP, Hooton TM. The efficacy of infection surveillance and control programs in preventing nosocomial infections in US hospitals. Am J Epidemiol 1985; 121:182–205.
12. Garner JS, Jarvis WR, Emori TG, Horan TC, Hughes JM. CDC definitions for nosocomial infections. Am J Infect Control 1988; 16:128–140.
13. Centers for Disease Control and Prevention. Guidelines for prevention of nosocomial pneumonia. Mor Mortal Wkly Rep 1997; 46(RR-1):1–79.
14. Mermel LA, Farr BM, Sherertz RJ, Raad II, O'Grady N, Harris JS, Craven DE. Guidelines for the management of intravascular catheter-related infections. Clin Infect Dis 2001; 32: 1249–1272.
15. O'Grady NP, Alexander M, Dellinger EP, Patchen DE, Gerberding JL, Heard SO, Maki DG, Masur H, McCormick RD, Mermel LA, et al. Guidelines for the prevention of intravascular catheter-related infections. Am J Inf Cont 2002; 30(8):476–489.
16. Boyce JM, Pittet D. Guideline for hand hygiene in health-care settings: recommendations of the Healthcare Infection Control Practices Advisory Committee and the HICPAC/SHEA/APIC/IDSA Hand Hygiene Task Force. Inf Cont Hosp Epidem 2002; 23(12 suppl):S3–S40.
17. Sehulster L, Chinn RY. Guidelines for environmental infection control in health-care facilities. Recommendations of CDC and the Healthcare Infection Control Practices Advisory Committee (HICPAC). Mor Mortal Wkly Rep Recomm Rep 2003; 52:1–42.
18. Tablan OC, Anderson LJ, Besser R, Bridges C, Hajjeh R. Centers for Disease Control and Prevention. Guidelines for preventing health-care–associated pneumonia, 2003: recommendations of CDC and the Healthcare Infection Control Practices Advisory Committee, 2003. http://www.cdc.gov/ncidod/hip/guide/CDCpneumo_guidelines.pdf Accessed 5/30/04.

19. Joint Commission on Accreditation of Health Care Organizations (JCAHO). Comprehensive accreditation manual for hospitals. Oakbrook Terrace, IL: JCAHO, 2004.

20. Richards MJ, Edwards JR, Culver DH, Gaynes RP. Nosocomial infection in medical intensive care units in the United States: national nosocomial infections surveillance systems. Crit Care Med 1999; 27:887–892.

21. Centers for Disease Control and Prevention. National Nosocomial Infections Surveillance (NNIS) System Report, data summary from January 1992 through June 2003, issued August 2003. Am J Infect Control 2003; 31:481–498.

22. Edmond MB, Wallace SE, McClish DK, Pfaller MA, Jones RN, Wenzel RP. Nosocomial bloodstream infections in United States hospitals: a three-year analysis. Clin Infect Dis 1999; 29:239–244.

23. Anonymous. Intensive Care Antimicrobial Resistance Epidemiology (ICARE) Surveillance Report, data summary from January 1996 through December 1997: a report from the National Nosocomial Infections Surveillance (NNIS) system. Am J Infect Control 1999; 27:279–284.

24. Weber DJ, Raasch R, Rutala WA. Nosocomial infections in the ICU: the growing importance of antibiotic-resistant pathogens. Chest 1999; 115(3 suppl): 34S–41S.

25. CDC. *Staphylococcus aureus* resistant to vancomycin—United States, 2002. Mor Mortal Wkly Rep 2002; 51:565–567.

26. CDC. Vancomycin-resistant *Staphylococcus aureus*—Pennsylvania, 2002. Mor Mortal Wkly Rep 2002; 51:902.

27. CDC. Vancomycin-resistant *Staphylococcus aureus*—New York, 2004. Mor Mortal Wkly Rep 2004; 53(15):322–323.

28. McGowan JE Jr. Antibiotic resistance in hospital bacteria: current modes for appearance or spread, and economic impact. Rev Med Micro 1991; 2: 161–169.

29. Archibald L, Phillips L, Monnet D, McGowan JE Jr, Tenover F, Gaynes R. Antimicrobial resistance in isolates from inpatients and outpatients in the United States: increasing importance of the intensive care unit. Clin Infect Dis 1997; 24:211–215.

30. Fridkin SK, Pear SM, Williamson TH, Galgiani JN, Jarvis WR. The role of understaffing in central venous catheter-associated bloodstream infections. Infect Control Hosp Epidemiol 1996; 17:150–158.

31. Robert J, Fridkin SK, Blumberg HM, Anderson B, White N, Ray SM, Chan J, Jarvis WR. The influence of the composition of the nursing staff on primary bloodstream infection rates in a surgical intensive care unit. Infect Control Hosp Epidemiol 2000; 21:12–17.

32. Phelps CE. Bug-drug resistance: sometimes less is more. Med Care 1989; 27:194–203.

33. Warren DK, Fraser VJ. Infection control measures to limit antimicrobial resistance. Critical Care Medicine 2001; 29(4 suppl):N128–N134.

34. Scheckler WE, Brimhall D, Buck AS, Farr BM, Friedman C, Garibaldi RA, Gross PA, Harris J, Hierholzer, WJ Jr, Martone WJ, et al. Requirements for infrastructure and essential activities of infection control and epidemiology in hospitals: a consensus panel report. Infect Control Hosp Epidemiol 1998; 19(2): 91–93.

35. Goldman DA, Weinstein RA, Wenzel RP, Tablan OC, Duma RJ, Gaynes RP, Schlosser J, Martone WJ. Strategies to prevent and control the emergence and

spread of antimicrobial-resistant microorganism in hospitals. A challenge to hospital leadership. J Am Med Assoc 1996; 275(3):234–240.

36. Shlaes DM, Gerding DN, John JF Jr, Craig WA, Bornstein DI, Duncan RA, Eckman MR, Farrer WE, Greene WH, Lorian V. Society for Healthcare Epidemiology of America and Infectious Diseases Society of America Joint Committee on the Prevention of Antimicrobial Resistance: guidelines for the prevention of anti-microbial resistance in hospitals. Clin Infect Dis 1997; 25:584–599.

37. Jarvis WR. Handwashing: the Semmelweis lesson forgotten? Lancet 1994; 344:1311–1312.

38. Larson EL. APIC guidelines for handwashing and hand antisepsis in health care settings. Am J Infect Control 1995; 23:251–269.

39. Simmons B, Bryant J, Neiman K, Spencer L, Arheart K. The role of handwashing in prevention of endemic intensive care unit infections. Infect Control Hosp Epidemiol 1990; 11:589–594.

40. Pittet D, Mourouga P, Perneger TV. Compliance with handwashing in a teaching hospital. Infection Control Program. Ann Intern Med 1999; 130: 126–130.

41. Voss A, Widmer AF. No time for handwashing!? Handwashing versus alcoholic rub: can we afford 100% compliance? Infect Control Hosp Epidemiol 1997; 18:205–208.

42. Pittet D, Hugonnet S, Harbarth S, Mouranga P, Sauvan V, Touveneau S, Perneger TV. Effectiveness of a hospital-wide programme to improve compliance with hand hygiene. Infection Control Programme. Lancet 2000; 356:1307–1312.

43. Eggimann P, Pittet D. Infection control in the ICU. Chest 2001; 120(6): 2059–2093.

44. Slaughter S, Hayden MK, Nathan C, Hu TC, Rice T, VanVoorhis J, Matushek M, Franklin C, Weinstein RA. A comparison of the effect of universal use of gloves and gowns with that of glove use alone on acquisition of vancomycin-resistant enterococci in a medical intensive care unit. Ann Intern Med 1996; 125:448–456.

45. Koss WG, Khalili TM, Lemus JF, Chelly MM, Margulies DR, Shabot MM. Nosocomial pneumonia is not prevented by protective contact isolation in the surgical intensive care unit. Am Surg 2001; 67:1140–1144.

46. Anonymous. Recommendations for preventing the spread of vancomycin resistance. Recommendations of the Hospital Infection Control Practices Advisory Committee (HICPAC). MMWR Recomm Rep 1995; 44:1–13.

47. CDC. Interim guidelines for prevention and control of Staphylococcal infection associated with reduced susceptibility to vancomycin. Mor Mortal Wkly Rep 1997; 46:624–628.

48. Centers for Disease Control and Prevention. Investigation and control of vancomycin-intermediate and resistant *Staphylococcus aureus*: A guide for health departments and infection control personnel. Atlanta, GA, 2003.

49. Muto CA, Jernigan JA, Ostrowsky BE, et al. SHEA guideline for preventing noso-comial transmission of multidrug-resistant strains of *Staphylococcus aureus* and *Enterococcus*. Infect Control Hosp Epidemiol 2003; 24:362–386.

50. O'Grady NP, Barie PS, Bartlett JG, Bleck T, Garvey G, Jacobi J, Linden P, Maki DG, Nam M, Pasculle W, et al. Practice guidelines for evaluating new fever in critically ill adult patients. Task Force of the Society of Critical Care Medicine and the Infectious Diseases Society of America. Clin Infect Dis 1998; 26: 1042–1059.

51. Pestotnik SL, Classen DC, Evans RS, Burke JP. Implementing antibiotic practice guidelines through computer-assisted decision support: clinical and financial outcomes. Ann Intern Med 1996; 124:884–890.

52. McGowan JE Jr. Do intensive hospital antibiotic control programs prevent the spread of antibiotic resistance? Infect Control Hosp Epidemiol 1994; 15: 478–483.

53. Gruson D, Hilbert G, Vargas F, Valentino R, Bebear C, Allery A, Bebear C, Gbikpi-Benissan G, Cardinaud JP. Rotation and restricted use of antibiotics in a medical intensive care unit: impact on the incidence of ventilator-associated pneumonia caused by antibiotic-resistant gram-negative bacteria. Am J Respir Crit Care Med 2000; 162:837–843.

54. Niederman MS, Mandell LA, Anzueto A, Bass JB, Broughton WA, Campbell GD, Dean N, File T, Fine MJ, Gross PA, et al. Guidelines for the management of adults with community-acquired pneumonia. Diagnosis, assessment of severity, antimicrobial therapy, and prevention. Am J Respir Crit Care Med 2001; 163:1730–1754.

55. Heyland DK, Cook DJ, Griffith L, Keenan SP, Brun-Buisson C. The attributable morbidity and mortality of ventilator-associated pneumonia in the critically ill patient. The Canadian Critical Trials Group. Am J Respir Crit Care Med 1999; 159:1249–1256.

56. Valles J, Artigas A, Rello J, Bonsoms N, Fontanals D, Blanch L, Fernandez R, Baigorri F, Mestre J. Continuous aspiration of subglottic secretions in preventing ventilator-associated pneumonia. Ann Intern Med 1995; 122: 179–186.

57. Chastre J, Fagon JY. Ventilator-associated pneumonia. Am J Respir Crit Care Med 2002; 165:867–903.

58. Centers for Disease Control and Prevention. National nosocomial infections surveillance (NNIS) report, data summary from October 1986–April 1997, issued May 1997. Am J Infect Control 1997; 25:477–487.

59. Walsh NM, Casano AA, Manangan LP, Sinkowitz-Cochran RL, Jarvis WR. Risk factors for Burkholderia cepacia complex colonization and infection among patients with cystic fibrosis. J Pediatr 2002; 141:512–517.

60. Stout JE, Yu VL. Legionellosis. N Engl J Med 1997; 337:682–687.

61. Collard HR, Saint S, Matthay MA. Prevention of ventilator-associated pneumonia: an evidence-based systematic review. Ann Intern Med 2003; 138:494–501.

62. Cook DJ, Kollef MH. Risk factors for ICU-acquired pneumonia. J Am Med Assoc 1998; 279:1605–1606.

63. van Nieuwenhoven CA, Buskens E, van Tiel FH, Bonten MJ. Relationship between methodological trial quality and the effects of selective digestive decontamination on pneumonia and mortality in critically ill patients. J Am Med Assoc 2001; 286:335–340.

64. Liberati A, D'Amico R, Pifferi S, Torri V, Brazzi L. Antibiotic prophylaxis to reduce respiratory tract infections and mortality in adults receiving intensive care. Cochrane Database Syst Rev 2004; CD000022.

65. Terpenning M, Bretz W, Lopatin D, Langmore S, Dominguez B, Loesche W. Bacterial colonization of saliva and plaque in the elderly. Clin Infect Dis 1993; 16(suppl 4):S314–S316.

66. Yoneyama T, Yoshida M, Ohrui T, Mukaiyama H, Okamoto H, Hoshiba K, Ihara S, Yanagisawa S, Ariumi S, Morita T. Oral care reduces pneumonia in older patients in nursing homes. J Am Geriatr Soc 2002; 50:430–433.

67. Girou E, Schortgen F, Delclaux C, Schortgen F, Delclaux C, Blot F, Lefort Y. Association of noninvasive ventilation with nosocomial infections and survival in critically ill patients. J Am Med Assoc 2000; 284: 2361–2367.

68. Girou E, Brun-Buisson C, Taille S, Lemaire F, Brochard L. Secular trends in nosocomial infections and mortality associated with noninvasive ventilation in patients with exacerbation of COPD and pulmonary edema. J Am Med Assoc 2003; 290:2985–2991.

69. Cook D, De Jonghe B, Brochard L, Brun-Buisson C. Influence of airway management on ventilator-associated pneumonia: evidence from randomized trials. J Am Med Assoc 1998; 279:781–787.

70. Holzapfel L, Chastang C, Demingeon G, Bohe J, Piralla B, Coupry A. A randomized study assessing the systematic search for maxillary sinusitis in nasotracheally mechanically ventilated patients. Influence of nosocomial maxillary sinusitis on the occurrence of ventilator-associated pneumonia. Am J Respir Crit Care Med 1999; 159:695–701.

71. Tambyah PA, Maki DG. Catheter-associated urinary tract infection is rarely symptomatic: a prospective study of 1497 catheterized patients. Arch Intern Med 2000; 160:678–682.

72. Patton JP, Nash DB, Abrutyn E. Urinary tract infection: economic considerations. Med Clin North Am 1991; 75:495–513.

73. Maki DG, Tambyah PA. Engineering out the risk of infection with urinary catheters. Emerg Inf Dis 2001; 7:1–6.

74. Garibaldi RA. Hospital-acquired urinary tract infections. In: Prevention and Control of Nosocomial Infection; 2nd ed. Baltimore: Williams & Wilkins, 1993: 600–613.

75. Garibaldi RA, Burke JP, Britt MR, Miller WA, Smith CB. Meatal colonization and catheter-associated bacteriuria. N Engl J Med 1980; 303:316–318.

76. Schaeffer AJ. Catheter-associated bacteriuria. Urol Clin North Am 1986; 13:735–747.

77. Kunin CM. Detection, prevention, and management of urinary tract infections. 3rd ed. Philadelphia: Lea and Febiger, 1979.

78. Sullivan NM, Sutter VL, Mims MM, Marsh VH, Finegold SM. Clinical aspects of bacteremia after manipulation of the genitourinary tract. J Infect Dis 1973; 127:49–55.

79. Bryan CS, Reynolds KL. Hospital-acquired bacteremic urinary tract infection: epidemiology and outcome. J Urol 1984; 132:494–498.

80. Centers for Disease Control and Prevention. National Nosocomial Infections Surveillance (NNIS) System Report, Data Summary from January 1990–May 1999, Issued June 1999. Am J Infect Control 1999; 27:520–532.

81. Wong ES. Guideline for prevention of catheter-associated urinary tract infections. Am J Infect Control 1983; 11:28–36.

82. Bronsema DA, Adams JR, Pallares R, Wenzel RP. Secular trends in rates and etiology of nosocomial urinary tract infections at a university hospital. J Urol 1993; 150:414–416.

83. Rabkin DG, Stifelman MD, Birkhoff J, Richardson KA, Cohen D, Nowygrod R, et al. Early catheter removal decreases incidence of urinary tract infections in renal transplant recipients. Transplant Proc 1998; 30:4314–4316.

84.   Warren JW. Catheter-associated urinary tract infections. Infect Dis Clin North Am 1997; 11:609–622.

85.   Kunin CM. Care of the urinary catheter. In: Urinary Tract Infections: Detection, Prevention and Management. 5th ed. Baltimore: Williams and Wilkins, 1997:227–299.

86.   Garibaldi RA, Mooney BR, Epstein BJ, Britt MR. An evaluation of daily bacteriologic monitoring to identify preventable episodes of catheter-associated urinary tract infection. Infect Control 1982; 3:466–470.

87.   Jarvis WR, Martone WJ. Predominant pathogens in hospital infections. J Antimicrob Chemother 1992; 29:19–24.

88.   Tambyah PA, Halvorson K, Maki DG. A prospective study of the pathogenesis of catheter-associated urinary tract infection. Mayo Clin Proc 1999; 74: 131–136.

89.   Stark RP, Maki DG. Bacteriuria in the catheterized patient. N Engl J Med 1984; 311:560–564.

90.   Pappas PG, Rex JH, Sobel JD, Filler SG, Dismukes WE, Walsh TJ, Edwards JE. Guidelines for treatment of candidiasis. Clin Infect Dis 2004; 38:161–189.

91.   Rello J, Ochagavia A, Sabanes E, Roque M, Mariscal D, Reynaga E, Valles J. Evaluation of outcome of intravenous catheter-related infections in critically ill patients. Am J Respir Crit Care Med 2000; 162:1027–1030.

92.   Crnich CJ, Maki DG. The promise of novel technology for the prevention of intravascular device-related bloodstream infection. I. Pathogenesis and short-term devices. Clin Infect Dis 2002; 34:1232–1242.

93.   Mermel LA. Prevention of intravascular catheter-related infections. Ann Intern Med 2000; 132:391–402.

93a. Donowitz LG, Wenzel RP, Hoyt JW. High risk of hospital-acquired infection in the ICU patient. Crit Care Med 1982; 10:355–357.

94.   Mermel LA, McCormick RD, Springman SR, Maki DG. The pathogenesis and epidemiology of catheter-related infection with pulmonary artery Swan-Ganz catheters: a prospective study utilizing molecular subtyping. Am J Med 1991; 91:197S–205S.

95.   Maki DG, Weise CE, Sarafin HW. A semiquantitative culture method for identifying intravenous-catheter-related infection. N Engl J Med 1977; 296: 1305–1309.

96.   Safdar N, Maki DG. The pathogenesis of catheter-related bloodstream infection with noncuffed short-term central venous catheters. Intensive Care Med 2004; 30:62–67.

97.   Herrmann M, Lai QJ, Albrecht RM, Mosher DF, Proctor RA. Adhesion of *Staphylococcus aureus* to surface-bound platelets: role of fibrinogen/fibrin and platelet integrins. J Infect Dis 1993; 167:312–322.

98.   Herrmann M, Suchard SJ, Boxer LA, Waldvogel FA, Lew PD. Thrombospondin binds to Staphylococcus aureus and promotes staphylococcal adherence to surfaces. Infect Immun 1991; 59:279–288.

99.   Gray ED, Peters G, Verstegen M, Regelmann WE. Effect of extracellular slime substance from Staphylococcus epidermidis on the human cellular immune response. Lancet 1984; 1:365–367.

100. Farber BF, Kaplan MH, Clogston AG. Staphylococcus epidermidis extracted slime inhibits the antimicrobial action of glycopeptide antibiotics. J Infect Dis 1990; 161:37–40.

101. Maki DG, Martin WT. Nationwide epidemic of septicemia caused by contaminated infusion products. IV. Growth of microbial pathogens in fluids for intravenous infusions. J Infect Dis 1975; 131:267–272.

102. Maki DG, Rhame FS, Mackel DC, Bennett JV. Nationwide epidemic of septicemia caused by contaminated intravenous products. Epidemiologic and clinical features. Am J Med 1976; 60:471–485.

103. Garcia CR, Johnston BL, Corvi G, Walker LJ, George WL. Intravenous catheter-associated Malassezia furfur fungemia. Am J Med 1987; 83:790–792.

104. Safdar N, Kluger DM, Maki DG. A review of risk factors for catheter-related bloodstream infection caused by percutaneously inserted, noncuffed central venous catheters: implications for preventive strategies. Medicine (Baltimore) 2002; 81:466–479.

105. Sherertz RJ, Ely EW, Westbrook DM, Gledhill KS, Streed SA, Kiger B, Flynn L, Hayes S, et al. Education of physicians-in-training can decrease the risk for vascular catheter infection. Ann Intern Med 2000; 132:641–648.

106. Eggimann P, Pittet D. Overview of catheter-related infections with special emphasis on prevention based on educational programs. Clin Microbiol Infect 2002; 8:295–309.

107. Mermel LA, Parenteau S, Tow SM. The risk of midline catheterization in hospitalized patients. A prospective study. Ann Intern Med 1995; 123:841–844.

108. Chaiyakunapruk N, Veenstra DL, Lipsky BA, Sullivan SD, Saint S. Vascular catheter site care: the clinical and economic benefits of chlorhexidine gluconate compared with povidone iodine. Clin Infect Dis 2003; 37:764–771.

109. Humar A, Ostromecki A, Direnfeld J, Marshall JC, Lazar N, Houston PC, Boiteau P, Conly JM. Prospective randomized trial of 10% povidone-iodine versus 0.5% tincture of chlorhexidine as cutaneous antisepsis for prevention of central venous catheter infection. Clin Infect Dis 2000; 31:1001–1007.

110. Maki DG, Ringer M. Evaluation of dressing regimens for prevention of infection with peripheral intravenous catheters. Gauze, a transparent polyurethane dressing, and an iodophor-transparent dressing. JAMA 1987; 258:2396–2403.

111. Eggimann P, Harbarth S, Constantin MN, Touveneau S, Chevrolet JC, Pittet D. Impact of a prevention strategy targeted at vascular-access care on incidence of infections acquired in intensive care. Lancet 2000; 355:1864–1868.

112. Goetz AM, Wagener MM, Miller JM, Muder RR. Risk of infection due to central venous catheters: effect of site of placement and catheter type. Infect Control Hosp Epidemiol 1998; 19:842–845.

113. Merrer J, De Jonghe B, Golliot F, Lefrant JY, Raffy Brigitte, Barre E, Rigaud JP, Casciani D, Misset B, Bosquet C, et al. Complications of femoral and subclavian venous catheterization in critically ill patients: a randomized controlled trial. JAMA 2001; 286:700–707.

114. Raad II, Hohn DC, Gilbreath BJ, Suleiman N, Hill LA, Bruso PA, Marts K, Mansfield PF, Bodey GP. Prevention of central venous catheter-related infections by using maximal sterile barrier precautions during insertion. Infect Control Hosp Epidemiol 1994; 15:231–238.

115. Timsit JF, Sebille V, Farkas JC, Misset B, Martin JB, Chevret S, Carlet J. Effect of subcutaneous tunneling on internal jugular catheter-related sepsis in critically ill patients: a prospective randomized multicenter study. JAMA 1996; 276:1416–1420.

116. Timsit JF, Bruneel F, Cheval C, Mamzer MF, Garrouste-Orgeas M, Wolff M, Misset B, Chevret S, Regnier B, Carlet J. Use of tunneled femoral catheters to prevent catheter-related infection. A randomized, controlled trial. Ann Intern Med 1999; 130:729–735.

117. Randolph AG, Cook DJ, Gonzales CA, Pribble CG. Ultrasound guidance for placement of central venous catheters: a meta-analysis of the literature. Crit Care Med 1996; 24:2053–2058.

118. Darouiche RO, Raad II, Heard SO, Thornby JI, Wenker OC, Gabrielli A, Berg J, Khardori N, Hanna H, Hachem R, et al. A comparison of two antimicrobial-impregnated central venous catheters. Catheter Study Group. N Engl J Med 1999; 340:1–8.

119. Veenstra DL, Saint S, Saha S, Lumley T, Sullivan SD. Efficacy of antiseptic-impregnated central venous catheters in preventing catheter-related bloodstream infection: a meta-analysis. JAMA 1999; 281:261–267.

120. Raad I, Darouiche R, Hachem R, Mansouri M, Bodey GP. The broad-spectrum activity and efficacy of catheters coated with minocycline and rifampin. J Infect Dis 1996; 173:418–424.

121. Maki DG, Cobb L, Garman JK, Shapiro JM, Ringer M, Helgerson RB. An attachable silver-impregnated cuff for prevention of infection with central venous catheters: a prospective randomized multicenter trial. Am J Med 1988; 85:307–314.

122. Anonymous. Antimicrobial Prophylaxis in Surgery. Med Lett 2001; 43:92–97.

123. Sheth NK, Franson TR, Rose HD, Buckmire FL, Cooper JA, Sohnle PG. Colonization of bacteria on polyvinyl chloride and Teflon intravascular catheters in hospitalized patients. J Clin Microbiol 1983; 18:1061–1063.

124. Maki DG, Ringer M. Risk factors for infusion-related phlebitis with small peripheral venous catheters. A randomized controlled trial. Ann Intern Med 1991; 114: 845–854.

125. Danzig LE, Short LJ, Collins K, Mahoney M, Sepe S, Bland L, Jarvis WR. Bloodstream infections associated with a needleless intravenous infusion system in patients receiving home infusion therapy. JAMA 1995; 273:1862–1864.

126. Do AN, Ray BJ, Banerjee SN, Illian AF, Barnett BJ, Pham MH, Hendricks KA, Jarvis WR. Bloodstream infection associated with needleless device use and the importance of infection-control practices in the home health care setting. J Infect Dis 1999; 179:442–448.

127. Groeger JS, Lucas AB, Thaler HT, Friedlander-Klar H, Brown AE, Kiehn TE. Infectious morbidity associated with long-term use of venous access devices in patients with cancer. Ann Intern Med 1993; 119:1168–1174.

128. McGee DC, Gould MK. Preventing complications of central venous catheterization. N Engl J Med 2003; 348:1123–1133.

129. Sesso R, Barbosa D, Leme IL, Sader H, Canziani ME, Manfredi S, Draibe S, Pignatari AC. Staphylococcus aureus prophylaxis in hemodialysis patients using central venous catheter: effect of mupirocin ointment. J Am Soc Nephrol 1998; 9:1085–1092.

130. Riu S, Ruiz CG, Martinez-Vea A, Peralta C, Oliver JA. Spontaneous rupture of polyurethane peritoneal catheter. A possible deleterious effect of mupirocin ointment. Nephrol Dial Transplant 1998; 13:1870–1871.

131. von Eiff C, Becker K, Machka K, Stammer H, Peters G. Nasal carriage as a source of Staphylococcus aureus bacteremia. Study Group. N Engl J Med 2001; 344(1):11–16.

132. Maki DG, Mermel LA, Kluger D, Narans L, Knasinski V, Parenteau S, Covington P. The efficacy of a chlorhexidine impregnated sponge (Biopatch) for the prevention of intravascular catheter-related infection— a prospective randomized controlled multicenter study [Abstract]. Interscience Conference on Antimicrobial Agents and Chemotherapy, Toronto, Ontario, Canada, 2000 (Abstract #1430).

133. Hoffmann KK, Weber DJ, Samsa GP, Rutala WA. Transparent polyurethane film as an intravenous catheter dressing. A meta-analysis of the infection risks. JAMA 1992; 267:2072–2076.

134. Yamamoto AJ, Solomon JA, Soulen MC, Tang J, Parkinson K, Lin R, Schears GJ. Sutureless securement device reduces complications of peripherally inserted central venous catheters. J Vasc Interv Radiol 2002; 13:77–81.

135. Bennett SN, McNeil MM, Bland LA, Arduino MJ, Villarino ME, Perrotta DM, Burwen DR, Welbel SF, Pegues DA, Stroud L, et al. Postoperative infections traced to contamination of an intravenous anesthetic, propofol. N Engl J Med 1995; 333:147–154.

136. Band JD, Maki DG. Steel needles used for intravenous therapy. Morbidity in patients with hematologic malignancy. Arch Intern Med 1980; 140:31–34.

137. Lai KK. Safety of prolonging peripheral cannula and i.v. tubing use from 72 hours to 96 hours. Am J Infect Control 1998; 26:66–70.

138. Eyer S, Brummitt C, Crossley K, Siegel R, Cerra F. Catheter-related sepsis: prospective, randomized study of three methods of long-term catheter maintenance. Crit Care Med 1990; 18:1073–1079.

139. Uldall PR, Merchant N, Woods F, Yarworski U, Vas S. Changing subclavian haemodialysis cannulas to reduce infection. Lancet 1981; 1:1373.

140. Cobb DK, High KP, Sawyer RG, Sable CA, Adams RB, Lindley DA, Pruett TL, Schwenzer KJ, Farr BM. A controlled trial of scheduled replacement of central venous and pulmonary-artery catheters. N Engl J Med 1992; 327:1062–1068.

141. Cook D, Randolph A, Kernerman P, Cupido C, King DB, Soukup C, Brun-Buisson C. Central venous catheter replacement strategies: a systematic review of the literature. Crit Care Med 1997; 25: 1417–1424.

142. Abi-Said D, Raad I, Umphrey J, Gonzalez V, Richardson D, Marts K, Horn D. Infusion therapy team and dressing changes of central venous catheters. Infect Control Hosp Epidemiol 1999; 20:101–105.

143. Maki DG, Stolz SS, Wheeler S, Mermel LA. A prospective, randomized trial of gauze and two polyurethane dressings for site care of pulmonary artery catheters: implications for catheter management. Crit Care Med 1994; 22:1729–1737.

144. Raad I, Umphrey J, Khan A, Truett LJ, Bodey GP. The duration of placement as a predictor of peripheral and pulmonary arterial catheter infections. J Hosp Infect 1993; 23:17–26.

145. Mermel LA, Maki DG. Infectious complications of Swan-Ganz pulmonary artery catheters. Pathogenesis, epidemiology, prevention, and management. Am J Respir Crit Care Med 1994; 149(4):1020–1036.

146. Rowley KM, Clubb KS, Smith GJ, Cabin HS. Right-sided infective endocarditis as a consequence of flow-directed pulmonary-artery catheterization. A clinicopathological study of 55 autopsied patients. N Engl J Med 1984; 311:1152–1156.

147. Martinez JA, Des Jardin JA, Aronoff M, Supran S, Nasraway SA, Snydman DR. Clinical utility of blood cultures drawn from central venous or arterial catheters in critically ill surgical patients. Crit Care Med 2002; 30:7–13.

148. Beutz M, Sherman G, Mayfield J, Fraser VJ, Kollef MH. Clinical utility of blood cultures drawn from central vein catheters and peripheral venipuncture in critically ill medical patients. Chest 2003; 123:854–861.

149. Brun-Buisson C, Abrouk F, Legrand P, Huet Y, Larabi S, Rapin M. Diagnosis of central venous catheter-related sepsis. Critical level of quantitative tip cultures. Arch Intern Med 1987; 147:873–877.

150. Sherertz RJ, Raad II, Belani A, Koo LC, Rand KH, Pickett DL, Straub SA, Fauerbach LL. Three-year experience with sonicated vascular catheter cultures in a clinical microbiology laboratory. J Clin Microbiol 1990; 28(1):76–82.

151. Siegman-Igra Y, Anglim AM, Shapiro DE, Adal KA, Strain BA, Farr BM. Diagnosis of vascular catheter-related bloodstream infection: a meta-analysis. J Clin Microbiol 1997; 35:928–936.

152. Farr BM. Catheters, microbes, time, and gold standards. Ann Intern Med 2004; 140:62–64.

153. Blot F, Nitenberg G, Chachaty E, Raynard B, Germann N, Antoun S, Laplanche A, Brun-Suisson C, Tancrede C. Diagnosis of catheter-related bacteraemia: a prospective comparison of the time to positivity of hub-blood versus peripheral-blood cultures. Lancet 1999; 354:1071–1077.

154. Raad I, Hanna HA, Alakech B, Chatzinikolaou I, Johnson MM, Tarrand J. Differential time to positivity: a useful method for diagnosing catheter-related bloodstream infections. Ann Intern Med 2004; 140:18–25.

155. Raad II, Hanna HA. Intravascular catheter-related infections: new horizons and recent advances. Arch Intern Med 2002; 162:871–878.

17

Practical Medical Ethics in Intensive Care

PAUL SCHNEIDER

VA Greater Los Angeles Healthcare System, Geffen School of Medicine at UCLA
Los Angeles, California, U.S.A.

I. Introduction

While I will try to present herein an overview of the most significant trends in the past few years as they relate to medical ethics in intensive care, truthfully, there is no specific ethic of intensive care. Of course, technologies that exist only in the critical care environment such as extracorporeal membrane oxygenation (ECMO) (1) and left ventricular assist devices (LVAD) (2) bring with themselves new dilemmas, new crises of conscience regarding their use. But the overwhelmingly more common problems encountered there relate to now standard forms of life-support, such as mechanical ventilation and dialysis—technologies employable not only outside of the critical care environment, but even at home for some patients. And of course, the sociocultural dynamics that create conflicts among doctors, patients, and surrogate decision-makers grow in a multistep process. So, one can imagine that the majority of ethical dilemmas, as they flower in the intensive care unit (ICU), truly germinated elsewhere—clinic, ward, and home. From this perspective, ethical problems, like icebergs, are partially covert and partially overt—partially potential and partially active—at any point in a patient's course.

When a patient is critically ill, and the stakes for cure versus death are higher, preexisting potential areas of conflict become more real and more active and, by necessity, must be dealt with and resolved to allow for any end to be reached. This is the true nature of an ethic of critical care: the need to create resolution from tensions brought about by severe medical illness as it interfaces with the possibility of cure—and a variably-conflicted social milieu—all in the face of a ticking clock.

In order to accomplish this task, the physician needs to be able to effectively utilize both his or her own knowledge and skills in medical ethics as well as those of ancillary personnel. It is my aim in this chapter to increase the specific knowledge and skills of the intensivist regarding these issues as well as to increase the understanding of when a bioethics consultant may be appropriately utilized. We will discuss the basic principles used to approach a bioethics problem as well as several critically important content areas within medical ethics, including informed consent, medical futility, withdrawal of life support, and understanding patients' advance directives. A discussion of brain death will be found in the chapter on Neurologic Problems in the ICU. It is my belief that medical ethics today should no longer be considered an unteachable or nebulous area, but a specific area like others in medicine in which expertise may be gained through study and practice.

II. The Approach to a Bioethics Problem

Within the framework of trying to address a medical ethics problem, one must first attempt to define the nature of the problem as exactly as possible. This is far from a trivial task in itself, and can only happen after an initial fact-finding period that typically involves hearing the opinions of all the major players in a case (family members, patient if possible, various staff members as appropriate).

Many cases are brought to ethics consultants' attention with the brief explanation that "something doesn't feel right about how we're treating Mr. Smith," or the similarly generic, "We'd like the ethics committee to review this case to make sure we're doing everything right." Analogous to how a cardiologist might evaluate any case with regards to coronary blood flow, electrical conduction, mechanical factors, and other complicating issues (e.g., anemia), the ethicist evaluates cases by using several "pillars" of bioethics. They are defined in Table 1.

The basic, prima facie meaning of each of the five pillars should be readily evident. To summarize briefly, Patient Autonomy versus Medical Paternalism is a spectrum in which the element of control varies between patient and doctor. In it lie issues of decision-making: Who decides what, for whom, and when? Who says what to whom? What rules regulate the relationship between patient and physician?

Beneficence and Nonmaleficence is also a spectrum in which we define the extent to which physicians go to do good and avoid harm for their patients. In this pillar we explore both the intent as well as the actions of the physician, mostly defining elements of practice and life that may distract or prevent us from providing ideal medical care to our patients. We also define the rules through which we establish respect for patients' basic human rights.

The pillar of Contextual Factors addresses what kinds of rules society has already made regarding the issue before us. There can be many layers of rules throughout society and medical practice that pertain to a certain conflict. Inherently, Contextual Factors vary widely in different practice settings, different nations, and different communities.

Table 1   The Principles of Medical Ethics and Their Ramifications

Patient autonomy versus medical paternalism	• Shared decision-making
	• Doctor–patient relationship
	• Boundary issues
	• Decisional-making capacity
	• Truth-telling
	• Advance directives, surrogate decision-makers
	• Code status
	• Informed consent
Beneficence and nonmaleficence	• Professionalism
	• Malpractice, impaired providers
	• Mode of care/goals of therapy
	• Clinical research
	• Informed consent
	• Conflicts-of-interest
	• Resident/student supervision
	• Managed-care
Contextual factors	• Law
	• Hospital policy
	• Codes of ethics (AMA, etc.)
	• Regulatory groups, professional societies
	• Organizational ethics
	• Employment issues
Sociocultural determinants	• Mistrust of the medical system
	• Alternative/complementary medicine
	• Folk-healing
	• Unreasonable expectations
	• Truth-telling
	• End-of-life care
Justice	• Access to care
	• Limitation of resources
	• Triage
	• Double-standards of care

Sociocultural Determinants help us understand how individual patients and healthcare providers can act as representatives of larger groups. Individuals' belief systems with regard to life, death, and healing are integrally tied to rearing and culturalization, dynamics which may be influenced by religion, affluence, education, literacy, ethnicity, and other factors.

The Principle of Justice defines the last pillar. To what extent is the patient treated fairly, with care being proportionate to need? To what extent does society aid or impede both organized medicine as well as individual practitioners to practice justly?

As a next step, one attempts to look at the issue at hand in light of these five pillars. Typically, most specific conflicts can be boiled down to one, two, or perhaps three areas, with one of them seeming most prominent. It is frequently enlightening to healthcare providers to learn that the problem they have been struggling with is, say, a basic problem in doctor–patient relationship issues, which is a subset of autonomy versus paternalism, with a complicating element of sociocultural determinants! Understanding this kind of description allows for the discourse that will ensue to happen with the appropriate intellectual foundation. By this I mean that at least the professionals involved in a bioethics dilemma (hopefully the patient and family, as well) will recognize that any individual conflict is really an expression of conflict(s) on a higher level: at the level of principles, and not just people. This understanding will help keep the discussion nonthreatening to the participants.

Once the dilemma has been interpreted in this manner, we are ready to move on to the task of attempting to resolve it. Now, complete resolution is an ideal, and not truly achievable in most cases, but usually a partial resolution—enough of a resolution to allow an impasse to be crossed—is. By way of experience, I have learned that while *all* parties need to be able to make some amount of compromise in order for resolution to be achieved, *some* parties are usually more amenable than others. Indeed, the last step in the approach to bioethical problems—conflict resolution—is much more about managing human emotions than it is about debating issues. One would then reasonably question the need for the step we completed previously: understanding the conflict on an intellectual level. I think the best answer to this is that both are necessary. Typically, once the conflict is understood at the rational level, the door is opened for work to begin at the emotional level, which is the true key to resolution. In my experience of most bioethics dilemmas, the barriers to consensus that a family harbors are negative emotions like guilt or abandonment—and these do not just vanish with any kind of intervention. One can address them intellectually, but the first major crack in them will occur at the emotional level. Addressing the emotional side of a medical case is something that many physicians are uncomfortable with, for a variety of reasons. In these situations, the best option is to ask your bioethics consultant to become involved in the case. Conflict mediation should be a routine skill that all bioethicists are comfortable with.

III. Informed Consent

First, let us dispel a myth. Informed consent does not exist to protect physicians from, or defend physicians in, lawsuits. This may be what many believe, but the evidence clearly shows that adequate disclosure of risks to patients prior to procedures does not indemnify physicians against future malpractice claims. So despite how some may attempt to use informed consent, it exists as a process intended to assure patients' human rights: the basic human rights of self-determination and freedom from harm. Indeed, it was only as a result of one of the great failures of modern medicine, that being Nazi medical experimentation during the holocaust, that the modern practice of informed consent became routine, first in clinical research, later in patient care (3). Second, informed consent is not a piece of paper with signatures on it. That is the documentation of informed consent. But the process of discussion which happened prior to those signatures, culminating in the patient's agreement to the intervention, is actually the informed consent. Likewise, if the same process had culminated in the patient refusing to have the proposed intervention, we would have an *informed refusal*. Both of these processes assume the patient to possess decisional-making capacity (DMC). DMC is the clinical equivalent of the legal construct of competence. Physicians do not assess competence, per se, judges do. Judges do not assess DMC, per se, physicians do. While these words are mostly clinically interchangeable, they are not legally interchangeable.

So what should be the practical approach to doing high-quality informed consent with patients? This will be a general discussion that should be lawful in most localities, but of course, the specifics will vary from state to state and hospital to hospital. First, determine if the procedure is elective or emergent. Emergent is usually defined as signifying imminent life or limb-threat, per general consensus. This is actually a high standard. It follows that many procedures that might be felt to be more urgent by physicians actually would not meet emergency status. This distinction is important because, in emergency situations, special rules apply with regard to lack of DMC. First, of course, informed consent should only even be attempted if there is time for it and the patient is stable. Second, DMC is not required as part of informed consent for emergency procedures in which the patient is unstable. In circumstances in which either there is no time to test for DMC or the patient lacks it, we operate under what is termed *presumed consent*, that is, it is appropriate to presume that all patients would want to undergo an emergency procedure in such circumstances. Of course, if you know the patient well enough to know that he/she would not have wanted it under these circumstances, you may not use presumed consent. Commonly, in presumed consent scenarios, hospital policies and local laws require that two physicians sign the consent form to attest to the fact that it is indeed an emergency. If a surrogate decision-maker is readily available, and there is time to discuss the procedure with him/her, that would be the preferred approach over a two-physician consent. It is appropriate to note that requirements regarding whether the two physicians must be licensed or not and whether they can be physicians in training or not vary. Proper surrogate decision-makers have the legal and ethical right to refuse an emergency procedure for the patient, with the famous exception of refusal based on religious grounds for a minor or incompetent adult. People have the right to die for their religion, but they do not have the right to make their children or their incompetent charges die for a religion that they likely do not fully understand.

If the procedure is elective, then it is expected that the informed consent process will include the physician's assessment of the patient's DMC. If you delegate the discussion to another employee in the medical office, in effect, you are entrusting the employee with not only adequate education of the patient but also adequate testing of DMC. In general, DMC is a higher standard than many physicians appreciate. Patients must be presented both the risks and benefits of the proposed intervention, any alternate interventions, and no intervention. It is required that the patient receive the information presented, process and understand it, and then communicate back (in any fashion) his/her choice. That's it! The signatures that follow, including the witness', are just documentation requirements. Likewise, documentation of DMC is not required usually. If you have the patient sign the document, it attests that you believed that the patient possessed DMC at the time.

In the situation of an elective procedure for which the patient lacks DMC, one should approach the appropriate surrogate decision-maker. Again, in this area, rules vary, but in the absence of an applicable living will or Durable-Power-of Attorney-for-Healthcare (DPAHC), convention holds the next-of-kin (NOK) the most appropriate. In many localities, in the absence of any contactable NOK, judicial approval for the procedure is the only recourse the physician can take. In the Veterans Affairs Healthcare System, it is recognized that for many patients who are estranged from their families, a close friend makes an acceptable surrogate decision-maker (Table 2). Bioethicists are also generally well-acquainted with the problem of being asked to make elective healthcare decisions for patients who lack DMC, lack an advance directive, lack a NOK, and lack any close friend. In these scenarios, the bioethicist should know whether he/she is locally empowered to make these kinds of decisions and, if not, to whom you should be referred for the legal counsel required to help you seek judicial approval of healthcare decisions. If the patient is expected to survive for longer than a few months, it may well be appropriate to seek judicial appointment of a conservator who will be empowered by the court to make medical decisions into the future. If not, the court will generally make the few decisions required without appointing a conservator.

IV. Medical Futility

The concept of medical futility more or less emerged in the late 1980s, reached its peak, and somewhat declined within a decade (4). Perhaps the classical example of a concept in medical ethics for which no consensus has been achieved, futility has become a great debate with only partial resolution. After more-or-less failed attempts at defining futility through quantitative and qualitative grounds, what emerged was, at best, a road-map that is helpful for dealing with cases of

Table 2   Order of Surrogate Decision Makers

The healthcare agent named in a valid durable power of attorney for healthcare
⇓
The legal guardian or conservator with medical powers
⇓
The spouse
⇓
An adult child (over 18 yr of age)
⇓
A parent
⇓
An adult sibling
⇓
A grandparent
⇓
An adult grandchild
⇓
A close friend
⇓
Bioethics committee and/or judge

Source: From Veterans Health Administration Informed Consent for Clinical Treatments and Procedures Handbook 2004.

medical futility through a process of dialogue and negotiation, that is, through the standard ethics committee consultative approach.

Schneiderman et al. (5) defined quantitative futility as follows: "when physicians conclude (either through personal experience, experiences shared with colleagues, or consideration of reported empiric data) that in the last 100 cases, a medical treatment has been useless, they should regard that treatment as futile," and qualitative futility as the situation in which treatment "merely preserves permanent unconsciousness or that fails to end a patient's total dependence on intensive medical care." As opposed to the concept of physiologic futility (e.g., it is physiologically futile to manage acute psychosis with psychotherapy; more in the realm of ICU medicine, it is physiologically futile to manage a severely bleeding peptic ulcer with an H2-blocker alone), the ideas of quantitative and qualitative futility leave much room open for debate. Indeed, the nature of futility can be cast as a nefarious struggle for decision-making power, a struggle over physician paternalism versus patient autonomy, or a veiled attempt to justify rationing. In general, futility has not been societally accepted enough to allow doctors to make unilateral judgments about when treatments can be withheld over patients' or surrogates' protests. Indeed, the courts have almost universally held (in the U.S.) in the favor of patients whose doctors have withheld treatment because of a perceived lack of potential medical benefit (6). This is not to say that futility as a concept has no place in medical thinking. It does. But it must be viewed as the contentious idea which it is—frequently morally-justified—but contentious nonetheless.

Inherent to the issue of qualitative futility are assumptions about the value that we assign to living different kinds of lives. Specifically, if a future lifetime is to be spent entirely in the ICU, is that life not worth living? Some groups argue that it is not within a physician's purview to judge what life is worth living and what life is not. In this view it is our mission to prolong life whenever possible, because of the essential sanctity of all life: that the last minute of life is as wondrous and sacred as the first minute of life. I would argue in response that not to judge a patient's quality-of-life, not to try to make some kind of assessment of what life we are prolonging for the patient through our interventions, is ultimately a disservice to the patient and an abandonment of our own sense of being moral agents. Neither choice is entirely right, yet to make no choice is also not right. This approach to assessing quality-of-life is justifiable because of the nebulous nature of the dividing line between life and death. Indeed, the disease burden that would have caused death in a patient 20 years ago might well be treatable now because of technological developments, but only treatable to the point that life is sustainable without achieving any of the other standardized goals of medicine (i.e., palliation of symptoms, rehabilitation of function, or cure of disease). Hence, our notions of what constitutes futility at any one point in time are, in reality, an ever-evolving function of technological factors, society's judgements about the goals of medicine, personal morals, and religious/spiritual factors. It is truly a moving target.

What about scenarios in which we can actually ask the conscious patient about his or her own perceptions of quality-of-life? Should our perceptions of a patient's quality-of-life ever outweigh the patient's own assessment? To think of the possibility of overruling a patient's request to sustain his/her own life is harrowing and should only even be considered under the worst circumstances of limited resources (e.g., battlefield triage when only the least injured can be saved). What is thankfully much more often the case is the scenario in which a dying patient asks to prolong his/her life through heroic measures in order to achieve some goal, typically to see a family member again, or to attend a family event. The general consensus within the ethics community is that these kind of requests are completely legitimate and that providing "futile" care in such a time-limited fashion is ethical.

Moreover, conscious patients in miserable clinical situations increasingly feel empowered to ask for their lives to be ended through voluntary starvation, termination of life support, physician-assisted suicide, or euthanasia. Actually, many patients prefer the notion of euthanasia to that of physician-assisted suicide, that is, they would prefer medical doctors to kill them by lethal injection over asking doctors to give them a prescription for a lethal dose of medication that they could fill at the pharmacy. The legal and ethical dimensions of this phenomenon go beyond the bounds of this chapter, but suffice it to say that these requests exist in our own caseloads and that one constructive way to view them is as patients' determinations of medical futility in their own cases. Needless to say, these requests should trigger bioethics consults. Physicians and nurses should not be expected to agonize about these kinds of dilemmas alone.

What has emerged as a nonrefutable tool in the management of all types of futility cases is a process of shared decision-making and negotiation, usually orchestrated by the medical ethics consultant. Various attempts to define and codify this process have been made, including a white paper on the subject by the National Ethics Committee of the Veterans Health Administration (7). Focusing on the issue of when Do-Not-Resuscitate orders might be ethically justified, even over a family's objections, the Paper made six recommendations (Table 3).

A somewhat newer approach, sometimes called "preventative ethics," has recently been studied in a multicenter, prospective, randomized, controlled trial (8). Five-hundred and fifty-one patients in the adult ICUs of seven hospitals were randomly assigned either to an a priori ethics consultation or usual care. The primary outcome measures were ICU days and life-sustaining treatments in those patients who did not survive to hospital discharge as well as those who did, as well as overall mortality rates in both groups. All patients were entered into the study after being identified by an ICU nurse as "patients in whom value-laden treatment conflicts were imminent or manifest that could lead to incompatible courses of action." These patients went on to receive an immediate ethics consultation (intervention group) versus usual care (ethics consultation only if specifically requested, in the usual fashion). Sixty-seven patients in the consultation group did not receive the intervention, while 77 in the usual-care group ultimately received an ethics consultation. Among those patients who received the intervention but did not survive to discharge from the hospital, compared with control patients, hospital days ($p = 0.01$), days spent in the ICU ($p = 0.03$), and days receiving ventilation ($p = 0.03$) were all reduced. These measures were deemed "nonbeneficial treatments." Mortality was not significantly different between the two groups. The authors concluded, "Hence, ethics consultations seem to be useful in resolving conflicts that may be inappropriately prolonging nonbeneficial or unwanted treatments at the end of life." The gist of preventative ethics, then, is to try to resolve conflicts before they get to the stage wherein medical futility is manifest.

One specific area within medical futility for which there is a large literature, as mentioned above, is cardiopulmonary resuscitation (CPR). Despite the publicity within the medical community of studies that show that CPR has extremely poor efficacy (perhaps qualifying for futility) for elderly, hospitalized patients (9), there are opposing views that maintain that the data is not actually so dreary. A meta-analysis conducted in 1993, utilizing 30 years of data, concluded that survival to discharge of elderly, in-hospital CPR patients was as high as 15% (10). Another interesting study that speaks to the public's initial lack of familiarity with CPR success rates, but ability to understand presented data, showed that while elderly patients might initially request CPR in 41% of

Table 3   Do-Not-Resuscitate Orders and Medical Futility

The NEC affirms the value of a procedural approach to resolving disputes over DNR orders based on medical futility and recommends the following:

1. Situations in which the physician believes that resuscitation is futile should be handled on a case by case basis through a predefined process that includes multiple safeguards to assure that patients' rights are fully protected, as detailed below.
2. Through a discussion with the patient or appropriate surrogate decision-maker, the physician should ascertain (to the extent possible) the patient's expressed or inferred wishes, focusing on the goals of care from the patient's perspective. For example, a patient who is imminently dying may want to be resuscitated in order to survive to see a relative arrive from out of town. Any determination that CPR is futile must be based on the physician's medical judgment that CPR cannot be reasonably expected to achieve the patient's goals.
3. The physician must thoroughly explain to the patient or surrogate the reasons for the medical futility determination and document this discussion in the medical record.
4. If the patient or surrogate disagrees with the DNR order, the physician must convene a meeting involving members of the health care team and the patient or surrogate. At this meeting, the reason for the disagreement must be thoroughly explored and discussed with the purpose of resolving the dispute. This discussion must be carefully documented in the medical record.
5. If the physician wishes to enter a DNR order despite the objection of the patient or surrogate, the physician must initiate and participate in a formal review process. If the patient suffers cardiopulmonary arrest before this process is completed, resuscitation must be attempted.
6. At a minimum, the review process should include the following steps:
   a. To assure that the medical futility determination is sound, a second physician must concur with the primary physician's medical futility determination and document the concurrence in the medical record.
   b. An individual or group designated by the facility (such as an Ethics Advisory Committee) must (1) discuss the situation with the involved parties in an attempt to reach a resolution, and (2) make a formal recommendation on the case.
   c. The patient or surrogate must be informed of the plan to enter the DNR order and the physician must offer to assist in the process of having the patient transferred to another physician or clinical site. Patients or their surrogates should have a reasonable time to seek transfer or court intervention before the order is written.
   d. Entering a DNR order over the objection of a patient or surrogate should be reserved for exceptionally rare and extreme circumstances after thorough attempts to settle or successfully appeal disagreements have been tried and failed. In all such cases, the Chief of Staff or a designee must authorize action on behalf of the institution.
   e. Legal Counsel should be informed of an involved in all cases in which conflicts over DNR orders cannot be resolved.

Abbreviations: NEC, National Ethics Committee; DNR, Do-Not-Resuscitate; CPR, cardiopulmonary resuscitation.
Source: From Ref. 7.

cases, after being informed about the general efficacy rates of CPR (10–17%), this rate drops to 22%. It drops to 5% when confronted with the 0–5% survival rate expected for individuals with a chronic illness and a life expectancy of less than one year (11). Interestingly, in a study of success rates of CPR as it appeared on the television programs *ER*, *Chicago Hope*, and *Rescue 911*, patients appear to have survived to hospital discharge in 67% of cases (12). This may speak to the public's higher request rates for CPR prior to receiving evidence-based information, as above.

Under the best of circumstances, in which patients' premorbid wishes regarding end-of-life care are known, reasoned decisions about forgoing CPR happen routinely, frequently allowing staff and physicians to feel good about caring for dying patients in the ICU. However, this is still not as common as might be wished. Many patients enter the ICU without such specific limits, and the ICU team must coordinate an approach to code status. Physicians often feel great consternation about discussing this issue with patients and, particularly, their families. In some circumstances, physicians feel reduced to doing what patients and/or surrogate decision makers want, that is, inappropriately coding dying patients, because it is felt that the confrontational nature of the discussion would be too much to go through in order to convince them otherwise. Of course, what frequently makes these discussions charged is the question of trust in the doctor–family–patient relationship. Historically, the doctor–patient relationship has been seen as a form of contract, in which each party cedes certain rights and responsibilities to the other. Many ethicists prefer to view this relationship as a covenant, that is, a special form of contractual relationship in which mutual trust provides the substrate for medical care (13). Unfortunately, this is frequently more of an ideal than a reality, especially with the noncontinuous nature of medical care as it is frequently practiced in major medical centers in America today, that is, the transfer of patients' care between different sets of doctors in different care settings. This very premise, which on the one hand promises patients increased physician expertise in specialized care settings, erodes trust through perceived abandonment and discontinuity. The ideal of the primary care physician as the glue that cements these various parts together and provides the element of continuity is, again, more of a reality in certain types of healthcare operations than others. Issues of the public's perception of the physician's conflict-of-interest with managed care organizations also contributes to this lack of trust. So this question of potentially forgoing CPR, an *ultimate* issue in healthcare, is approached from the standpoint of a frequently uneasy doctor–patient–family relationship. Therein lies the crux of most CPR-related ethical dilemmas.

V. Withdrawal of Life-Support

In my role as a medical ethics consultant, I frequently ask house-officers to define what mode of care they are using to treat an individual patient. After an initial quizzical look, many people will ask me what I mean. Basically, the issue boils down to one of intent. Is it the doctor's intent to *cure* a medical illness, to *care* for a chronic problem, or to *palliate* an incurable condition (14)? While this might seem simple initially, it is indeed quite complex, for many reasons. First, these modes do not exist in isolation; we actually combine them in various ways. We try to cure an acute infection while caring for the patient's underlying diabetes. We try to palliate a patient dying of metastatic carcinoma while curing a new pneumonia. But one mode should seem prominent in any individual patient scenario. Secondly, care modes frequently default to cure when challenged by discontinuity of clinical coverage, by fear of malpractice, or by ineffective communication, i.e., doctors often take the position of "security" in these situations, which is that "more aggressive care is better care." Thirdly, many young resident physicians are blinded to the issue of care mode because of an absorption into the minutiae of clinical data they are asked to manage, or "not seeing the forest for the trees."

Typically, the decision to withdraw life-support comes close on the heels of a decision to change the care mode from cure to palliate. Now the reason that this is so important is that some burdens might be acceptable to the patient in a *cure* scenario (such as the risk of allergic reaction to antibiotics, or of minor tracheal irritation from short-term mechanical ventilation), but the magnification of risks and discomforts that happen with very ill patients receiving long-term cure therapy creates burdens that are unacceptable to many, if not most.

Withdrawing life-support means different things in different situations. Sometimes it means turning off a mechanical ventilator. It also may mean stopping antibiotics in some circumstances or allowing them as a palliative measure in others. Additionally, the switch to palliative care may well happen at the same time as termination of life-support, and so other things, like opiate analgesics, may have to be added. Palliative care consultants, who are available in many hospitals, are a valuable resource in facilitating this transition, both philosophically and mechanistically. My gestalt feeling that doctors and nurses generally understood what to do in withdrawal of life-support was shattered one day when a surgical intern called me to discuss a case involving turning off the ventilator on a patient dying in the SICU. He wanted to know, "What is the dose?" I asked him, "The dose of what?" and he replied, "Well, of morphine." I replied that we frequently used a morphine drip to titrate for dyspnea or agitation, but that we would not have to use it in his patient's case because the patient was comatose and not likely to experience discomfort. He replied, "Oh, I thought we give a really big morphine dose at the end, to sort of help it along." Needless to say, understanding may not be as complete as I expected.

Opiate therapy at the end of life is best understood through "The Principle of Double-Effect." Already appreciated by theologians of the middle ages (15), this concept clarifies that while administering opiates to dying patients both relieves symptoms as well as hastens death, the physician is relieved of guilt (or originally, sin) because his intent was the former and not the latter. Of course, the reality of the situation may be quite different from this over-simplification of the philosophical/theological construct. Indeed, it may well be the intent of many doctors and nurses to hasten death, as well as to ease suffering. One could argue that the two effects are so intertwined that the idea of intending one and not the other is impossible and artificial. The actual under-pinnings of the rule are quite philosophically complex (16), requiring that the intervention satisfy four criteria to be acceptable: (1) the physician's intervention must be morally good (easing suffering); (2) the physician must intend ease-of-suffering and not death; (3) death must not be the means through which the end of ease-of-suffering is sought; (4) the suffering must be so great that relief of it justifies something as terrible as death. In the end, it is the individual's own moral sense that determines if the principle of double-effect for him/her is more of a mental exercise used to rationalize hastening death, or more of a reflection of reality.

A particularly useful set of guidelines, entitled "Withdrawing Intensive Life-Sustaining Treatment—Recommendations for Compassionate Clinical Management," was published in the New England Journal of Medicine in 1997 (17). Serving as a primer of palliative care during withdrawal of life-support, these guidelines address such issues as optimal use of opiates and sedatives, use of antimicrobials, withdrawal of artificial nutrition and hydration, and counseling and support for the family. See Tables 4 and 5 regarding management of symptoms that may occur during withdrawal of mechanical ventilation and, more rarely, withdrawal of artificial fluids and nutrition.

Of course, withdrawal of life support is not an all-or-none phenomenon; it is a process. There is no consensus approach as to how or when which aspects of life support should be withdrawn, or in what order. There are some principles that are helpful, however:

1. The patient's goals, as best they can be known (either through direct communication with a conscious patient or through reading the living will of a noncommunicative patient) or guessed (by a

Table 4 Possible Regimen for Conscious Patients Requesting Sedation for Ventilator Withdrawal[a]

Indication	Treatment
Before withdrawal	Bolus dose of 2–4 mg of midazolam
Distress during weaning	Bolus dose of 5–10 mg of morphine, followed by continuous morphine infusion (50% of bolus dose/hr)
Further distress	Repeat bolus dose. Increase infusion rate correspondingly

[a]These doses are for patients who were not previously taking anxiolytic drugs or opioids: if a tolerance for these drugs is established, higher doses will be needed.
Source: From Ref. 17 and Massachusetts Medical Society, 1997.

Table 5 Management of Symptoms that Occasionally Complicate the Withdrawal of Artificial Nutrition and Hydration

Symptom	Management
Thirst (rare)	Sips of fluids (patients commonly take much less than required for physiologic volume replacement)
Dry mouth (common)	Glycerine swabs, ice chips, sips of fluid; review medication list for any that cause dry mouth
Dry mouth (if aggravated by glycerine or lemon swabs)	Artificial saliva, petroleum-jelly, lip balm
Mouth debris or poor hygiene	Nonalcoholic mouthwashes, dilute hydrogen peroxide
Oral inflammation	Diphenhydramine liquid, viscous lidocaine; antimonilial therapy
Pain, restlessness (rare)	Morphine or benzodiazepines in titrated doses
Nausea (rare)	Antiemetic drugs

Source: From Ref. 17 and Massachusetts Medical Society, 1997.

surrogate-decision-maker exercising substituted judgment for a patient, that is, "trying to think with the patient's brain") should guide end-of-life care. This ensures the primacy of patient autonomy among the various pillars of medical ethics. Let us take the example of a diabetic patient with end-stage kidney disease who, during a hospitalization for the treatment of pneumonia and sepsis, competently decides that he wants to stop dialysis. This gentleman is terribly bothered by the years of needle sticks that he has had to endure and wants them to stop now. He has been poorly compliant with dialysis as an outpatient, but he feels forced into the treatments while in the ICU. He does not want lab tests anymore and he does not want to go to dialysis anymore, even though his pneumonia is clearing. He feels that his current life is worse than death. Q—Should you follow his request? A—Yes, he has made a legal and valid request. Q—What about if he is depressed? A—Yes, unless he is so depressed that his ability to understand and communicate the risks and benefits of stopping are impaired. You may, and perhaps should, try to convince him to accept a psychiatric evaluation and a trial of an antidepressant medication prior to stopping. Q—Should you stop both dialysis and lab draws, or maybe just one or the other first? A—Stopping just one or the other makes little sense because it would represent a half-way step towards accomplishing his goal, and nothing is to be gained by doing so.

2. Many physicians and families prefer to withdraw therapies in ascending order of perceived moral difficulty. This is mostly used to palliate

the guilt of the living rather than the suffering of the dying, but this is defensible in situations wherein the suffering of the dying is *not* prolonged. For example, let us say that an elderly patient with disseminated malignancy has been treated for ARDS with mechanical ventilation, antibiotics, pressors, intravenous fluids, and NG tube feedings for two weeks. He is now comatose after cardiopulmonary arrest that happened on day 3 of his hospitalization. His son finds his living will that requests termination of life-support in the setting of incurable illness or permanent unconsciousness. You are told by the consulting neurologist that his prognosis for neurologic recovery is grave. The son does not want to let you extubate his father, even though you explain the meaning of the living will. Q—Would it be acceptable to pose to the son that stopping pressors and/or antibiotics should be the next step? A—Yes it would be. Stopping either or both of these would likely allow him to die in accordance with his wishes, and if it did not, one could quickly move to withdrawing mechanical ventilation or food/fluids—either of which is more morally charged for many.

3. Unnecessary, burdensome interventions should be stopped, and tender-loving-care should be given. As in 1 above, routine lab draws have little-to-no place in the care of a patient who is undergoing termination of life support. Painful, routine turning and care of decubiti should be stopped, unless perhaps the patient actually requests them. Extra lines, tubes, and monitors should be removed. Nursing and other staff who conscientiously object to withdrawal of life support should be given the opportunity to opt out, with other staff taking their place. Spiritual and emotional support and guidance should be offered to family, patient, and staff, as appropriate. In the words of a colleague, Dr Bruce Zawacki, "We should not so much be searching for how to treat a patient at the end-of-life, but how to love a person at the end-of-life."

Specifically, regarding termination of mechanical ventilation, theoretically two methods exist: terminal weaning (titrating the ventilator down to off) versus abrupt discontinuation. Additionally, the endotracheal tube may be left in place or removed. While none of these approaches is ethically superior, it is nearly universal practice to remove the endotracheal tube and to abruptly stop the ventilator. However, some authors advocate that it may be appropriate to leave the tube in place in cases in which it is anticipated that there will be problems with pulmonary toilet. Additionally, there are strong reasons against using neuromuscular blocking agents during withdrawal of mechanical ventilation. Further guidelines on this subject by separate authors delineate that neuromuscular blockers should never be introduced at the time of extubation and should be withdrawn in patients already on them. The one ethical exception would be in the patient in which the reversal process is expected to take so long that "... the burdens to the patient and family of waiting for the neuromuscular blockade to diminish to a reversible level exceed the benefits of allowing better assessment of the patient's comfort and the possibility of interaction with loved ones" (18).

VI. Advance Directives

Typically, the phrase *advance directive* is used to denote any of the following three documents: A Durable Power of Attorney for Healthcare (DPA-HC), a living will, or a statement of treatment preferences. A DPA-HC allows a patient to formally designate who should be asked to make medical treatment decisions for the patient should he/she become unable to do so for him/herself. While it is frequently practice to automatically turn to the NOK when a patient does not have decisional-making capacity, it should be more widely understood that it is incumbent upon physicians to check first for the presence of a DPA-HC. Should one exist, it is mandatory to approach the DPA-HC initially, to the exclusion of the NOK. All of the requirements that are normally applied to patients regarding ability to comprehend a medical problem and make decisions about it should be required of the DPA-HC; that is, if the DPA-HC does not seem to possess decisional-making capacity in your discussion with him/her, it is incumbent on you to find someone else. Likewise, many patients create DPA-HC documents without discussing their choice with the proposed individual. Needless to say, this can come as quite of a surprise to the DPA-HC. The DPA-HC should be allowed to indicate whether or not they feel comfortable making healthcare decisions for the patient. Should they not, they should be allowed to delegate another individual who would. Moreover, the DPA-HC is required to demonstrate substituted-judgment. This means that the DPA-HC can demonstrate to you that he/she is capable of considering the treatment decision in the light of what the competent patient would have wanted for him/herself. This is indeed a difficult thing for mere acquaintances to do, or for people who have conflicts-of-interest regarding keeping the patient alive (e.g., the wife of a comatose patient who continues to collect a monthly pension check as long as the patient is kept alive). It should be recognized that a DPA-HC is not required for a NOK to make decisions for an incapacitated patient. Within most healthcare systems in the U.S., though, a DPA-HC would be required for a lover or friend to serve as the surrogate-decision maker, legally. Within the VA healthcare system, however, all that is required is a written statement from the potential surrogate defining the nature of the relationship with the patient and testifying to the fact that he/she can and is willing to serve as a surrogate decision maker. It is a matter of principle that a close friend is frequently a better surrogate than an estranged relative. DPA-HCs may either be executed in a lawyer's office, done at home by the patient on preprinted stationary, or completed in the hospital with the assistance of hospital staff.

Living wills are typically executed with the assistance of an attorney, though again, this is not required. They usually consist of several paragraphs, typically stating that in the occasion of patients being unable to speak for themselves, and of terminal illness or permanent unconsciousness, they wish to forego life-sustaining treatment. A set of treatment preferences would typically be tacked on to this, wherein specific guidance about use of artificial nutrition/hydration, use of antibiotics, pressors, or any other specific intervention could be mentioned. It is expected, and usually explicitly stated, that the DPA-HC should be guided by any living will and/or treatment preferences if they exist. This is one more requirement that the DPA-HC should be expected to meet.

A recent study demonstrated that what is really important in seriously-ill patients' treatment preferences is not so much the specific intervention (like insertion of a PEG tube) but the level of burden of the proposed intervention and the likelihood of an adverse outcome (such as severe cognitive impairment or death) (19). These factors must be understood when interpreting the typical set of treatment preferences that patients write down. In other words, it is appropriate to use commonsense in interpreting the frequently rigid statements that are listed in treatment-preference documents. A bioethics consultant may be helpful in this regard. As a specific example, one could ethically write a Do-Not-Resuscitate order for a nursing home patient with nosocomial pneumonia and coma in the ICU if there was a treatment preference in the medical record that stipulated that in the face of life-threatening illness, the patient did not want to receive life-support. This type of decision-analysis is very appropriate for referral to your hospital ethics committee or consultant.

References

1. Montgomery VL, Strotman JM, Ross MP. Impact of multiple organ system dysfunction and nosocomial infections on survival of children treated with extracorporeal membrane oxygenation after heart surgery. Crit Care Med 2000; 28(2):526–531.
2. Bramstedt KA, Wenger NS. When withdrawal of life-sustaining care does more than allow death to take its course: the dilemma of left ventricular assist devices. J Heart Lung Trans 2001; 20(5):544–548.
3. Jonsen AR, Veatch RM, Walters L. Source Book in Bioethics: A Documentary History. Georgetown University Press: The Nuremberg Code, 1998:11.
4. Helft PR, Siegler M, Lantos J. The rise and fall of the futility movement. N Engl J Med 2000; 343:293–296.
5. Schneiderman LJ, Jecker NS, Jonsen AR. Medical futility: its meaning and ethical implications. Ann Intern Med 1990; 112:949–954.
6. Daar JF. Medical futility and implications for physician autonomy. Am J Law Med 1995; 21:221–240.
7. Cantor MD, Braddock C, Derse AR, Edwards DM, Logue GL, Nelson W, Prudhomme AM, Pearlman RA, Reagan JE, Wlody GS, Fox E. Do-Not-Resuscitate Orders and Medical Futility—A Report by the National Ethics Committee of the Veterans Health Administration. December 2000.

8. Schneider LJ, Gilmer T, Teetzel JD, Dugan DO, Blustein J, Cranford R, Briggs KB, Komatsu GI, Goodman-Crews P, Cohn F, Young EWD. Effect of ethics consultations on nonbeneficial life-sustaining treatments in the intensive care setting: a randomized controlled trial. J Am Med Assoc 2003; 290(9):1166–1172.

9. Raffet GE, Teasdale TA, Luchi RJ. In-hospital cardiopulmonary resuscitation. J Am Med Assoc 1988; 260.

10. Schneider AP, Nelson DJ, Brown DD. In-hospital cardiopulmonary resuscitation: a 30-year review. J Am Board Fam Pract 1993; 6(2):91–101.

11. Murphy DJ, Burrows D, Santilli S, Kemp AW, Tenner S, Kreling B, Teno J. The influence of the probability of survival on patients' preferences regarding cardiopulmonary resuscitation. New Engl J Med 1994; 330:545–549.

12. Diem SJ, Lantos JD, Tulsky JA. Cardiopulmonary resuscitation on television – miracles and misinformation. New Engl J Med 1996; 334:1578–1582.

13. Crenshaw R, Rogers DE, Pellegrino ED, Bulger RJ, Lundberg GD, Bristow LR, Cassel CK, Barondess JA. Patient-physician covenant. J Am Med Assoc 1995; 273(19):1553.

14. Jonsen AR, Siegler M, Winslade WJ. Clinical Ethics: A Practical Approach to Ethical Decisions in Clinical Medicine. 2 ed. New York: Prentice Hall, 1982.

15. Mangan JT. An historical analysis of the principle of double effect. Theol Studies 1949; 10:41–61.

16. Quill TE, Dresser R, Brock DW. The rule of double-effect—a critique of its role in end-of-life decision making. New Engl J Med 1997 Dec; 337:1768–1771.

17. Brody H, Campbell MI, Faber-Langendoen K, Ogle KS. Withdrawing intensive life-sustaining treatment—recommendations for compassionate clinical management. New Engl J Med. 1997; 336:652–657.

18. Truog RD, Burns JP, Mitchell C, Johnson J, Robinson W. Pharmacologic paralysis and withdrawal of mechanical ventilation at the end of life. New Engl J Med 2000; 342:508–511.

19. Fried TR, Bradley EH, Towle VR, Allore H. Understanding the treatment preferences of seriously ill patients. New England Journal of Medicine 2002; 346:1061–1066.

18

The Electronic Intensive Care Unit

SANJAY VADGAMA and GUY W. SOO HOO

Pulmonary and Critical Care Section,
West Los Angeles Healthcare Center
  VA Greater Los Angeles
  Healthcare System, and Geffen
  School of Medicine at UCLA
Los Angeles, California, U.S.A.

I. Introduction

Optimal management of hospitalized and critically ill patients requires close monitoring and ongoing assessment of their status. An extraordinary amount of data is generated daily for each patient that in turn must be assimilated and distilled to direct the most appropriate course of therapy. The sheer volume of data and information has increased the reliance on the computer and associated applications. While no electronic medium can ever replace the human element in patient care, these devices have achieved a near-indispensable status that will only increase in the future. It is only fitting that in a book devoted to the practical aspects of pulmonary and critical care management, and as an acknowledgment of their importance, that a section is devoted to this arena.

The electronic era has already become quite entrenched in medical care, although this may not be immediately recognized by the casual observer. Bedside monitors and telemetry units have taken advantage of advances in microprocessor capability to improve on simple monitoring capabilities. Most monitoring systems have the ability to recognize characteristic changes in cardiac rhythm (atrial and ventricular dysrhythmias) to generate an alarm. In addition, there are programs that allow monitoring of ST-segment elevation and other ischemic changes. These programs automate continuous monitoring to some extent, with a tendency to err on the conservative side, and verification is still required by medical staff. Other advances allow computerized readings of ECG

595

(electrocardiogram) tracings, automated blood pressure readings, and devices that continuously monitor previously manually-obtained clinical parameters (respiratory rate, heart rate, temperature, oxygen saturation, etc.). The technology has now progressed beyond these basic tasks, and it is important for the clinician to be aware of available technology, its role in patient management, and its current capabilities and limitations. The following will provide an overview of the current status of computers and electronic applications in the management of patients in the intensive care unit (ICU).

II. The Electronic Medical Record

A patient's medical records are essential in the delivery of appropriate healthcare and even more important in the ICU setting. In the ICU, patients are frequently unstable, obtunded, or intubated, and therefore not able to provide an accurate past medical history nor information about their healthcare database (current or past medications, allergies, and other important clinical information). The patient's medical records become invaluable in assisting with diagnostic and therapeutic treatment plans.

It is well documented that a patient's traditional paper medical record is often missing crucial elements. This frequently involves laboratory or radiology reports, occurring in up to 20% of charts, but also includes important narrative sections of the medical record (1). In an outpatient setting, up to 30% of patients may be seen without their medical record. Even in those with records, information desired for the visit may not be able to be located in up to 80% of the charts (2). This often leads to repeat studies and inevitable delays in management. This experience is well documented in the outpatient arena. These issues are further compounded in critically ill patients, where there needs to be nearly immediate decisions in management.

It is clear that traditional paper-based medical records can no longer meet the needs of health care providers in the ICU. In addition to missing data and records, data may be misfiled or misplaced, and paper records are often illegible. Access is limited to a single provider, and there can be difficulty in locating the chart as it passes through several hands for processing. These limitations of the traditional paper-based medical records can result in inferior and inefficient care, and they contribute to repeated or unnecessary medical investigations and higher costs.

This is compounded when one realizes that ICU patients generate tremendous amounts of paperwork. A single patient can produce over a thousand pieces of information daily (3), from continuous monitoring of vital signs to frequent changes in management and medications required by the patient's changing clinical requirements. With a paper-based chart, this voluminous amount of data may be difficult to locate expediently and vary from minutes to hours (4). The complexity further increases as up to 236 separate categories of data may need to be reviewed prior to bedside clinical decision making (5).

While it seems intuitive that converting these paper-based records to a computerized or electronic form would solve some of the aforementioned issues, the process of developing a comprehensive, functional electronic medical record has been daunting and remains a work in progress. Whereas the information contained in a traditional medical record is paper-based and the only medium by which data is processed, the electronic record must be able to handle a diverse range of electronic data sources, ranging from text-based material to graphics and digital files. The evolution of computer technology has mandated that current systems also be able to assess archived materials, permit data sharing, facilitate interaction, and permit transactions (orders) between separate users, through both local intranet networks and the World Wide Web or Internet. These needs tax both equipment (hardware) and software and create separate problems unique to computers and the electronic medical record (EMR). In addition, the EMR requires both coordination of process automation and systems integration that has to be seamless and fault proof for every user, despite varying levels of sophistication (6).

The Institute of Medicine has defined the computer-based EMR as "an electronic patient record that resides in a system specifically designed to support users by providing accessibility to complete and accurate data, alerts, reminders, clinical decision support systems, links to medical knowledge, and other aids." It is considered essential technology. It is noteworthy that this conclusion was from a book published in 1991, recent by most standards, but dated with respect to the computer timeline (7). Table 1 provides an overview and compares the differences between the traditional paper chart and the EMR. The advantage in function and utility is clearly with the EMR. It is worthwhile to further examine some of the key aspects of the electronic medical record as well as some barriers to its implementation.

III. Implementation

While a laudable concept, the implementation of the EMR into healthcare has been relatively limited when compared to the pace of technology. The progress of the computer age can be better appreciated when one realizes that the first commercially available computers did not appear until 1951. They were large machines, filling rooms, subject to failure, and impractical except for large institutions (8). The personal desktop computer was introduced by International Business Machines (IBM) in 1981. The use of handheld computers were reported as early as 1985, but the widespread use of these devices did not start until the mid-1990s (9). The Internet was originally a Department of Defense networking experiment funded by the Advanced Research Project Agency (ARPA), and four institutions joined to the ARPANET network in 1969 (10). However, it remained a research tool until 1991 when a rudimentary program was released that

Table 1   Comparison of Differences Between Types of Patient Charts

	Traditional paper chart	Electronic medical record
Costs		
Materials	Inexpensive (paper)	Expensive (hardware/software)
Maintenance	More time consuming	More efficient, better organization
Retrieval	Can be tedious	Nearly instantaneous
Storage	Large space requirement	Much smaller space requirement
Accessibility		
Real time	Limited to a single provider	Access by multiple providers
Privacy	Protected by limited access to chart	Potential for abuse by unauthorized users, even with password protection
Quality of chart information		
Timeliness	Subject to filing delays	Nearly real-time access
Reports	May be missing or misfiled	More likely to be complete
Legibility	Subject to illegibility	Legibility issues nonexistent
Comparison of data	Tedious, requires complete records	Rapid, facilitated by electronic medical record
Trending	Not possible, requires additional charting	Possible with some programs
Integration of different information medium	Not possible	Possible with some programs (written, graphic, digital, etc.)
Potential for errors		
Patient ID	Potential for misidenfication	Reduced by unique identifiers
Charting	Potential for human error	Reduced by automated data acquisition and oversight, but still possible due to human element
Technical requirements		
	None	Hardware
		Software
		Interface requirements between computer and data source
		Information technology staff
Resource information and decision support		
References	Requires access of outside source	Often accessible on-line and available during the user session
Decision support	Requires access of outside source	Often accessible on-line and available during the user session

broadened access, but this was limited to text files. It was not until 1994 that a Web browser with graphics user interface (GUI) was available (11).

The use of computers in medicine mirrors this timeline of development. The use of a computer to assist in diagnostic evaluations was reported in 1961

(12). The use of computers to monitor patients and physiologic variables with both measured and computer-calculated output was described in 1966 (13). However, along with this technologic advance was resistance by staff because of its intrusion into usual work patterns and the added work required for implementation. While the system was eventually accepted, this lesson should not be lost on others who wish to implement new technology.

Despite over 40 years of exposure, the use of the EMR in the U.S. falls woefully short of experience in other countries. In a report from 2002, it was noted that only 17% of U.S. primary care physicians had used a EMR, compared to 58% of their counterparts in the U.K. and 90% in Sweden (14). There can be many barriers to successful implementation of an EMR that span from the trivial to what seems insurmountable. The level of healthcare provider computer expertise and sophistication is always a consideration, but this should dissipate with time as the collective computer savvy increases.

The dizzying array of data input devices and languages further increases the complexity of implementation. The current computer landscape is much simpler now, but one might recall an array of different and sometime incompatible operating systems (MS-DOS®, Mac-OS®, Windows®, IBM OS®, and variants of UNIX and Linux). In a similar fashion there are also a multitude of medical standard interfaces [HL 7 (Health Level 7), DICOM (Digital Imaging Communications in Medicine)], not to mention coding for clinical diagnoses and concepts [ICD-10 (International Disease Classification), CPT (Current Procedural Terminology), SNOMED (Systemized Nomenclature Medicine), and LOINC (Logical Observation Identifier Name Codes)]. The complexity has reached a point that resulted in a project called Unified Medical Language System, a composite of 40 vocabularies, half a million biologic concepts, and over 1 million descriptors designed to facilitate communications between computer programs and devices (15,16). The optimal system needs to be sufficiently comprehensive to meet these requirements, and flexible enough to handle new technology as well as legacy (archival) data. Files may be text, coded, or mixed in structure and may also include graphics and images. It is not surprising that conflicts may arise between hardware and software, especially when older hardware may not have the physical requirements to handle new software.

However, even more important than hardware and software issues is the change from the culture of the paper chart to the electronic chart (17,18). The most successful systems in current use are locally created where there is input between the developer and end-user (19,20). A dedicated information technology section is crucial for success. Systems that are imported to other institutions without an investment in culture change are less likely to be successfully integrated into daily use (21). Once staff have committed to an EMR, there remain a few areas that will aid in successful implementation of the system. The most important requirement involves the ease of access and charting. As might be expected, the degree of acceptance is dependent on the type of interaction between the healthcare provider and the computer interface or workstation. Something as trivial as an extra window or a few extra seconds to access the proper window may impact utilization. Data entry by physicians (notes, orders) seems to be a major obstacle. Fundamental skills would include typing and the ability to use a mouse, something that cannot be taken for granted, especially among older healthcare providers. Voice-recognition and pen-stylet interfaces may facilitate this obstacle. A separate section will deal with the subject of physician order entry.

Charting requirements for nursing staff are mixed. It would seem intuitive that computerized charting would decrease the time requirement for nursing staff. White and Hemby (22) reported about half an hour less time per 12 hour shift spent in data management, with accordingly more time spent on patient care, after implementation of a computerized system. Others have also reported upwards of a 20% decrease in manual charting time with a computerized system (23,24). However, in a more detailed analysis, Pierpont and Thilgen were not able to document an actual time reduction in data management. In their analysis, nurses decreased their data gathering time from 7% to 4% and charting from 17% to 10%, but then spent an additional 10% on the terminal, with a net effect of no difference between the pre- and post-computer period. The amount of time spent in other patient care activities was also unchanged (25). Issues of patient severity, complexity, and the software and hardware are all factors in this type of analysis and may make a valid comparison difficult. However, it is clear is that staff do spend less time in charting with a computerized system.

It should be clear by now that charting and progress notes form only a portion of the complete EMR. Additional components have been added on a regular basis, both in response to increased technologic capabilities and in response to patient care needs. As the record becomes more comprehensive, there is also greater vulnerability given greater dependence on the electronic record, need for archival and back-up systems, and potential for accidental loss of data and security breaches.

IV. Information Security and Privacy

As more health care providers move from paper files to EMRs, issues of confidentiality become more complex. EMRs appear to present new threats to maintaining the privacy of patient-identifiable medical records. An EMR can be called up instantaneously by someone with access to the data system and the relevant password. Although a paper record can be photocopied and faxed, it is less easy to distribute widely and requires physical possession for accessibility. Computerized records systems are "black boxes" to many health professionals who are otherwise familiar with traditional records systems; they fear losing control of the systems and rely on computer experts who may not have internalized the privacy-related ethics of the medical profession. Proposals to link all medical records systems so that patient data can be accessed wherever and whenever patients require medical services raise the prospect that access to one portion of one record may afford unintended access to all records on an individual.

EMRs also raise ethical issues pertaining to healthcare insurance. In the traditional, fee-for-service model of health care delivery, patient records would be produced and retained by the physician or other provider of services. The patient's health insurer would be given access to selected records needed for claims review. Disclosure of the records requires patient authorization, although, typically, patients execute these authorizations automatically and in blanket fashion. In a managed care organization, the provider of care and the insurer, in some sense, are the same entity. Any medical information in the possession of the provider also is held by the insurer.

The fear here is that the insurer will gain access to medical records that the patient and the provider would not normally transmit and that the insurer will use the data to take action adverse to the patient's interest, such as limiting benefits or terminating the patient's insurance coverage. Similarly, patient information can be transmitted to another party for unrelated purposes. In a well-publicized incident, patient prescription records that included information on nicotine replacement products were sent to a marketing firm who in turn used the patient list to send advertisements about a new oral smoking cessation product (26). This should not be surprising given the many other intrusions and information that is acquired by frequented Web sites (27).

In 1996, Congress passed the Health Insurance Portability and Accountability Act (HIPAA). This was originally designed to protect workers from losing their health insurance when they changed jobs. The scope was expanded to include protection of sensitive health information. However, Congress did not meet the initial self-imposed deadline of August 21, 1999. Additional modifications and comments were received, but it was not until April 14, 2001 that guidelines started a phase-in period. Full compliance of the regulations was not required until April 14, 2003, with the deadline for small health plans one year later on April 14, 2004 (28). HIPAA regulations require that comprehensive policies and procedures be established to safeguard electronic health records and patient confidentiality (29,30). All forms or medical records are protected (paper, electronic, and verbal).

The main elements of the regulations require healthcare organizations to provide a notice about patients' rights and how their personal health information can be used. Patients are usually asked to sign a form that they have received this information. Patients have a right to their medical records, to obtain copies, to be able to restrict access to their records as well as obtain information on who has accessed their records, and also to request that records be corrected. The regulations help clarify who has legal right to an individual's confidential medical record.

The type of protected information includes the patient's name, age, employer, address, telephone number, birth dates, hospitalization dates, social security number, medical device number, and anything else that can be used to identify the patient. This protection became especially pertinent when one realizes that a birth date, gender, and zip code will uniquely identify 87% of the U.S. population (31). This can identify a patient even if the name and social security number are not known. The regulations include measures to provide security against potential breaches. Health care organizations and record makers and keepers are required to implement a set of technical steps to protect the security of medical records. There are both financial penalties and prison time for those who release sensitive information to unauthorized organizations or for inappropriate purposes.

There are numerous ways in which this information can be restricted and protected. There may be physical restriction to workstations or patient menus. Password-protected entry into the system provides another barrier. Although passwords can limit access to records, this provides imperfect protection. Passwords can be "uncovered" accidentally, released inadvertently, and unfortunately shared. The concept of "strong" passwords includes the use of capitalized letters, numbers, and characters. Passwords can also be "discovered" with relatively minimal effort and must be changed regularly to afford the best protection.

Technical steps being touted include unique patient and access identifiers; "audit trails," which are electronic methods of detecting and recording the identities of anyone who accesses a record; encryption of external transmissions of record information; appointment of internal information security officers with responsibility to police record-keeping practices; and "firewalls," which are electronic barriers that isolate records systems from unauthorized access or penetration. These features are of special importance, especially as there are increasing numbers of commercially-available systems (not developed in-house) that need to provide these types of safeguards for patients.

The issue of privacy is of primary importance with respect to research using patient records and health information. There must be a balance between the use of information that may improve general public health or be of public benefit without breaching patient privacy. The criteria for the use of electronic medical records for the purpose of research, clinical care, and quality improvement are the same as those applying to paper records. With respect to research, the HIPAA regulations do close some gaps in privacy protection. Health information may be used without the patient's permission provided there is a waiver from the Institutional Review Board. The criteria for waiver include findings that (1) the use or disclosure involves no more than minimal risk; (2) research could not be practically conducted without the waiver; (3) privacy risks are reasonable in relation to anticipated benefits; (4) there is a plan to destroy patient identifiers unless there is some overriding health or research justification; and (5) there are written assurances that the data is not disclosed to others except for research oversight or other research that also qualifies for the waiver (32). The use of EMRs for local quality improvement, such as identifying bacterial resistance patterns in the ICU, would not require institutional review board approval and may not require patient consent. The line between research and quality improvement is, however, not well established.

V. Computerized Physician Order Entry

The Institute of Medicine's National Roundtable on Health Care Quality was one of three reports that critically addressed health care quality in the U.S. They raised concerns about the prevalence of poor quality care and issues of patient safety and made suggestions on improvement (33–35). The three reports recognized the potential for information technology as an important agent of change (36). A key feature of technology was the ability to transform the process of a physician's order from a paper-based, labor-intensive, often tedious, multistep process to one that was electronic, seamless, and allowed simultaneous access and initiation by multiple parties.

Computerized physician order entry (CPOE) refers to a variety of computer-based systems for ordering medications, communicating requests for tests, treatments, and consultations. There has been an evolution from rudimentary systems that only permitted basic data entry or requests. Most CPOE systems now include or interface with clinical decision support systems, also refered to as computer decision support systems (CDSS), to allow cross-checking across several databases (37). CPOE ensures orders are standardized, legible, and complete. CDSSs can perform multiple functions depending upon the level of sophistication; these include drug allergy checks, drug–drug interaction, drug–laboratory or drug–disease checks, dose calculations, monitoring and documenting adverse events, interaction with treatment guidelines, and clinical reminders. The Leapfrog Group, a coalition of the country's largest employers established to improve the quality of healthcare, has also identified computerized physician order entry as one of the three important steps needed to substantially improve patient safety (38).

CPOE has many potential advantages. Healthcare organizations are able to standardize their practice, incorporate clinical decision support, improve communication between all health care providers, and provide data for research management and quality improvement. CPOE with CDSSs have been shown to reduce both medication errors and adverse medication events (39–41). Features such as patient specific dosing recommendations (39,42,43), reminders to monitor drug levels (44), and reminders to choose the appropriate medication (19,22,24) promote the safe use of medications (39,42,44). Studies have also demonstrated an increase in the rates of ordering the appropriate prophylactic medications and vaccinations (45).

The greatest impetus for CPOE has been the recognition that medication errors and adverse drug events are an enormous, yet preventable, medical problem. An estimated 44,000 to 98,000 patients in the U.S. die each year as a result of medical errors, with over half due to medication errors (33). It is estimated that 777,000 persons per year are affected adversely by adverse drug events (ADEs) (46,47). The estimated annual additional cost associated with preventable ADEs occurring in a large tertiary care hospital is $2.8 million, and the cost associated with all ADEs is $5.6 million. These estimates do not include costs of injuries to patients, malpractice costs, or the costs of less serious medication errors or admissions related to ADEs (46,48,49). About 28% of ADEs are related to a medication error, and of preventable ADEs, 56% occur during drug ordering (50).

It follows that CPOEs, in conjuction with CDSSs, would be able to reduce medications errors and, in turn, reduce ADEs. Although intuitive, the published data is somewhat sparse in this arena. In a meta-analysis of the impact of CPOEs and CDSSs, only five trials met the authors' criteria for review (51). Only two specifically addressed clinical outcomes as measured by ADEs and medication errors (40,52). It should be noted that ADEs are relatively infrequent events to begin with, and most studies are underpowered to detect differences in ADEs. However, with different study designs, these investigators identified a 55% and 86% decrease in nonintercepted serious medical errors. The ADEs rate decreased 17% and 25% per 1000 patient days but did not achieve statistical significance. The penetration of CPOE into hospitals has been slow, with recent surveys demonstrating CPOE in only 4–16% of hospitals (53–55). It should also be noted that some of these systems have limited capabilities, with restriction primarily to order entry, and only about 10% of hospitals have a comprehensive order entry package (55). With the exception of one system that will be discussed in detail, most of these systems have been developed "in-house," with commercially available packages still quite limited.

CPOE has been shown to improve efficiency also. The introduction of CPOE for diagnostic tests in an ICU was associated with an improved timeliness of "stat" laboratory and imaging tests (56). The reduction in time can be quite impressive. In this medical-surgical ICU, the authors found that the median times for "stat" laboratory results (from ordering to results in hand) decreased from 148 to 74 minutes and imaging from 97 to 30 minutes. For critically ill patients, this becomes an important factor when providing rapid and appropriate management.

Although it has been shown that more time is taken writing orders using the CPOE, less time is taken processing them (57). In a before-and-after evaluation, ordering using CPOE increased from 2% to 9% of total work time, but with an additional time savings of 2%, for a net increase of only 5%. Presumably, there would be less time spent dealing with inquiries from nursing or pharmacy with overall increased efficiency. Studies have also demonstrated a reduction in overall hospital costs and length of stay in ICU patients (39) and general medicine wards (58). Improvements in safety with fewer adverse events would also reduce hospital and healthcare costs.

VI. Computer Decision Support Systems

Closely related, but separate from computerized physician order entry, are computer decision support systems (CDSS) that can also help optimize patient care. These are intricately linked with medications since many of the decisions in patient care involve a choice of medications. However, these systems also facilitate guideline implementation, patient care, and areas that do not involve medications (59,60).

Their potential in identifying the optimal dose and frequency of dosing is obvious. This is especially pertinent in patients with renal insufficiency who require some adjustment because of decreased creatinine clearance. Over 600 medications have been identified that need some modification in patients with renal failure, and experience with a CDSS has been reported (43). Fifteen percent of medication orders required an adjustment by the computer because of renal insufficiency. The appropriateness of medication prescribing, whether by dose or frequency, improved significantly on the order of 24–69%. Other areas of application include dosing of anticoagulants, aminoglycosides, other antibiotics, and theophylline (39,51,61–66). Unfortunately, these studies were underpowered to conclusively demonstrate definitive results, but it was clear that the computer-based systems resulted in fewer patients developing toxicity, excess serum levels, or bleeding.

These CDSSs can also be interactive and provide more assistance than just correcting the dose or frequency of a medication. Guidelines can be written into a program to generate physician alerts for intervention or to provide sufficient interaction that can assist with medication choices as well as patient management. This can help minimize errors and variations in care and, therefore, standardize an approach to a particular condition or disease. This is often referred to as protocol-driven care and does run some risk of inflexibility. On the other hand, patients can be quite variable in their presentation, and management may not be possible using a protocol driven program.

Antibiotic prescribing may be one area that would be most amenable to this type of support. Antibiotics are one of the most expensive items in healthcare, comprising between 20–50% of health expenditures (67). Yet, up to half of antibiotic use may be inappropriate or unwarranted (68,69). The Latter Day Saint's Hospital in Salt Lake City, Utah, includes an antibiotic management program imbedded in their computer decision support systems also referred to as clinical decision support systems (CDSS) (70). The program focuses the use prophylactic (pre-operative) antibiotics, empiric use for suspected infection and therapeutic use for established infections. The program used local consensus guidelines and antibiograms to provide information to the provider about antibiotics choices and dosing. In addition, it also monitors the need for changes due to serum levels, comorbidities (renal function), culture results, and transition to oral agents as well as monitoring for adverse drug effects. Although the proportion of patients who were administered antibiotics increased, there was a 25% decrease in antibiotic costs, 23% reduction in antibiotic resistance, 30% decline in ADEs, and improvement in the timeliness of prophylactic antibiotics for surgery from 40% to 99% without any change in antibiotic resistance patterns or length of stay. These impressive results may be unique to LDS Hospital given its long standing and sophisticated computer system, but this provides a glimpse of the possibilities with this type of program.

Management of mechanically ventilated patients is another arena in which the CDSSs have been described (60). Developed at LDS Hospital, this involves a paper flow diagram and computer-based program for the respiratory management of patients with acute respiratory distress syndrome (ARDS), covering aspects of respiratory evaluation (mechanics), oxygenation, ventilation, weaning, and extubation. They determined that the protocol was able to control management and decision making 95% of the time in their patients. It should be emphasized that the clinician was still able to override the protocol recommendations, although this was rarely done. They were able to demonstrate a survival of 66% in their patients compared to a mortality rate of 33% in historical controls. They subsequently performed a multicenter trial involving 200 ARDS patients in 10 centers using their CDSS. Although the mortality rate between protocol-driven and standard care patients was about the same (26%), there was a lower incidence of multiorgan system dysfunction and barotraumas with protocol patients (71). Similar experience was reported in using the protocol to manage trauma-associated ARDS patients. The protocol was able to be implemented successfully, but no differences in mortality were noted between those treated with the protocol (72). As with any internally developed program, its utility is limited to its successful application at other sites. While this type of program can be incorporated in other hospitals, the efficacy of this particular program remains to be determined. However, it is clear that there will only be more of these types of CDSSs that will come into use in the future.

Electronic medical records in the ICU have been shown to improve information access, both retrieval of patient information and nursing documentation (73,74), decision support, alerts and critical pathways, support for clinical research, data quality and quality of care, and compliance with the Joint Commission on the Accreditation of Healthcare Organization (JCAHO) and other related organizations (22). They have been endorsed for use by several organizations and are clearly the future of medical care despite their slow adoption into medical care. One system will be described in more detail.

VII. The Veterans Health Administration EMR

Despite a relatively weak presence in the healthcare market, there has been a virtual explosion of vendors of EMR software and systems as this has clearly emerged as a top priority item (75). These programs have targeted both office-based and hospital-based operations, offering general and subspecialty-based packages (emergency rooms, anesthesiology). In addition to physician and nursing charting, coding, billing, scheduling, and prescription management are necessary elements of the package. These proprietary packages run the gamut of expense, but added costs include software licensing fees, support staff, staff training, and hardware. Installation limited to respiratory care and ventilator management can be in the $150,000–$250,000 range for a 400-bed hospital, with annual recurring costs of 10–25% for support (76). Of course, less expensive packages may not be lacking in features. Many of the oldest EMR systems in use were internally developed and therefore created and molded to address specific needs. These function well at their local sites but are often the product of several thousands of hours of development and require an extensive support staff (19,20). It is not clear how well these systems may function at disparate sites. However, there is a system with a national, multisite presence that has evolved with computer technology. This system primarily serves the Veterans Administration.

The Veterans Health Administration (VHA) is the nation's largest integrated healthcare system, consisting of 163 medical centers, more than 850 ambulatory care and community-based clinics, and 137 nursing homes serving 4 million patients each year (77). Over 180,000 healthcare professionals are employed at VHA, with an additional 80,000 students and residents in healthcare fields receiving training on an annual basis. All sites are computerized and, with proper authorization, are able to access a veteran's EMR. This clearly represents the largest integrated EMR system with the greatest number of users in the U.S. and, most likely, the world.

Work on the system began in the late 1970s as part of a project to computerize the text portion of the patient record. The project started in 1977, and despite minimal administrative support, programmers gradually added modules that included information on admission, discharge and transfer, scheduling, pharmacy, laboratory reports, radiology, dietetics, pulmonary function testing, and mental health. These were incorporated using a basic database and lexicon. In 1982, the VHA fully committed to building an electronic healthcare architecture called Decentralized Hospital Computer Program (DHCP). The program was implemented at eight sites nationwide that year. By 1985, DHCP was installed at 169 sites. Other applications, including fiscal, supply, medical records, nursing, surgery and medical center management, were installed in 1989 (78).

The system continued to evolve in conjunction with technologic advances. Implementation of a visual layer led to a change in the name of the system in 1996 to the Veterans Health Information Systems and Technology (VistA). There are currently 99 separate packages in the VistA system, of which 55 represent clinical applications with the others involved in administration, finance and infrastructure. One of the most visible packages is the Computerized Patient Record System (CPRS), which was also released starting in 1996. This represented an advance on several fronts with a shift in focus from a departmental approach to a patient-centered approach. This included the release of a health summary application that allowed consolidation of several elements of patient care. The introduction of CPRS also represented a shift to GUI programming. This represented a shift from paper-based charting to computer-based charting. Providers could enter electronic progress notes and orders. This change also coincided with a shift from primarily inpatient care to outpatient-based care. This represented a major improvement and advance from DHCP, which had served primarily as a depository of information.

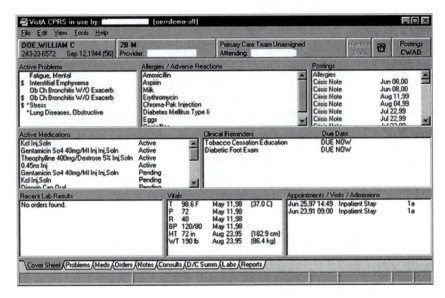

Figure 1   An example of a CPRS cover sheet. This provides a snapshot of the patient's active problems, medications, vital signs, and clinical reminders.

CPRS integrates several programs with a tabular chart format that is intuitive and easy to navigate. It provides a single interface, allowing staff to order lab tests, medications, diets, radiology tests, and procedures (Fig. 1). It also provides a record of a patient's allergies and adverse drug reactions, and it has the ability to request and track consults, enter progress notes and procedures notes, and discharge summaries. CPRS improves efficiency and safety through features such as order checking for potential drug to drug interactions, out of range values, duplicates, and maximum order frequency. Orders are integrated with progress notes, results, and procedures. Quick orders and order sets save time, and clinical reminders which meet Clinical Guidelines improve quality of care. The system automatically time-stamps each entry and can generate an electronic trail of every interaction. While orders can be entered only by one provider at a time, the chart can be viewed simultaneously by literally dozens of healthcare providers, so that an order that requires more than one provider to be fulfilled can reach all involved parties virtually instantaneously. Passwords and electronic signatures provide security for patients and also allow another electronic trail. Computer installation eliminates the need for dedicated workstations.

A crucial requirement of any healthcare system is the ability to retrieve past records. This is even more important in the VA system, which encompasses a great number of sites not only within a geographic area, but also nationwide. Of course, records are limited to the extent that patients use the VA as their sole healthcare provider, but this is a limitation of any system. The remote view package is an especially useful option that has further facilitated care.

This provides an electronic link to all VA facilities and allows the retrieval of patient data from any VA facility in the country where the patient may have been treated. Retrieval is completed in seconds, usually no more than a minute from the time of request. The remote data view feature reduces the likelihood of duplicating tests or prescribing incompatible medications, further enhancing patient care and safety.

The other advantage lies in the management of patients who come from out of the area for care. The advantage of this feature can be illustrated by two recent examples at our facility. One involved a patient with clinically metastatic lung cancer with a large pleural effusion. Unfortunately, he was not able to provide much information about his prior care. He had been treated in Denver, and using remote view to access his records allowed providers to determine his diagnosis, past treatment (which included chest tube drainage), and that he had not undergone pleurodesis. In a different case, another patient presented with chest pain and bleeding, along with a request for narcotics, and provided a very complex medical history of a collagen vascular disorder and a hypercoagulable state with multiple scars noted on his body. Admission in another era might have prompted a host of tests and procedures (79) before discovery. However, he was recognized by staff who had treated him at an outside VA facility, which raised suspicions. Eventually, access to his records revealed a man with suspected Munchausen's disorder. He had been hospitalized in over 30 VA facilities nationwide with similar complaints. Unfortunately, he left this facility before his diagnosis could be confirmed, which was a common pattern. The remote view option provided revealing insight into his behavior and allowed a refocus on psychiatric issues.

Advances in CPRS technology now incorporate VistA imaging, which provides a multimedia online patient record that integrates the traditional medical chart information with medical images, including radiographs, pathology slides, video images, EKG tracings, images from invasive procedures (cardiology, gastroenterology, etc.), wound photos, and anything else that can be placed in a digital file (Fig. 2). Consent forms and other written documents can be scanned into the medical record. Work is also in place to eventually permit electronic signatures or digital signatures similar to those used by credit card agencies that would create a truly paperless medical record.

Proper identification of patients is crucial for patient safety and to avoid medical errors. In another advance, the bar code medication administration (BCMA) package is a bedside feature that generates a computerized medication administration record. Key elements of the system are mobile laptop computers that accompany the nurse to the bedside, handheld scanners, patient unique wristband bar codes, and bar codes for staff and medications. When medications are administered, the patient's wristband is scanned along with the medication and employee identification card, and this information is transmitted wirelessly to the electronic medical administration record. This provides confirmation of the patient and medication with exact documentation of the time of administration.

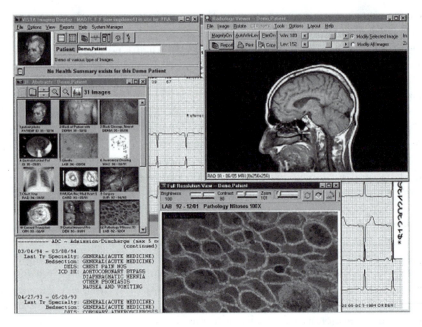

Figure 2 An example of the VistA Imaging System. VistA Imaging handles high quality image data from many specialties, including cardiology, pulmonary and gastrointestinal medicine, pathology, radiology, hematology, and nuclear medicine.

This will alert the provider to errors in patient or medication and provide an electronic log that can be used to confirm administration or omission of medications. This technology has also expanded to laboratory specimens, blood products, and other areas that require exact patient identification. This package was developed in the VA system starting in 1994 and has been in place nationwide since 2000. It is currently the model for healthcare bar code technology. It has virtually eliminated medication errors, decreasing by 70% with BCMA technology at one VA (78). The laptops also double as mobile workstations, usually for checking of laboratory studies or notes, as the wireless transmission makes access to the system slower than through a designated workstation.

The ease of use and powerful capabilities of VistA and CPRS are obvious to the healthcare providers who are fortunate to use this system. In addition to the VA, the list of outside organizations who have adopted this system is growing. Included are other governmental healthcare agencies, such as the Department of Defense and their military hospitals and Indian Health Service. National users include the Texas Cancer Data Center, Eastern and Western State Hospital, Washington, and HealthPartners, Minneapolis. International users include Helsinki University Hospital, University of Wurzburg, Germany, National Cancer Institute, Cairo, and hospitals in Columbia and Pakistan. Questions frequently arise as to adoption of the system or components by other healthcare entities. VistA software, including the VistA imaging software, is available through the Freedom of Information Act with a few exceptions that primarily involve privacy and financial applications. Demonstration software can be accessed at http://www.va.gov/vista/. A monograph that further details all of the capabilities can be obtained by request from VistAMonograph@med.va.gov. The 2004 version of the monograph lists the cost of both VistA and the imaging software at $50.70. It is important to note that while the software may be inexpensive, the technical infrastructure required for proper operation can be daunting. Realizing that the system may be beyond the capabilities and scope of many healthcare organizations, a version of the software called VistA Lite is under development. An office based version called Vista-office EHR is being developed in collaboration with the Centers for Medicare and Medicaid with more information available at www.vista-office.org.

Health eVet–VistA will be the next generation of Veterans Health Information Systems. Preliminary versions were launched in November 2003. The goal will be to move from a facility centric model to a person/data centric system. Veterans and their families will be able to access key portions of their EMR, track personal health metrics such as blood pressure, blood glucose and cholesterol, and have access to a Health Education Library and health assessment tools. Encrypted data will be stored in secure eVaults. A Health Data Repository (HDR) will create a true longitudinal healthcare record that includes data from VA and non-VA sources. This also represents a shift from the original focus of electronic data, which was the medical record, to information that encompasses not only known medical details but also information that involves the total health of the patient. This end result of this effort is an electronic health record (EHR), which will represent full integration of all aspects of patient health. This health data system will also help support research and population analysis, facilitate patient access to data, and improve the sharing of information as well as data quality and data security.

The Institute of Medicine recently described the key components of an EHR (80). These core capabilities were presented in a recent report with a goal of widespread implementation set for 2010. However, all of these requisite features are already in place and functional in VistA. These elements are highlighted in Table 2 and can be used to form the basis of any EHR system.

VIII. Clinical Information Systems

The prior sections have dealt primarily on the EMR from the perspective of the healthcare provider. The focus has been on generated reports, images, provider charting, and orders. Equally important in the electronic ICU are advances in the clinical information systems (CIS) that further incorporate data acquisition and charting to form a complete and paperless EMR.

The evolution of computers in medical care has been outlined in an earlier section. The first reported use of computers in the ICU was in 1964 at the University of Southern California Medical School Shock Research Unit at

Table 2 Core Capabilities of the Electronic Health Record Located in VistA/CPRS

Core capability	VistA/CPRS function or feature
Health information and data	Organization by tabs and sheets Diagnoses, allergies, lab results, medications Specified location for important data (advance directives) Ability to locate specific notes by group or title
Result management	Rapid access to current and past results Worksheet function allows composite view of results Data sorting by a variety of strategies Graphing function for selected laboratory results
Order management	Computerized physician order entry Includes medications, consultations, diagnostic studies
Decision support	Pharmacy screens with alerts, reminders General reminders and alerts for other conditions Links to guideline recommendations and best practices On line access to references and other databases
Electronic communication and connectivity	Consultation and test results alerts to providers Electronic mail
Patient support	Health eVet Home monitoring system under implementation
Adminstrative processes	Computerized administrative tools Scheduling, generation of appointment letters
Reporting	Current and past reports (archival and legacy data) Remote view feature to locate information at off sites Disease surveillance and patient safety

Los Angeles County Hospital. Clinical data such as arterial and venous pressures, electrocardiograms, body temperature and urinary outputs were collected. Data was displayed in graphic and tabular form (13,81). This represented a major advance in the capabilities of the physician in the monitoring of the patient. Physiologic variables could be monitored more frequently and, in some cases, continuously.

First generation information systems were introduced in the early 1970s. Central microcomputers collected and automatically displayed data from a patient's monitors to bedside terminals. Healthcare providers could enter data such as laboratory results, medications, nursing, and physician notes. However, these systems were difficult to use, relatively crude systems with complex menus. They were not suitable for widespread use and, therefore, not adopted in the vast majority of ICUs. However, the features that permitted frequent or continuous monitoring of certain physiologic variables, such as electrocardiographic tracings, arterial and central venous pressures (through intravascular catheters), and pulmonary artery pressures with calculated hemodynamic parameters, soon became the standard in critical care.

Second generation systems were introduced in the late 1980s. These systems had graphical interfaces, with point-and-click capability, and were more user friendly. Second generation systems now comprise the majority of CIS currently in use (82). They represent the electronic equivalent to the bedside flow sheet, which is also their standard presentation format. Data from bedside monitors is automatically displayed onto the flow sheet. Staff needs to verify the accuracy of the data before it becomes incorporated into the medical record, but charting time is obviously reduced. Annotations and corrections are possible with an electronic audit trail. This includes physiologic patient data, such as blood pressure, heart rate, respiratory rate and oxygenation, but also information from ventilators, infusion pumps, and urinometers. Charting of medications, nursing assessments, and physicians notes is also possible. A laboratory link allows review of laboratory values, enabling the user to determine trends and the effects of treatments. The second generation systems run on a network of personal computers known as clients. These clients allow the user to access patient information anywhere a network connection is available. This therefore allows access to data from outside of the ICU. The patient data is maintained on server databases, which are accessed by the client personal computers.

A third generation of systems has since been developed and adopted in a few institutions. These systems utilize Microsoft Windows®, as opposed to the UNIX system used by many previous systems. They have several advantages over the second generation systems. Its Windows interface is familiar to millions of users as is the Windows operating system with software that allows access to existing Windows applications, such as word processors and spreadsheets (81). The other major advance is the ability to incorporate relational databases into their software. This was invented in 1970 and transformed the approach to data management (83). A relational database represents data that is organized in structured tables that can then be accessed or reconstructed without having to reorganize the database. The standard application program interface to the relational database is structured query language (SQL), which is used both to query the database and generate reports. A major advantage is that new data can be incorporated by adding another table instead of changing the software. The medical record is composed of a vast array of both structured (laboratory) and unstructured (text) data and can be difficult to access. The relational database is a powerful business tool and in medical care allows generation of consolidated reports for one patient or trends in patient management and outcome (84). This feature is limited in part by information retrieval software technology, and this aspect of these systems has yet to be fully utilized by end-users (85).

Third generation systems provide similar clinical functions to the second generation systems; however, they also allow voice recording as an input into transcription, direct access to informational databases, remote access over the internet, criteria-based alarms to clinician via e-mail, fax, or pager, and tools for clinical pathways analysis.

Institutions are able to integrate and adapt systems according to their requirements. The CareVue® system at Cedars–Sinai Medical Center in Los Angeles, California, is one such example. This employs the standard CareVue functions, such as connectivity to bedside monitors, links to laboratory, radiology and pharmacy. The standard CareVue databases are configured to allow the data to be used for clinical, administrative, and research purposes. They also devised a system which continuously analyzes data exported from the CareVue system for the occurrence of exceptional or life-threatening clinical events. A configurable rule-based system was created to detect and act on such events. When detected, the system formats an alerting message, dials a modem, and transmits the message, which appears on the screen of a Palm® Personal Digital Assistant (PDA) carried by designated clinicians (86,87).

There are an increasing number of vendors of commercially available clinical information systems. Some, like CareVue®, have undergone acquisition by several parent firms over their existence (Hewlett-Packard → Agilent → Phillips) or represent products of mergers, e.g., Centricity Enterpise CIS® (GE Marquette). Others systems include CareSuite® (Picis), Essentris Critical Care® (Clinicomp), Sunrise Critical Care® (Eclipsys), and Soarian® Clinical Access and Infinity Chartassist® (Siemens). These systems can vary in some features but all incorporate standard features, such as flow sheet charting, progress notes, health report forms (laboratory, ventilator, etc.), and medication administration records. Some allow more flexibility in configuration of reports than others, and technological advances include the ability to archive data and interface with other entities, such as a digital picture archiving and communication system (PACS). The move to this electronic capability improves efficiency, reduces errors, and has the potential for overall improvement in patient care (88,89). However, there are no comprehensive health technology assessments of these systems (90). Cost is always a consideration, and these systems are expensive, ranging from $10,000 to $25,000 per bed, with recurring costs that exceed $100,000 per year. The return on investment should be in favor of these systems, but the initial start-up costs may remain prohibitive (91).

It is anticipated that future iterations of these systems will have even greater access to information systems, including the Internet, and have wireless capability. Their scope will further expand beyond monitoring, charting, and compilation of data. They will integrate composite medical care data to improve workflow and the quality of care. They will also be involved in all aspects of patient care, such as finances and storage of old documents, including legacy (paper) materials, to complete a truly paperless EHR.

IX. Medicine and the Internet

It is fair to conclude that nothing has changed the world over the past decade as much as access to the Internet. What was once limited to an elite few has now become available to virtually everyone on this planet through an increasing number of smaller and more portable devices. It is estimated that over 100 million people in the U.S. access the Internet monthly, and the worldwide number is obviously much higher. At its simplest level, it represents a global collection of networks that facilitates communications between computers connected to those networks. It allows anyone who can access the network the ability to interact with anyone or any computer that is also connected to this giant network. Transmission of data travels through routers based on a Transmission Control Protocol/Internet Protocol (TCP/IP) and occurs in milliseconds. Web browsers allow Web sites to be accessed by their unique address or uniform resource locator (URL), and advances have allowed all types of files (text, graphic, audio, and video) to be viewed. With the power of endless communication also comes the vulnerability of attack by any number of computer viruses that can originate from any other computer on this vast network.

The practice of medicine has not been exempt from the influence of the Internet (10). The greatest change has been the method of communication with other physicians and healthcare providers. Whereas once medical information and advances were promulgated through lectures and meetings with limited access or through print journals, information is now available worldwide, with minimal delay if any at all (seconds). Access to the information is available not only to healthcare providers, but also patients and their families. Patients have equal access to many journals or to news organizations that synthesize the information for general use. Communication is also facilitated by electronic mail (e-mail), mailing lists, and newsletters. In some instances, physicians and patient can communicate by e-mail, undergo some evaluation by off-site providers, and have medications prescribed or renewed, all through the Internet.

The most compelling example of the power and influence of the Internet on Medicine is the recent elucidation of Severe Acute Respiratory Syndrome (SARS) (92–96). This was a new infectious respiratory pathogen that was recognized, with the infecting organism identified and control measures in place literally in weeks of its first reports. Initial cases were noted in late February 2003. An index case was hospitalized on March 4, with the recognition that healthcare workers were falling ill beginning March 10, and within two weeks, a full fledged epidemic was evident. News of this epidemic was disseminated through multiple health care agencies, with the World Health Organization taking the lead with frequently updated Web pages. A full written report on this index case and infected healthcare workers was available as an electronic publication on April 7. This was a remarkably rapid response to a new illness, facilitated through the electronic medium, but it also raised questions as to whether the response was fast enough for public health (97). By comparison, while an outbreak of Legionairre's disease was recognized in the summer of 1976, the offending organism was not identified until a year later (98,99).

Internet use amongst physicians continues to grow, estimated at 89% in 2001 and 96% in 2002, with 90% of physicians using the Internet to research clinical issues (100). An increasing number of Web sites are aimed at healthcare providers, patients, and their relatives. A not unusual comment these days is that patients often have access to just-published information before the physician can review and digest the data. The Internet is changing the way information is accessed and applied. With increasing technology, search engines are able to retrieve enormous volumes of references on almost any subject instantly. It is important to note that these results of searches are based on algorithms that focus on relevancy of the Web site to the key word(s) entered in the request. This involves ranking sites based on links from other Web sites. Needless to say, this results in identification of the most popular sites, but not necessarily the most important sites. The search results may differ greatly dependent of the term entered and the algorithm used to locate that term. It should be noted that some sites may not even have any input from healthcare professionals.

The volume of available information has raised concerns about the quality of the information (101–103). Patients may receive erroneous information or be falsely reassured, leading to delays in appropriate therapy. The quality of scientific information may be suspect. One report felt that up to a third of the scientific information found on the Internet was inaccurate or misleading and up to 90% was unreferenced (104). A significant number of Web sites are not peer-reviewed or associated with governing bodies such as the American Medical Association or the British Medical Association (105,106). Eysenbach and colleagues reviewed a total of 79 studies which in turn evaluated almost 6000 Websites and over 1300 Webpages. Vast differences in methodology limit some conclusions, but 70% of the studies found quality to be an issue. It is more difficult to determine the number of inaccurate Web sites because of differences in criteria used to define accuracy, but somewhere between 15% and 38% of sites had inaccuracies identified.

The American Medical Association has published guidelines for medical and health information Web sites (107). These principles were developed for their own Web sites, but are a useful benchmark for all health-related Web sites. They caution about the need for constant review and revision given the rapidity of changes in this field. They list four basic principles that cover the conduct with respect to content, principles for advertising and sponsorship, privacy and confidentiality, and e-commerce. Key points include the need to review content for quality, dates and sources of editorial comment, review of external links prior to posting, clear disclosures of relationship to advertisements including financial support, warnings about entry to other sites, privacy disclosures, use of "cookies," specifically persistent "cookies," which are permanent files, and confidentiality.

Despite the caution raised by many, there are many excellent sources of information available. A list of informative critical care and general medical

Table 3 Examples of General Medicine and Critical Care Web sites

Category	Web site
Online literature database	
PubMed	http://www.ncbi.nlm.nih.gov/entrez/query.fcgi
Ovid	http://www.ovid.com/site/index.jsp
Journals	
Am J Respir Crit Care	http://ajrccm.atsjournals.org/
Anesthesia and Intensive Care	http://www.aaic.net.au/
Annals of Internal Medicine	http://www.annals.org/
British Medical Journal	http://bmj.bmjjournals.com/
Chest	http://www.chestjournal.org/
JAMA	http://jama.ama-assn.org/
Lancet	http://www.thelancet.com/
The New England Journal of Medicine	http://nejm.org/
Respiratory Care	http://www.rcjournal.com/
Thorax	http://thorax.bmjjournals.com/
Other organizational sites	
Centers for Disease Control	http://www.cdc.gov/
European Respiratory Society	http://www.ersnet.org/ers/default.aspx
Medical Letter	http://www.medletter.com/
Society of Critical Care Medicine	http://www.sccm.org/
World Health Organization	http://www.who.int/en/
Medical information sites	
DocMD	http://docmd.com/
Medscape	http://www.medscape.com/
PDR	http://www.pdr.net/
Virtual Hospital	http://www.vh.org/
Journal repositories	
Highwire Press	http://highwire.stanford.edu/
Free Medical Journals	http://www.freemedicaljournals.com/
Medical Journals	http://www.medical-journals.com/
MedBioWorld	http://www.medbioworld.com/index.html

Notes: 1. Many sites provide online access as part of the cost of the subscription. 2. An increasing number of journals release full-text articles to all six months to a few years after publication date.

Web sites is shown in Table 3. Web sites associated with national healthcare organizations and professional societies are likely to be the most reliable sources on the Internet. The list is by no means comprehensive but should provide the reader with a good starting point to information.

Other features available via the Internet include paging. Many pager companies now offer Web-based services for sending text messages from any Internet-connected personal computer to its pagers. High-speed access methods now offer real-time video and voice communications. The Internet of the future will serve as a repository for individual health-related information that, under the appropriate conditions, can be accessed by healthcare providers. This can only facilitate and improve the quality of patient care. However, secure control over privacy and confidentiality issues will be paramount before this can occur.

X. Handheld Devices in the ICU

For busy critical care physicians, it can be difficult to keep up with the wealth of information now available, not only in journals, but also Internet sites. Multiple medications with numerous potential interactions, optimal utilization of medical/hospital resources, and tracking patients require more efficient methods of handling and processing information. Reducing delays in implementing new advances by improving access to the most current guidelines at the point of care may lead to improved patient outcomes, optimal bed utilization, and reduced cost (108,109).

With advances in technology, point-of-care access to current medical information is now possible (110), and studies with mobile computerized carts have been shown to be more likely to incorporate evidence based medicine into clinical practice (111).

The other major advance in the computer era is the continued reduction in size and increased capacity of electronic devices. Handheld devices, also known as PDAs, can provide a portable, integrated platform for point-of-care clinical reference, patient management, and data communication. These devices are now equipped with processors and memory capacity once reserved for high-end desktop computers and at a fraction of the cost. Physician use of PDAs continues to grow, from 15% in 1999 to 26% in 2001, with an estimated 50% of all doctors using PDAs by 2004 or 2005 (112,113). Entering medical students at the Geffen School of Medicine at UCLA are required to have a PDA for use. In one survey, almost 80% of resident physicians reported daily use of PDAs, most likely to access medical references, with the highest use among trainees in internal medicine (112). Common uses of PDAs are summarized in Table 4 (114).

PDAs can be broadly divided into two categories according to their operating system, the Palm® OS (Palm Inc. Santa Clara CA) or Windows® CE, also known as Pocket PC® (Microsoft, Seattle). Currently the Palm® system is

Table 4   Examples of Common Uses of Personal Digital Assistants (PDAs)

Point of care assistance	Drug information, clinical guidelines, decision aids, patient education
Patient information	Patient teaching, clinical results
Administrative functions	Electronic prescribing, coding, tracking schedules
Research activities	Data collection, participant education
Medical education	Lecture notes, presentations, photographs, and diagrams

the more popular system with more medical software applications available. Unfortunately, these two operating systems do not interface well. Key considerations prior to purchase include choosing the platform that best interfaces with the hospital healthcare informatics, platforms used by colleagues (allows sharing of programs), and the available software that best fits intended use (115). PDAs also include some basic functions, such as an address book, scheduler, calculator, to-do list, and memo functions.

A great deal of medical software is now available for PDAs, ranging from pharmacopoeias to medical calculators, textbooks to patient tracking software. Many applications require software known as document readers to view certain text files or documents downloaded from the Internet. Examples of document readers are shown in Table 5. Various software applications allow access to Internet-based literature. Examples include Avantgo®, JournalToGo®, and Highwire®. Journal Web sites can be accessed via the Internet and connected to the handheld device during each synchronization, allowing access to both abstracts and full articles from relevant medical journals (116). Highwire® Press also offers many peer-reviewed journals, including the British Medical Journal, in handheld downloadable format. Other features allow tracking of journal contents, abstracts, and citations, all of which can be updated during regular synchronization of the handheld computer with the computer or Internet. Searches for medical literature are also possible through the popular Ovid® search engine, which has software for the handheld that retrieves journal abstracts for reviewing with each synchronization.

There are an increasing number of textbooks and handbooks available in handheld format. Examples include Griffith's 5-Minute Clinical Consult 2005®, Harrison's Manual of Medicine, and The Washington Manual™ of Medical Therapeutics. Table 5 lists some examples of publishers through which these can be purchased. Adatia and Bedard (117) recently reviewed several general medical reference programs, comparing the major titles available, the advantages, disadvantages, and relative cost of available software. Numerous programs can be carried in a PDA, and regular updates are possible with synchronization. In addition, wireless capabilities may eventually eliminate even that connection to a network. These programs vary in price, but most are in the $50–$100 range and can be downloaded from the Internet, often with a time-limited use license.

Pharmacopoeias, or drug information bases, are very popular programs, ideally suited for handheld devices. They offer comprehensive drug lists, both adult and pediatric drug dosing, drug interactions, common side effects, and retail prices (116). Currently there are many programs available. Ten core databases have recently been evaluated for both the Palm and Pocket PC applications (118). ePocrates® is an example of one of the most popular handheld drug databases available for both Palm and Pocket PC platforms. Originally launched in 1999, ePocrates offers several applications, including a free drug reference guide. For a fee, it offers enhanced applications, combining the drug formulary with extensive disease, diagnostic, and laboratory references, with an integrated

Table 5 Handheld Medical Applications and Their Web sites

Category	Web site
Links to medical software sites	
Handango	http://www.handango.com/
DocMD	http://www.docmd.com/pdasoftware
Palmgear	http://www.palmgear.com
Skyscape	http://www.skyscape.com
PDACortex	http://www.pdacortex.com/
Document readers	
Documents to Go	http://www.dataviz.com
iSilo	http://www.isilo.com
Mobipocket	http://www.mobipocket.com/en/
Access to Medical Literature	
Avantgo	http://www.avantgo.com
JournalToGo	http://www.journaltogo.com
Ovid at hand	http://www.ovid.com
Highwire	http://www.highwire/stanford/edu
Drug reference applications	
ePocrates	http://www.epocrates.com/
Micromedex	http://www.micromedex.com/
Lexidrug	http://www.lexi.com
Infectious disease applications	
Hopkins antibiotic guide	http://www.hopkins-abxguide.org/
ePocrates ID	http://www.epocrates.com
Sanford Guide	http://www.sanfordguide.com
Infectious Diseases Notes	http://www.pdamedsolutions.com
Calculators	
Medcalc	http://www.freewarepalm.com/
ICUmath	http://www.freewarepalm.com/
ABGPro	http://www.stacworks.com
MedMath	http://smi-web.stanford.edu/people/pcheng/medmath/
Patient Tracking Software	
Patient tracker	http://www.handheldmed.com/
Patient Keeper	http://www.patientkeeper.com/
Assorted Medical applications	http://www.freewarepalm.com/

infectious diseases treatment guide and other tools. Many applications are updated regularly and data transferred during synchronization ensuring current and accurate information. With so many new medications being approved and marketed, it can be virtually impossible for physicians to keep abreast of possible drug interactions. Drug information databases as well as specific drug interaction software are likely to increase prescriber awareness of adverse reactions and reduce medication errors. The accuracy, comprehensiveness, and ease of use several of the drug interaction software applications used with PDAs have also been recently reviewed (119).

Along with drug formularies, there are many infectious disease applications currently available for handheld devices. Popular examples include eProcrates ID®, The Sanford Guide, John Hopkins Division of Infectious Diseases Antibiotic guide, and Infectious Diseases Notes (previously Infectious Diseases and Antimicrobial Notes). The advantages and disadvantages of these four applications have recently been reviewed in detail (120). Such applications provide point-of-care information allowing antibiotic information to be retrieved by anatomical site, pathogen, or drug for diagnostic or therapeutic use. These applications also include dosing, adverse events, and drug interactions. Content to all of these programs is regularly updated and can be transferred to the PDA during the synchronization process.

Several medical calculator applications are also available (Table 5). Increasing numbers of programs, often written by healthcare professionals, are geared toward the ICU healthcare professional. Many are free and can be downloaded from the Internet, including ICUmath, which offers 52 adult ICU applications using 82 medical equations divided into groups, such as pulmonary, chemistry, and cardiac, and scores which include the Glasgow Coma Scale and Apache II. Other freeware programs include Medformula, MedMath, and MedCalc, all examples of medical calculators, often with overlapping programs. Such applications are likely to become increasingly popular amongst healthcare professionals in the ICU, where large amounts of data are constantly generated and need to be accurately analyzed, often using complex equations. Specialized programs are also available that address a specific element of medical care. These include programs with self-explanatory titles such as Advanced Cardiac Life Support, Anoxic Brain Injury Prognosis, Eponyms, Lung Injury Score, PE Paths, Pneumonia Severity Index, and TB Treatment Guidelines. Through a wireless connection, the medical literature can be searched using PubMed on Tap.

Patient tracking software may improve patient data management and sign over between physicians at shift change. Applications such as Patient Follower or ProfileMD Classic are freeware that help keep up with patients and their database. Patient Tracker is another similar program that was also once freeware. It is a program that allows the user to enter patient demographics, laboratory results, medications, radiology, and laboratory results. Data can be transferred between PDA users by either directly beaming the information or via a database during synchronization. It now has iterations that allow placement on a desktop, use from a workstation, or use through a wireless connection to a hospital network. It only follows that the PDA can be used to access not just a server-based network, but a Web-based system as well (121). The latter refinements will further solidify the use of the PDA and reflect the continued consolidation of technology into medical care. Table 5 lists examples of patient tracking applications. Additional PDA applications include dictionaries and billing, with charting and notes emerging as the next area of application.

Handheld devices may also be integrated into the training of residents, documenting patient contact and educational experiences, and facilitating communication between physician teams (122,123). The PDA can also be used to log clinical procedures as a tool to ensure adequate educational experience (124,125).

In the ICU, PDAs have been shown to be a feasible means of providing point-of-care access to medical reference material, potentially improving clinical decision making, and initial studies have shown the introduction of handheld computers to ICU physicians to be well received (126,127). The most valuable role was found to be access to medical reference information and drug dosing.

Acceptance of new technology is variable. Barriers to acceptance of handheld devices may include lack of familiarity with the technology, inadequate training, and issues concerning the device itself, such as size, limited memory, and battery life. There will always be concern and some uncertainty in placing large amounts of vital information into a single device that may be subject to physical loss or accidental erasure. Privacy issues remain the same as with any electronic-based system, and control decreases with increasing portals of entry into a system as well as expansion to wireless capability. With e-mail capabilities, there is also the risk of acquiring disabling computer viruses. Back-up systems are even more crucial in this area, especially in the event of a power failure or anything else that may disrupt the network or computer system.

Nevertheless, the use of these devices will only grow. Despite some disadvantages, their benefits far outweigh any negative elements. With continuing advances in technology and improvement in training, handheld computers will undoubtedly become an essential medical tool.

XI.   National Health Information Infrastructure

Recognizing the importance and potential of current and evolving health information technology on medical care, the U.S. government has helped to coordinate the development of a National Health Information Infrastructure (NHII). This initiative is voluntary and has broad objectives, including improvement in patient safety, improvement in health care quality, creating the ability to detect patterns that might be related to bioterroism, and to provide better information to healthcare consumers to allow informed personal healthcare decisions. It is important to note that the NHII will NOT be a centralized database of medical records or a government regulation. Its goal is to unite both public and private stakeholders in the development of this agenda. The three major beneficiaries of the NHII would be the users of this information, namely patients, healthcare providers, and public health organizations (128,129). The first conference was held in 2003 and, in July 2004, a 10-year

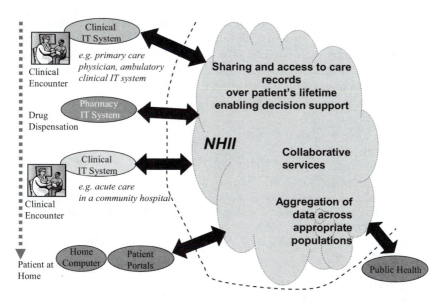

Figure 3 Schematic of the points of contact and types of interaction recommended for the National Health Information Infrastructure (NHII). *Source*: Adapted from material at http://aspe.hhs.gov/sp/nhii/.

plan for implementation was announced. Their report can be viewed in detail at their website: http://aspe.hhs.gov/sp/nhii/. A framework for action was presented as well as key strategies. These include goals to inform clinical practice (implementing EHRs into clinical practice using incentives, reducing the risk of investment, and expanding to rural and underserved areas), interconnect clinicians (requiring an interoperable infrastructure through regional collaborations with a national health information network), personalize care (consumer-centric information and personal health records), and to improve population health (unifying databases, accelerating research, and disseminating evidence). Key goals of the health information system include continuity of health records over a patient's lifetime, collaborative services, integration of knowledge for decision support, and aggregation of population health information. Figure 3 further outlines the structure of the points of contact of the NHII and its types of interaction.

XII. Summary

The intent of this overview was to provide a glimpse of the current impact of computers and computer technology in patient care. This is a constantly changing and evolving area, and some of the content runs the risk of being dated even prior to publication. The Internet provides the means to access the most current information, but it carries a risk for inaccurate or misleading information for the unsophisticated. Nevertheless, it is clear that the medical field is moving towards a complete and comprehensive EHR. These efforts will be facilitated by the NHII initiative. While these advances may never be considered in the same light as a new ventilator or medication, it is destined to become an integral part of medical management and play an invaluable role in patient care.

References

1. Tufo HM, Speidel JJ. Problems with medical records. Med Care 1971; 9(6): 509–517.
2. Tang PC, Fafchamps D, Shortliffe EH. Traditional medical records as a source of clinical data in the outpatient setting. Proc Annu Symp Comput Appl Med Care 1994; 575–579.
3. Clemmer TP, Gardner RM. Data gathering, analysis, and display in critical care medicine. Respir Care 1985; 30(7):586–601.
4. McDonald CJ, Tierney WM. Computer-stored medical records. Their future role in medical practice. J Am Med Assoc 1988; 259(23):3433–3440.
5. East TD. Computers in the ICU: panacea or plague? Respir Care 1992; 37(2):170–180.
6. Shortliffe EH. The evolution of electronic medical records. Acad Med 1999; 74(4):414–419.
7. Dick RS SEe. The Computer Based Patient Record: An Essential Technology for Health Care. Washington, DC: National Academic Press, 1991.
8. Tegtmeyer K, Ibsen L, Goldstein B. Computer-assisted learning in critical care: from ENIAC to HAL. Crit Care Med 2001; 29(suppl 8):N177–N182.
9. Hess D, Maxwell C, Agarwal NN, Silage DA. Applications of a hand-held computer in critical care medicine. Respir Ther 1985; 15(4):25–28.
10. Varon J, Marik PE. Critical care and the World Wide Web. Crit Care Clin 1999; 15(3):593–604, vii.
11. Weigle CG, Markovitz BP, Pon S. The Internet, the electronic medical record, the pediatric intensive care unit, and everything. Crit Care Med 2001; 29(suppl 8): N166–N176.
12. Lipkin M, Engle RL Jr, Davis BJ, Zworykin VK, Ebald R, Sendrow M, Berkley C. Digital computer as aid to differential diagnosis. Use in hematologic diseases. Arch Intern Med 1961; 108:56–72.
13. Shubin H, Weil MH. Efficient monitoring with a digital computer of cardiovascular function in seriously ill patients. Ann Intern Med 1966; 65(3):453–460.
14. Bodenheimer T, Grumbach K. Electronic technology: a spark to revitalize primary care? J Am Med Assoc 2003; 290(2):259–264.
15. Lindberg DA, Humphreys BL, McCray AT. The unified medical language system. Methods Inf Med 1993; 32(4):281–291.
16. Humphreys BL, Lindberg DA, Schoolman HM, Barnett GO. The unified medical language system: an informatics research collaboration. J Am Med Inform Assoc 1998; 5(1):1–11.
17. Clemmer TP, Spuhler VJ. Developing and gaining acceptance for patient care protocols. New Horiz 1998; 6(1):12–19.

18. Clemmer TP, Spuhler VJ, Berwick DM, Nolan TW. Cooperation: the foundation of improvement. Ann Intern Med 1998; 128(12 Pt 1):1004–1009.

19. McDonald CJ, Overhage JM, Tierney WM, Dexter PR, Martin DK, Suico JG, Zafar A, Schadow G, Blevins L, Glazemer T, et al. The Regenstrief Medical Record System: a quarter century experience. Int J Med Inform 1999; 54(3):225–253.

20. Safran C, Sands DZ, Rind DM. Online medical records: a decade of experience. Methods Inf Med 1999; 38(4–5):308–312.

21. Clemmer TP, Spuhler VJ, Oniki TA, Horn SD. Results of a collaborative quality improvement program on outcomes and costs in a tertiary critical care unit. Crit Care Med 1999; 27(9):1768–1774.

22. White C, Hemby C. Automating the bedside. Healthc Inform 1997; 14(2):68,70,74.

23. Allen D, Davis M. A computerized CIS enhances bedside intensive care. Nurs Manage 1992; 23(7):112I–112J,112N,112P.

24. Hammond J, Johnson HM, Ward CG, Varas R, Dembicki R, Marcial E. Clinical evaluation of a computer-based patient monitoring and data management system. Heart Lung 1991; 20(2):119–124.

25. Pierpont GL, Thilgen D. Effect of computerized charting on nursing activity in intensive care. Crit Care Med 1995; 23(6):1067–1073.

26. Lo B, Alpers A. Uses and abuses of prescription drug information in pharmacy benefits management programs. J Am Med Assoc 2000; 283(6):801–806.

27. Appelbaum PS. Threats to the confidentiality of medical records—no place to hide. J Am Med Assoc 2000; 283(6):795–797.

28. Gostin LO. National health information privacy: regulations under the Health Insurance Portability and Accountability Act. J Am Med Assoc 2001; 285(23):3015–3021.

29. Bovi AM. Ethical guidelines for use of electronic mail between patients and physicians. Am J Bioeth 2003; 3(3):W–IF2.

30. Ward SR. Health smart cards: merging technology and medical information. Med Ref Serv Q 2003; 22(1):57–65.

31. Lamberg L. Confidentiality and privacy of electronic medical records: psychiatrists explore risks of the "information age". J Am Med Assoc 2001; 285(24):3075–3076.

32. Gostin LO. National health information privacy: regulations under the Health Insurance Portability and Accountability Act. J Am Med Assoc 2001; 285(23):3015–3021.

33. Kohn LCJ, Donaldson ME. To Err is Human. Building a Safer Health System. Washington, DC: National Academy Press, 1999.

34. Chassin MR, Galvin RW. The urgent need to improve health care quality. Institute of Medicine National Roundtable on Health Care Quality. J Am Med Assoc 1998; 280(11):1000–1005.

35. Institute of Medicine. Crossing the Quality Chasm: A New Health System for the 21st Century. Washington, DC: National Academy Press, 2000.

36. Kuperman GJ, Gibson RF. Computer physician order entry: benefits, costs, and issues. Ann Intern Med 2003; 139(1):31–39.

37. Schiff GD, Rucker TD. Computerized prescribing: building the electronic infrastructure for better medication usage. J Am Med Assoc 1998; 279(13):1024–1029.

38. The Leapfrog Group for Patient Safety. Computer Physician Order Entry. Leapfrog Group, 1–3. 2004. 11-3-2004. http://www.leapfroggroup.org/media/file/Leapfrog-Computer_Physician_Order_Entry_Fact_Sheet.pdf. (Accessed 11/3/04).

39. Evans RS, Pestotnik SL, Classen DC, Clemmer TP, Weaver LK, Orme JF Jr, et al. A computer-assisted management program for antibiotics and other antiinfective agents. N Engl J Med 1998; 338(4):232–238.

40. Bates DW, Leape LL, Cullen DJ, Laird N, Petersen LA, Teich JM, et al. Effect of computerized physician order entry and a team intervention on prevention of serious medication errors. J Am Med Assoc 1998; 280(15):1311–1316.

41. Bates DW, Teich JM, Lee J, Seger D, Kuperman GJ, Ma'Luf N, Boyle D, Leape, L. The impact of computerized physician order entry on medication error prevention. J Am Med Inform Assoc 1999; 6(4):313–321.

42. Teich JM, Merchia PR, Schmiz JL, Kuperman GJ, Spurr CD, Bates DW. Effects of computerized physician order entry on prescribing practices. Arch Intern Med 2000; 160(18):2741–2747.

43. Chertow GM, Lee J, Kuperman GJ, Burdick E, Horsky J, Seger DL, Lee R, Mekala A, Song J, Komaroff AL, Bates DW. Guided medication dosing for inpatients with renal insufficiency. J Am Med Assoc 2001; 286(22): 2839–2844.

44. Overhage JM, Tierney WM, Zhou XH, McDonald CJ. A randomized trial of "corollary orders" to prevent errors of omission. J Am Med Inform Assoc 1997; 4(5):364–375.

45. Dexter PR, Perkins S, Overhage JM, Maharry K, Kohler RB, McDonald CJ. A computerized reminder system to increase the use of preventive care for hospitalized patients. N Engl J Med 2001; 345(13):965–970.

46. Classen DC, Pestotnik SL, Evans RS, Lloyd JF, Burke JP. Adverse drug events in hospitalized patients. Excess length of stay, extra costs, and attributable mortality. J Am Med Assoc 1997; 277(4):301–306.

47. Cullen DJ, Sweitzer BJ, Bates DW, Burdick E, Edmondson A, Leape LL. Preventable adverse drug events in hospitalized patients: a comparative study of intensive care and general care units. Crit Care Med 1997; 25(8):1289–1297.

48. Classen DC. Clinical decision support systems to improve clinical practice and quality of care. J Am Med Assoc 1998; 280(15):1360–1361.

49. Bates DW, Spell N, Cullen DJ, Burdick E, Laird N, Petersen LA, Small SD, Sweitzer BJ, Leape LL. The costs of adverse drug events in hospitalized patients. Adverse Drug Events Prevention Study Group. J Am Med Assoc 1997; 277(14):307–311.

50. Bates DW, Cullen DJ, Laird N, Petersen LA, Small SD, Servi D, Laffel G, Sweitzer BJ, Shea BF, Hallisey R. Incidence of adverse drug events and potential adverse drug events. Implications for prevention. ADE Prevention Study Group. J Am Med Assoc 1995; 274(1):29–34.

51. Kaushal R, Shojania KG, Bates DW. Effects of computerized physician order entry and clinical decision support systems on medication safety: a systematic review. Arch Intern Med 2003; 163(12):1409–1416.

52. Bates DW, Teich JM, Lee J, Seger D, Kuperman GJ, Ma'Luf N, Boyle D, Leape L. The impact of computerized physician order entry on medication error prevention. J Am Med Inform Assoc 1999; 6(4):313–321.

53. Ash JS, Gorman PN, Hersh WR. Physician order entry in U.S. hospitals. Proc AMIA Symp 1998; 235–239.

54. Pedersen CA, Schneider PJ, Santell JP. ASHP national survey of pharmacy practice in hospital settings: prescribing and transcribing—2001. Am J Health Syst Pharm 2001; 58(23):2251–2266.

55. Ash JS, Gorman PN, Seshadri V, Hersh WR. Computerized physician order entry in U.S. hospitals: results of a 2002 survey. J Am Med Inform Assoc 2004; 11(2): 95–99.

56. Thompson W, Dodek PM, Norena M, Dodek J. Computerized physician order entry of diagnostic tests in an intensive care unit is associated with improved timeliness of service. Crit Care Med 2004; 32(6):1306–1309.

57. Shu K, Boyle D, Spurr C, Horsky J, Heiman H, O'Connor P, Lepore J, Bates DW. Comparison of time spent writing orders on paper with computerized physician order entry. Medinfo 2001; 10(Pt 2):1207–1211.

58. Tierney WM, Miller ME, Overhage JM, McDonald CJ. Physician inpatient order writing on microcomputer workstations. Effects on resource utilization. J Am Med Assoc 1993; 269(3):379–383.

59. Bates DW, Gawande AA. Improving safety with information technology. N Engl J Med 2003; 348(25):2526–2534.

60. Morris AH. Computerized protocols and bedside decision support. Crit Care Clin 1999; 15(3):523–45, vi.

61. Burton ME, Ash CL, Hill DP Jr, Handy T, Shepherd MD, Vasko MR. A controlled trial of the cost benefit of computerized bayesian aminoglycoside administration. Clin Pharmacol Ther 1991; 49(6):685–694.

62. Evans RS, Classen DC, Pestotnik SL, Lundsgaarde HP, Burke JP. Improving empiric antibiotic selection using computer decision support. Arch Intern Med 1994; 154(8):878–884.

63. Casner PR, Reilly R, Ho H. A randomized controlled trial of computerized pharmacokinetic theophylline dosing versus empiric physician dosing. Clin Pharmacol Ther 1993; 53(6):684–690.

64. Hurley SF, Dziukas LJ, McNeil JJ, Brignell MJ. A randomized controlled clinical trial of pharmacokinetic theophylline dosing. Am Rev Respir Dis 1986; 134(6):1219–1224.

65. Mungall DR, Anbe D, Forrester PL, Luoma T, Genovese R, Mahan J, LeBlanc S, Penney JB. A prospective randomized comparison of the accuracy of computer-assisted versus GUSTO nomogram—directed heparin therapy. Clin Pharmacol Ther 1994; 55(5): 591–596.

66. White RH, Hong R, Venook AP, Daschbach MM, Murray W, Mungall DR, Coleman RW. Initiation of warfarin therapy: comparison of physician dosing with computer-assisted dosing. J Gen Intern Med 1987; 2(3):141–148.

67. Shah ND, Vermeulen LC, Santell JP, Hunkler RJ, Hontz K. Projecting future drug expenditures—2002. Am J Health Syst Pharm 2002; 59(2):131–142.

68. Kunin CM, Johansen KS, Worning AM, Daschner FD. Report of a symposium on use and abuse of antibiotics worldwide. Rev Infect Dis 1990; 12(11):12–19.

69. Maki DG, Schuna AA. A study of antimicrobial misuse in a university hospital. Am J Med Sci 1978; 275(3):271–282.

70. Pestotnik SL, Classen DC, Evans RS, Burke JP. Implementing antibiotic practice guidelines through computer-assisted decision support: clinical and financial outcomes. Ann Intern Med 1996; 124(10):884–890.

71. East TD, Heermann LK, Bradshaw RL, Lugo A, Sailors RM, Ershler L, Wallace CT, Morris AH, McKinley B, Marquez A, et al. Efficacy of computerized

decision support for mechanical ventilation: results of a prospective multi-center randomized trial. Proc AMIA Symp 1999; 251–255.

72. McKinley BA, Moore FA, Sailors RM, Cocanour CS, Marquez A, Wright RK, Tonnesen AS, Wallace CJ, Morris AH. Computerized decision support for mechanical ventilation of trauma induced ARDS: results of a randomized clinical trial. J Trauma 2001; 50(3):415–424.

73. Brimm JE. Computers in critical care. Crit Care Nurs Q 1987; 9(4):53–63.

74. Manzano JL, Villalobos J, Church A, Manzano JJ. Computerized information system for ICU patient management. Crit Care Med 1980; 8(12):745–747.

75. Bates DW, Ebell M, Gotlieb E, Zapp J, Mullins HC. A proposal for electronic medical records in U.S. primary care. J Am Med Inform Assoc 2003; 10(1):1–10.

76. Howard WR. Development of an affordable data collection, reporting, and analysis system. Respir Care 2003; 48(2):131–137.

77. Graham G, Nugent L, Strouse K. Information every where: how the EHR transformed care at VHA. J AHIMA 2003; 74(3):20–24.

78. Brown SH, Lincoln MJ, Groen PJ, Kolodner RM. VistA—U.S. Department of Veterans Affairs national-scale HIS. Int J Med Inform 2003; 69(2–3):135–156.

79. Justus PG, Kreutziger SS, Kitchens CS. Probing the dynamics of Munchausen's syndrome. Detailed analysis of a case. Ann Intern Med 1980; 93(1):120–127.

80. Institute of Medicine. Key Capabilities of an Electronic Health Record System: Letter Report. Washington, DC: National Academy Press, 2003.

81. Seiver A. Critical care computing. Past, present, and future. Crit Care Clin 2000; 16(4):601–621.

82. Sado AS. Electronic medical record in the intensive care unit. Crit Care Clin 1999; 15(3):499–522.

83. Codd EF. A relational model of data for large shared data banks. 1970. MD Comput 1998; 15(3):162–166.

84. Delaney DP, Zibrak JD, Samore M, Peterson M. Use of relational database management system by clinicians to create automated MICU progress note from existent data sources. Proc AMIA Annu Fall Symp 1997; 7–11.

85. Fisk JM, Mutalik P, Levin FW, Erdos J, Taylor C, Nadkarni P. Integrating query of relational and textual data in clinical databases: a case study. J Am Med Inform Assoc 2003; 10(1):21–38.

86. Shabot MM. The HP CareVue clinical information system. Int J Clin Monit Comput 1997; 14(3):177–184.

87. Shabot MM, LoBue M. Real-time wireless decision support alerts on a Palmtop PDA. Proc Annu Symp Comput Appl Med Care 1995; 174–177.

88. Fraenkel DJ, Cowie M, Daley P. Quality benefits of an intensive care clinical information system. Crit Care Med 2003; 31(1):120–125.

89. Kundel HL, Seshadri SB, Langlotz CP, Lanken PN, Horii SC, Nodine CF, Polansky M, Feingold E, Brikman I, Bozzo M, et al. Prospective study of a PACS: information flow and clinical action in a medical intensive care unit. Radiology 1996; 199(1):143–149.

90. Adhikari N, Lapinsky SE. Medical informatics in the intensive care unit: overview of technology assessment. J Crit Care 2003; 18(1):41–47.

91. Snyder-Halpern R, Wagner MC. Evaluating return-on-investment for a hospital clinical information system. Comput Nurs 2000; 18(5):213–219.

92. Lee N, Hui D, Wu A, Chan P, Cameron P, Joynt GM, Ahuja A, Yung MY, Leung CB, To KF, et al. A major outbreak of severe acute respiratory syndrome in Hong Kong. N Engl J Med 2003; 348(20):1986–1994.

93. Tsang KW, Ho PL, Ooi GC, Yee WK, Wang T, Chan-Yeung M, Lam WK, Sefo WH, Yam LY, Cheung TM, et al. A cluster of cases of severe acute respiratory syndrome in Hong Kong. N Engl J Med 2003; 348(20):1977–1985.

94. Drazen JM, Campion EW. SARS, the Internet, and the Journal. N Engl J Med 2003; 348(20):2029.

95. Ksiazek TG, Erdman D, Goldsmith CS, Zaki SR, Peret T, Emery S, Tong S, Urbani C, Comer JA, Lim W, et al. A novel coronavirus associated with severe acute respiratory syndrome. N Engl J Med 2003; 348(20):1953–1966.

96. Peiris JS, Yuen KY, Osterhaus AD, Stohr K. The severe acute respiratory syndrome. N Engl J Med 2003; 349(25):2431–2441.

97. Gerberding JL. Faster... but fast enough? Responding to the epidemic of severe acute respiratory syndrome. N Engl J Med 2003; 348(20):2030–2031.

98. McDade JE, Shepard CC, Fraser DW, Tsai TR, Redus MA, Dowdle WR. Legionnaires' disease: isolation of a bacterium and demonstration of its role in other respiratory disease. N Engl J Med 1977; 297(22):1197–1203.

99. Fraser DW, Tsai TR, Orenstein W, Parkin WE, Beecham HJ, Sharrar RG, Harris J, Mallison GF, Martin SM, McDade JE et al. Legionnaires' disease: description of an epidemic of pneumonia. N Engl J Med 1977; 297(22):1189–1197.

100. Podichetty V, Penn D. The progressive roles of electronic medicine: benefits, concerns, and costs. Am J Med Sci 2004; 328(2):94–99.

101. Risk A, Petersen C. Health information on the internet: quality issues and international initiatives. J Am Med Assoc 2002; 287(20):2713–2715.

102. Impicciatore P, Pandolfini C, Casella N, Bonati M. Reliability of health information for the public on the World Wide Web: systematic survey of advice on managing fever in children at home. Br Med J 1997; 314(7098):1875–1879.

103. Crocco AG, Villasis-Keever M, Jadad AR. Two wrongs don't make a right: harm aggravated by inaccurate information on the Internet. Pediatrics 2002; 109(3): 522–523.

104. Allen ES, Burke JM, Welch ME, Rieseberg LH. How reliable is science information on the web? Nature 1999; 402(6763):722.

105. Winker MA, Flanagin A, Chi-Lum B, White J, Andrews K, Kennett RL, De Angelis CD, Masacchio RA. Guidelines for medical and health information sites on the internet: principles governing AMA web sites. American Medical Association. J Am Med Assoc 2000; 283(12):1600–1606.

106. Eysenbach G, Powell J, Kuss O, Sa ER. Empirical studies assessing the quality of health information for consumers on the world wide web: a systematic review. J Am Med Assoc 2002; 287(20):2691–2700.

107. Winker MA, Flanagin A, Chi-Lum B, White J, Andrews K, Kennett RL, De Angelis CD, Masacchio RA. Guidelines for medical and health information sites on the internet: principles governing AMA web sites. American Medical Association. J Am Med Assoc 2000; 283(12):1600–1606.

108. Pronovost PJ, Rinke ML, Emery K, Dennison C, Blackledge C, Berenholtz SM. Interventions to reduce mortality among patients treated in intensive care units. J Crit Care 2004; 19(3):158–164.

109. Pronovost PJ, Angus DC, Dorman T, Robinson KA, Dremsizov TT, Young TL. Physician staffing patterns and clinical outcomes in critically ill patients: a systematic review. J Am Med Assoc 2002; 288(17):2151–2162.

110. Bates DW, Gawande AA. Improving safety with information technology. N Engl J Med 2003; 348(25):2526–2534.

111. Sackett DL, Straus SE. Finding and applying evidence during clinical rounds: the "evidence cart". J Am Med Assoc 1998; 280(15):1336–1338.

112. Barrett JR, Strayer SM, Schubart JR. Assessing medical residents' usage and perceived needs for personal digital assistants. Int J Med Inform 2004; 73(1): 25–34.

113. Physicians' use of handheld personal computing devices increases from 15% in 1999 to 26% in 2001. Taylor H, Leitman R, eds. Harris Interactive 1[25]: 1–4. 8-15-2001. 12-27-0004. www.harrisinteractive.com/news/allnewsbydate.asp? NewsID = 345 (Accessed 12/27/04).

114. McAlearney AS, Schweikhart SB, Medow MA. Doctors' experience with handheld computers in clinical practice: qualitative study. Br Med J 2004; 328(7449):1162.

115. Adatia FA, Bedard PL. "Palm reading": 1. Handheld hardware and operating systems. Canad Med Assoc J 2002; 167(7):775–780.

116. Fischer S, Stewart TE, Mehta S, Wax R, Lapinsky SE. Handheld computing in medicine. J Am Med Inform Assoc 2003; 10(2):139–149.

117. Adatia F, Bedard PL. "Palm reading": 2. Handheld software for physicians. Canad Med Assoc J 2003; 168(6):727–734.

118. Clauson KA, Seamon MJ, Clauson AS, Van TB. Evaluation of drug information databases for personal digital assistants. Am J Health Syst Pharm 2004; 61(10): 1015–1024.

119. Barrons R. Evaluation of personal digital assistant software for drug interactions. Am J Health Syst Pharm 2004; 61(4):380–385.

120. Miller SM, Beattie MM, Butt AA. Personal digital assistant infectious diseases applications for health care professionals. Clin Infect Dis 2003; 36(8): 1018–1029.

121. Chen ES, Mendonca EA, McKnight LK, Stetson PD, Lei J, Cimino JJ. PalmCIS: a wireless handheld application for satisfying clinician information needs. J Am Med Inform Assoc 2004; 11(1):19–28.

122. Sullivan L, Halbach JL, Shu T. Using personal digital assistants in a family medicine clerkship. Acad Med 2001; 76(5):534–535.

123. Lei J, Stetson PD, Chen ES, McKnight LK, Mendonca EA, Cimino JJ. Structured data entry of cross-coverage notes using a PDA. Medinfo 2004; 2004(CD):1712.

124. Martinez-Motta JC, Walker R, Stewart TE, Granton J, Abrahamson S, Lapinsky SE. Critical care procedure logging using handheld computers. Crit Care 2004; 8(5): R336–R342.

125. Hammond EJ, Sweeney BP. Electronic data collection by trainee anaesthetists using palm top computers. Eur J Anaesthesiol 2000; 17(2):91–98.

126. Lapinsky SE, Weshler J, Mehta S, Varkul M, Hallett D, Stewart TE. Handheld computers in critical care. Crit Care 2001; 5(4):227–231.

127. Lapinsky SE, Wax R, Showalter R, Martinez-Motta JC, Hallett D, Mehta S, Burry L, Stewart TE. Prospective evaluation of an internet-linked handheld computer critical care knowledge access system. Crit Care 2004; 8(6):R414–R421.

128. Yasnoff WA, Humphreys BL, Overhage JM, Detmer DE, Brennan PF, Morris RW, Middleton B, Bates DW, Fanning JP. A consensus action agenda for achieving the national health information infrastructure. J Am Med Inform Assoc 2004; 11(4):332–338.

129. Detmer DE. Building the national health information infrastructure for personal health, health care services, public health, and research. BMC Med Inform Decis Mak 2003; 3(1):1.

Index